I0044593

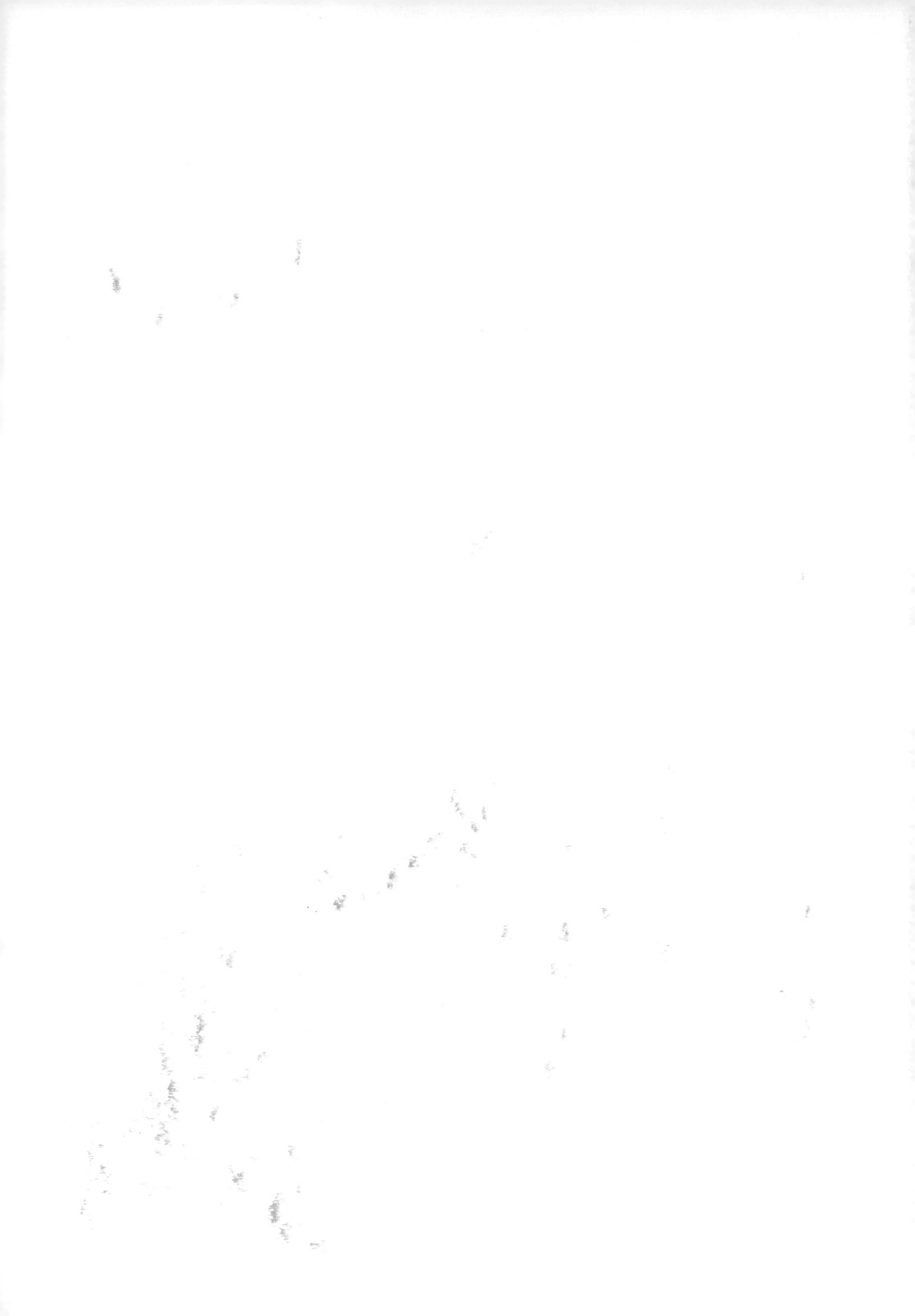

Essentials of Urology

Essentials of Urology

Edited by Ezra Martin

hayle
medical

New York

Hayle Medical,
750 Third Avenue, 9th Floor,
New York, NY 10017, USA

Visit us on the World Wide Web at:
www.haylemedical.com

© Hayle Medical, 2019

This book contains information obtained from authentic and highly regarded sources. Copyright for all individual chapters remain with the respective authors as indicated. All chapters are published with permission under the Creative Commons Attribution License or equivalent. A wide variety of references are listed. Permission and sources are indicated; for detailed attributions, please refer to the permissions page and list of contributors. Reasonable efforts have been made to publish reliable data and information, but the authors, editors and publisher cannot assume any responsibility for the validity of all materials or the consequences of their use.

ISBN: 978-1-63241-779-4

Trademark Notice: Registered trademark of products or corporate names are used only for explanation and identification without intent to infringe.

Cataloging-in-Publication Data

Essentials of urology / edited by Ezra Martin.
    p. cm.
Includes bibliographical references and index.
ISBN 978-1-63241-779-4
1. Urology. 2. Genitourinary organs--Diseases. I. Martin, Ezra.
RC871 .E87 2019
616.6--dc23

Contents

Preface

The area of study which deals with the diseases related to the male and female urinary-tract system and male reproductive organs is known as urology. Pediatric urology, reconstructive urology and female urology are some of the significant sub-fields of urology. Pediatric urology deals with the urological disorders in children. Some of the disorders which come under the scope of this discipline include enuresis, cryptorchidism and vesicoureteral reflux. Reconstructive urology deals with the restoration of both the structure and function of the genitourinary tract in males. The sub-field of urology dealing with overactive bladder, pelvic organ prolapse and urinary incontinence is known as female urology. This book is compiled in such a manner, that it will provide in-depth knowledge about the theory and practice of urology. Some of the diverse topics covered herein address the varied branches that fall under this category. This book will prove to be immensely beneficial to students, doctors and researchers in this field.

Significant researches are present in this book. Intensive efforts have been employed by authors to make this book an outstanding discourse. This book contains the enlightening chapters which have been written on the basis of significant researches done by the experts.

Finally, I would also like to thank all the members involved in this book for being a team and meeting all the deadlines for the submission of their respective works. I would also like to thank my friends and family for being supportive in my efforts.

Editor

A prospective and randomized comparison of rigid ureteroscopic to flexible cystoscopic retrieval of ureteral stents

Dehui Lai[1*†], Meiling Chen[1†], Shifang Zha[2] and Shawpong Wan[3]

Abstract

Background: Flexible cystoscopy has become an accepted alternative for stent retrieval. However, it is associated with higher cost. Some reports have described experiences of using rigid ureteroscope to retrieve ureteral stents. We compared rigid ureteroscopic to flexible cystoscopic retrieval of ureteral stents in a prospective and randomized clinical trial.

Methods: Three hundred patients treated with ureteral stents between July 2012 and July 2013 were accrued in this study. These patients were divided into two groups using the random number table method. Group A, with 162 patients, had stents removed with a flexible cystoscope and Group B, with 138 patients, had stents removed with a rigid ureteroscope. All procedures were performed under topical anesthesia by the same urologist. Patients in each group were compared in terms of preoperative, perioperative, and postoperative data. Postoperative data were collected using telephone interview on the postoperative day two. The postoperative questionnaire used included three items: hematuria, irritable bladder symptoms, and pain scores.

Results: All the stents were retrieved successfully. No statistical differences were noted between the two groups in terms of gender, age, laterality and duration of the stents, operative time, postoperative hematuria, irritable bladder symptoms, and pain scores. The per-use cost of instrument was much higher for the flexible cystoscopic group, RMB 723.1 versus 214.3 (USD 107.9 versus 28.2), $P < 0.05$.

Conclusion: Ureteral stent retrieval using rigid ureteroscope under topical anesthesia is as safe and effective as flexible cystoscope but with a much lower cost to patients.

Keywords: Ureteral stents, Stent retrieval, Cost-effectiveness

Background

Ureteral stents are frequently used in minimally invasive procedures for the upper urinary tract diseases. It may alleviate temporary postoperative obstruction in the ureter from trauma and swelling [1, 2]. It can also be used as a means of passive preoperative ureteral dilation. Conventionally, the indwelling ureteral stents present for a longer period are retrieved using a rigid cystoscope and grasping forceps in adults under topical anesthesia as out-patient. The procedure can be painful and may cause urethral injury in men. Recently, flexible cystoscopy has become an accepted alternative for stent retrieval. However, flexible cystoscope is associated with higher cost and may not be readily available in developing countries [3, 4]. Some reports have described experiences of using rigid ureteroscope to retrieve ureteral stents, especially in the occasional situations such as migrated or retained stents [4–6]. There has been no study published comparing the outcome between using a flexible cystoscope and a rigid ureteroscope for the

* Correspondence: dehuilai@hotmail.com
†Equal contributors
[1]Urology Department, Fifth Affiliated Hospital, Guangzhou Medical University, 621 Gangwan Road, Huangpu District, Guangzhou 510700, China
Full list of author information is available at the end of the article

ureteral stent removal. In this prospective and randomized clinical trial, we intend to investigate this issue.

Methods

Patient cohorts

This prospective and randomized trial was approved by the Ethics Committee of the Fifth Affiliated Hospital of the Guangzhou Medical University. From July 2012 to July 2013, 300 adult patients with unilateral 6 Fr. double-J ureteral stents were accrued for the study. Patients with residual stones, chronic renal failure, diabetes, solitary kidney, history of sepsis, febrile infection, or migrated stents were excluded. Written informed consent was obtained for all participants. Using the random number table, patients were separated into two groups based on the method of stent retrieval. Group A of 162 patients had stents removed using a 16 French Karl Storz flexible cystoscope. Group B of 138 patients had stents removed using a 8.0/9.8 French Richard Wolf ureteroscope. All patients underwent urinalysis and KUB prior to the procedure.

Procedures and Data collection

All the stents were removed by a single urologist to minimize the variables. First, 2% lidocaine gel was instilled into the urethra and held for 5 min to implement topical anesthesia. Next either a flexible cystoscope or a rigid ureteroscope was introduced into the urethra under direct vision and advanced to the bladder per group assignment. The ureteral stents were removed using either flexible foreign body forceps for the flexible cystoscopic method or the four Fr. rigid grasping forceps for the rigid ureteroscopic method.

The clinical data assessed includes the duration of the stent placement, laterality of the stent, reason for the stent placement, operative time, perioperative and postoperative pain, postoperative hematuria, and irritable bladder symptoms. Operative time was calculated from the insertion of the endoscope to the completion of the stent removal. A visual analogue pain scale (VAS) was used to assess the intensity of the pain. The perioperative and postoperative pain scales were evaluated immediately after the procedure and 48 h after the procedure by telephone. Postoperative macroscopic hematuria lasting more than 1 day after the procedure were recorded. Irritable bladder symptoms included four items: pain in the bladder, dysuria, urinary frequency and urgency. These data were acquired just before the procedure and at 48 h follow up after the procedure by telephone.

The calculated cost of the instruments included the cost of endoscopes, grasping forceps, and maintenance. Per-use cost of the instruments for both groups was appraised and compared.

Statistical analyses

Statistical analysis was performed using the SPSS 17.0® for Windows®. Continuous variables were compared using the Student-t and the Wilcoxon tests. Univariable analysis was conducted using the Pearson χ^2 statistics or Fisher's exact test for the categorical data. P values <0.05 were considered statistically significant.

Results

All stents were successfully removed under topical anesthesia in both groups. There were no statistical differences noted between the two groups in terms of age, gender, laterality of the stent, and the reasons for the stent placement (Table 1).

Duration of the stent, operative time, perioperative and postoperative pain scores, and data for postoperative macroscopic hematuria and irritable bladder symptoms are shown by gender (Tables 2 and 3). The mean operative time was shorter for the ureteroscopic group in both sexes. There was no statistically significant difference between the two groups in both perioperative and postoperative pain scores. When compared to the female patients, the mean perioperative pain score was higher for men in both groups.

All patients were discharged 20–30 min after the procedure. No one required analgesics, antibiotics, or hospitalization. Follow-up data was available in 91.4% of the cohorts in Group A and 90.5% in Group B. Four male patients (20.3%) in Group A and 18 (26.4%) in the Group B had postoperative macroscopic hematuria for more than 1 day, $p = 0.395$; whereas only five female patients (6.3%) in Group A and five (8.8%) in group B experienced macroscopic hematuria for more than 1 day, $p = 0.742$. These patients were treated with 5 mg adrenosin once a day and the hematuria ceased in 3 to 5 days.

Table 1 Demographic, characteristics of patient, stent laterality, and reason for stent placement

	Flexible cystoscope group ($N = 162$)	Ureteroscope group ($N = 138$)	P
Gender, no.			
Male/Female	77/85	74/64	0.293
Mean age ± SD, (range in years)	40.1 ± 10.3, (20–79)	39.6 ± 11.1, (19–68)	0.79
Stent laterality, Left/Right	90/72	73/65	0.645
Causes of stent placement			
MPCNL	97	84	0.996
Ureteroscopic lithotripsy	41	37	
Shock wave lithotripsy	7	5	
Hydronephrosis			
Ureteral stricture	11	8	
Pregnancy	2	1	
Open surgery	4	3	

Table 2 Days from stent placement to removal, perioperative and postoperative characteristics of male patients

Variable	Flexible cystoscope group (N = 77)	Ureteroscope group (N = 74)	P
Duration of stent placement mean ± SD, range in days	28.6 ± 9.4,14–32	29.9 ± 9.5,14–36	0.652
Operative time, mean ± SD, range in minutes	3.4 ± 0.8,2.8–4.2	2.7 ± 0.9,2.4–3.5	0.203
VAS score for perioperative pain, mean ± SD, range	3.1 ± 1.8,3–6	4.3 ± 0.9,3–8	0.103
VAS score for postoperative pain, mean ± SD, range	2.4 ± 1.1,1–4	3.1 ± 1.2,1–5	0.324
Patients lost at follow up, n (%)	8 (10.4)	6 (8.1)	0.629
Postoperative macroscopic hematuria, n (%)			
More than 1 day	14 (20.3)	18 (26.4)	0.395
Postoperative irritable bladder symptoms, n (%)	19 (29.2)	23 (33.8)	0.425

The rates of postoperative irritable bladder symptoms were higher in the ureteroscopic group, especially for men, but there was no statistically significant difference between the two groups. No one required hospitalization due to the postoperative complications. Two forceps and two flexible cystoscopes were damaged during the procedure in Group A. The deflection lever on one of the scopes was severed and the damage on the other was the outer rubber sheath. No ureteroscope and only one pair of grasping forceps was damaged in Group B. The per-use cost for the instrument was much higher in Group A than Group B, RMB 723.1 (USD 107.9) versus RMB 214.3 (USD 28.2) respectively.

Discussion

Since first introduced in 1967, ureteral stents have been widely used in the urological surgery [5, 7]. As a foreign body, it is generally removed in 3 days to 4 weeks after its insertion. The conventional method for the retrieval

Table 3 Duration of the stents, perioperative and postoperative characteristics of female patients

Variable	Flexible cystoscope group (N = 85)	Ureteroscope group (N = 64)	P
Duration of stents, mean ± SD, range, days	27.6 ± 6.5,16–29	28.8 ± 10.5,14–31	0.703
Operative time, mean ± SD, range, minutes	3.0 ± 0.6,2.2–3.5	2.3 ± 0.6,1.5–2.7	0.062
VAS score of perioperative pain, mean ± SD, range	2.5 ± 1.2, 2–6	3.1 ± 1.9, 3–8	0.234
VAS score of postoperative pain, mean ± SD, range	2.3 ± 1.2, 1–4	2.8 ± 1.4, 1–4	0.325
Patients lost at follow up, n (%)	6 (7.1)	7 (10.9)	0.406
Postoperative macroscopic hematuria, n (%)			
More than 1 day	5 (6.3)	5 (8.8)	0.742
Postoperative irritable bladder symptoms, n (%)	6 (7.6)	6 (10.5)	0.382

is using the widely available rigid cystoscope and grasping forceps. Various non-endoscopic techniques for the stent retrieval have also described. A tethered nylon string attached to the end of the stent is frequently used for stents intended to be used for a short duration. Magnets, wire loops, and crochet hook–like retrievers have also been tried but not widely used [8–13]. With the introduction of flexible cystoscopes, the flexible cystoscopic stent removal has become a preferred method in the more affluent countries. However, flexible cystoscope is more expensive and is less readily available in many places around the world.

Haluk et al. described using rigid ureteroscopy for ureter stent retrieval as an alternative that can be less expensive than the flexible cystoscope and may be less painful than the rigid cystoscope [4]. We have been routinely using both the rigid ureteroscope and the flexible cystoscope for the stent retrieval in our center. However, to our knowledge, there has never been a study comparing the clinical data for these two surgical modalities.

Previous studies have shown that using a flexible cystoscope to remove ureteral stent offer the advantage of being less painful in the male patient [14]. In the present study, we found that the perioperative and postoperative VAS for patients whose ureteral stent were removed using ureteroscopy were similar to those removed using flexible cystoscopy for both genders. In our opinion, because of its small caliber, rigid ureteroscopy can be an acceptable alternative for ureteral stent retrieval with less discomfort.

Irritable bladder symptoms and hematuria are the most common problems following flexible cystoscopy [15]. Donoghue et al. [16] and Kortman et al. [17] reported that 37% and 35.3% of men had pain over the bladder after flexible cystoscopy, respectively. 5% of the patients still had dysuria at 48 h postoperatively [15]. Dysuria is usually associated with trauma to the mucosa. Both rigid ureteroscopy and flexible cystoscopy tend to cause less trauma to the urethra than the rigid cystoscope. In our study, 3.4% of Group A and 3.2% of Group B experienced dysuria at postoperative day two, $P > 0.05$. There was no statistically significant difference between the two groups. Most of the dysuria resolved after 48 h without treatment.

Hematuria is the most common cause for hospital admission after stent removal [15]. No one in our study required hospitalization due to hematuria. Due to strong aversion to macroscopic hematuria in the Chinese culture, we routinely treat patients complaining of macroscopic hematuria with oral hemostatics for 3 to 5 days, a more aggressive therapy than in other countries. We found the incidence of hematuria and other postoperative complications were similar for both groups.

Flexible cystoscopes are more expensive and less durable than rigid cystoscopes. In addition, the per-use cost including the sterilization is higher than the per-use cost for the rigid scope. The deflection tip and outer bending rubber are the most common sites for damage. In a retrospective study by McGill et al., the mean failure time for flexible cystoscope was 134.6 procedures [18]. In this study, the per-use cost of the instrument was much higher in flexible cystoscopic group (RMB 723.1 or USD 107.9) than for the ureteroscope group (RMB 214.3 or USD 28.2). Two flexible cystoscopes were damaged during the 162 procedures. The flexible foreign body, forceps, was also more prone to breakage. In an in-vitro study, the maximum extraction force for the flexible graspers was only 1.3 kg [19]. Two flexible forceps were damaged during this study. The mean usage was 56.6 times. Moreover, a stone basket was occasionally required due to an inaccessible angle; this further escalated the cost. By contrast, no rigid ureteroscopes and only one pair of ureteroscopic grasping forceps were damaged after the 138 procedures.

The ureteroscopic method can be a reasonable alternative for the ureteral stent retrieval. The rigid ureteroscope, with its relatively low cost, is generally available in most of the hospitals and most of the urologists are proficient with its use. In fact, ureteroscopic extractions of stones have been widely performed even in lower income countries during the last two decades [20, 21].

The main limitation of this study is that it was a single-center study with a relatively small sample size. There would be unavoidable inherent bias. A multi-center prospective randomized controlled study with a larger sample size would be more ideal.

Conclusion

Ureteral stent retrieval using a ureteroscope under topical anesthesia is as safe and effective as using a flexible cystoscope but at a lower cost. Rigid ureteroscopes may also be more available than flexible cystoscopes.

Abbreviations
KUB: Kidneys, ureters, and bladder x-ray; RMB: Ren Min Bi; USD: United States dollar; VAS: Visual analogue pain scale

Acknowledgements
None.

Funding
No funding was obtained for this study.

Authors' contributions
Experiment conception and design: DHL. Performance of the experiments: DHL, MLC, SFZ. Data analysis: DHL, MLC. Contribution of reagents/materials/analysis tools: DHL, MLC. Manuscript writing and editing: DHL, MLC, SPW. All authors read and approved the final manuscript.

Competing interests
The authors declare that they have no competing interests.

Declarations
The paper adhered to the CONSORT guidelines.

Author details
[1]Urology Department, Fifth Affiliated Hospital, Guangzhou Medical University, 621 Gangwan Road, Huangpu District, Guangzhou 510700, China. [2]Urology, Citic Huizhou Hospital, Huizhou, Guangdong, China. [3]Urology, First People's Hospital of Xiaoshan, Hangzhou, Zhejiang, China.

References
1.   Aravantinos E, Gravas S, Karatzas AD, et al. Forgotten, encrusted ureteral stents: a challenging problem with an endourologic solution. J Endourol. 2006;20(12):1045–9.
2.   Taylor WN, McDougall IT. Minimally invasive ureteral stent retrieval. J Urol. 2002;168:2020–3.
3.   Simonato A, Galli S, Carmignani G. Simple, safe and inexpensive retrieval of JJ stents with a flexible cystoscope. Br J Urol. 1998;81:490–49.
4.   Söylemez H, Sancaktutar AA, Bozkurt Y, et al. A cheap minimally painful and widely usable alternative for retrieving ureteral stents. Urol Int. 2011;87(2):199–204.
5.   Murthy KV, Reddy SJ, Prasad DV. Endourological management of forgotten encrusted ureteral stents. Int Braz J Urol. 2010;36(4):420–9.
6.   Jeong H, Kwak C, Lee SE. Ureteric stenting after ureteroscopy for ureteric stones: a prospective randomized study assessing symptoms and complications. BJU Int. 2004;93:1032–4.
7.   Zimskind PD, Fetter TR, Wilkerson JL. Clinical use of long-term indwelling silicone rubber ureteral splints inserted cystoscopically. J Urol. 1967;97:840–4.
8.   Figueroa TE. Retrieval of ureteral stents in children. Tech Urol. 1995;1:45–7.
9.   Schulman CC WT, Zlotta AR. Single-J ureteral stent with a distal suture. In: Yachia D, editor. Stenting the Urinary System. Oxford: Isis Medical Media; 1998. p. 161–4.
10. Wetton CW, Gedroyc WM. Retrograde radiological retrieval and replacement of double-J ureteric stents. Clin Radiol. 1995;50:562–5.
11. Vesey SG, Athmanathan N. A computerized ureteric stent retrieval system. Br J Urol. 1996;78:156.
12. Cowan NC, Cranston DW. Retrograde radiological retrieval and replacement of double-J ureteric stents. Clin Radiol. 1996;51:305–6.
13. Kawahara T, Ito H, Terao H, et al. Ureteral stent retrieval using the crochet hook technique in females. PLoS One. 2012;7(1):e29292.
14. Jeong YB, Doo AR, Park HS, Shin YS. Clinical significance of ureteral stent removal by flexible cystoscopy on pain and satisfaction in young males: a prospective randomised control trial. Urolithiasis. 2016;44(4):367–70.
15. Erkal S. Patients' experiences at home after day case cystoscopy. J Clin Nurs. 2007;16(6):1118–24.
16. Donoghue J, Pelletier D, Duffield C, Torres M. Australian men's experience of cystoscopic day surgery Part 2. Ambulatory Surg. 1998;6:189–96.
17. Kortman BBM, Sonke GS, D'ancona FCH, et al. The tolerability of urodynamic studies and flexible cysto-urethroscopy used in the assessment of men with lower urinary tract symptoms. Br J Urol Int. 1999;84:449–53.

Canadian Men's perspectives about active surveillance in prostate cancer: need for guidance and resources

Margaret Fitch[1], Kittie Pang[1], Veronique Ouellet[2], Carmen Loiselle[3], Shabbir Alibhai[4], Simone Chevalier[3], Darrel E. Drachenberg[5], Antonio Finelli[4], Jean-Baptiste Lattouf[2,6], Simon Sutcliffe[7], Alan So[8], Simon Tanguay[3], Fred Saad[2,6]* and Anne-Marie Mes-Masson[2,9]

Abstract

Background: In prostate cancer, men diagnosed with low risk disease may be monitored through an active surveillance. This research explored the perspectives of men with prostate cancer regarding their decision-making process for active surveillance to identify factors that influence their decision and assist health professionals in having conversations about this option.

Methods: Focus group interviews (*n* = 7) were held in several Canadian cities with men (*N* = 52) diagnosed with prostate cancer and eligible for active surveillance. The men's viewpoints were captured regarding their understanding of active surveillance, the factors that influenced their decision, and their experience with the approach. A content and theme analysis was performed on the verbatim transcripts from the sessions.

Results: Patients described their concerns of living with their disease without intervention, but were reassured by the close monitoring under AS while avoiding harmful side effects associated with treatments. Conversations with their doctor and how AS was described were cited as key influences in their decision, in addition to availability of information on treatment options, distrust in the health system, personality, experiences and opinions of others, and personal perspectives on quality of life.

Conclusions: Men require a thorough explanation on AS as a safe and valid option, as well as guidance towards supportive resources in their decision-making.

Keywords: Active surveillance, Prostate cancer, Decisions making, Focus group, Low risk disease

Background

Prostate cancer, the most commonly diagnosed cancer in Canadian men, accounted for 21,600 new cancer diagnoses in 2016 (Canadian Cancer Statistics, 2016). PCa consumes a significant amount of treatment resources [1], initiating efforts to distinguish men with high risk disease who require therapeutic intervention to avert premature death and disability. For men with low risk disease, interventional therapy is neither required nor appropriate to ensure a lifespan uncompromised by cancer or by the therapeutic consequences (reviewed in [2]).

Presently, men with low risk PCa are given the option of 'active surveillance' (AS). With AS, practitioners delay curative treatment until there are indications that the disease is progressing. Very low- or low-risk localized PCa is defined to include tumor stage (T1c, prostate-specific antigen [PSA] detected or T2a, small palpable nodule); PSA value (less than 10 ng/mL); Gleason score ($\leq$ 6); and extent of disease in biopsy (<3 biopsy cores positive and $\leq$50% cancer in any cores) [3] (reviewed in [4, 5]). With the advent of PSA screening, more low risk cancers have been detected along with recommendations of AS.

* Correspondence: fred.saad@umontreal.ca
[2]Institut du cancer de Montréal and Centre de recherche du Centre hospitalier de l'Université de Montréal, 900 St Denis St, Montreal, QC, Canada
[6]Department of Surgery Université de Montréal, 2900 Edouard Montpetit Blvd, Montreal, QC, Canada
Full list of author information is available at the end of the article

Patients and practitioners have expressed discomfort with the option of AS as a significant proportion of patients may be understaged given the intrinsic sampling error of prostate biopsies [6]. Investigation is underway to identify biomarkers that accurately detect truly low risk disease for patients with a grade 6 cancer or even those with Gleason score 7 [1, 7]. This would enlarge the pool of individuals for whom AS would be considered an appropriate approach.

The Canadian PCa Biomarker Network team investigated the uptake of AS in Canada in 2010 [8]. AS is widely practiced across Canada, but important regional differences exist in its use for reasons that remain unknown. Additionally, there is little systematic understanding about the factors that influence the acceptance of and adherence to AS in PCa in Canada.

The uptake of AS is dependent upon patient, clinical, and societal factors that influence the individual's decision about a regimen of AS. While prevailing public messages about cancer advocate immediate treatment, AS infers that curative treatment is applied only when the disease progresses to a clinically significant stage. Thus, men who consider AS must decide if they can live with their disease without receiving any treatment or intervention at all, or for some time.

Methods

This research explored the perspectives of men with PCa regarding their decision-making process for AS. Understanding men's perspectives on following a regimen of AS would help clinicians in providing clear information and meaningful discussions on treatment options and supportive care.

The study utilized a qualitative descriptive design [9] and recruited men from PCa programs in Montreal, Toronto, Winnipeg, Vancouver, and Thunder Bay. These programs provided access to urologists, medical oncologists and radiation oncologists. Candidates for AS had low grade, localized PCa and were informed about the study by a clinician providing their care. A local research coordinator contacted and informed interested individuals on study details and the arrangements for participation upon consent. Research ethics approval was obtained from each of the participating sites including the Centre de recherche du centre hospitalier de l'Université de Montréal, the McGill University Health Centre, Cancer Care Manitoba, the University Health Network and the University of British Columbia.

Participants either attended one focus group or engaged in a single interview if they were unable to attend the group session. The focus groups and interviews were facilitated by qualified personnel and were conducted in the language preferred by the participants (MF all English, CL all French). All sessions were attended by three other team members who assisted with the logistics, note-taking, and clarification of questions from the participants. Sessions and interviews were audio-recorded and transcribed verbatim.

Focus groups and interview guides were developed for the study and covered the same topic. Participants were asked to describe their experiences in being diagnosed, hearing about AS, deciding their course of action, communicating their decision with others, seeking information, being on AS, and deciding whether to stay on the regime or not. Questions were open-ended and probes were inserted only for clarification purposes.

Analysis

The transcripts were subjected to a qualitative description analysis [9]. Four team members (MF, KP, AMM, VO) read transcripts independently, taking marginal notes about the content. Team members shared their perspectives on all content identified and designed a content-coding framework based on shared perspectives. The content-coding framework contained a list of topics and definitions regarding what type of data belonged in each of those topic categories. Two members (MF, KP) used this framework to code all transcripts from the focus groups and interviews, and then reviewed the coded categories in-depth before summarizing the content for each category with an identified key theme (i.e., commonly held perspectives by the participants). The analysis was presented to three other team members who reviewed the clarity and relevance of the findings (two team members had attended the group sessions while the other was a clinician who interacted with the men considering AS). The resulting consensus about the findings provided the basis for this manuscript which focuses on decision-making about AS.

Results
Patient characteristics

Seven focus groups were held with locations in Montreal (one English and one French), Toronto (two groups), Winnipeg, Vancouver, and Thunder Bay. Nine men engaged in one-on-one interviews. A total of 52 men participated, ranging in age from 53 to 81 years (mean = 67.8; median = 68). Among them, 70.8% had completed post-secondary education or above. Participants with PCa had been living with their disease since diagnosis for 1 to 16 years (median = 3). Table 1 presents the number of men who were on, or had been on an AS regime. Overall, the participants who had been on AS reflected an average of 3.4 years of experience with the approach (range of 1 to 15 years). These data were self-reported by men on the demographic questionnaire.

Table 1 Participant Characteristics

Treatment decision-making stage	Number of participants (out of 52)
Diagnosed with prostate cancer and presently under active surveillance	38
Diagnosed with prostate cancer and withdrew from active surveillance	
-for reasons of disease progression	0
-for reasons other than disease progression	1
Diagnosed with prostate cancer and decided to undergo surgery or radiation at the beginning	9
Diagnosed with prostate cancer and currently deciding about treatment	2
Declined to provide data	2

Perspectives shared by participants

Four main themes emerged from the analysis of data. Each are described below, drawing from relevant content categories and illustrated by patient quotes in Table 2. The findings captured a range of perspectives from men on being diagnosed with PCa, seeking relevant information and communication, and making decisions on their course of action. Participants varied in their viewpoints and understandings about AS. Factors that influenced their decision-making on AS have implications for clinical practice.

Theme: an important decision is needed at a time of emotional upset and uncertainty

Consent for AS was recognized as an important decision that required careful consideration within a context of emotional upset and uncertainty. The emotional upheaval arose during the assessment of a diagnosis, in hearing the diagnosis, and upon request for a decision without sufficient information and understanding.

Obtaining a definite diagnosis can take time Few participants had symptoms before their diagnosis. Most had been followed by their family doctors with regular PSA testing prior to observing a rise in levels. Subsequent referral to a surgeon or urologist usually resulted in a biopsy. The diagnosis was based on, at minimum, one biopsy result. However, it was not unusual for the men to undergo more than one test and to wait for various lengths of time for a definite diagnosis.

Hearing the definite diagnosis is a shock Participants acknowledged that they were shocked and upset at hearing the PCa diagnosis, even though they understood that tests were performed to detect the disease. They indicated feeling numb, overwhelmed, frightened, and uncertain about the future, questioning whether the results were correct and why this had happened to them.

Having little information about PCa causes uncertainty Many participants stated that they knew very little about PCa and its treatment at diagnosis. They did not understand what caused the disease, their risk of death, how the cancer was treated, what treatment options were available, or the impact of various treatment approaches. Those who knew something about the disease were drawing on experiences of family members or friends. Essentially, they perceived cancer as a fatal illness and experienced uncertainty about their situation and fear for their mortality.

Being told it is your decision to make was surprising Many participants were dismayed when they discovered that they had the final say on their treatment. They had anticipated that the physician or surgeon would provide clear direction on which treatment option to pursue. They were surprised in the variety of options, feeling startled and, to some extent, frustrated when they realized that they had a significant role in the decision-making instead of principally complying with the best course of action from an expert. Many wondered on how to make a good decision without adequate information.

Theme: information is necessary on a number of topics before a decision can be made about AS

The participants cited the need for information as a critical element in making their decision about AS. Important components included understanding the information on a number of topics, searching for the information by oneself, and applying and detecting the relevant information to one's own situation. Participants' experiences varied across these components in terms of fulfilling their needs.

Information is needed on PCa, treatment options, benefits, side effects and AS Participants listed a range of topics to comprehend before making an informed decision about AS. Understanding the disease, the various options for treatment, and the anticipated outcomes and side effects of each option were commonly cited. The men sought for knowledge of topics in general and an understanding of facts related to their own situation. In particular, they needed to understand AS and its intended benefits. Most had not heard of AS and had initially interpreted it as doing nothing to combat a feared disease.

There is a need to actively seek information Once they had learned their diagnosis, participants felt that actively seeking information was critical for making an informed decision. For some, this step came naturally whereas others searched for information because they

Table 2 Representatives quotes from main theme content categories

Main Theme	Contributing content categories	Illustrative quote examples
An important decision is needed at a time of emotional upset and uncertainty	Obtaining a definite diagnosis can take time	*I had a physical with my family physician and he ordered a PSA test. The test revealed a slightly higher level...I was referred. I think I went through a number of PSA tests and they sort of bounced around, up and down, and eventually reached the stage where Dr. X concluded a biopsy was in order. The first biopsy revealed, out of ten samples, that eight were OK and two were inconclusive. I think we did another one or two PSA tests and it kept rising, which resulted in another biopsy. And this time one of the samples revealed cancer.*
	Hearing the definite diagnosis is a shock	*I felt I'd been hit by a truck.* *Why me? Why did this happen to me? And now? What do I do?*
	Having little information about prostate cancer causes uncertainty	*It's amazing that you don't really know about prostate cancer until you are diagnosed; like, why would I want to know about it?* *I really didn't know anything about prostate cancer or even what the prostate was...I wasn't sure what was going on.*
	Being told it is your decision to make was surprising	*He said, 'You have to decide what you want to do.' I was, like sort of, 'You tell me what to do.' You know? That's what I found difficult...he didn't say, 'You definitely need this or that.' He said, 'Well, what did you decide?' Me, I said, 'Well what are the choices? What would you recommend?...What would you tell your brother?'*
Information is necessary on a number of topics before a decision can be made about active surveillance	Information is needed on prostate cancer, treatment options, expected impacts/benefits, side effects, and active surveillance	*For example, I went into the biopsy without any idea what I was going into...you should prepare people better for what's ahead.* *I had not heard about active surveillance before at all... when I first got cancer, and before I read up on active surveillance, I must admit, well, I thought I got cancer, get it out right away. What the hell am I doing walking around with it? It never crossed my mind, I guess I never thought of something growing so slowly that it's not going to, it will never effect you...but that's what's going through my mind a lot now.*
	There is a need to actively seek information	*The first thing I did when I got home was go on the Internet. You need to explore all the options so when push comes to shove and you need to cross that bridge, at least you are better armed to make an informed decision.* *I had really wished there had been a group like this that I could sit down and talk about making decisions. I felt quite isolated, that I had to go out and search for people.*
	There is a need to check with different sources of information	*I talked with everyone I could. It felt like I had all the time I needed to make a decision, and that I could make the best one for me. I just needed to know the options for me and the possible impacts in my situation before I made it.* *I did a ton of reading and I spoke to a ton of people who had had it. It didn't confuse me but it didn't necessarily help me sort if all out.*
	It is important to sort out what information is relevant to the individual's own situation	*There is a lot of information out there, but I do not know how accurate it is.* *I had to sort out what applied to me, to my disease and situation. It was hard to know just from everything I read and had heard.*
Disease status and quality of life are important factors for men in deciding about active surveillance	Various factors are taken into consideration in making a final decision about active surveillance	*I took it all into account [the doctor, the reading, talking to my wife]...weighed all the facts, gathered my evidence, all the information, and then made an informed decision.* *For me, it was a combination of factors...weighing them out and coming to a logical conclusion.*

Table 2 Representatives quotes from main theme content categories *(Continued)*

Main Theme	Contributing content categories	Illustrative quote examples
		Understanding of the disease and potential for harm:
		• *I was told it was small and low grade…a little level of cancer.*
		• *They told me it is mild…and that the tumor cells are slow growing…it won't likely get me before something else.*
		Understanding of active surveillance and potential for benefit:
		• *My first reaction to the concept [active surveillance], which came right at the beginning from the urologist, that's really doing nothing. So I am not sure that's the right thing to do…but he laid it all out…and as I researched it, and got into it, it is doing something. It's actually monitoring in a quite regular basis. I got comfortable with that.*
		• *It's not about doing nothing, you are doing something. You are monitoring and going to catch it in time if it gets bigger. I will have time to act.*
		Side effects of treatment
		• *If I could go another 10 years without an operation, I'd feel good about that, about not having one. I'm 67 now.*
		• *I did a lot of reading and found a lot of negative things about the surgery.*
		Wanting to be rid of cancer
		• *As soon as I found out that I got it, I thought, 'What the hell, I gotta get rid of this' cause, you know, in everybody's mind cancer isn't good for you.*
		• *I said, 'If I got it, might as well get rid of it…get it over with.'*
		Past experiences with family/friends
		• *I have a brother who is 15 years younger than me and he had his prostate removed. His cancer was small too. But he couldn't live with it…but I can. I'm 64. Maybe if I was younger I'd have had it out too*
		• *My father had treatment for prostate cancer and his life was never the same again. I didn't want that for me. I am too young.*
		Medical opinion
		• *I had four doctors that have more or less indicated to me that it is not a major thing [to wait].*
		• *It was my doctor's decision. But I was very relieved that I did not have to go under the knife, you know.*
		• *I am beginning to fear surgery but, definitely, if the doctors all said, 'Listen, you've got to get it out,' I will definitely go for surgery when the time comes, if it happens to come, I will do it.*
		Age and health status
		• *I have sort of decided that I am not going to do anything rash. I just turned 80 so it's not as if I am in my 50's. So I decided the best thing is just to go through with it, to do the surveillance.*
		• *I was more or less on [the idea that] the less aggressive form of action would be better for me right now… postpone as long as we can. Fifty-seven is too young to go under the knife.*
		• *I am young, I can deal with it [surgery] now and recovery will be quicker than if I wait and do something when I was in later years.*
		Emotional toll over time
		• *Any time you have a bit of an issue you would think, ah, maybe it's because I have prostate cancer, so I decided to get it out, taken care of at that time.*
		• *You have to learn to live with the fact you have cancer, at least a little bit of it, and that it may never get you.*
		• *I decided I don't want to live with this [prostate cancer] anymore…I am tired. So, let's do it [treatment].*

Table 2 Representatives quotes from main theme content categories *(Continued)*

Main Theme	Contributing content categories	Illustrative quote examples
		Family viewpoints • *My wife said, 'You need to be treated. I want you to be here.' But for me, active surveillance sounded fine.* • *But my two daughters said, 'Dad, don't fool around with it. Deal with it.' There was family pressure. So I made a decision to go with radiation, stop what was there.* • *My wife was involved too…it wasn't just my decision. We are together on that…but she wanted me to be treated!* **Not enough information to decide** • *I have read so much and talked to a lot of people, and the information is really not clear. That's why I am on active surveillance. I feel I don't have all the information [to decide about treatment].*
	Disease status is an important consideration/factor for men	**Choosing active surveillance** *I have no symptoms…it is a very small cancer. It's not aggressive. So I decided that was the course for me. I would take active surveillance. I am not afraid of dying.* *At my age, there's this notion that one could die before you die of prostate cancer, you die of other causes.* **Staying on active surveillance** *It's been 7 years and I feel fine…as long as my numbers are good, my exams are good, I am going to stay on active surveillance.* *If I was ever going to have another biopsy, and there were shown major changes in the amount of cancer in the biopsy bits, and if the doctor suggested that well maybe we should consider an operation, I mean that is the kind of information you want to hear to help you make a decision on it.*
	Quality of life is an important consideration/factor for men	**Choosing active surveillance** • *I told him I am not interested in anything of [treatment]. It's about quality of life…I don't have symptoms now, so I am going to wait.* • *Treatment is scary, in terms of side effects on things… the side effects of the hormone drug I might have to take are huge. I think with radiation as well.* **Choosing treatment** • *If I live for another 35 years, I would like it to be a good quality I don't want to deal with cancer…me? I would just do it [treatment]. So I said, 'Don't wait, let's just do it.*
	There is a need to balance what is important to you	*Some of these treatments have pretty drastic after effects, ah, you would have to live with them. So you have to weigh it all out.* *You sort of balance the things about invasive surgery, you know, and what else is happening to your body from other causes. If you are pretty healthy then you want to stay that way. If it gets serious, then I will think of the alternatives. You kind of have to figure out what you need for surviving and what you need for quality of life. It just seemed to me that active surveillance gave me options. I did not have a lot of disease and, who knows, if I wait for treatment until I really need it, there could be other things available.*
Conversations with doctor(s) have significant influences on men in their decision-making about active surveillance	Conversations with doctors can be helpful or add to a patient's distress	*I talked with the surgeon and really just had one option offered to me. I was not satisfied with that, I wanted to have all of my options explained. So I went to another doctor.* *To be frank with you, I had my GP tell me, 'You know, it's a long term thing. Don't worry about it'…he told me not to worry about it. So I am taking him at face value and I am not overly concerned.* *So at this point, in talking with two urologists and a radiologist, I've decided, well, I think they helped me decide, that the thing to do was, ah, not to do anything too drastic but to maintain surveillance of the growth.*

Table 2 Representatives quotes from main theme content categories *(Continued)*

Main Theme	Contributing content categories	Illustrative quote examples
		I have to say I was a little apprehensive before I talked with Dr. X and the radiologist...I was quite impressed because they were quite conservative in their approach. That kind of reinforced my thinking because I was a little bit apprehensive about going through any kind of radiation treatment or something like that.
		There is no doubt about it, you turn to the physician and depend on what he is telling you what is right for your situation. He can certainly sway you one way of the other.
	Confidence and trust are of importance	*What persuaded me most was the reaction of the medical staff. They didn't seem to be overly excited about the whole thing.*
		I talked with the first urologist and then with two other doctors, and I was sort of reassured. I mean I may need treatment sometime, that may happen, but for the moment I've decided to do surveillance
		He has high credentials. So you know he knows what he is doing...keeping up to date...pleasant....his reputation.
		Trusting the doctor is the answer.
		This guy has a way of talking with you. He explains. He shows you...but he leaves you, it's your decision.
		I listen to him. I have been with him for more than 11 years. I do what he says, he knows better than me.
		I listened to what the doctors had to say. There were slight variations, but not much. There's some consensus there.
	The ideal process from a patient's perspective allows for tailored discussion and reflection	*You have to help people prepare for what they are heading into.*
		You need to give them an honest appraisal of their status. They can govern themselves...it is important that you let them know it is mild and slow progressing...it is a different type of cancer.
		Dissemination of information is very important on a direct basis...you give as much information as you can.
		The person [who goes on active surveillance] wants to know, if I go on this regime of just testing every so often, am I at risk? Will it get past the threshold of danger, you now, before we find out?...having time to act if something begins to change, is there time to act? That's critical. That's what makes action surveillance safe for us.

wanted to confirm the information from their physicians or felt that it was incomplete. Others wanted a second or third opinion, input from other cancer patients, or assistance in understanding what they were reading. A commonly held perspective was that one had to be self-reliant in educating themselves and could not solely rely upon the information received from health care professionals.

There is a need to check with different sources of information Participants utilized different sources for their information search and were generally encouraged to do so by their physicians. The internet was the most cited resource, followed closely by the advice from health care professionals, family members and friends. Men found it helpful when cancer centres provided information packages or referrals to local PCa peer groups. Different sources offered input on different topics; while some provided factual information, others offered the

opportunity for discussion, particularly among peers who had been through a similar situation.

It is important to sort out what information is relevant to the individual's situation Men expressed concern about the reliability of information from various sources, the amount of searching they had to do without guidance from health care professionals, the large amount of information available, and the wide variation in suggested treatment approaches for PCa. Participants expressed surprise and frustration on the lack of agreement between treatment guidelines and indicated the benefits of talking with a knowledgeable individual who could apply information that was specific to their own situation. Men found it helpful in knowing that they could take time to reflect on what they were learning and how it applied to them, and not feel pressured to make an immediate decision.

Theme: disease status and quality of life are important factors for men in deciding about AS

Disease status and quality of life emerged as the most important factors to consider in the decision for AS. Participants sought a wide range of information, but acknowledged that primary influences included the nature of their disease and the quality of life they wanted. These same factors applied for men who selected AS or those who elected to pursue interventional treatment, but the interpretation and application to a man's situation varied. For example, age could be used to argue for pursuing immediate surgery (e.g., recover more quickly) or electing to wait (e.g., too young to live with potential impotence).

Various factors are taken into consideration for a final decision about AS Participants described a range of factors they considered when deciding their course of action. These included understanding their disease and its treatment, their risk of death, AS and its intention, treatment side effects, age and health status (both now and later), the desire to be cancer-free, medical opinion, past experiences with cancer, family perspectives, and the emotional toll of living with cancer. Factors were prioritized differently based on the individual's life experience and situation.

Disease status is an important consideration/factor for men Men considered their disease status as a key factor when selecting either a course of AS or interventional treatment. The type and size of tumor and risk for death from the cancer were significant pieces of information. Prior to their diagnosis, the participants had not understood that low grade or slow growing PCa did not require interventional treatment. Most had not heard of AS and were introduced to the idea as an option for low grade disease by their physicians. Although some confused interchangeably the terms 'watchful waiting', 'routine follow-up care' post-surgery and AS, participants described AS as appropriate for low grade disease; they understood the delay in treatment and its side effects while being closely monitored, and that interventional treatment was applied when it became necessary. Treatment was described as necessary if the disease progressed and the physician indicated that action was required. However, waiting offered the possibility of new treatment approaches being available at a future date as well as avoidance of an operation and disturbing side effects. Comfort with an AS approach was based on the idea of being closely monitored with reliable tests, and acting in a timely fashion when required.

Quality of life is an important consideration/factor for men The issue of side effects emerged prominently in discussions about quality of life. Both radiation and surgery for PCa were seen as having significant side effects with potential to impact a person's relationships, sexuality, functioning, and emotional well-being. Avoiding side effects was seen as desirable by participants and figured highly in their decision-making about AS. Once they were reassured that their health was not at greater risk on AS with access to treatment in a timely fashion if required, men viewed AS as a preferred option. The subsequent challenge was living with the idea of cancer in their bodies and not dwelling on that fact on a daily basis. Given that most of the participants were not experiencing symptoms, avoiding side effects became a clear choice for quality of life.

There is a need to balance what is important to you Participants described how they came to realize that the decision about treatment was largely their responsibility. However, this realization emerged only after seeking information and discussion with health care professionals, family members and others. In the final analysis, they needed to identify and give due consideration to what was important to them, and balance various considerations for their life situation. In particular, the men reflected that the idea of AS was different from the public cancer messages about early diagnosis and prompt treatment. They, alongside family and friends, had to come to terms with understanding this difference. More often than not, family and friends were encouraging the men to the treat the cancer.

Theme: conversations with doctors have significant influences on men in their decision–making about AS

Almost without exception, participants spoke of conversations with doctors as significant for them and in their decision-making. Many men relied on the physician/surgeon for clear direction on which treatment option to pursue. This included helping them understand the benefits and consequences of various treatments, and what the best approach would be for them, given their situation.

Conversations with doctors can be helpful or add to a patient's distress Participants described wide variation in the nature of conversations with physicians. Variation existed in the duration of the conversations, the clarity of information provided, the personal care and concern that was expressed, consistency of information from different doctors, who was involved in the conversational exchange, the number of treatment options and specific effects discussed, and the active encouragement to seek other opinions. While some participants were entirely satisfied with the exchange and felt well informed and supported afterwards, others found these conversations were less than helpful and experienced heightened frustration and uncertainty.

Confidence and trust are of importance Participants expressed a high sense of confidence and trust in the physicians and their viewpoints. For many, this confidence emerged from conversations held, the relevance and clarity of the information provided by the physician, opportunities to openly question and discuss test results and options, and the attention paid to the men's individual preferences. For others, the confidence emerged from having known the doctor over many years or knowing the physician's reputation.

The ideal process from a patient's perspective allows for tailored discussion and reflection Participants readily identified important characteristics of an ideal process for holding conversations about AS. These included easy access to information, having time for conversational exchange, providing clear and honest information, providing information relevant to the individual's situation, delivering the information with sensitivity and compassion, including family members, supporting the conversation with written information, and providing reliable web-site addresses for personal follow-up. Clearly, participants viewed broad access to information as an important feature, but emphasized that information should be tailored or applied to the individual's particular situation, preferences, and values. Access to relevant understandable information was of paramount importance in assisting men with their decisions and in preparing for what was ahead.

Discussion

In this qualitative study, a wide-ranging discussion about patients' decision-making process regarding AS showed that selecting AS was not an isolated decision but involved the entire experience of confronting the reality of having cancer.

A number of participants' perspectives have been reported previously: emotional upheaval at diagnosis and surprise at the PSA elevation with no symptoms (reviewed in [10, 11]); lack of knowledge about PCa and its treatment, and lessening of anxiety once men understood more about their situation and available choices [12] (reviewed in [11, 13, 14]); influence of emotional anxiety on treatment decision-making [15, 16]; variation in preferences for involvement in decision-making, including the desire of some men for a passive role [17–19]; the need to search for information and the frustration of searching on their own [19]; the need for support from others (reviewed in [20]); the participants' view about the significance of the physician's role in the decision-making process [12, 18, 19, 21, 22] (reviewed in [11, 13, 20]); and the differences in the provision of information from different cancer programs or providers [23].

Unique to this study was the insight into the ways men approached decision-making regarding AS. At the onset of their experience, they were unfamiliar with AS and following a course of AS ran counter to the men's original preconceptions about cancer and treatment. They identified a need to shift their thinking about what actions to take. Once men had relevant information, understood the actual degree of risk for themselves, and perceived the opportunity to avoid treatment side effects, some became more open to the idea of AS.

Understanding that their disease was low risk, combined with the notion of avoiding treatment side effects, were strong incentives for those who opted for AS. Enduring treatment side effects was perceived as reducing their quality of life. This aligns with a questionnaire analysis [15] and a study reporting analysis of internet conversations showing an increased awareness of quality of life and associated comfort with AS [24]. In contrast to participants in a reported phone survey analysis, patients from our focus groups felt well-informed on the possible side effects of treatments [25]. They also emphasized the comfort in being closely monitored, as reported in other studies [12, 21]. Close monitoring would allow for future treatment intervention in a timely fashion, if necessary. This idea was important for the men and contributed to their ease in handling the sense of risk.

For those who opted not to follow a course of AS, many talked about their capacity to undergo immediate treatment, based on their age or physical status, or feeling a pressure to deal with the cancer, which emerged from their internal sense of risk from the disease or from commentary by family members. The desire to be cancer-free or to reduce their risk or on-going worry, influenced their final decision to pursue surgery or radiation treatment. These findings also aligned with other recent reports [12, 15, 21, 26, 27]. Anxiety was a reason not to adhere initially to AS but was also a factor that influenced the decision for a radical treatment after a period of time on AS (reviewed in [20, 28]).

Most participants consulted a number of individuals, either for information or for support, while deciding about AS. Variation existed in whom they consulted, what input they sought, and the helpfulness of responses they received. In particular, family members and friends were consulted frequently. However, they were often unaware of PCa treatment options and had to adjust their ideas about the low risk nature of the disease, as did the men. Other health care professionals, including family physicians, were also consulted regarding AS. Participants found that these practitioners did not always have the necessary information on AS. Finally, a few men had the opportunity to meet with a support group for men diagnosed with PCa; those that attended meetings found the conversations with peers informative.

Ultimately, the role of the physician in the decision-making process was significant to the participants; they referred to this person for advice and direction. Confidence and trust was engendered primarily through the manner in which conversations unfolded and the way questions were answered. Fundamentally, men sought for clarity in information and forthright conversations about their risks from PCa (now and in the future), and time for discussion about their unique situation. Inconsistency in information from one practitioner to another, or one treatment guideline to another, was distressing for these men, as were hurried conversations with medical technical language. These findings are in line with those reported previously where the increased number of visits to the specialist rendered the treatment decision more difficult for men [25] and raised more concerns by patients in regards to the unbiased recommendation of treatment by their specialists [24].

Implications for practice and future research

With one exception (the Thunder Bay group), all focus groups were held in metropolitan academic centres where PCa care was delivered within specialized clinical programs. Nonetheless, men identified variation in their access to relevant, meaningful information about PCa, treatment options, and AS. This raises questions about the process for providing information to men and their family members and emphasizes the need for standardization across the country. Ultimately, the content should be clear and comprehensive, and the delivery should include multiple types of formats and easy access. Where possible, the opportunity to discuss the information in relevance to an individual's situation could be deemed valuable to those interested.

We isolated several factors that men took into consideration when deciding their PCa treatment. Conversations with clinicians need to include dialogue about these factors with as much clarity as possible. In particular, tools for decision-making (i.e., decision boards) around AS could be designed and tested. This concept was assessed and deemed helpful by low risk PCa patients [29]. However, based on a systemic review, the majority of decision-aid tools are lacking important information for PCa treatment decisions or do not provide sufficient elements to favor shared decision-making by both the patient and the health care provider (reviewed in [30–32]). Organizing the opportunity for more than one conversation with time to make decisions would likely be of benefit to men, and allow clarification of facts and anticipated implications of one course of action over another. Follow-up studies could include interrogating the universality of specific findings of our

qualitative study, using a more quantitative questionnaire-based approach, to more fully understand the patient-centered decision making process around active surveillance.

Acknowledgements
We thank all participants who shared with us their experience with their PCa journey. We are grateful to Paula Sitarik, Lucie Hamel, Maureen Palmer, Kathy Li, who generously provided their assistance during the study. We also thank Jacqueline Chung for careful reading and editing of this manuscript.

Funding
This research was part of the pan-Canadian initiative named the Canadian PCa Biomarker Network and funded by the Terry Fox Research Institute.

Authors' contributions
Participate in the conception and initial design: FS, AMMM, SS, MF, VO. Participate in the acquisition: MF, KP, VO, CL, SC, DEC, AF, JBL, AS, ST, FS, AMMM Participate in the analysis and interpretation: MF, KP, VO, SA, FS, AMMM. Participate in the drafting and/or revision of the manuscript: MF, KP, VO, CL, SA, SC, DEC, AF, JBL, SS, AS, ST, FS, AMMM. All authors read and approved the final manuscript.

Competing interests
The authors declare that they have no competing interests.

Author details
[1]Sunnybrook Health Sciences Centre, 2075 Bayview Ave, Toronto, ON, Canada. [2]Institut du cancer de Montréal and Centre de recherche du Centre hospitalier de l'Université de Montréal, 900 St Denis St, Montreal, QC, Canada. [3]McGill University and McGill University Health Centre, 1001 Decarie Blvd, Montreal, QC, Canada. [4]University Health Network, 610 University Ave, Toronto, ON, Canada. [5]Manitoba Prostate Centre, 675 McDermot Ave, Winnipeg, MB, Canada. [6]Department of Surgery Université de Montréal, 2900 Edouard Montpetit Blvd, Montreal, QC, Canada. [7]Terrry Fox Research Institute, 675 West 10th Avenue, Vancouver, BC, Canada. [8]Vancouver Prostate Centre, 2660 Oak St, Vancouver, BC, Canada. [9]Department of Medicine, Université de Montréal, 2900 Edouard Montpetit Blvd, Montreal, QC, Canada.

References
1. Raldow AC, Zhang D, Chen MH, Braccioforte MH, Moran BJ, D'Amico AV. Risk group and death from prostate cancer: implications for active surveillance in men with favorable intermediate-risk prostate cancer. JAMA Oncol. 2015;1(3):334–40.
2. Sternberg IA, Vela I, Scardino PT. Molecular profiles of prostate cancer: to treat or not to treat. Annu Rev Med. 2016;67:119–35.
3. National Comprehensive Cancer Network. Clinical Practive Guidelines in Oncology - Prostate Cancer. https://www.nccn.org/professionals/physician_gls/pdf/prostate.pdf.
4. Bruinsma SM, Bangma CH, Carroll PR, Leapman MS, Rannikko A, Petrides N, Weerakoon M, Bokhorst LP, Roobol MJ, Movember GAPc. Active surveillance for prostate cancer: a narrative review of clinical guidelines. Nat Rev Urol. 2016;13(3):151–67.
5. Tosoian JJ, Carter HB, Lepor A, Loeb S. Active surveillance for prostate cancer: current evidence and contemporary state of practice. Nat Rev Urol. 2016;13(4):205–15.
6. Dinh KT, Mahal BA, Ziehr DR, Muralidhar V, Chen YW, Viswanathan VB, Nezolosky MD, Beard CJ, Choueiri TK, Martin NE, et al. Incidence and predictors of upgrading and up staging among 10,000 contemporary patients with low risk prostate cancer. J Urol. 2015;194(2):343–9.
7. Ting F, van Leeuwen PJ, Delprado W, Haynes AM, Brenner P, Stricker PD. Tumor volume in insignificant prostate cancer: increasing the threshold is a safe approach to reduce over-treatment. Prostate. 2015;75(15):1768–73.

8. Timilshina N, Ouellet V, Alibhai SM, Mes-Masson AM, Delvoye N, Drachenberg D, Finelli A, Jammal MP, Karakiewicz P, Lapointe H, et al. Analysis of active surveillance uptake for low-risk localized prostate cancer in Canada: a Canadian multi-institutional study. World J Urol. 2016;35(4):595-03.
9. Thorne S. Data analysis in qualitative research. Evid Based Nurs. 2000;3:68–70.
10. Glaser AP, Novakovic K, Helfand BT. The impact of prostate biopsy on urinary symptoms, erectile function, and anxiety. Curr Urol Rep. 2012;13(6):447–54.
11. Kazer MW, Psutka SP, Latini DM, Bailey DE Jr. Psychosocial aspects of active surveillance. Curr Opin Urol. 2013;23(3):273–7.
12. Volk RJ, McFall SL, Cantor SB, Byrd TL, Le YC, Kuban DA, Mullen PD. It's not like you just had a heart attack': decision-making about active surveillance by men with localized prostate cancer. Psychooncology. 2014;23(4):467–72.
13. van den Bergh RC, Korfage IJ, Bangma CH. Psychological aspects of active surveillance. Curr Opin Urol. 2012;22(3):237–42.
14. Venderbos LD, van den Bergh RC, Roobol MJ, Schroder FH, Essink-Bot ML, Bangma CH, Steyerberg EW, Korfage IJ. A longitudinal study on the impact of active surveillance for prostate cancer on anxiety and distress levels. Psychooncology. 2015;24(3):348–54.
15. van den Bergh RC, van Vugt HA, Korfage IJ, Steyerberg EW, Roobol MJ, Schroder FH, Essink-Bot ML. Disease insight and treatment perception of men on active surveillance for early prostate cancer. BJU Int. 2010;105(3):322–8.
16. de Bekker-Grob EW, Bliemer MC, Donkers B, Essink-Bot ML, Korfage IJ, Roobol MJ, Bangma CH, Steyerberg EW. Patients' and urologists' preferences for prostate cancer treatment: a discrete choice experiment. Br J Cancer. 2013;109(3):633–40.
17. Hurwitz LM, Cullen J, Elsamanoudi S, Kim DJ, Hudak J, Colston M, Travis J, Kuo HC, Porter CR, Rosner IL. A prospective cohort study of treatment decision-making for prostate cancer following participation in a multidisciplinary clinic. Urol Oncol. 2015;34(5):233.e17-25.
18. Davison BJ, Goldenberg SL. Patient acceptance of active surveillance as a treatment option for low-risk prostate cancer. BJU Int. 2011;108(11):1787–93.
19. Davison BJ, Breckon E. Factors influencing treatment decision making and information preferences of prostate cancer patients on active surveillance. Patient Educ Couns. 2012;87(3):369–74.
20. Luke A Robles, Shihning Chou, Owen J Cole, Akhlil Hamid, Amanda Griffiths and Kavita Vedhara Psychological and Social Factors influencing Patients' Treatment Selection for Localised Prostate Cancer, Advances in Prostate Cancer, Dr. Gerhard Hamilton (Ed.), InTech. 2013. Available from: https://www.intechopen.com/books/advances-in-prostate-cancer/psychological-and-social-factors-influencing-patients-treatment-selection-for-localised-prostate-can.
21. O'Callaghan C, Dryden T, Hyatt A, Brooker J, Burney S, Wootten AC, White A, Frydenberg M, Murphy D, Williams S, et al. 'What is this active surveillance thing?' Men's and partners' reactions to treatment decision making for prostate cancer when active surveillance is the recommended treatment option. Psychooncology. 2014;23(12):1391–8.
22. Orom H, Homish DL, Homish GG, Underwood W 3rd. Quality of physician-patient relationships is associated with the influence of physician treatment recommendations among patients with prostate cancer who chose active surveillance. Urol Oncol. 2014;32(4):396–402.
23. Tombal B, Baskin-Bey E, Schulman C. Access to information and expectations of treatment decisions for prostate cancer patients–results of a European survey. Eur J Cancer Care (Engl). 2013;22(2):210–8.
24. Mishra MV, Bennett M, Vincent A, Lee OT, Lallas CD, Trabulsi EJ, Gomella LG, Dicker AP, Showalter TN. Identifying barriers to patient acceptance of active

surveillance: content analysis of online patient communications. PLoS One. 2013;8(9):e68563.
25. Dogan C, Gultekin HM, Erdogan SM, Ozkara H, Talat Z, Erozenci AN, Obek C. Patient decision making prior to radical prostatectomy: what is and is not involved. Am J Mens Health. 2015. Epub ahead of print.
26. Anandadas CN, Clarke NW, Davidson SE, O'Reilly PH, Logue JP, Gilmore L, Swindell R, Brough RJ, Wemyss-Holden GD, Lau MW, et al. Early prostate cancer–which treatment do men prefer and why? BJU Int. 2011;107(11):1762–8.
27. Devos J, Van Praet C, Decaestecker K, Claeys T, Fonteyne V, Decalf V, De Meerleer G, Ost P, Lumen N. Cognitive factors influencing treatment decision-making in patients with localised prostate cancer: development of a standardised questionnaire. Acta Clin Belg. 2015;70(4):272–9.
28. Simpkin AJ, Tilling K, Martin RM, Lane JA, Hamdy FC, Holmberg L, Neal DE, Metcalfe C, Donovan JL. Systematic review and meta-analysis of factors determining change to radical treatment in active surveillance for localized prostate cancer. Eur Urol. 2015;67(6):993–1005.
29. Chabrera C, Font A, Caro M, Areal J, Zabalegui A. Developing a decision aid to support informed choices for newly diagnosed patients with localized prostate cancer. Cancer Nurs. 2015;38(1):E55–60.
30. Adsul P, Wray R, Spradling K, Darwish O, Weaver N, Siddiqui S. Systematic review of decision aids for newly diagnosed patients with prostate cancer making treatment decisions. J Urol. 2015;194(5):1247–52.
31. Lin GA, Aaronson DS, Knight SJ, Carroll PR, Dudley RA. Patient decision aids for prostate cancer treatment: a systematic review of the literature. CA Cancer J Clin. 2009;59(6):379–90.
32. Violette PD, Agoritsas T, Alexander P, Riikonen J, Santti H, Agarwal A, Bhatnagar N, Dahm P, Montori V, Guyatt GH, et al. Decision aids for localized prostate cancer treatment choice: systematic review and meta-analysis. CA Cancer J Clin. 2015;65(3):239–51.

3

Comparison of radiofrequency ablation and partial nephrectomy for tumor in a solitary kidney

Wu Xiaobing, Gong Wentao, Liu Guangxiang, Zhang Fan, Gan Weidong, Guo Hongqian and Zhang Gutian[*]

Abstract

Background: To estimate oncologic and functional outcomes for radiofrequency ablation (RFA) versus partial nephrectomy (PN) for tumors in a solitary kidney.

Methods: Nineteen patients with sporadic renal cell carcinoma in a solitary kidney were treated with RFA, and 21 patients were treated with PN between November 2008 and September 2015. Basic demographic information including age, gender, operative and pathological data, complications, renal function, oncological outcomes, was obtained for each patient. Statistical analysis was done to test for the correlation of clinical and pathological features, renal function outcomes, as well as oncological outcomes of RFA and PN. All statistical tests were 2-sided, and p-value < 0.05 was considered significant. Statistical analyses were performed using SPSS 19.0.

Results: No significant differences were indicated between the RFA and PN with respect to mean patient age, tumor size, as well as intraoperative or postoperative complications. The mean length of hospitalization ($P = 0.019$) and mean operative time ($P = 0.036$) was significantly shorter in RFA, with the median estimated blood loss being greater in PN ($P = 0.001$). The mean serum creatinine level 24 h following operation were significantly higher than preoperative creatinine in PN ($P = 0.009$), but did not reach statistical significance in RFA. Local recurrence were detected in only 1 patient (5%) in PN and 3 patients (18.75%) in RFA ($P = 0.4$). One patient developed pulmonary metastasis and one exhibited tumor persistence in RFA, none were present in PN.

Conclusions: Radiofrequency Ablation and Partial Nephrectomy for Tumors in a Solitary Kidney were all safe and effective, with each method having distinct advantages. It is the decision of the patient and urologist to pick the best approach.

Keywords: Radiofrequency ablation, Partial nephrectomy, Solitary kidney, Oncologic and functional outcomes

Background

The incidence of renal cell carcinoma (RCC) continues to increase because of the widespread use of modern imaging examination, with an increasing number of patients with no urological symptoms being examined. Radical nephrectomy (RN) used to be regarded as the gold standard for the treatment of RCC for many years; recently, nephron-sparing surgery (NSS) was recommended particularly for tumors in a solitary kidney by a number of researchers and specialists. Tumors in a solitary kidney represent a challenging population where tumor control with maximal nephron preservation is essential. RN for tumors in a solitary kidney could lead to permanent hematodialysis; open partial nephrectomy (OPN) was regarded as the gold standard therapy for non-metastatic tumors in a solitary kidney, and laparoscopic partial nephrectomy (LPN) for tumor in a solitary kidney was feasible [1]. Radiofrequency ablation (RFA) was also considered as an approach to RCC [2]. Both PN (partial nephrectomy) and RFA (radiofrequency ablation) could be used for tumors in a solitary kidney. This study aimed to evaluate oncologic and functional outcomes for RFA versus PN for tumors in a solitary kidney, thus helping patients decide on the suitable surgery.

* Correspondence: zgt6810@aliyun.com
Nanjing University Medical School Affiliated Nanjing Drum Tower Hospital, Nanjing 210008, China

Methods

Patients

The Nanjing Drum Tower Hospital Urologic Oncology Database, which was approved by the Institutional Review Board, was retrospectively reviewed. Nineteen patients with RCC in a solitary kidney were treated with RFA, and 21 patients were treated with PN between November 2008 and September 2015. Patients with confirmed single or multiple tumors in an anatomical (congenital or acquired) or functional solitary kidney shown in the CT or MRI of the urinary tract were selected. Patients presenting with bilateral metastasis or have a history of hereditary RCC or a family history of RCC were excluded from analysis. One patient in the PN group and 3 patients in the RFA group who had metastasis preoperatively and received palliative therapy (via oral medication) were subsequently excluded from our analysis.

Surgical methods

Approaches to RFA include percutaneous and laparoscopic procedures; these surgical techniques for RFA have been described in previous studies [3, 4]. In the present study, the Cool-tip RFA system was used; all RFAs were conducted by the same experienced physician, and all cases followed the protocol provided by the system manufacturer. During RFA, ultrasound localization was conducted to locate endophytic tumors and ensure that the tumors were completely ablated; ablation cycles depended on tumor size. Renal biopsies were not obtained for every patient who received RFA.

Approaches to PN include open or laparoscopic surgery (LPN and RPN); the surgical techniques have been previously described [5–7]. After clamping of the renal artery during PN, the tumor was excised sharply outside the zone of a 0.5 cm peritumoral margin. The wound was sutured, and the collecting systems were closed when necessary.

Recorded variables and follow-up

Follow-up data was collected up to March 2016. The recorded variables included the following: patient age, gender, tumor size, R.E.N.A.L. nephrometry score, operative time, estimated blood loss (EBL), intraoperative and postoperative complications, length of hospitalization, pathologic outcomes, and serum creatinine. Postoperative follow-up included the follow-up period, recurrence, and metastasis. Complications were classified as intraoperative and postoperative. Intraoperative complications included significant injury to an adjacent organ, major vessel, ureter or pleura, and conversion to open surgery or transfusion (> 2 units). Post-operative complications included serious infection (requiring antibiotics), urine leakage, hemorrhage (requiring second surgery to stop bleeding). The R.E.N.A.L. nephrometry scoring system comprises the tumor size, tumor depth, proximity to the collecting system, tumor positioning in the anterior/posterior plane, and tumor location with regard to polarity; this system was used to measure the comorbidity in patients with renal tumors [8].

For RFA and PN, these data were obtained at 3 months, 12 months, and yearly thereafter; patients were contacted via outpatient review and telephone.

Statistical methods

Descriptive statistics are presented as the mean ± SD, median, and range or percentage. Demographic and clinical characteristics were analyzed using Student's t-tests for continuous variables and the chi-square test for categorical variables. The survival curve was generated using the Kaplan–Meier method, and differences between 2 groups were assessed using the log-rank test. All statistical tests were 2-sided, and p-value < 0.05 was considered significant. Statistical analyses were performed using SPSS 19.0.

Results

A total of 20 patients in the PN group and 16 patients in the RFA group satisfied the selection criteria. Demographic and clinical characteristics are presented in Table 1. No significant differences were indicated between the RFA and PN with respect to mean patient age, tumor size, as well as intraoperative or postoperative complications. The tumor complexity of the RFA group was similar to that of the PN group ($p = 0.56$). PN was associated with a greater median EBL (377 vs. 65.6 mL; $p = 0.001$). The mean length of hospitalization (12 vs. 17 d; $p = 0.019$) and mean operative time (145 vs. 199.8 min; $p = 0.036$) were significantly shorter in the RFA group. Mean renal artery blocking time was 25.2 min in the PN group, whereas no hilar clamping was necessary in the RFA group. Intraoperative (23.8% vs. 5.6%; $p = 0.13$) and postoperative complications (19.0% vs. 11.1%; $p = 0.41$) tended to be higher in the PN group; similarly, total complications were higher (42.8% vs. 16.7%; $p = 0.096$), but no significant difference was determined.

Renal function outcomes are presented in Table 2. The mean serum creatinine level (120.4 μmol/L) was significantly higher 24 h post-operatively than preoperatively (91.4 μmol/L) in the PN group ($p = 0.01$). In the RFA group, mean serum creatinine level (108.5 μmol/L) trended to higher 24 h post-operatively than preoperatively (94.9 μmol/L); however, no significant difference was indicated ($p = 0.06$). Three months post-operatively,

Table 1 Demographic and clinical characteristics

	RFA	PN	P value
Patients	16	20	
Procedures	18	21	–
Male/female	11/5	15/5	0.48
Mean age(years)(range)	59.6(36–79)	62.1(41–83)	0.55
Left/right	10/8	13/8	0.47
Tumor size (cm) (range)	3.4(1.5–6.0)	3.6(1.5–6.0)	0.5
Median EBL (mL) (range)	65.6(20–200)	377(20–1200)	0.001
Surgical approach, n (%)			
Percutaneous	7	–	–
Laparoscopic	7	11	–
Open	2	9	–
Mean operative time (min) (range)	145.0(50–260)	199.8(60–440)	0.036
Mean length of stay (days) (range)	12(6–28)	17(9–42)	0.019
renal artery blocking time (min)	–	25.2	–
complications (%)	3(16.7)	9(42.8)	0.096
Intra-operative complications	1(5.6)	5(23.8)	0.13
Postoperative complications	2(11.1)	4(19.0)	0.41

the mean serum creatinine level in each group showed no significant increase ($p = 0.26$; $p = 0.45$). No dialysis was needed for either group during the follow-up period.

Oncologic outcomes are listed in Table 3. In the PN group, no incidence of positive surgical margins was reported. Mean follow-up was 26.1 months in the PN group and 33.7 months in the RFA group ($p = 0.25$). In the PN group, 18 cases were identified as RCC: 1 was papillary, and 2 were chromophobe. In the RFA group, 14 cases were identified as RCC, and four were not specified. Local recurrence was detected in only one patient (5%) in the PN group and three patients (18.75%) in the RFA group ($p = 0.1$). Overall, one of 16 patients (6.25%) in the RFA group had incomplete ablation; the patient was successfully re-ablated 8 months later and remained cancer-free. In addition, one patient developed multiple metastasis in the RFA group, where none was reported in the PN group. Table 4 presents detailed information on recurrence; no deaths were reported.

Figure 1a, b show the comparative outcomes for the local recurrence-free survival (RFS) and the metastasis-free survival (MFS) for PN group vs. RFA group. No significant difference between the two groups was indicated.

Discussion

Tumor in a solitary kidney poses a distinct challenge for maintaining adequate renal function and providing oncologic control. PN is regarded as the gold standard treatment in patients with tumor in a solitary kidney [9], whereas RFA is an optional surgical procedure [10]. Both PN and RFA present certain advantages. Compared with PN, RFA showed easier recovery, less surgical trauma, less EBL, and a shorter length of hospitalization, thereby reducing recovery time and costs. These results were confirmed by Lotan Y and Cadeddu JA [11]. As shown in the study by Johnson DB et al. [12], RFA is a safe procedure with a low total complication rate (11.1%), which is similar to our findings (16.7%). Matsumoto ED et al. [13] indicated that tumors were successfully ablated in 100% of the cases when tumors < 3.7 cm and not centrally located. The total complication rate of PN seemed higher than that of RFA; however, no significant difference was found. This result is in agreement with the study by Wang Shangqian et al. [14], which demonstrated that total complications in PN treatment showed no difference from that in the RFA treatment. Similar to RFA, PN is

Table 2 Renal function data

Mean serum creatinine (μmol/L)(range)	Pre-operation	24 h following operation	3 mon after operation	P1	P2
PN group	91.4(53–174)	120.4(75–209)	102.3(50–200)	0.01	0.26
RFA group	94.9(66–113)	108.5(80–154)	98.7(70.6–120)	0.06	0.45

P1: 24 h following operation vs. pre-operation in each group; P2: 3 months after operation vs. pre-operation in each group

Table 3 Oncological outcome

	PN	RFA	P value
No. patients	20	16	
Procedures	21	18	–
Tumor histology, n (%)			
Clear cell	18	14	
Papillary	1	0	
Chromophobe	2	0	–
Not specified	0	4	
Positive surgical margins	0	–	
Mean follow-up (months)	26.1 ± 16.2	33.7 ± 22.9	0.25
Tumor persistence	0	1(6.25)	0.4
Local recurrence (%)	1(5)	3(18.75)	0.1
Metastasis	0	1(6.25)	0.4
Deaths	0	0	–

a potentially safe method for a tumor in a solitary kidney.

Mean serum creatinine was significantly higher 24 h post-operatively than preoperatively in PN ($p = 0.01$), although this finding was not observed in RFA. Several studies indicated that RFA was better than PN because of the lower complication rate, particularly with respect to renal functional impairment. Johnson DB et al. [12] found that only 2% of patients with impaired renal function were examined again after RFA. Possible causes included the following: First, renal artery block was required in PN, which could impede renal function, whereas no hilar clamping was necessary in RFA. Research has shown that warm ischemia time > 30 min would cause irreversible damage to renal function [15]. Second, surgical trauma in PN was greater than that in RFA, which could aggravate damage to the kidney. Moreover, more renal parenchyma might be excised in PN. Three months post-operatively, no significant increase in the mean serum creatinine level was observed in PN, and neither PN nor RFA groups needed dialysis. PN and RFA exerted almost no effect on middle-term renal function. This finding suggested that both PN and RFA were safe procedures for a tumor in a solitary

kidney. Jeffery W et al. [16] showed that adequate hydration, use of mannitol, minimization of the duration of renal ischemia, and involvement of a nephrologist in the perioperative care benefited the renal function.

No incidence of positive surgical margins was reported in PN in our database. Jeffery W et al. [16] showed that the positive surgical margin rate was 15%. The low positive surgical margin rate in the present study could improve by ultrasonic location when necessary during PN. Occurrence of positive margins predicts recurrence; research has shown that positive margin increases the risk of local recurrence as well as metastasis [17]. During follow-up, we observed 1 case (5%) of local recurrence in the PN group vs. 3 cases (18.75%) in the RFA group ($p = 0.1$). The local recurrent rate tended to be higher in the RFA group than in the PN group; however, no significant difference was indicated.

Our data and analysis showed that 2-year local RFS, MFS, and OS were statistically similar for RFA and PN. This finding was in agreement with the study by Ephrem O. Olweny et al. [18], who reported that 5-year OS and CSS, 5-year local RFS, MFS, and overall DFS were statistically similar for RFA and PN. Owing to its low local recurrent rate and long-term RFS, PN was an effective technique for tumor in a solitary kidney [1]. This finding was consistent with the data obtained in the current study, given that RFA obtained oncologic outcomes similar to those of PN. Therefore, both RFA and PN are effective approaches for the treatment of tumor in a solitary kidney.

The present study has certain limitations. (i) The study is a retrospective, nonrandomized design, which shows potential for selection bias and additional confounders. (ii) The small sample size weakened the statistical power of our analyses. (iii) Various methods for RFA (percutaneous, laparoscopic, open) and PN (open, laparoscopic, robot) could potentially influence our analyses. (iv) 4 patients being treated without a biopsy in the RFA group might make a difference to the recurrence rates. (v)The follow-up period was not sufficiently long to estimate long-term oncological and functional outcomes. Further evaluations require more cases and longer follow-ups.

Table 4 Details on recurrences

	Recurrence type	n	Detection and treatment details
RFA	Local recurrence	3	One recurred on CT 8 months, re-ablated, now NED; the other two recurrence identified on CT at 12 months, then re-ablated, now NED.
	Metastatic recurrence	1	Two neoplasm were observed; then developed multiple metastasis at 13 months.
PN	Local recurrence	1	One detected at 6 months, being observed; then tried ablation in other hospital; still had segmental tumor residue, but was steady.

RFA radiofrequency ablation, *PN* partial nephrectomy, *NED* no evidence of disease, *CT* computer tomography

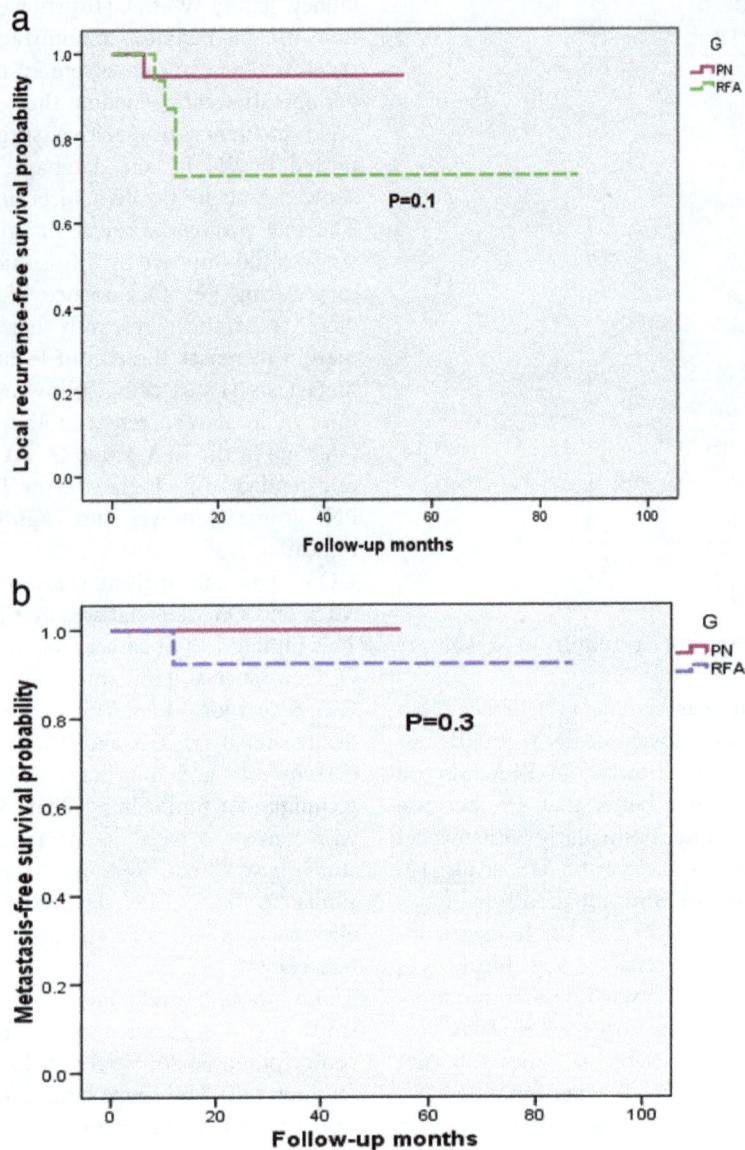

Fig. 1 a and **b** local recurrence-free survival and metastasis-free survival for RFA versus PN

Conclusion

Our data showed that the oncological and functional outcomes of RFA and PN were similar, meaning that both RFA and PN are a safe and effective approach, which procedure is chosen depends on the common choice of patients and urologists. With the development of minimally invasive technology and the use of robots tumors that were difficult to excise once, such as in the renal pelvis or with huge size, can be successfully removed from a solitary kidney. For this reason an increasing number of specialists tend to select LPN or RPN (robotics-assisted partial nephrectomy). For patients who were old or whose physical health was poor, we prefer to recommend RFA.

Abbreviations
CSS: Cancer-specific survival; DFS: Disease-free survival; EBL: Estimated blood loss; LPN: Laparoscopic partial nephrectomy; MFS: Metastasis-free survival; NSS: Nephron-sparing surgery; OPN: Open partial nephrectomy; OS: Overall survival; PN: Partial nephrectomy; RCC: Renal cell carcinoma; RFA: Radiofrequency ablation; RFS: Recurrence-free survival; RN: Radical nephrectomy; RPN: Robotics-assisted partial nephrectomy

Acknowledgements
The authors thank all our participants for their gracious participation in this study.

Funding
Not applicable.

Authors' contributions
WXB: Project development, Data Collection, Manuscript writing; ZGT: Project development, Data analysis, Manuscript revision; GWT: Data collection; LGX: Data analysis; GWD: Manuscript revision; ZF: Data collection, Data analysis; GHQ: Manuscript revision. All authors read and approved the final manuscript.

Competing interests
The authors declare that they have no competing interest.

References
1. Fergany AF, Saad IR, Woo L, Novick AC. Open partial nephrectomy for tumor in a solitary kidney: experience with 400 cases. J Urol. 2006;175:1630–3.
2. Chang X, Liu S, Zhang F, et al. Radiofrequency ablation versus partial Nephrectomy for clinical T1a renal-cell carcinoma: long-term clinical and oncologic outcomes based on a propensity score analysis. J Endourol. 2015;29(5):518–25.
3. Chiou YY, Hwang JI, Chou YH, et al. Percutaneous radiofrequency ablation of renal cell carcinoma. J Chin Med Assoc. 2005;68(5):221–5.
4. Chang X, Ji C, Zhao X, et al. The application of R.E.N.A.L. nephrometry scoring system in predicting the complications after laparoscopic renal radiofrequency ablation. J Endourol. 2014;28:424–9.
5. Nor Azhari MZ, Tan YH, Sunga PA, et al. Laparoscopic partial nephrectomy for renal tumours: early experience in Singapore general hospital. Ann Acad Med Singap. 2009;38(7):576–80.
6. Kaouk JH, Khalifeh A, Hillyer S, et al. Robot-assisted laparoscopic partial nephrectomy: step-by-step contemporary technique and surgical outcomes at a single high-volume institution. Eur Urol. 2012;62(3):553–61.
7. Sukumar S, Rogers CG. Robotic partial nephrectomy: surgical technique. BJU Int. 2011;108:942–7.
8. Kutikov A, Uzzo RG. The R.E.N.A.L. nephrometry score: a comprehensive standardized system for quantitating renal tumor size, location and depth. J Urol. 2009;182:844–53.
9. La Rochelle J, Shuch B, Riggs S, et al. Functional and oncological outcomes of partial nephrectomy of solitary kidneys. J Urol. 2009;181(5):2037–43.
10. Ljungberg B, Cowan NC, Hanbury DC, et al. EAU guidelines on renal cell carcinoma: the 2010 update. Eur Urol. 2010;58(3):398–406.
11. Lotan Y, Cadeddu JA. A cost comparison of nephron sparing surgical techniques for renal tumour. BJU Int. 2005;95(7):1039–42.
12. Johnson DB, Solomon SB, Su LM, et al. Defining the complications of cryoablation and radio frequency ablation of small renal tumors: a multi-institutional review. J Urol. 2004;172(3):874–7.
13. Matsumoto ED, Johnson DB, Ogan K, et al. Short-term efficacy of temperature-based radiofrequency ablation of small renal tumors. Urology. 2005;65(5):877–81.
14. Wang S, Qin C, Peng Z, et al. Radiofrequency ablation versus partial nephrectomy for the treatment of clinical stage 1 renal masses: a systematic review and meta-analysis. Chin Med J. 2014;127(13):2497–503.
15. Orpiglia F, Renard J, Billia M, et al. Is renal warm ischemia over 30 minutes during laparoscopic partial nephrectomy possible? One-year results of a prospective study. Eur Urol. 2007;52(4):1170–8.
16. Saranchuk JW, Touijer AK, Hakimian P, et al. Partial nephrectomy for patients with a solitary kidney: the memorial Sloan-Kettering experience. BJU Int. 2004;94(9):1323–8.
17. Khalifeh A, Kaouk JH, Bhayani S, et al. Positive surgical margins in robot-assisted partial nephrectomy: a multi-institutional analysis of oncologic outcomes (leave no tumor behind). J Urol. 2013;190(5):1674–9.
18. Olweny EO, Park SK, Tan YK, et al. Radiofrequency ablation versus partial Nephrectomy in patients with solitary clinical T1a renal cell carcinoma: comparable oncologic outcomes at a minimum of 5 years of follow-up. Eur Urol. 2012;61(6):1156–61.

4

The validation of the Dutch SF-Qualiveen, a questionnaire on urinary-specific quality of life, in spinal cord injury patients

Sarah H. M. Reuvers[1*], Ida J. Korfage[2], Jeroen R. Scheepe[1], Lisette A. 't Hoen[1], Tebbe A. R. Sluis[3] and Bertil F. M. Blok[1]

Abstract

Background: Optimizing the patients' quality of life is one of the main goals in the urological management of spinal cord injury (SCI) patients. In this study we validated the Dutch SF-Qualiveen, a short questionnaire that measures the urinary-specific quality of life, in SCI patients. No such measure is yet available for this patient group.

Methods: In 2015–2016 SCI patients with urinary symptomatology who visited the outpatient clinics of Urology at the Erasmus Medical Centre and Rehabilitation at Rijndam Revalidation completed the SF-Qualiveen and UDI-6 during the visit and 1–2 weeks later. The UDI-6, a urinary tract symptom inventory, served as gold standard. Controls, recruited from the Otolaryngology outpatient clinic, completed the questionnaires once. Content-, construct-, and criterion validity and reliability (internal consistency and reproducibility) of the SF-Qualiveen were determined.

Results: Fifty seven SCI patients and 50 controls were included. 12 SCI patients asserted that the SF-Qualiveen covered their bladder problems (good content validity). Patients' SF-Qualiveen scores being positively associated with severity of urinary symptoms and patients' scores being higher than those of controls indicated good construct validity. The positive association that was found between SF-Qualiveen and UDI-6 in patients ($r = 0.66$–0.67, $P < 0.001$) and controls ($r = 0.63$, $P < 0.001$) confirmed good criterion validity. Internal consistency (Cronbach's alpha 0.89–0.92) and reproducibility (intraclass correlation coefficient 0.94) of the SF-Qualiveen were good.

Conclusions: The Dutch SF-Qualiveen is a valid and reliable tool to measure the urinary-specific quality of life in SCI patients.

Keywords: Patient reported outcome measure, Urinary bladder, neurogenic, Validation studies, Quality of life, Surveys and questionnaires

Background

Spinal cord injury (SCI) causes urological dysfunction in 70–84% of patients [1]. The type of detrusor and/or sphincter dysfunction depends on the localization of the SCI and the damage to the spinal cord. Clinical presentation can vary from urinary incontinence to inability to empty the bladder [2].

More than two thirds of SCI patients in the Netherlands reported bladder regulation problems as one of their most frequent health problems [3]. Bladder problems were perceived as a major secondary impairment and as having the greatest impact on social life [3]. Bladder problems in patients with SCI were found to be associated with a lower quality of life [4]. Optimizing the quality of life is considered one of the most important aspects in the urological management of patients with neuro-urological dysfunction due to SCI [5].

Currently, there is no validated measure available in the Netherlands to evaluate the urinary-specific quality of life in SCI patients. The Qualiveen-30 [6] and its short version, the SF-Qualiveen [7], are measures that evaluate urinary-specific quality of life in patients with neurological

* Correspondence: s.reuvers@erasmusmc.nl; sarahreuvers@yahoo.com
[1]Department of Urology, Erasmus MC, Wijtemaweg 80, Room Na 1724, 3015, CN, Rotterdam, The Netherlands
Full list of author information is available at the end of the article

disorders. The Qualiveen-30 has been validated in both multiple sclerosis (MS) and SCI patients [6, 8], but is not available in Dutch. Based on data of MS patients only, the eight most responsive items of the Qualiveen-30 were used to create the SF-Qualiveen [7]. The SF-Qualiveen has been validated in English [7], French [7] and Dutch [9] for MS patients, but not yet for SCI patients. Although the neuro-urological dysfunction in MS and SCI patients is similar in some aspects, its clinical presentation and the influence on the quality of life might differ due to dissimilarities between the two diseases (e.g. the onset of disease is acute in SCI vs. progressive in MS; SCI often entails a total loss of sensation of the lower body, while MS entails an altered sensibility, but often no total loss of sensibility). For this reason, it is essential to evaluate the validity and reliability of the SF-Qualiveen in SCI patients before its use can be recommended as a measurement tool in the management of Dutch SCI patients to optimize their quality of life.

Methods
Design and subjects
The research protocol (MEC-2014-534) was reviewed by the local medical research ethics committee, which concluded that the rules as stated in the Dutch Medical Research Involving Human Subjects Act did not apply to this study. The study was conducted at the Urology outpatient clinic of the Erasmus University Medical Center (Erasmus MC), Rotterdam, the Netherlands and at the Rehabilitation outpatient clinic at Rijndam Rehabilitation, Rotterdam, the Netherlands. In August and September 2015 face-to-face interviews were conducted with SCI patients with urinary symptomatology to assess content-validity of the Dutch translated version of the SF-Qualiveen. Between late September 2015 and May 2016 adult patients with SCI and urinary symptomatology were included. We intended to invite all eligible consecutive patients who visited the outpatients clinics to participate. Exclusion criteria were cognitive impairment, Dutch language difficulties, recent malignant tumors, symptomatic urinary tract infections, and (foreseen) change of (bladder-specific) treatment within the test-retest period. After having provided written informed consent, participants completed the SF-Qualiveen and the Urinary Distress Inventory-6 (UDI-6) at the outpatient clinic (test) and 1 to 2 weeks later at home (re-test). Clinical characteristics of included patients were retrieved from their medical charts.

We used earlier collected data of a control group, that was recruited at the Otolaryngology outpatient clinic in 2016 [9]. Exclusion criteria for this group were cognitive impairment, Dutch language difficulties and neuro-urological dysfunction. The control patients had provided written informed consent and completed the measures once.

Measures
The SF-Qualiveen is a measure that evaluates the urinary-specific quality of life in neuro-urological patients. Table 1 shows the eight questions of the questionnaire. Each item is scored on an ordinal Likert scale ranging from 0 (no impact) to 4 (high impact). The total score is the mean of the eight separate scores [7]. The SF-Qualiveen consists of four domains, each containing two questions: bother with limitations (question 1 and 2), fears (question 3 and 4), feelings (question 5 and 6) and frequency of limitations (question 7 and 8).

The Dutch UDI-6 is a validated Dutch measure [10], but has not been specifically validated in a neuro-urological patient group. The questionnaire (six questions) assesses the severity of urinary tract symptoms. It consists of three domains: irritative, stress and obstructive/discomfort urinary symptoms [11]. We chose this measure as a gold standard in the absence of a perfect gold standard for this patient group.

Validation process
The cross-cultural adaptation of the SF-Qualiveen into Dutch by our group was previously described [9]. In short; two forward-translations of the SF-Qualiveen from English to Dutch, and one backward translation were followed by consensus meetings between translators and clinicians. Standardized guidelines for linguistic validation were followed [12]. *Content validity* was assessed by face-to-face interviews with SCI and MS patients [13]. The goal of these interviews was to confirm that the translated version of the SF-Qualiveen used clear wording and that it was a complete measure.

In the current study, predefined hypotheses on *construct validity* were assessed:

1. We hypothesized that SF-Qualiveen scores of patients would be positively associated with the severity of urinary symptoms (UDI-6 domains irritative, stress and obstructive/discomfort urinary symptoms and total score).

Table 1 Questions of the SF-Qualiveen

1. In general, do your bladder problems complicate your life?
2. Are you bothered by the time spent passing urine or realizing catheterization?
3. Do you worry about your bladder problems worsening?
4. Do you worry about smelling of urine?
5. Do you feel worried because of your bladder problems?
6. Do you feel embarrassed because of your bladder problems?
7. Is your life regulated by your bladder problems?
8. Can you go out without planning anything in advance?

2. We hypothesized that scores of the SF-Qualiveen in the patient group would be higher than scores in the control group.

Criterion validity was determined by assessing the relationship between the SF-Qualiveen and the UDI-6 as a gold standard. *Floor and ceiling effects* were presumed to be present if more than 15% of respondents achieved the highest or lowest possible score. Therefore, percentages of respondents with the highest and lowest possible score were calculated. A floor effect was to be expected in the control group.

The *internal consistency* of the SF-Qualiveen questions, i.e. whether the questions measure the same underlying construct, was determined by calculating Cronbach's alpha. The *reproducibility* of the SF-Qualiveen was determined by calculating the intraclass correlation coefficient (ICC) for agreement of the repeated measurements. The *limits of agreement* (LOA) were determined. In general, differences in scores within the LOA can be interpreted as measurement error [14].

A post hoc subgroup analysis was performed to investigate construct- and criterion validity, internal consistency and reproducibility of the Dutch SF-Qualiveen in different subgroups based on level of SCI, ASIA (American Spinal Injury Association) Impairment Scale and manner of bladder emptying.

Statistical analyses

We aimed to include at least 50 patients and 50 controls to comply with the guidelines for validation of questionnaires [13]. For the face-to-face interviews we aimed to include at least 10 SCI patients.

For the statistical analyses we used SPSS version 21. Descriptive results are presented as mean ± standard deviations for continuous data and counts and percentages for discrete data. Student's T-tests were used to assess differences between groups for continuous variables and Chi-Square tests for categorical variables. Associations between variables were assessed using the Pearson's correlation coefficient in case of a linear association. Cronbach's alpha's were calculated to determine the internal consistency. Cronbach's alpha's between 0.7 and 0.95 were considered good [13]. The LOA were calculated as the mean change in scores of repeated measurements ±1.96 x standard deviation (SD) of the changes [14]. ICCs of 0.7 or higher were considered to represent good reproducibility [13]. Statistical significance was assumed at a *p*-value of less than 0.05.

Results

66 SCI patients completed the questionnaires at baseline ('test'). Seven patients did not return the second questionnaires while one declined further participation. The mean SF-Qualiveen score (test) of these patients was 1.81 ± 0.65. One patient was diagnosed with a malignant tumor and excluded. In total, 57 SCI patients completed the second questionnaires (retest) on average 12.7 (±9.0) days after the first questionnaires and were included in the analyses. Characteristics of the study groups are displayed in Table 2. Most patients had a thoracic SCI, required a wheelchair for mobility and were dependent upon catheterization (intermittent or indwelling) to empty their bladder. The 50 controls were significantly younger than the SCI patients. The proportion of males and females was similar in both groups.

Validation process

Following the translation of the SF-Qualiveen into Dutch, 12 SCI patients and 11 MS patients were interviewed to assess *content validity*. The translated SF-Qualiveen was distributed to the patients. Thereafter, patients were asked whether the questions covered all the bladder problems that affected their quality of life. Both patient groups agreed on the importance of the questions and found it a complete measure that covered the broad range of bladder problems that they experienced. Furthermore, patients found the Dutch version clear and easy to complete.

The predefined hypotheses on *construct validity* were confirmed:

1. Positive significant associations were found between both the total UDI-6 and the different domains of the UDI-6 which measure the severity of irritative, stress and obstructive/discomfort urinary symptoms and the total SF-Qualiveen scores in the patient group. (Table 3) The hypothesis that SF-Qualiveen scores of patients would be positively associated with the severity of urinary symptoms was confirmed.
2. The mean of the total scores of the SF-Qualiveen for the patient group was 1.81 ± 0.99 for the test and 1.80 ± 1.08 for the re-test while the control group reported a mean score of 0.34 ± 0.59 (*P* < 0.001). In an older subgroup of controls >40 years (*n* = 27, mean age 53.9 years) the mean total SF-Qualiveen score was 0.51. A significant difference in mean SF-Qualiveen scores between the patient group and the control group >40 years was found (P < 0.001).

A significant positive association between the SF-Qualiveen and the UDI-6 was found in both the patient (Table 3) and control group (*r* = 0.632 and P < 0.001). *Criterion validity* was hereby found to be good. *Floor and ceiling effects* were not found in the patient group for the total SF-Qualiveen score (Test: no patients had the lowest or highest possible score. Re-test: 2% of the patients had the lowest and 2% had the highest possible

Table 2 Clinical characteristics

		Patients	Controls	P-value
N		57	50	
Age at examination		53.2 ± 14.6	42.3 ± 14.2	<0.001
Sex	Male	37 (64.9%)	26 (52.0%)	0.176
	Female	20 (35.1%)	24 (48.0%)	
Years after SCI		13.1 ± 12.8		
Level of SCI	Cervical	15 (26.3%)		
	Thoracic	31 (54.4%)		
	Lumbar	11 (19.3%)		
ASIA Impairment Scale	A	23 (40.3%)		
	B	5 (8.8%)		
	C	7 (12.3%)		
	D	20 (35.1%)		
		Missing: 2 (3.5%)		
Mobility	Fully ambulatory	4 (7.0%)		
	Limited walking	16 (28.1%)		
	Wheelchair only	35 (61.4%)		
		Missing: 2 (3.5%)		
Manner of bladder emptying	(normal) voiding	5 (8.8%)		
	Abdominal pressure	1 (1.8%)		
	Total incontinence	1 (1.8%)		
	Intermittent catheterization	27 (47.4%)		
	Indwelling catheter	22 (38.6%)		
		Missing: 1 (1.8%)		

Results are presented as mean ± standard deviations for continuous data and counts and percentages for discrete data. ASIA Impairment Scale, American Spinal Injury Association Impairment Scale (A: Complete, B: Sensory incomplete, C: Motor incomplete - half of key muscle functions below the neurological level of injury have a muscle grade less than 3, D: Motor incomplete - at least half of key muscle functions below the neurological level of injury have a muscle grade > 3) [16]; SCI, Spinal Cord Injury

score). As expected, a floor effect was found in the control group for the total SF-Qualiveen score: 50% of the controls had the lowest possible score. No ceiling effect was found in the control group (none had the highest possible score).

Cronbach's alpha's of 0.89 (test) and 0.92 (re-test) indicated good *internal consistency* for the total SF-Qualiveen. (Table 4) The domains 'bother with limitations' and 'feeling' showed good internal consistency as well. Internal consistency of the domains 'fears' and 'frequency of limitations' was moderate. The ICCs for the repeated measurements of the test and re-test for the

SF-Qualiveen total score and domain scores showed good *reproducibility* (Table 5). Table 5 shows the *limits of agreement* (LOA) as well. Differences between −0.72 and 0.70 can be interpreted as not clinically important.

In Table 6 the results of the post hoc subgroup analyses based on level of SCI, ASIA Impairment Scale and manner of bladder emptying are shown. Most subgroups showed a positive significant association between the SF-Qualiveen total scores and the UDI-6 score and a significant difference in mean SF-Qualiveen scores compared to the control group, indicating good criterion and construct validity. Cronbach's alpha's of >0.79 and

Table 3 Correlations between severity of urinary symptoms (UDI-6 domain scores) – and SF-Qualiveen total scores in patient group

	Test	Re-test
UDI-6 – total score	$r = 0.663$ and $P < 0.001$	$r = 0.673$ and $P < 0.001$
Severity of irritative urinary symptoms	$r = 0.596$ and $P < 0.001$	$r = 0.543$ and $P < 0.001$
Severity of stress urinary symptoms	$r = 0.451$ and $P < 0.001$	$r = 0.424$ and $P = 0.001$
Severity of obstructive/discomfort urinary symptoms	$r = 0.521$ and $P < 0.001$	$r = 0.630$ and $P < 0.001$

Pearson's correlation coefficients were determined to assess the relationship between variables. UDI-6, Urinary Distress Inventory-6

Table 4 Internal consistency – Cronbach's alpha (n = 57 SCI patients)

	Test	Re-test
SF-Qualiveen total score	0.89	0.92
SF-Qualiveen domains:		
Bother with limitations	0.87	0.90
Fears	0.53	0.73
Feeling	0.80	0.84
Frequency of limitations	0.55	0.75

SCI Spinal Cord Injury

ICCs >0.86 confirmed good internal consistency and reproducibility for the different subgroups.

Discussion

In this study we introduced the SF-Qualiveen in a SCI patient group. We showed good content-, construct- and criterion validity, internal consistency and reproducibility of the SF-Qualiveen in this patient group. We conclude that the SF-Qualiveen can be used in the Netherlands to evaluate the urinary-specific quality of life in SCI patients.

The ICCs of the repeated measurements in this study (ranging from 0.79 to 0.94) showed good reproducibility for the total SF-Qualiveen and the separate domains, although they were somewhat lower than the ICCs found in the French and English SF-Qualiveen validation study in MS patients (0.88 to 0.94) [7]. The ICCs as found in the present study are comparable to the Dutch validation study of the SF-Qualiveen in MS patients (0.72 to 0.90) [9]. The Dutch SF-Qualiveen showed to be a reliable instrument for SCI patients.

Internal consistency for the total SF-Qualiveen was good. Cronbach's alpha's of 0.53 to 0.75 for the separate domains 'fears' and 'frequency of limitations' showed moderate internal consistency. This is consistent with results from the Dutch validation study of the SF-Qualiveen in MS patients [9]. Internal consistency was not described in the French and English validation study of the SF-Qualiveen. These study results indicate that the four domains of the Qualiveen-30 cannot be confirmed in the SF-Qualiveen, probably due to the small number of questions (two) in every domain. This strengthens the previous recommendation of Reuvers et

Table 5 Reproducibility of SF-Qualiveen

	ICC	LOA
SF-Qualiveen total score	0.94	−0.72 to 0.70
Bother with limitations	0.90	−1.12 to 1.00
Fears	0.92	−0.97 to 0.99
Feeling	0.87	−1.27 to 1.23
Frequency of limitations	0.79	−0.72 to 0.70

ICC Intraclass Correlation Coefficient, *LOA* Limits of Agreement

al. [9] to not use the separate domains of the SF-Qualiveen, but only the total SF-Qualiveen.

The results of the subgroup analyses suggest that the Dutch SF-Qualiveen has equal measurement properties for SCI patients with different levels of SCI, ASIA Impairment statuses and manners of bladder emptying. Not finding a statistical significant correlation between the SF-Qualiveen scores and UDI-6 scores in the ASIA group B (n = 5) and C (n = 7) and the group without catheter usage (n = 7) could be explained by the lack of statistical power in the small patient groups due to the post hoc analysis.

Most SCI patients experience bladder problems as a consequence of damage to the spinal cord [1, 3]. These bladder problems have a negative effect on patients' quality of life [4]. In the urological management of SCI patients optimization of the quality of life is an important aspect as mentioned in the EAU guidelines [5]. Therefore, it is essential for healthcare professionals to be informed about a patients' present urinary-specific quality of life. The SF-Qualiveen is now available to objectively assess this topic in the Dutch SCI population. Only after being informed about present urinary-specific quality of life, an optimal treatment plan can be defined.

For the future we suggest that urology and rehabilitation departments in the Netherlands implement the Dutch-version SF-Qualiveen in the urological management of SCI patients. The Dutch SF-Qualiveen is now available as a measurement tool. Further research should be aimed at determining its responsiveness to treatment. Once this has been established as sufficient, the Dutch SF-Qualiveen may be used to evaluate the effect of treatments on the urinary-specific quality of life in clinical and research settings.

A question that arises is if we can recommend the use of the SF-Qualiveen in all neuro-urological patients. D'Ancona et al. [15] included, next to 33 SCI and eight MS patients, 10 patients with meningomyelocele (MMC) in the validation study of the Portuguese Qualiveen-30. Results of the different patient groups were not separately described. The authors state that MMC patients would have the same concerns regarding urinary-specific quality of life as SCI and MS patients. However, there might be a difference in the experience of patients with congenital neurological diseases such as MMC compared to patients with acquired diseases like SCI and MS. Therefore, it would be valuable to study the usefulness of the SF-Qualiveen in congenital neurological patients.

It is questionable if our Dutch version SF-Qualiveen validated in the Netherlands can be used in other Dutch speaking countries such as Belgium and South-Africa. Although the language is technically the same, wording and expressions can be different as well as cultural

Table 6 Subgroup analyses

		Patient numbers	Mean total SF-Qualiveen scores	Cronbach's alpha	ICC	Correlation between SF-Qualiveen scores and UDI-6 scores	Patients' SF-Qualiveen scores compared to controls
Level of SCI	Cervical	15 (26%)	1.68–1.68	0.93–0.96	0.95	$r = 0.853$, $p < 0.001$ $r = 0.788$, $p < 0.001$	$p < 0.001$
	Thoracic	31 (55%)	1.77–1.75	0.88–0.91	0.95	$r = 0.552$, $p = 0.001$ $r = 0.547$, $p = 0.001$	$p < 0.001$
	Lumbar	11 (19%)	2.11–2.15	0.79–0.80	0.89	$r = 0.686$, $p = 0.02$ $r = 0.769$, $p = 0.006$	$p < 0.001$
ASIA Impairment Scale	A	23 (40.3%)	1.58–1.50	0.88–0.92	0.94	$r = 0.585$, $p = 0.003$ $r = 0.650$, $p = 0.001$	$p < 0.001$
	B	5 (8.8%)	2.18–2.48	0.80–0.88	0.92	$r = 0.895$, $p = 0.040$ $r = 0.597$, $p = 0.287$	$p < 0.001$
	C	7 (12.3%)	1.70–1.57	0.83–0.82	0.86	$r = 0.715$, $p = 0.071$ $r = 0.677$, $p = 0.095$	$p < 0.001$
	D	20 (35.1%)	2.04–2.11	0.90–0.92	0.96	$r = 0.706$, $p < 0.001$ $r = 0.709$, $p < 0.001$	$p < 0.001$
	Missing: 2						
Manner of bladder emptying	No catheter use	7 (12%)	1.36–1.21	0.87–0.91	0.94	$r = 0.707$, $p = 0.076$ $r = 0.817$, $p = 0.025$	$p < 0.001$
	Intermittent catheterization	27 (47%)	2.19–2.20	0.89–0.88	0.92	$r = 0.571$, $p = 0.002$ $r = 0.518$, $p = 0.006$	$p < 0.001$
	Indwelling catheter	22 (39%)	1.47–1.48	0.85–0.93	0.95	$r = 0.743$, $p < 0.001$ $r = 0.768$, $p < 0.001$	$p < 0.001$
	Missing: 1						

ASIA Impairment Scale American Spinal Injury Association Impairment Scale, *ICC* Intraclass Correlation Coefficient

habits. Therefore, we recommend a new validation process before introducing the Dutch SF-Qualiveen in other Dutch language countries.

A strength of this study was the homogeneous patient group of SCI patients. Study results therefore provide a clear view of the validity and reliability of the SF-Qualiveen in this patient group. Furthermore, as this study was conducted at the outpatient clinics of urology of a general hospital and rehabilitation clinic, the SF-Qualiveen may be considered suitable for the use in both settings.

A limitation of the study was that eight of 66 patients (12.1%) were excluded because they did not complete the second questionnaire. This may have introduced a selection bias. However, the SF-Qualiveen scores (test) of these patients were similar to those of the included patients. Therefore, the selection bias may not be an important issue. Another limitation is that no other validated urinary-specific quality of life measure for neuro-urological patients is available to serve as a perfect gold standard to determine the criterion validity of the SF-Qualiveen. In the absence of a perfect gold standard, we chose the UDI-6, a urinary tract symptom inventory, which may have been suboptimal. In addition, criticism could be raised on the age difference between the patient and control group. To investigate one of the hypotheses on construct validity, we used data of a control group. We hypothesized that scores of the SF-Qualiveen in the patient group would be higher than scores in the control group. As a consequence of using earlier collected data, the age of the patient and control group were not matched and we found a statistical significant age difference between the groups. However, we did not expect this age difference to influence outcomes. We assumed that non-neuro-urological patients of the control group, regardless of their age, would have lower scores on a measure that evaluates the urinary-specific quality of life (developed for the use in neuro-urological patients) than the neuro-urological patient group. This expectation was strengthened by the fact that we also found a statistical significant difference in SF-Qualiveen scores between the patient group and the older control group (>40 years).

Conclusions

From this study we can conclude that the Dutch SF-Qualiveen is valid and reliable to measure the urinary-specific quality of life in SCI patients. This short questionnaire, which is easy to complete, can be a valuable instrument. We suggest to use the total Dutch SF-Qualiveen for evaluation of the urinary-specific quality of life in SCI patients.

Abbreviations

Erasmus MC: Erasmus University Medical Center; ICC: Intraclass correlation coefficient; LOA: Limits of agreement; MMC: Meningomyelocele; MS: Multiple sclerosis; SCI: Spinal cord injury; SD: Standard deviation; SUI: Stress urinary incontinence; UI: Urinary incontinence

Acknowledgements

Elaine Utomo is thanked for her help with the initiation of this study and Floris van Zijl and Toscane Noordhoff are thanked for their help with the inclusion of patients and controls.

Funding

No funding.

Authors' contributions

SR concept and design, data acquisition, data analysis and interpretation, drafting of the manuscript. IK concept and design, data analysis and interpretation, revision of the manuscript. JS concept and design, data acquisition, revision of the manuscript. LH concept and design, revision of the manuscript. TS data acquisition, revision of the manuscript. BB concept and design, data acquisition, revision of the manuscript. All authors read and approved the final manuscript.

Competing interests

The authors declare that they have no competing interests.

Author details

[1]Department of Urology, Erasmus MC, Wijtemaweg 80, Room Na 1724, 3015, CN, Rotterdam, The Netherlands. [2]Department of Public Health, Erasmus MC, Rotterdam, The Netherlands. [3]Department of Rehabilitation, Rijndam Rehabilitation, Rotterdam, The Netherlands.

References

1. McKinley WO, Jackson AB, Cardenas DD, DeVivo MJ. Long-term medical complications after traumatic spinal cord injury: a regional model systems analysis. Arch Phys Med Rehabil. 1999;80(11):1402–10.
2. Madersbacher H. The various types of neurogenic bladder dysfunction: an update of current therapeutic concepts. Paraplegia. 1990;28(4):217–29.
3. Bloemen-Vrencken JH, Post MW, Hendriks JM, De Reus EC, De Witte LP. Health problems of persons with spinal cord injury living in the Netherlands. Disabil Rehabil. 2005;27(22):1381–9.
4. Ku JH. The management of neurogenic bladder and quality of life in spinal cord injury. BJU Int. 2006;98(4):739–45.
5. Groen J, Pannek J, Castro Diaz D, Del Popolo G, Gross T, Hamid R, Karsenty G, Kessler TM, Schneider M, t Hoen L, et al. Summary of European Association of Urology (EAU) guidelines on neuro-urology. Eur Urol. 2016; 69(2):324–33.
6. Costa P, Perrouin-Verbe B, Colvez A, Didier J, Marquis P, Marrel A, Amarenco G, Espirac B, Leriche A. Quality of life in spinal cord injury patients with urinary difficulties. Development and validation of qualiveen. Eur Urol. 2001; 39(1):107–13.
7. Bonniaud V, Bryant D, Parratte B, Guyatt G. Development and validation of the short form of a urinary quality of life questionnaire: SF-Qualiveen. J Urol. 2008;180(6):2592–8.
8. Bonniaud V, Parratte B, Amarenco G, Jackowski D, Didier JP, Guyatt G. Measuring quality of life in multiple sclerosis patients with urinary disorders using the Qualiveen questionnaire. Arch Phys Med Rehabil. 2004;85(8):1317–23.
9. Reuvers SH, Korfage IJ, Scheepe JR, Blok BF. The urinary-specific quality of life of multiple sclerosis patients: Dutch translation and validation of the SF-Qualiveen. Neurourol Urodyn. 2016;
10. Utomo E, Korfage IJ, Wildhagen MF, Steensma AB, Bangma CH, Blok BF. Validation of the urogenital distress inventory (UDI-6) and incontinence impact questionnaire (IIQ-7) in a Dutch population. Neurourol Urodyn. 2015; 34(1):24–31.
11. Uebersax JS, Wyman JF, Shumaker SA, McClish DK, Fantl JA. Short forms to assess life quality and symptom distress for urinary incontinence in women: the incontinence impact questionnaire and the urogenital distress inventory. Continence program for women research group. Neurourol Urodyn. 1995;14(2):131–9.
12. Guillemin F, Bombardier C, Beaton D. Cross-cultural adaptation of health-related quality of life measures: literature review and proposed guidelines. J Clin Epidemiol. 1993;46(12):1417–32.
13. Terwee CB, Bot SD, de Boer MR, van der Windt DA, Knol DL, Dekker J, Bouter LM, de Vet HC. Quality criteria were proposed for measurement properties of health status questionnaires. J Clin Epidemiol. 2007;60(1):34–42.
14. Bland JM, Altman DG. Statistical methods for assessing agreement between two methods of clinical measurement. Lancet. 1986;1(8476):307–10.
15. D'Ancona CA, Tamanini JT, Botega N, Lavoura N, Ferreira R, Leitao V, Lopes MH. Quality of life of neurogenic patients: translation and validation of the Portuguese version of Qualiveen. Int Urol Nephrol. 2009;41(1):29–33.
16. Kirshblum SC, Burns SP, Biering-Sorensen F, Donovan W, Graves DE, Jha A, Johansen M, Jones L, Krassioukov A, Mulcahey MJ, et al. International standards for neurological classification of spinal cord injury (revised 2011). J Spinal Cord Med. 2011;34(6):535–46.

5

Extraperitoneal laparoscopic resection for retroperitoneal lymphatic cysts: initial experience

Yichun Wang[1†], Chen Chen[1†], Chuanjie Zhang[1†], Chao Qin[2*] and Ninghong Song[2*]

Abstract

Background: To assess the safety and efficacy of laparoscopic retroperitoneal resection for retroperitoneal lymphatic cysts.

Methods: A retrospective analysis was conducted based on clinical data from eight patients with hydronephrosis caused by retroperitoneal lymphatic cysts. All patients underwent laparoscopic retroperitoneal lymphatic cyst resection and received postoperative follow-up. A follow-up ultrasound was performed postoperatively every 6–12 months to evaluate the recovery of the hydronephrosis.

Results: All operations were successful, and their postoperative pathological results revealed lymphatic cyst walls. The operation time ranged from 43 to 88 min (mean: 62 min), with a blood loss of 20 to 130 mL (mean: 76 mL), and the length of hospital stay was 3 to 6 days (mean: 4.5 days). Within the follow-up of 12 to 36 months (mean: 28.5 months), great relief was detected in all eight cases, and no recurrence was found. Moreover, complications such as renal pedicle or renal pelvis injury were not observed.

Conclusions: Laparoscopic retroperitoneal lymphatic cyst resection is an effective treatment for retroperitoneal lymphatic cysts and has the advantages of being minimally invasive, producing less intraoperative blood loss and leading to a quick recovery. This treatment thus deserves further studies.

Keywords: Hydronephrosis, Lymphatic cyst, Laparoscope

Background

Lymphatic cysts are a rare lymphatic-vessel-generated disease that have a thick fibrotic wall lacking epithelial lining [1], and they generally occur following congenital lymphatic system heteroplasia or surgical procedures such as pelvic or retroperitoneal operations [2, 3]. There are no typical manifestations, and they are mostly diagnosed incidentally with physical examination or surgery [4]. Retroperitoneal lymphatic cysts are particularly uncommon and usually appear near the renal, retrocolon and cauda pancreatis [5, 6]. They do not cause any symptoms at first. When a cyst becomes sufficiently large, it could constrict the neighboring anatomic structures and cause symptoms such as lower abdominal pain, obstructive uropathy, lower lymphoedema, bowel obstruction and venous thrombosis [7–10]. Most patients come to the hospital for the presence of an abdominal mass. It is difficult to make a definite diagnosis before the operation. However, by using X-ray, computed tomography (CT), ultrasound, and other techniques, doctors could make a presumptive diagnosis. The narrow and deep retroperitoneal space increases the difficulty of the operation, so an open operation is always the first choice. However, with the development of laparoscopic techniques, laparoscopic retroperitoneal lymphatic cyst resection has become an optional choice and possesses advantages such as short hospitalization duration, less pain and short recovery time. It is a quite promising minimally invasive surgery [11]. From December 2011 to January 2014, 8 patients underwent laparoscopic retroperitoneal lymphatic cyst resection.

* Correspondence: qinchao@njmu.edu.com; songninghong@126.com
†Equal contributors
²Department of Urology, The First Affiliated Hospital of Nanjing Medical University, 300 Guangzhou Road, Nanjing 210029, China
Full list of author information is available at the end of the article

Methods

Clinical information

From December 2011 to January 2014, 8 male patients with hydronephrosis caused by retroperitoneal lymphatic cysts were admitted to our hospital. Routine preoperative written informed consent was obtained from all patients involved in this study. The indication for laparoscopic retroperitoneal lymphatic cyst resection in this study was hydronephrosis accompanied by the obvious obstructive factor of a retroperitoneal lymphatic cyst. The patients' ages ranged from 38 to 85 (mean of 57). Of all the cases, one patient had undergone an appendectomy in 2001, and the others declared no medical history of trauma or surgery. Two patients suffered waist discomfort. The diameter of the cyst ranged from 7.5 cm to 12.0 cm (mean of 9.7 cm). The degree of hydronephrosis was described according to ultrasound (Table 1). The preoperative serum creatinine levels were in the normal range. All patients underwent preoperative examination, including ultrasound, enhanced CT scan, and intravenous urography (IVU) combined with other laboratory examinations, and were diagnosed with retroperitoneal lymphatic cyst with hydronephrosis (Figs. 1 and 2). The follow-up was 12–36 months. During the follow-up, ultrasound examination was performed every 6 months to monitor the development of hydronephrosis in the first year. Thereafter, ultrasound was performed every 12 months.

Operation procedure

All patients were given general anesthesia through the trachea; then, a unilateral ureteral stent was inserted to identify and preserve ureter function during the operation. After introducing the ureteral sent, the patient was placed in the unaffected lateral position and tilted up to the waist bridge. A 2.0-cm incision was made to the inferior of the 12th rib in the posterior axillary line. Various muscular layers were bluntly divided until the peritoneum could be accessed. Then, a homemade balloon inflated with 700 mL of gas was inserted to create a retroperitoneal space. Using a forefinger, 0.5-cm, 0.5-cm, and 1.0-cm incisions were made into the inferior of rib in the anterior axillary line, near the crista iliaca, and 2 cm superior of crista iliaca in the midaxillary line, respectively. A 10-mm trocar was placed, and a pneumoperitoneum was created with a pressure of 10 mmHg. Then, the retroperitoneal fat was dissociated along the musculi psoas major until the diaphragm was reached. Subsequently, the perirenal fascia was exposed and incised from the anterior and lower renal poles. The musculi psoas major was exposed to find the ureter along the interior of the musculi psoas major. The cyst behind the renal pelvis was carefully circumferentially dissected from the ureter, surrounding vessels and adhesions. A titanium clip was used when the surrounding adhesions were difficult to dissociate. After successful dissociation, a small incision was made into the surface of the cyst to decompress the cyst. The liquid content was clear without evidence of bile, blood or chyle. Then, the cyst wall was excised completely and sent for pathological examination. Bleeding was then checked, and a drainage tube was inserted in the upper section of the renal surrounding. The ureteral stent was unsheathed 1 month after discharge from the hospital. Follow-up was performed regularly.

Results

In these cases, all operations were completed successfully, with no injury of the renal hilus or collection system, no conversions to open surgery and no intraoperative blood transfusion. The operation time ranged from 43 to 88 min (mean: 62 min). The blood loss was 20–130 mL (mean: 76 mL). The perioperative hospitalization time was 3–6 days (mean: 4.5 days). The histopathologic results included lymphatic cyst with fibrous capsule walls (Fig. 3). The follow-up was 12–36 months (mean of 28.5 months). During the follow-up, no complications such as lymphatic fistula, renal pedicle or renal pelvis injury were observed. The hydronephrosis in all patients had resolved, and no recurrence was observed. The waist discomfort of two of the patients decreased (Table 2).

Discussion

Retroperitoneal lymphatic cysts involve one or more chamber cysts with clear or chylous fluid. Most cysts are large but have no symptoms in the early stage; this is related to the anatomical characteristics of the retroperitoneal space, which is full of deep and large gaps. At the same time, the retroperitoneal lymphatic cyst grows slowly and shows no invasiveness. However, when the cyst grows too large, it could trigger some symptoms, such as infection, bleeding in the cyst, and constriction of the tissues, or even flatulence and hydronephrosis.

Table 1 Preoperative demographic data and information about patients

Patient	Age	Cyst side	Cyst diameter (cm)	Hydronephrosis stage	Symptom
1	38	Right	7.5	Mild	No symptom
2	67	Right	9.3	Moderate	No symptom
3	46	Left	8.2	Mild	No symptom
4	42	Right	8.7	Moderate	No symptom
5	72	Left	10.6	Severe	Waist discomfort
6	56	Left	12.0	Moderate	No symptom
7	85	Right	11.6	Severe	No symptom
8	52	Right	9.7	Severe	Waist discomfort

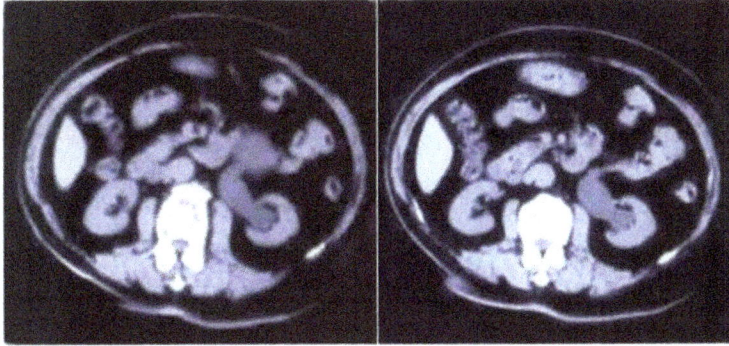

Fig. 1 CT:Moderate hydronephrosis

Patients can occasionally palpate a painless mass on the abdomen [12]. The disease is easy to misdiagnose [13] and must be distinguished from other abdominal cysts, such as liver cysts, renal cysts, pancreas cysts, ovarian cysts, cystic teratoma and tumor cystic lesions [14]. Some studies revealed that retroperitoneal cysts could lead to the compression of the adjacent organs [15, 16]. Once a cyst is enlarged, it could compress the junction of the renal pelvis and ureter, which could result in obstruction, retention of urine and hydronephrosis. If the kidney does not contain a substantial lesion, the surgeon only needs to remove the cyst to relieve the hydronephrosis.

Several methods for the management of lymphatic cyst with various results have been proposed, including conservative observation, percutaneous catheter drainage with or without sclerotherapy and internal marsupialization. In the research of William E. Braun [17], the authors observed three cases of spontaneously drained lymphatic cysts over 1–2 weeks and adopted conservative observation treatment in three cases after renal transplantation. Their results hinted that there could be an alternative for managing asymptomatic or mildly symptomatic cases. This therapeutic schedule is based on the phenomenon that some surgically derived lymphatic cysts may cause minimal symptoms and spontaneously disappear over 1 year [17]. However, the background for this management is based mainly on

surgically derived lymphatic cysts due to the destruction of lymphatic channels. Lymphatic vessels could regenerate over the time, and this process may explain the disappearance of some lymphatic cysts. In our research, most patients had no surgical or traumatic experience, and these cases are supposed to be classified as congenitally generated, which means that they may not be remediated without medical intervention [4]. Additionally, long-term obstruction of the ureter may lead to the deterioration of renal function, and should therefore be resolved in a timely manner. Among these therapies, many research institutions have adopted percutaneous catheter drainage because of its safety and efficacy. However, according to Jae-Kyu Kim [18], recurrence can be observed in 13% of patients after the first successful drainage procedure in the 6-month follow-up period. It has a long treatment duration: the mean duration of treatment ranges from 10 to 20 days, which increases patient inconvenience [1]. Additionally, during percutaneous catheter drainage, patients should undergo at least two lymphographic procedures, which have an associated radiation exposure. Internal marsupialization surgery also has limitations because it can only drain the sterile content into the peritoneal cavity and is not applicable for infected lymphatic cysts [19, 20]. The effect of retroperitoneal lymphatic cyst surgery is encouraging. During the surgery, the exact dissociation of all the adhesions around the cyst should be done carefully

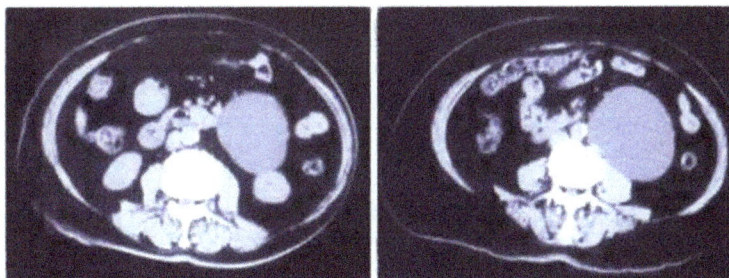

Fig. 2 Retroperitoneal lymphatic cyst

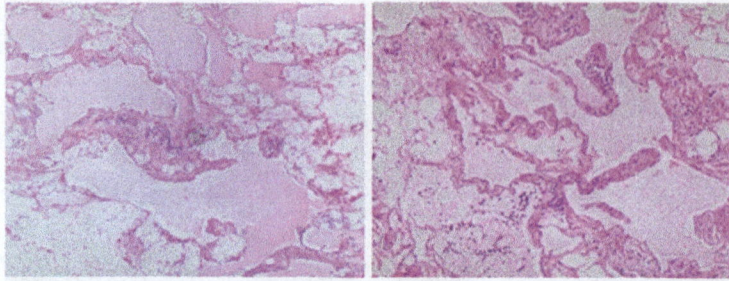

Fig. 3 Postoperative pathology: lymphatic cyst, fibrous capsule wall

to ensure that all cyst walls are excised and thereby avoid recurrence. In our study, all patients had hydronephrosis that might have been caused by the obstruction, so we used minimally invasive surgery to remove the obstruction of the ureter. Laparoscopic surgery is safer, produces less pain after operation, produces less blood loss and leads to shorter hospitalization durations [11]. Laparoscopic retroperitoneal cystectomy can be done via two approaches: abdominal or retroperitoneal. This choice is based on the skill of the surgeon and the location of the cyst. Most retroperitoneal cysts grow near the dorsal side of the kidney, so the operation could be performed via the retroperitoneal approach, especially since the invention of the retroperitoneal balloon dilator, which provides surgeons with a clear view of the retroperitoneal structure and can create sufficient operation space. The retroperitoneal approach could avoid both injury to abdominal organs and abdominal contamination and could decrease the complications of bowel paralysis, adhesion and ejaculatory disorders [21]. The restrictions of laparoscopy because of a medical history of abdominal surgery, injury or infection could be overcome, and the damage to the pancreas and splenic vessels that can potentially occur when the pancreas is dissociated and turned over via a transperitoneal approach could also be avoided. In recent years, many domestic and foreign units have carried out retroperitoneal laparoscopic lymphatic cyst resection [11], and the effects of this operation are encouraging.

In our study, all patients underwent laparoscopic retroperitoneal lymphatic cyst resection via a retroperitoneal approach. All operations were successful. According to the treatment experience of our center, the main treatment regimen included the following steps: 1. The patients underwent a CT scan to determine the size of the cyst and the location of the renal pelvis and renal pedicle vessels. 2. During the operation, the surgeon paid attention to the retroperitoneal space, the liver, the duodenum, the colon, the pancreas, the spleen, the vena cava and other organs and vessels. To prevent bleeding, blunt dissection was performed. Where necessary, an ultrasonic knife was utilised to cut the adjacent tissue. 3. A drainage tube was placed in the case of hydronephrosis. 4. Intraoperative monitoring of blood oxygen saturation and carbon dioxide levels was used. This study is encouraging, but its application has some restrictions: The operation and equipment costs are high, we included only patients with hydronephrosis caused by retroperitoneal lymphatic cysts, and the number of the cases was limited. We need further research to validate this method.

Conclusions

This study showed that laparoscopic retroperitoneal lymphatic cyst resection, with the advantages of being minimally invasive, producing less pain and having a short recovery time, may be an alternative method to cure hydronephrosis caused by retroperitoneal lymphatic cysts.

Table 2 Intraoperative and postoperative patient data

Patient	Age (year)	Hydronephrosis stage	Cyst diameter (cm)	Operative time (min)	Blood loss (mL)	Hospitalization time (days)	Follow-up (months)
1	38	Mild	7.5	43	20	3	18
2	67	Moderate	9.3	56	40	5	36
3	46	Mild	8.2	49	35	4	12
4	42	Moderate	8.7	62	79	5	24
5	72	Severe	10.6	88	130	6	36
6	56	Moderate	12.0	66	107	4	30
7	85	Severe	11.6	70	100	5	36
8	52	Severe	9.7	59	98	4	36

Abbreviations
CT: Computed tomography; IVU: Intravenous urography

Acknowledgements
The authors would like to thank all our participants in this study.

Funding
This work was supported by Jiangsu Province's Key Provincial Talents Program (Su Wei Ke Jiao [2016] No.22), the Jiangsu Province "Six Talent Peaks Project" (WSN-011, WSN-020), the Priority Academic Program Development of Jiangsu Higher Education Institutions (PAPD), the Program for Provincial Initiative Program for Excellency Disciplines of Jiangsu Province, and the National Natural Science Foundation of China [grant number 81672531, 81,372,757].

Authors' contributions
CQ and NHS conceived of the study. YCW, CC and CJZ participated in the design, analysis and drafted the manuscript of the study. They contributed equally to the study, and all authors gave final approval for the manuscript and agree to be accountable for all aspects of the work herein.

Competing interests
The authors declare that they have no competing interests.

Author details
[1]The First Clinical Medical College, Nanjing Medical University, Nanjing, China. [2]Department of Urology, The First Affiliated Hospital of Nanjing Medical University, 300 Guangzhou Road, Nanjing 210029, China.

References
1. Karcaaltincaba M, Akhan O. Radiologic imaging and percutaneous treatment of pelvic lymphocele. Eur J Radiol. 2005;55(3):340–54.
2. Touska P, Constantinides VA, Palazzo FF. A rare complication: lymphocele following a re-operative right thyroid lobectomy for multinodular goitre. BMJ Case Rep. 2012. doi:10.1136/bcr.02.2012.5747.
3. Mikou F, Elkarroumi M, Sefrioui O, Morsad F, Ghazli M, Matar N, Moumen M. Pelvic lymphocele: report of a case and review of the literature. J Gynecol Obstet Biol Reprod (Paris). 2002;31(8):779–82.
4. Ge W, Yu DC, Chen J, Shi XB, Su L, Ye Q, Ding YT. Lymphocele: a clinical analysis of 19 cases. Int J Clin Exp Med. 2015;8(5):7342–50.
5. Urs AB, Shetty D, Praveen RB, Sikka S. Diverse clinical nature of cavernous lymphangioma: report of two cases. Minerva Stomatol. 2011;60(3):149–53.
6. Braunert M, Wiechmann V, Born K, Plato R, Lamesch P. Omentum minus cystic lymphangioma: report of a case and a literature review. Zentralbl Chir. 2011;136(2):175–7.
7. Ebadzadeh MR, Tavakkoli M. Lymphocele after kidney transplantation: where are we standing now? Urol J. 2008;5(3):144–8.
8. Radosa MP, Diebolder H, Camara O, Winzer H, Mothes A, Runnebaum IB. Small-bowel obstruction caused by duodenal compression of a paraaortic lymphocele. Onkologie. 2011;34(7):391–3.
9. Haeberlin A, Fuster DG. Abdominal pain, emesis and dyspnea after kidney transplantation. Nephrology (Carlton). 2015;20(8):582–3.
10. Fuller TF, Kang SM, Hirose R, Feng S, Stock PG, Freise CE. Management of lymphoceles after renal transplantation: laparoscopic versus open drainage. J Urol. 2003;169(6):2022–5.
11. Ahn KS, Han HS, Yoon YS, Kim HH, Lee TS, Kang SB, Cho JY. Laparoscopic resection of nonadrenal retroperitoneal tumors. Arch Surg. 2011;146(2):162–7.
12. Martin-Perez E, Tejedor D, Brime R, Larranaga E. Cystic lymphangioma of the lesser omentum in an adult. Am J Surg. 2010;199(2):e20–2.
13. Dong B, Zhou H, Zhang J, Wang Y, Fu Y. Diagnosis and treatment of retroperitoneal bronchogenic cysts: a case report. Oncol Lett. 2014;7(6): 2157–9.
14. Thaler M, Achatz W, Liebensteiner M, Nehoda H, Bach CM. Retroperitoneal lymphatic cyst formation after anterior lumbar interbody fusion: a report of 3 cases. J Spinal Disord Tech. 2010;23(2):146–50.
15. Sarkar D, Gulur D, Patel S, Nambirajan T. An unusual presentation of a retroperitoneal cyst. BMJ Case Rep. 2014. doi:10.1136/bcr-2014-206284.
16. Mirsadeghi A, Farrokhi F, Fazli-Shahri A, Gholipour B. Retroperitoneal bronchogenic cyst: a case report. Med J Islam Repub Iran. 2014;28:56.
17. Braun WE, Banowsky LH, Straffon RA, Nakamoto S, Kiser WS, Popowniak KL, Hewitt CB, Stewart BH, Zelch JV, Magalhaes RL, et al. Lymphoceles associated with renal transplantation: report of fifteen cases and review of the literature. Proc Clin Dial Transplant Forum. 1973;3:185–9.
18. Kim JK, Jeong YY, Kim YH, Kim YC, Kang HK, Choi HS. Postoperative pelvic lymphocele: treatment with simple percutaneous catheter drainage. Radiology. 1999;212(2):390–4.
19. Livingston WD, Confer DJ, Smith RB. Large lymphoceles resulting from retroperitoneal lymphadenectomy. J Urol. 1980;124(4):543–6.
20. Gill IS, Hodge EE, Munch LC, Goldfarb DA, Novick AC, Lucas BA. Transperitoneal marsupialization of lymphoceles: a comparison of laparoscopic and open techniques. J Urol. 1995;153(3 Pt 1):706–11.
21. LeBlanc E, Caty A, Dargent D, Querleu D, Mazeman E. Extraperitoneal laparoscopic para-aortic lymph node dissection for early stage nonseminomatous germ cell tumors of the testis with introduction of a nerve sparing technique: description and results. J Urol. 2001;165(1):89–92.

6

Comparison of the efficacy and safety of URSL, RPLU, and MPCNL for treatment of large upper impacted ureteral stones: a randomized controlled trial

Yunyan Wang[†], Bing Zhong[†], Xiaosong Yang[†], Gongcheng Wang, Peijin Hou and Junsong Meng[*]

Abstract

Background: There are three minimally invasive methods for the management of large upper impacted ureteral stones: mini-percutaneous nephrolithotomy (MPCNL), transurethral ureteroscope lithotripsy (URSL), and retroperitoneal laparoscopic ureterolithotomy (RPLU). This study aimed to compare MPCNL, URSL, and RPLU, and to evaluate which one is the best choice for large upper impacted ureteral stones.

Methods: Between January 2012 and December 2015, at the Department of Urology, Huai'an First People's Hospital, 150 consecutively enrolled patients with a large upper impacted ureteral stone (>15 mm) were included. The patients were randomly divided (1:1:1) into the MPCNL, URSL, and RPLU groups. The primary endpoint was success of stone removal measured 1 month postoperatively and the secondary endpoints were intraoperative and postoperative parameters and complications.

Results: Fifteen patients needed auxiliary ESWL after URSL, and 3 patients after MPCNL, but none after RPLU. The stone clearance rate was 96% (48/50) in the MPCNL group and 72% (33/46) in the URSL group. In the RPLU group the stones were completely removed and the stone clearance rate was 100% (48/48) ($P = 0.021$ vs. URSL; $P = 0.083$ vs. MPCNL). Operation-related complications were similar among the three groups (all $P > 0.05$). Hospital stay was shorter in the URSL group compared with MPCNL ($P = 0.003$). Operation time was the shortest with URSL and the longest with MPCNL (all $P < 0.05$).

Conclusions: MPCNL and RPUL are more suitable for upper ureteral impacted stones of >15 mm. URSL could be considered if the patient is not suitable for general anesthesia, or the patient requests transurethral uretroscopic surgery.

Keywords: Ureteral calculi, Ureteroscopy, Nephrostomy, Percutaneous, Laparoscopy

Background

Urinary lithiasis, where stones known as calculi form in the urinary system, is a common problem for more than 12% of the population [1], that is increasingly prevalent in many populations [2–4]. The definition of an impacted ureteral stone is one that stays in the same location at least for 2 months and results in ureteral obstruction [5]. Such stones can cause pain and lead to hydronephrosis or urinary tract infections, which may result in loss of renal function [6]. Generally, the transverse diameter of an impacted ureteral stone is longer than the ureter caliber. Other characteristics such as a large volume, anomalous shape, and uneven density, will result in ureteral obstruction, nephrohydrosis, and pyonephrosis. Secondary infection and the immune response to foreign material resulting from chronic oppression, pathological lesions such as ureteral polyps, and stricture also occur in the stone site [7].

* Correspondence: hayywyy1322@163.com
[†]Equal contributors
Department of Urology, Huai'an First People's Hospital, Nanjing Medical University, No. 6 West Beijing Road, Huai'an, Jiangsu 223300, China

Therefore, these stones require interventions for their removal. Various treatment modalities are available, from open ureterolithotomy to modern endourologic procedures [8].

Before the 1980s, the majority of large upper ureteral stones required open operation for their removal [9]. With the development of minimally invasive techniques, various treatment options have become available such as extracorporeal shock wave lithotripsy (ESWL), ureteroscopic lithotripsy (URSL), percutaneous nephrolithotomy (PCNL), as well as retroperitoneal ureterolithotomy (RPUL), all with different efficacy rates [10].

In most cases, ESWL is the first line choice for upper ureteral stones that do not pass spontaneously, but for large ureteral impacted stones, ESWL has been less successful [11]. Therefore, the debate over the optimal treatment for larger stones of 15 mm diameter or more remains [8]. When the stones are located in a high position and are close to the renal pelvis there is a risk of the stones returning to the pelvis, which results in the failure of URSL [12]. Both PCNL and mini-PCNL (MPCNL) have been used more often to treat upper ureteral stones in recent years [13]. With the improvement of laparoscopic techniques and equipment, retroperitoneoscopic ureterolithotomy (RPUL) has also become a popular choice [6].

All these mini-invasive treatment approaches can be used to treat impacted upper ureteral stones, but how to select one and what is their efficiency remains controversial. A meta-analysis by Torricelli et al. [14] showed that the outcomes of RPUL were more favorable than for semi-rigid ureteroscopic lithotripsy, making it the treatment of choice when flexible ureteroscopy is not available. PCNL has been reported to have the same efficacy as laparoscopic pyelolithotomy, but to be associated with better operative parameters [15]. Therefore, the aim of this study was to compare three minimally invasive methods; URSL, MPCNL and RPUL to evaluate which one is the best choice for large upper ureteral stones (>15 mm) in terms of efficacy and safety.

Methods
Clinical materials
From January 2012 to December 2015, 150 consecutive patients with upper ureteral stones who were referred to the department of Urology, Huai'an First People's Hospital (Huai'an, Jiangsu Province) were included in the study.

The inclusion criteria were patients with a single upper ureteral stone (located below the ureteropelvic junction to the superior aspect of sacroiliac joint); the stone was >15 mm along its longest diameter as revealed by kidney-ureter-bladder (KUB) abdominal plain film. The exclusion criteria were those patients with a history of any intervention operation on the corresponding ureter, radiolucent stones, active infection, or urinary tract abnormalities, coagulopathy, or pregnancy, as well as those patients requiring simultaneous treatment of a kidney stone. The patients all agreed to enter the study, and this study was approved by the Ethic Committee of Huai'an First People's Hospital, Nanjing Medical University (IRB-PJ2012–015-01). A written informed consent was obtained from all subjects prior to the start of the trial.

In addition to routine history and clinical examinations, the investigations included assessment of the hemoglobin and serum creatinine values, full coagulation profile, ultrasonography, and KUB plain film. Excretory urography was performed if the serum creatinine was normal. Urine specimens were obtained for culture. A sensitive antibiotic was given to the patients with positive cultures to control the infection before surgical intervention.

The patients included in the study were randomly divided (1:1:1) into three groups by use of a computer generated random number table.

Procedures
All procedures were performed by the same physician.

URSL
The patient was under spinal or general anesthesia and placed in the lithotomy position. An 8 to 9.8 F rigid ureteroscope (Richard Wolf GmbH, Knittlingen, Germany) was used for uteroscopy and access was provided by retrograde insertion of a 0.038-in. floppy tip guide wire over which the ureteroscope was introduced into the ureter without dilating the ureteral orifice. The stones were fragmented with a holmium YAG laser through the ureteroscope. A double-J stent was placed in cases with large residual stones, significant mucosal edema, stone impaction, or probable ureteral trauma. The stent was removed when the patient was stone-free on follow-up evaluation as an outpatient.

MPCNL
Under general anesthesia, the patient was placed in the lithotomy position and an external 5 Fr or 6 Fr ureteral catheter was inserted to the target ureter under direct ureteroscopic vision. Then the patient was rotated to the prone position with a pack under the ipsilateral hemipelvis. An ultrasound-guided percutaneous puncture was made by the urologist with an 18-gauge puncture needle being pushed into the designated calyx. A flexible guide wire was then inserted through the calyceal puncture into the renal pelvis and across the ureteropelvic junction into the ureter. An 8 Fr fasical dilator was employed initially, and the caliber was increased

gradually by progressive 2 Fr fascial dilators along the guide wire, until the percutaneous nephrostomy tract was dilated to 18 Fr. A matched peel-away sheath was inserted into the renal collecting system. All the stones were fragmented with a Swiss lithoclast used as the sole device for using a 2.4 F (0.8-mm thick), 668-mm-long probe and stone debris were flushed out by a water flow produced by an endoscopic perfusion pump (EMS - Electro medical Systems S.A., Nyon, Switzerland). At the end of the procedure, a 5 Fr double-J stent was indwelled via the percutaneous access with the assistance of the guide wire. All the percutaneous tracts were inserted with a 16 Fr silastic nephrostomy tube.

RPLU

Under general endotracheal anesthesia, the patients were placed in the lateral decubitus position. A skin incision was made at the tip of the 12th rib and the aponeurosis was bluntly perforated under safe control of both hands. A retroperitoneal working space was created with a self-made expansion balloon that was inserted by pushing the peritoneum forward. Approximately 800 ml of sterile saline solution was injected into the dissection balloon through the transparent channel. The retroperitoneal space was bluntly dissected and the dissection balloon was removed. A 5- or 10-mm trocar was then inserted under the subcostal margin in the anterior axillary line. A 10-mm trocar was also placed above the iliac crest in the midaxillary line and this space was filled with CO_2 pneumoretroperitoneum for the laparoscope (Karl Storz Endoskope, Tuttlingen, Germany). Within the retroperitoneal space the psoas muscle and other important landmarks were easily recognized. The Gerota's fascia was incised parallel to the psoas muscle. Renal vessels were clearly visible as pulsing. Extraperitoneal adipose tissue was removed and the ureter was recognized on the psoas muscle. The stone location could be identified by a conspicuous bulge as the ureter was dissected. The ureteral wall was longitudinally incised by a cold knife over the bulge and the stone was extracted and removed through the first port. An indwelling double-J ureteral stent was placed through the incision. Intracorporeal suturing was used to close the ureteral incisions with 4–0 absorbable sutures.

Appraisal methods

Radiologists were blind to patient data during all follow-up examinations. All the patients accepted the KUB plain film examination within 3 days of their procedure. ESWL on residual stone was performed 1 week after surgery in the URSL group, and 2 weeks after surgery in the MPCNL group. For these patients, KUB plain film examination was performed again within 3 days after their procedure.

The primary outcome was whether treatment was successful. Successful treatment was defined as complete removal of the target stones or the presence of peripheral small insignificant gravel (<4 mm in diameter) [16]. According to the Chinese guidelines of medicine, stones of <4 mm are considered to be able to pass by themselves. Therefore, obtaining fragments <4 mm was considered successful [16]. If the residual stone diameter was >4 mm, then auxiliary ESWL treatment was undertaken.

One month after surgery, the patient returned to the hospital to remove the double-J stent and to be re-examined by KUB film. Stone clearance was defined as the absence of stone debris on the KUB film, and the stone clearance rate was calculated.

The secondary outcomes were intraoperative and postoperative parameters and complications. Complications arising intraoperatively and postoperatively, and hospitalization days after surgery were assessed. The Clavien method was used for the classification of surgical complications [17]. The patients were followed up at 6 and 12 months to ensure that there was no novel stone or stenosis.

Statistical analysis

No power calculation was performed before beginning the trial and the sample size was based on convenience. Nevertheless, a post hoc power analysis based on the primary outcome revealed that our experiment had a 95% power to detect the differences in the primary outcome with a two-tailed $\alpha = 0.05$. SPSS 16.0 (IBM Corp., Armonk, NY, USA) was used for statistical analysis. The continuous or categorical data are presented as mean ± standard deviation (SD), frequency, percentile, and range, as appropriate. For normally distributed continuous variables, analysis of variance (ANOVA) was used to detect differences among the groups and the Tukey's post hoc test was used. Variables in the contingency table were analyzed by the χ^2 test (or the Fisher exact test). $P < 0.05$ indicated statistical significance.

Results
Baseline data

There were 88 men and 62 women. None of the patients withdrew from the study (Fig. 1). The detailed characteristics of the patients are presented in Table 1 and Fig. 1 shows the patient flowchart. There were no statistically significant differences among the three groups for stone size and nephrohydrosis extent (both $P > 0.05$; Table 1). All patients were followed up at 6 and 12 months.

All procedures in the MPCNL group were completed at the first attempt. Four patients failed to undergo the designated procedure in the URSL group because the ureteroscope could not approach the stone location. One of these patients then underwent URSL successfully

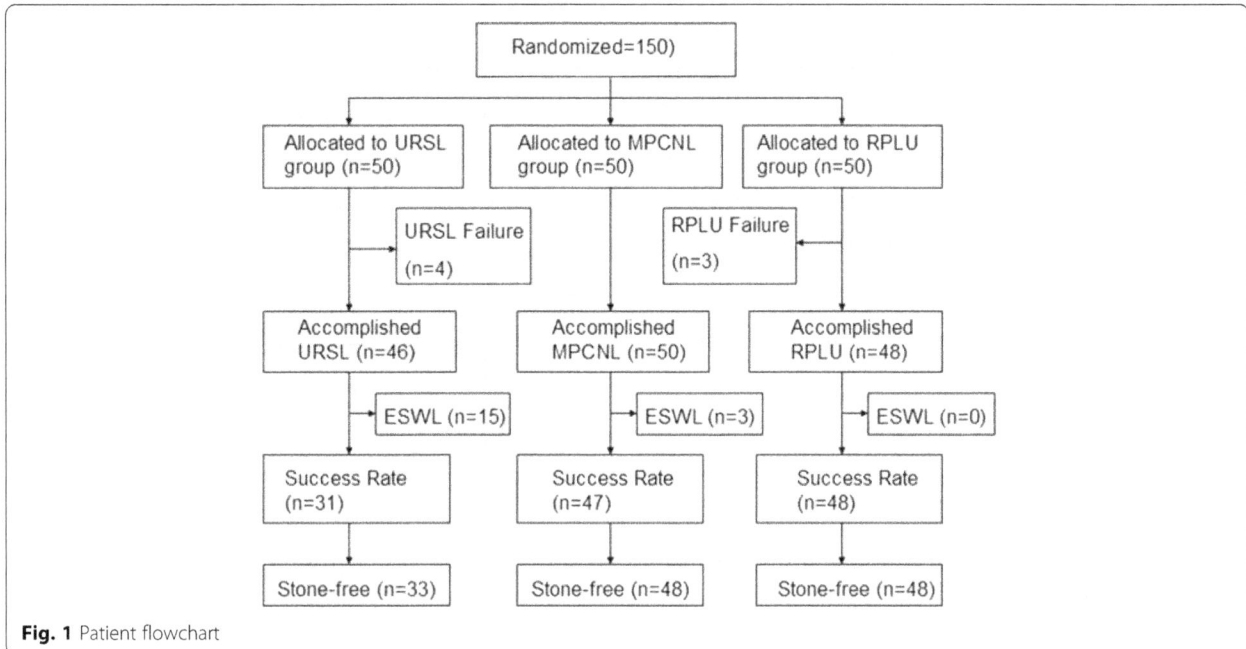

Fig. 1 Patient flowchart

5 days after placing the double-J stent. The other three patients underwent open surgery to remove the stone. Two patients in the RPLU group failed to undergo the procedure because the stone returned to the renal pelvis and the stone was removed by open surgery. These six cases of failure to perform the procedure at the first attempt were not included in the statistics data of stone clearance rate. ESWL on the residual stone was performed 1 week after surgery in URSL group (n = 15), and 2 weeks after surgery in MPCNL group (n = 3).

Primary endpoint

The successful treatment rate was 31/50 (62%) in the URSL group, 47/50 (94%) in the MPCNL group, and 48/50 (96%) in the RPUL group. The differences were not significant among the three groups (Table 2), but differences of stone clearance rate 1 month after operation among the three groups were statistically significant (P < 0.05). Auxiliary ESWL was required in a large number of patients in the URSL group (n = 15), but only in three patients in the MPCNL group and in none in the RPUL group.

Secondary endpoints

There were no statistically significant differences in the length of major axis and surface area of stones as well as in the complications and morbidity (P > 0.05). The mean operation time was significantly different among the groups; the shortest was in the URSL group at 55.7 ± 23.9 min and the longest was in the MPCNL group at 125.6 ± 41.2 min (P < 0.05). A similar result was found with the length of hospital stay: a significantly shorter time was needed after URSL (2.5 ± 1.3 days) than after RPUL (4.3 ± 2.2 days) and the longest hospital stay was after MPCNL (6.8 ± 2.6 days, all P < 0.05).

Adverse effects or complications

There were no severe complications in any of the patients. In the URSL group, the main postoperative complications were stone fragment migration, perforation, and ureteral stricture. In the MPCNL group, bleeding occurred in five cases and three of them needed a blood transfusion. Three cases had fever because of urosepsis. In the RPUL group, six complications

Table 1 Baseline characteristics of the included patients

Variable	URSL group	MPCNL group	RPUL group	P value[a]	P value[b]	P value[c]
	N = 50	N = 50	N = 50			
Mean age (years)	42 ± 14	41 ± 15	44 ± 11	0.769	0.385	0.581
Male/female	28/22	31/19	29/21	0.274	0.162	0.469
Side (left / right)	26/24	27/23	29/21	0.481	0.376	0.583
Mean stone size (mm)	16.8 ± 2.1	19.3 ± 1.8	18.8 ± 1.4	0.677	0.943	0.876
Hydronephrosis (mm)	35.8 ± 5.5	40.2 ± 7.8	38.4 ± 6.9	0.264	0.573	0.815

[a]URSL vs. MPCNL; [b]URSL vs. RPUL; [c]MPCNL vs. RPUL

Table 2 Patient outcomes after the procedure

Variable	URSL group	MPCNL group	RPUL group	P value[a]	P value[b]	P value[c]
Success rate	31/50 (62%)	47/50 (94%)	48/50 (96%)	<0.001	<0.001	0.698
Mean operation time (min)	55.7 ± 23.9	125.6 ± 41.2	99.5 ± 34.6	<0.001	0.027	0.012
Hospital stay after surgery (d)	2.5 ± 1.3	6.8 ± 2.6	4.3 ± 2.2	0.003	0.056	0.063
Auxiliary ESWL after 3 days	15/46 (32.6%)	3/50 (6%)	0/48 (0%)	<0.001	<0.001	<0.001
Stone-free rate after 1 month	33/46 (72%)	48/50 (96%)	48/48 (100%)	0.035	0.021	0.083

[a]URSL vs. MPCNL; [b] URSL vs. RPUL; [c] MPCNL vs. RPUL

occurred, including abdominal distention caused by peritoneal rupture, subcutaneous emphysema, and urine leakage (Table 3).

Discussions

There are many treatments for impacted upper ureteral stones, including URSL, MPCNL, and RPLU. Because impacted stones usually are wrapped around or adhere to an ureteral polyp, ESWL is often not effective [18]. Indeed, White et al. reported that if upper ureteral stone diameter was smaller than 10 mm, stone clearance rate by ESWL was 69%, however; when the diameter was larger than 10 mm, it was 59% [18]. It was also reported that when upper ureteral stones are larger than 10 mm, stone clearance rate by ESWL was only 42% [19].

Each method has its pros and cons. Indeed, RPUL takes a long time, but has more chance of success and a lower requirement for ESWL; it also results in fewer complications, but the surgeons have to be adept at local anatomy [10]. PCNL has a good efficacy, but may result in large surgical trauma and bleeding, complicating the recovery of the patients and prolonging hospitalization [10, 20]. URSL is not as effective as RPUL and PCNL, and is prone to move the calculi upward; nevertheless, the surgical trauma by URSL is minimal, leading to short recovery [10, 21]. A meta-analysis by Torricelli et al. [14]

showed that the outcomes of RPUL were more favorable than for semi-rigid ureteroscopic lithotripsy, making it the treatment of choice when flexible ureteroscopy is not available.

Ureteroscopic surgery is a minimally invasive procedure, which has a good acceptance for patients and the patients restore quickly after operation. In this study the success rate was 62% and the stone clearance rate was 72% 1 month after operation in the URSL group. The success rate was previously reported to be 35–87% by URSL [22, 23]. Usually, general anesthesia is required in MPCNL and RPLU, while URSL can be performed under spinal anesthesia. So, URSL is especially appropriate for patients who are not suitable for general anesthesia.

However, there are several disadvantages with URSL when dealing with impacted upper ureteral stones. Firstly, the stone clearance rate is relatively low. In most cases, the stones are large and near to renal pelvis. During URSL, the stone and its debris are inclined to return to the renal pelvis under the flushing fluid, resulting in residual stones. Secondly, ESWL is often needed as auxiliary treatment after surgery. Chen et al. [24] reported that ESWL as an auxiliary procedure was 16%. In our study, as an auxiliary procedure, the ESWL treatment rate was 32.6%.

Table 3 Complications and adverse events

Variable	URSL group	MPCNL group	RPUL group	P value[a]	P value[b]	P value[c]
Grade I						
Pain	6/46(13%)	8/50(16%)	9/48(18%)	0.276	0.027	0.795
Fever	2/46(4.3%)	3/50(6%)	2/48(4.2%)	0.735	0.658	0.743
Nausea/vomiting	2/46(4.3%)	1/50(2%)	3/48(6%)	0.273	0.342	0.042
Urine leakage	0/46(0%)	0/50(0%)	3/48(6%)	NS	<0.001	<0.001
Grade II						
Minor pelvic/ureter perforation	3/46(6.5%)	0/50(0%)	0/48(0%)	<0.001	<0.001	NS
Urinary tract infection	1/46(3%)	1/50(2%)	0/48(0%)	NS	<0.001	<0.001
Ureteral stricture	2/46(4.3%)	0/50(0%)	0/48(0%)	<0.001	<0.001	NS
Grade III						
Blood transfusion	0/46(0%)	3/50(6%)	0/48(0%)	<0.001	NS	<0.001
Grade III - V	0/46(0%)	0/50(0%)	0/48(0%)	NS	NS	NS

[a]URSL vs. MPCNL; [b]URSL vs. RPUL; [c] MPCNL vs. RPUL; *NS* No Significance

In this study, there were two cases of ureteral stricture postoperatively in the URSL group, which may correlate with long-term obstruction, chronic inflammation and polyp proliferation. Moreover, the holmium laser crushed the stone at an identical spot during the operation time, which would aggravate the ureter mucosal membrane damage, inevitably resulting in occurrence of ureteral stricture. For these patients, we suggest that the double-J stent indwelling time should be increased to 8–12 weeks. Regarding the obvious polyp proliferation cases, urotroscopy was required to detect ureteral stricture when the double-J stent was removed.

With the improvement of endoscopy and lithotripsy instruments in the last decade, PCNL, instead of open surgery, has already become an option for minimally invasive lithotripsy for kidney stones and is gradually being adopted for upper ureteral stones [11, 25]. Karami [26] and colleagues compared URSL and PCNL in 70 cases of upper ureteral impacted stones >1 cm. The results showed that the stone clearance rate was 96% in the PCNL group, while the stones of 32% patients in the URSL group returned to the renal pelvis and needed ESWL after surgery. The authors thought that PCNL was the first choice for these kinds of stones. A similar conclusion was drawn in another study of 53 patients who underwent either PCNL or URSL. The stone-free rate at 1-month follow-up was 95.4% in the PCNL group and 58% in the URSL group, and eight patients had upward migrating stones during the URSL procedure; they were treated by ESWL [27]. Out results show that the stone clearance rate was 96% 1 month after surgery in the MPCNL group. We found similar results when comparing URSL and MPCNL, but the complications in the groups were similar. In our opinion, intrapoerative puncture is not difficult for cases of moderate or severe hydronephrosis resulting from upper ureteral impacted stones.

RPLU was first reported by Gaur [28] in 1994. As we know, RPLU has many merits, such as high stone-free rate, less blood loss, less incision pain, and shorter hospitalization time [29]. Therefore, RPLU should be considered for safe and effective treatment for reducing ureteral obstruction in selected patients with large proximal ureteric stones [6, 15, 30, 31]. In this study, the stone-free rate was 100% 3 days after operation in the RPLU group.

We realized that RPLU should be selected for upper ureteral stones when they are combined with mild hydronephrosis, when the ureteropelvic junction is angled, or when it is difficult for PCNL to arrive at the stone position. If the stone is near to the UPJ and hydronephrosis is obvious, the possibility of stones going back into the renal pelvis during the operation increases greatly, which will affect the success rate of the RPLU procedure. In this study, there was no ureteral stricture after RPLU during the long-term follow-up, which might contribute to ureter incision going along the ureteral axis and little heat damage of the ureteral mucosal membrane. However, impacted stones might adhere to the ureteral wall so closely that it is difficult to identify the ureter and remove the stone using RPLU [27]. Therefore, RPLU should only be conducted by urologists who have mastered the subtle skills needed for the laparoscopic technique.

This study has some limitations. The sample was from one single center. Although it was larger than many studies, it remains quite small. Studies from multiple centers would provide more weight to these results. There was no postoperative CT examination 1 month after the operation when the stone clearance rate was calculated. The follow-up of 6–12 months was quite short, so we cannot provide any comparison of recurrence rates or long term complications between the groups.

Conclusions

In our opinion, MPCNL and RPUL are more suitable for upper ureteral impacted stones with a diameter of >15 mm. URSL could be considered if the patient is not suitable for general anesthesia, or the patient requests transurethral uretroscopic surgery.

Abbreviations
CTU: computed tomography urography; ESWL: Extracorporeal shock wave lithotripsy; KUB: kidney-ureter-bladder; MPCNL: mini-percutaneous nephrolithotomy; PCNL: percutaneous nephrolithotomy; RPLU: retroperitoneal laparoscopic ureterolithotomy; SD: standard deviation; UPJ: ureteropelvic junction; URSL: ureteroscope lithotripsy

Acknowledgements
Not applicable.

Funding
Not applicable.

Authors' contributions
YYW and JSM participated in designing protocol of the study. YYW, BZ and GCW drafted the manuscript. YYW and PJH critically revised the manuscript. YYW, XSY, PJH and JSM collect the data of the study. All the authors read and approved the final manuscript.

Competing interests
The authors declare that they have no competing interests.

References

1. Brener ZZ, Winchester JF, Salman H, Bergman M. Nephrolithiasis: evaluation and management. South Med J. 2011;104:133–9.
2. Turney BW, Reynard JM, Noble JG, Keoghane SR. Trends in urological stone disease. BJU Int. 2012;109:1082–7.
3. Scales CD Jr, Curtis LH, Norris RD, Springhart WP, Sur RL, Schulman KA, et al. Changing gender prevalence of stone disease. J Urol. 2007;177:979–82.
4. Matlaga BR, Schaeffer AJ, Novak TE, Trock BJ. Epidemiologic insights into pediatric kidney stone disease. Urol Res. 2010;38:453–7.
5. Roberts WW, Cadeddu JA, Micali S, Kavoussi LR, Moore RG. Ureteral stricture formation after removal of impacted calculi. J Urol. 1998;159:723–6.
6. Yasui T, Okada A, Hamamoto S, Taguchi K, Ando R, Mizuno K, et al. Efficacy of retroperitoneal laparoscopic ureterolithotomy for the treatment of large proximal ureteric stones and its impact on renal function. Springerplus. 2013;2:600.
7. Mugiya S, Ito T, Maruyama S, Hadano S, Nagae H. Endoscopic features of impacted ureteral stones. J Urol. 2004;171:89–91.
8. Kadyan B, Sabale V, Mane D, Satav V, Mulay A, Thakur N, et al. Large proximal ureteral stones: ideal treatment modality? Urol Ann. 2016;8:189–92.
9. Muslumanoglu AY, Karadag MA, Tefekli AH, Altunrende F, Tok A, Berberoglu Y. When is open ureterolithotomy indicated for the treatment of ureteral stones? Int J Urol. 2006;13:1385–8.
10. Liu Y, Zhou Z, Xia A, Dai H, Guo L, Zheng J. Clinical observation of different minimally invasive surgeries for the treatment of impacted upper ureteral calculi. Pak J Med Sci. 2013;29:1358–62.
11. Bozkurt IH, Yonguc T, Arslan B, Degirmenci T, Gunlusoy B, Aydogdu O, et al. Minimally invasive surgical treatment for large impacted upper ureteral stones: Ureteroscopic lithotripsy or percutaneous nephrolithotomy? Can Urol Assoc J. 2015;9:E122–5.
12. Shao Y, Wang DW, Lu GL, Shen ZJ. Retroperitoneal laparoscopic ureterolithotomy in comparison with ureteroscopic lithotripsy in the management of impacted upper ureteral stones larger than 12 mm. World J Urol. 2015;33:1841–5.
13. Ferakis N, Stavropoulos M. Mini percutaneous nephrolithotomy in the treatment of renal and upper ureteral stones: lessons learned from a review of the literature. Urol Ann. 2015;7:141–8.
14. Torricelli FC, Monga M, Marchini GS, Srougi M, Nahas WC, Mazzucchi E. Semi-rigid ureteroscopic lithotripsy versus laparoscopic ureterolithotomy for large upper ureteral stones: a meta - analysis of randomized controlled trials. Int Braz J Urol. 2016;42:645–54.
15. Li S, Liu TZ, Wang XH, Zeng XT, Zeng G, Yang ZH, et al. Randomized controlled trial comparing retroperitoneal laparoscopic pyelolithotomy versus percutaneous nephrolithotomy for the treatment of large renal pelvic calculi: a pilot study. J Endourol. 2014;28:946–50.
16. Lee JW, Park J, Lee SB, Son H, Cho SY, Jeong H. Mini-percutaneous Nephrolithotomy vs retrograde Intrarenal surgery for renal stones larger than 10 mm: a prospective randomized controlled trial. Urology. 2015;86:873–7.
17. Dindo D, Demartines N, Clavien PA. Classification of surgical complications: a new proposal with evaluation in a cohort of 6336 patients and results of a survey. Ann Surg. 2004;240:205–13.
18. White W, Klein F. Five-year clinical experience with the Dornier Delta lithotriptor. Urology. 2006;68:28–32.
19. Park H, Park M, Park T. Two-year experience with ureteral stones: extracorporeal shockwave lithotripsy v ureteroscopic manipulation. J Endourol. 1998;12:501–4.
20. Liu GH, Wu SD, Gu NQ, He XP. Ureteroscopy pneumatic lithotripsy for 38 cases of ureteral calculi and severe hydronephrosis. J Guangxi Med Uni. 2012;29:632–3.
21. Wu CF, Chen CS, Lin WY, Shee JJ, Lin CL, Chen Y, et al. Therapeutic options for proximal ureter stone: extracorporeal shock wave lithotripsy versus semirigid ureterorenoscope with holmium:yttrium-aluminum-garnet laser lithotripsy. Urology. 2005;65:1075–9.
22. Lee YH, Tsai JY, Jiaan BP, Wu T, Yu CC. Prospective randomized trial comparing shock wave lithotripsy and ureteroscopic lithotripsy for management of large upper third ureteral stones. Urology. 2006;67:480–4. discussion 4
23. Mugiya S, Ozono S, Nagata M, Takayama T, Nagae H. Retrograde endoscopic management of ureteral stones more than 2 cm in size. Urology. 2006;67:1164–8. discussion 8
24. Chen CS, Wu CF, Shee JJ, Lin WY. Holmium:YAG Lasertripsy with semirigid ureterorenoscope for upper-ureteral stones >2 cm. J Endourol. 2005;19:780–4.
25. Basiri A, Tabibi A, Nouralizadeh A, Arab D, Rezaeetalab GH, Hosseini Sharifi SH, et al. Comparison of safety and efficacy of laparoscopic pyelolithotomy versus percutaneous nephrolithotomy in patients with renal pelvic stones: a randomized clinical trial. Urol J. 2014;11:1932–7.
26. Karami H, Arbab AH, Hosseini SJ, Razzaghi MR, Simaei NR. Impacted upper-ureteral calculi >1 cm: blind access and totally tubeless percutaneous antegrade removal or retrograde approach? J Endourol. 2006;20:616–9.
27. Juan YS, Li CC, Shen JT, Huang CH, Chuang SM, Wang CJ, et al. Percutaneous nephrostomy for removal of large impacted upper ureteral stones. Kaohsiung J Med Sci. 2007;23:412–6.
28. Gaur DD, Agarwal DK, Purohit KC, Darshane AS, Shah BC. Retroperitoneal laparoscopic ureterolithotomy for multiple upper mid ureteral calculi. J Urol. 1994;151:1001–2.
29. Gaur DD, Trivedi S, Prabhudesai MR, Madhusudhana HR, Gopichand M. Laparoscopic ureterolithotomy: technical considerations and long-term follow-up. BJU Int. 2002;89:339–43.
30. Wang Y, Hou J, Wen D, OuYang J, Meng J, Zhuang H. Comparative analysis of upper ureteral stones (> 15 mm) treated with retroperitoneoscopic ureterolithotomy and ureteroscopic pneumatic lithotripsy. Int Urol Nephrol. 2010;42:897–901.
31. Saad KS, Youssif ME, Al Islam Nafis Hamdy S, Fahmy A, El Din Hanno AG, El-Nahas AR. Percutaneous Nephrolithotomy vs retrograde Intrarenal surgery for large renal stones in pediatric patients: a randomized controlled trial. J Urol. 2015;194:1716–20.

Tubeless versus standard percutaneous nephrolithotomy: an update meta-analysis

Yang Xun[1], Qing Wang[1], Henglong Hu[1], Yuchao Lu[1], Jiaqiao Zhang[1], Baolong Qin[1], Yudi Geng[2] and Shaogang Wang[1]* ⓘⅮ

Abstract

Background: To update a previously published systematic review and meta-analysis on the efficacy and safety of tubeless percutaneous nephrolithotomy (PCNL).

Methods: A systematic literature search of EMBASE, PubMed, Web of Science, and the Cochrane Library was performed to confirm relevant studies. The scientific literature was screened in accordance with the predetermined inclusion and exclusion criteria. After quality assessment and data extraction from the eligible studies, a meta-analysis was conducted using Stata SE 12.0.

Results: Fourteen randomized controlled trials (RCTs) involving 1148 patients were included. Combined results demonstrated that tubeless PCNL was significantly associated with shorter operative time (weighted mean difference [WMD], −3.79 min; 95% confidence interval [CI], −6.73 to −0.85; $P = 0.012$; $I^2 = 53.8\%$), shorter hospital stay (WMD, −1.27 days; 95% CI, −1.65 to −0.90; $P < 0.001$; $I^2 = 98.7\%$), faster time to return to normal activity (WMD, −4.24 days; 95% CI, −5.76 to −2.71; $P < 0.001$; $I^2 = 97.5\%$), lower postoperative pain scores (WMD, −16.55 mm; 95% CI, −21.60 to −11.50; $P < 0.001$; $I^2 = 95.7\%$), less postoperative analgesia requirements (standard mean difference, −1.09 mg; 95% CI, −1.35 to −0.84; $P < 0.001$; $I^2 = 46.8\%$), and lower urine leakage (Relative risk [RR], 0.30; 95% CI 0.15 to 0.59; $P = 0.001$; $I^2 = 41.2\%$). There were no significant differences in postoperative hemoglobin reduction (WMD, −0.02 g/dL; 95% CI, −0.04 to 0.01; $P = 0.172$; $I^2 = 41.5\%$), stone-free rate (RR, 1.01; 95% CI, 0.97 to 1.05; $P = 0.776$; $I^2 = 0.0\%$), postoperative fever rate (RR, 1.05; 95% CI, 0.57 to 1.93; $P = 0.867$; $I^2 = 0.0\%$), or blood transfusion rate (RR, 0.79; 95% CI, 0.36 to 1.70; $P = 0.538$; $I^2 = 0.0\%$). The results of subgroup analysis were consistent with the overall findings. The sensitivity analysis indicated that most results remained constant when total tubeless or partial tubeless or mini-PCNL studies were excluded respectively.

Conclusions: Tubeless PCNL is an available and safe option in carefully evaluated and selected patients. It is significantly associated with the advantages of shorter hospital stay, shorter time to return to normal activity, lower postoperative pain scores, less analgesia requirement, and reduced urine leakage.

Keywords: Percutaneous nephrolithotomy, PCNL, Tubeless, Update, Meta-analysis

Background

As a common urological disease, the prevalence rates for urinary stones vary from 1% to 20%. In countries with a high standard of life such as Canada or the United States of America (USA), renal stone prevalence is notably high (>10%) [1]. Urinary stones can cause renal function injury, which has a great impact on public health. With the advances of surgical technology, less invasive procedures such as percutaneous nephrolithotomy (PCNL) have gradually become a preferred therapy for urinary stone in the last two decades [2, 3]. Using a nephrostomy tube for drainage has been considered the standard procedure after PCNL [4]. Since Bellman first introduced tubeless PCNL in 1997 [5], the interest and enthusiasm of this surgical procedure had been widespread. PCNL without postoperative nephrostomy tube placement is defined as tubeless PCNL. When neither a nephrostomy tube nor a ureteral stent is used, the

* Correspondence: sgwangtjm@163.com
[1]Department of Urology, Tongji Hospital, Tongji Medical College, Huazhong University of Science and Technology, No.1095 Jiefang Avenue, Wuhan, China
Full list of author information is available at the end of the article

procedure is commonly regarded as total tubeless PCNL [6]. A large number of studies on tubeless PCNL have been performed and several previously published systematic reviews have reported its efficacy and safety [4, 7–9]. However, the available evidence is still currently inconclusive because of the limited quality and quantity of the analyzed randomized controlled trials (RCTs). More rigorously designed RCTs are required to collect better evidence to support the use of tubeless PCNL. Furthermore, tubeless PCNL has not been generally accepted in clinical medicine, probably due to concerns of urine leakage, obstruction by residual stone fragments, or requirement for repeat access [10]. Since 1997, several RCTs [11–24] have been performed to compare the safety and effectiveness of tubeless and standard PCNL, including five high-quality RCTs published after 2012 [20–24]. These latest publications need to be included in an updated review to explore the most recent evidence on the use of tubeless PCNL. Therefore, we performed a meta-analysis to update previously published systematic reviews on the efficacy and safety of tubeless PCNL.

Methods
Literature search
We performed a systematic literature search of Medline (using PubMed as the search engine), Web of Science databases, EMBASE (using Ovid as the search engine) and the Cochrane Library to confirm relevant studies in accordance with Cochrane standards, and PRISMA (Preferred Reporting Items for Systematic Reviews and Meta-Analyses) guidelines [25] in November 2016 and updated in March 2017. There were no strict restrictions of year or language in the searching process. The search was performed with the following terms in combination to identify relevant studies: ("total tubeless" or "tubeless") and ("percutaneous nephrolithotomy" or "percutaneous lithotripsy" or "PCNL" or "PNL" or "PCN"). Two authors screened all the citations and abstracts independently. All potentially eligible studies involving comparison of the tubeless and standard PCNL were included.

Selection criteria
Inclusion criteria were: (1) RCTs; (2) studies published in English; (3) studies comparing tubeless and standard PCNL; (4) patients included in the studies were suited to PCNL, with no ureteric obstruction, no significant bleeding during the surgery, and no major collecting-system injury or normal renal function; (5) the nephrostomy tube placed at the completion of the procedure in the standard PCNL group; (6) patients included in the tubeless PCNL group were contraindicated from using a nephrostomy tube, however those with a double-J stent or external ureteral catheter could be considered; (7) studies reported at least one of the following clinical

outcomes: operative time, hospital stay, postoperative hemoglobin drop, postoperative analgesic requirement, return to normal activity, postoperative pain score, stone free rate, or major complications.

The exclusion criteria included: (1) pediatric patients under 14 years of age; (2) non-RCTs; (3) patients who underwent bilateral simultaneous PCNL; (4) patients with staghorn stones, congenital urinary tract anomalies, serious urinary infection, solitary functioning kidneys, or kidneys with prior open surgery.

Two reviewers completed the selection process independently.

Data extraction
Data extraction and quality evaluation were carried out by two reviewers. The information including study name, authors, publication year, country, study design, interventions, size of the drainage tube, number of patients, age, gender, stone burden, and clinical outcomes of interest (stone-free rate, operative time, hospital stay, return to normal activity, postoperative hemoglobin drop, postoperative analgesic requirements, postoperative pain score (VAS), blood transfusion, fever, urine leakage) were extracted from each included study. With the purpose of reducing the heterogeneity of the different studies and to make them easier to describe and understand, operative time was reported in minutes as a unit for all studies. Pain score was transformed by using linear 100 mm (the range of 0–100) visual analogue scale (VAS) (0 no pain, 100 maximum intolerable pain) uniformly [26]. In order to perform the sensitivity analysis, the type of drainage was also extracted from each study.

Assessment of quality
The criteria provided by the Oxford Center for Evidence-Based Medicine [27] was used to assess the level of evidence for all studies. The risk of bias for each RCT included was evaluated by two reviewers independently, according to the Cochrane Collaboration's tool [28]. The tool includes six aspects: random sequence generation, allocation concealment, blinding of participants and personnel, blinding of outcome assessment, incomplete outcome data, selective reporting, and other biases. The risk of bias was analyzed via the Cochrane Review Manager (REVMAN 5.3). Disagreements were resolved by discussion.

Statistical analysis
A meta-analysis was conducted to compare the effectiveness and safety of tubeless PCNL with standard PCNL. All statistical analyses were performed using Stata software (Stata SE 12.0). We chose statistical analysis methods and size effects based on data types and evaluation purposes. Relative risk (RR) was used for dichotomous data, while

continuous data was evaluated using weighted mean difference (WMD) or standardized mean difference (SMD). If continuous data was presented as means and range, the methodology described by Hozo et al. was used for calculating the standard deviations (SD) [29]. All the results were reported with 95% confidence intervals (95% CI). The heterogeneity of included studies were evaluated via the chi-square test and quantified by measuring I^2 value. When I^2 values did not exceeded 50%, the fixed-effect model was used to calculate pooled estimates. However, if an I^2 value exceeded 50% and could not be resolved by subgroup analysis, which indicated significant heterogeneity among the included studies, the random-effect model was used. The Z-test was used to determine the pooled effects, and P-value <0.05 was considered to be statistically significant. Forest plots were carried out to express the results of the meta-analysis. Influence analysis was performed to evaluate the effect of the included studies on the inter-study heterogeneity. The publication bias was assessed by Begg's test. Furthermore, sensitivity analysis was carried out to detect the influence of the total tubeless, partial tubeless, and standard PCNL studies on the overall effect.

Results

Study characteristics

Based on the inclusion and exclusion criteria, 14 RCTs [11–24] were finally included in our meta-analysis, and consisted of 576 patients who underwent tubeless PCNL and 572 patients who underwent standard PCNL. The process used for literature search and study selection is shown in Fig. 1. The studies included five RCTs [16–19, 24] which compared total tubeless PCNL with standard PCNL and nine RCTs [11–15, 20–23] which discussed partial tubeless PCNL. Table 1 shows the basic characteristics of the studies. The characteristics of the stones, including stone burden, stone location, and stone composition are summarized in Table 2. Age, sex ratio, and all stone characteristics described were comparable for the tubeless and standard PCNL groups in each study. The sex ratio was not reported in one study [11] and three studies [13, 18, 22] did not mention the size of the drainage tube. Other baseline characteristics which may have affected the outcome measures, such as body mass Index (BMI) [11, 13, 18, 19, 23], stone side [16, 19, 23, 24], number of punctures [10, 12, 22, 23], subcostal and supracostal punctures [13, 14, 17], and auxiliary procedures [13, 14, 18, 19, 21, 22, 24] were also reported in some studies. All data was also comparable between the two groups for each study.

Quality assessment

Table 1 shows that the level of evidence for each included study was graded Level 2. Fig 2A generalizes the results relative to the risk of bias for each randomized controlled study. As for the allocation concealment, five studies [11, 15, 17, 18, 21] did not describe the concealed method. Four studies [12, 13, 19, 20] were considered to have high risk of bias resulting from of the use of a random numbers table. There was a high risk of

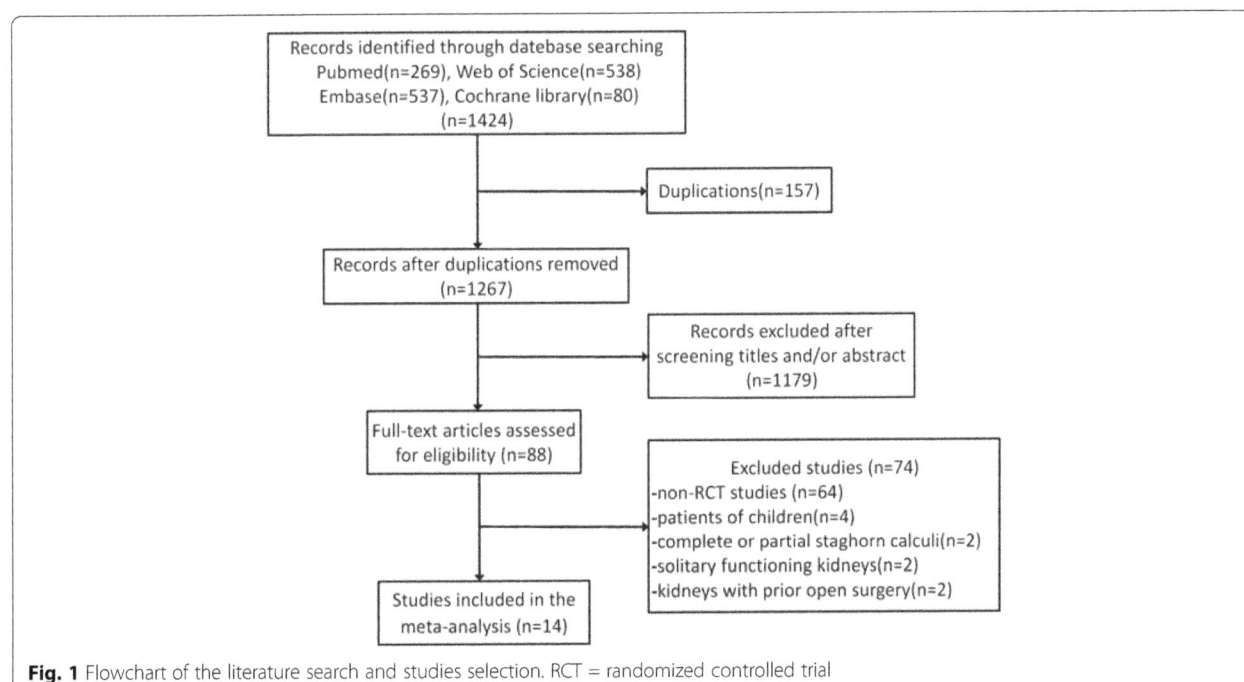

Fig. 1 Flowchart of the literature search and studies selection. RCT = randomized controlled trial

Table 1 The basic characteristics and methodological quality of included studies

Study	year	nation	study design	Level of evidence	PCNL (tubeless/standard)	Drainage (Size of tube)	Sample size	Age(Year)	Sex (M/F)	Outcome measures
Kumar	2016	India	RCT	Level 2	Total tubeless	–	56	36.20 ± 13.32	33/23	1, 2, 3, 4, 5,
					Nephrostomy tube	18F	57	36.00 ± 11.82	31/26	6, 7, 8, 9, 10
Sebaey	2016	Egypt	RCT	Level 2	External ureteric catheter	6F	40	40.6 ± 11.9	31/9	1, 2, 3,
					Nephrostomy tube	14F	40	46.1 ± 18.4	27/13	5, 6, 10
Zhao	2016	American	RCT	Level 2	Double-J ureteral stent	–	15	54.7 ± 12.2	9/6	1, 2, 3, 5,
					Nephrostomy tube	8F/10F	15	58.3 ± 17.6	8/7	6, 8, 9
Agrawal	2014	India	RCT	Level 2	Double-J ureteral stent	5F/26cm	83	33 (18–55)	62/21	1, 3, 4, 5,
					Nephrostomy tube	12F	83	31 (21–57)	59/24	6, 7, 8, 9, 10
Lu	2013	China	RCT	Level 2	External ureteric catheter	F5	16	43.81 ± 18.89	6/10	1, 2, 3,
					Nephrostomy tube+ Double-J ureteral stent	F16 + F6	16	46.25 ± 22.37	7/9	5, 9, 10
Chang	2011	Taiwan	RCT	Level 2	Total tubeless	–	68	59.22 ± 12.44	51/17	1, 2, 3, 4,
					Nephrostomy tube + Double-J ureteral stent	F20 + F7	63	58.70 ± 10.85	50/13	5, 6, 7, 10
Aghamir	2011	Iran	RCT	Level 2	Total tubeless	–	35	38.4 ± 11.7	23/12	1, 2, 3, 4,
					Nephrostomy tube + Double-J ureteral stent	NA	35	40 ± 11.95	21/14	5, 6, 8
Istanbulluoglu	2009	Turkey	RCT	Level 2	Total tubeless	–	45	47.48 ± 13.04	25/20	1, 2, 3, 5,
					Nephrostomy tube	14F	45	43.91 ± 14.44	24/21	6, 8, 9, 10
Crook	2008	The United Kingdom	RCT	Level 2	Total tubeless	–	25	53	15/10	1, 3, 5, 6, 8
					Nephrostomy tube	26F	25	52	19/6	
Singh	2008	India	RCT	Level 2	Double-J ureteral stent	NA	30	31 (14–55)	14/16	1, 2, 3, 4,
					Nephrostomy tube	22F	30	34 (17–55)	15/15	5, 6, 7, 8, 10
Shah	2008	India	RCT	Level 2	Double-J ureteral stent	6F	33	44.18 ± 13.13	20/13	1, 2, 3, 5,
					Nephrostomy tube	8F	32	46.69 ± 12.46	21/11	6, 7, 8, 9, 10
Agrawal, Madhu S	2008	India	RCT	Level 2	Double-J ureteral stent	6F/26cm	101	33 (18–55)	76/25	1, 3, 4, 5,
					Nephrostomy tube	16F	101	31 (21–57)	76/25	6, 7, 8, 9, 10
Tefekli	2007	Turkey	RCT	Level 2	External ureteric catheter	5F	17	38.4 ± 12.3	8/9	1, 2, 3,
					Nephrostomy tube	14-F	18	41.3 ± 14.7	11/7	5, 6
Choi	2006	American	RCT	Level 2	Double-J ureteral stent	6F	12	52.9 ± 14	NA	2, 3, 4,
					Nephrostomy tube	8.2F	12	47 ± 16	NA	6, 7, 8

RCT Randomized Controlled Trial, *PCNL* Percutaneous Nephrolithotomy, *NA* Not Available (Insufficient Information Provided)
1, Stone-free rate; 2, Operative time; 3, Hospital stay; 4, Return to normal activity; 5, Postoperative hemoglobin drop; 6, Postoperative analgesic requirements; 7, Postoperative pain scores; 8, Blood transfusion; 9, Fever; 10, Urine leakage

Table 2 The basic characteristics of stones

Study	PCNL (tubeless/standard)	Stone burden	Stone location	Stone composition
Kumar	TB	30.2 ± 4.6 mm	Pelvic (35) Calyceal (15) Pelvic + Calyceal (6)	NA
	SD	29.5 ± 4.2 mm	Pelvic (20) Calyceal (24) Pelvic + Calyceal (13)	NA
Sebaey	TB	1.82 ± 0.36 cm	Renal pelvis (9) Lower calyx (25) Middle calyx (5) Upper calyx (1)	NA
	SD	1.91 ± 0.37 cm	Renal pelvis (8) Lower calyx (25) Middle calyx (5) Upper calyx (2)	NA
Zhao	TB	259.0 mm^2	NA	Primarily calcium oxalate (53.3%) Mixed calcium (26.7%) Primarily uric acid (20%) Struvite (0%)
	SD	276.6 mm^2	NA	Primarily calcium oxalate (40%) Mixed calcium (20%) Primarily uric acid (33.3%) Struvite (6.7%)
Agrawal	TB	3.8 (1.0–5.7) cm^2	NA	NA
	SD	3.6 (1.1–5.3) cm^2	NA	NA
Lu	TB	3.11 ± 0.62 cm	NA	NA
	SD	3.29 ± 0.54 cm	NA	NA
Chang	TB	Length 24.74 ± 2.69 mm Width 16.40 ± 3.65 mm	NA	Struvite + apatite (8–11.8%) Uric acid (0%) Whewellite (30–44.1%) Whewellite + apatite (13–19.1%) Weddellite (17–25%)
	SD	Length 24.86 ± 2.78 mm Width 15.29 ± 4.50 mm	NA	Struvite + apatite (7.9%) Uric acid (3.2%) Whewellite (38.1%) Whewellite + apatite (30.2%) Weddellite (20.6%)
Aghamir	TB	2.81 ± 0.59 cm^2	NA	NA
	SD	2.87 ± 0.62 cm^2	NA	NA
Istanbulluoglu	TB	448.93 ± 249.13 mm^2	lower calyx (26) pelvis (11) multiple calyces(6) upper ureter (1) upper calyx (1)	NA
	SD	453.35 ± 165.97 mm^2	lower calyx (14) pelvis (19) multiple calyces (10) upper ureter (2)	NA
Crook	TB	17.5 mm	NA	NA
	SD	21.6 mm	NA	NA
Singh	TB	750 mm^2	Superior (9) middle (12) inferior calices (9)	mixture of calcium oxalate monohydrate /calcium oxalate dihydrate stones (71%) calcium phosphate (7%) carbonate apatite (7%)
	SD	800 mm^2	Superior (9) middle (15) inferior calices (7)	magnesium ammonium phosphate hexahydrate (7%) pure calcium oxalate monohydrate (7%) xanthine (1%)

Table 2 The basic characteristics of stones *(Continued)*

Study	PCNL (tubeless/standard)	Stone burden	Stone location	Stone composition
Shah	TB	535.36 ± 543.39 mm^2	NA	Calcium oxalate monohydrate (60.6%) Calcium oxalate dihydrate (18.18%) Calcium phosphate (3.03%) Struvite (12.12%) Uric acid (6.06%) Cystine (0%)
	SD	495.91 ± 445.92 mm^2	NA	Calcium oxalate monohydrate (53.12%) Calcium oxalate dihydrate (28.12%) Calcium phosphate (0%) Struvite (9.37%) Uric acid (6.25%) Cystine (3.12%)
Agrawal, Madhu S	TB	3.8 (1–5.7) cm^2	NA	calcium oxalate (87%) struvite (7%) uric acid (1%)
	SD	3.6 (1.1–5.3) cm^2	NA	calcium oxalate (84%) struvite (9%) uric acid (3%)
Tefekli	TB	3.0 ± 0.7 cm^2	Renal pelvis (6) Lower pole calyx (11)	NA
	SD	3.1 ± 0.9 cm^2	Renal pelvis (9) Lower pole calyx (9)	NA
Choi	TB	28.5 ± 15.4 mm	NA	NA
	SD	26.8 ± 13.5 mm	NA	NA

TB Tubeless Percutaneous Nephrolithotomy, *SD* Standard Percutaneous Nephrolithotomy, *NA*, Not Available (Insufficient Information Provided)

attrition bias in two studies [16, 22] due to the absence of SD. Two studies [16, 20] had a high risk of selective reporting bias because detailed explanation for some important outcomes was lacking.

Publication bias
The publication bias was evaluated via Begg's test. The Begg's funnel plot of the hospital stay which was included in almost all studies is shown in Fig. 2B. The results of the Begg's test for other factors are summarized in Table 3. Only postoperative pain score appeared to have a publication bias.

Influence analysis
For research indexes in which the I^2 value exceeded 50%, such as the operative time, hospital stay, return to activities, and postoperative pain scores (VAS), influence analysis has been assessed to screen studies which have a significant effect on heterogeneity. The results are shown in Fig. 3.

Meta-analysis
Operative time
Eleven studies [11–14, 17–20, 22–24] assessed the operative time. Due to the lack of SD reported, two studies [13, 22] were excluded from the data combination. Analysis of the final nine studies showed that tubeless PCNL required less operative time than standard PCNL with a statistically significant difference (WMD, –3.79 min; 95% CI, –6.73 to –0.85; $P = 0.012$; I^2 = 53.8%) (Fig. 4A).

Hospital stay
Hospital stay was measured in 14 studies [11–24]. Of these, 11 studies [11–15, 17–19, 21, 23, 24] were analyzed except for three trials [16, 20, 22], which did not report SD values. The pooled result showed the tubeless PCNL group was charged with a shorter hospital stay than the standard PCNL group (WMD, –1.27 days; 95% CI, –1.65 to –0.90; $P < 0.001$; I^2 = 98.7%) (Fig. 4B).

Return to normal activity
Seven studies [11, 13, 15, 18, 19, 21, 24] assessed the time to return to normal activity between two groups. Meta-analysis of these studies via a random effect model showed that the tubeless PCNL group required a shorter time to return to normal activity than the standard PCNL group (WMD, –4.24 days; 95% CI, –5.76 to –2.71; P < 0.001; I^2 = 97.5%) (Fig. 4C).

Postoperative hemoglobin drop
The mean (SD) estimated blood loss, reported by Choi et al. [11], was 72.73 (52.71) mL and 105 (68) mL in the tubeless PCNL group and the standard PCNL group, respectively. No statistical differences were found between

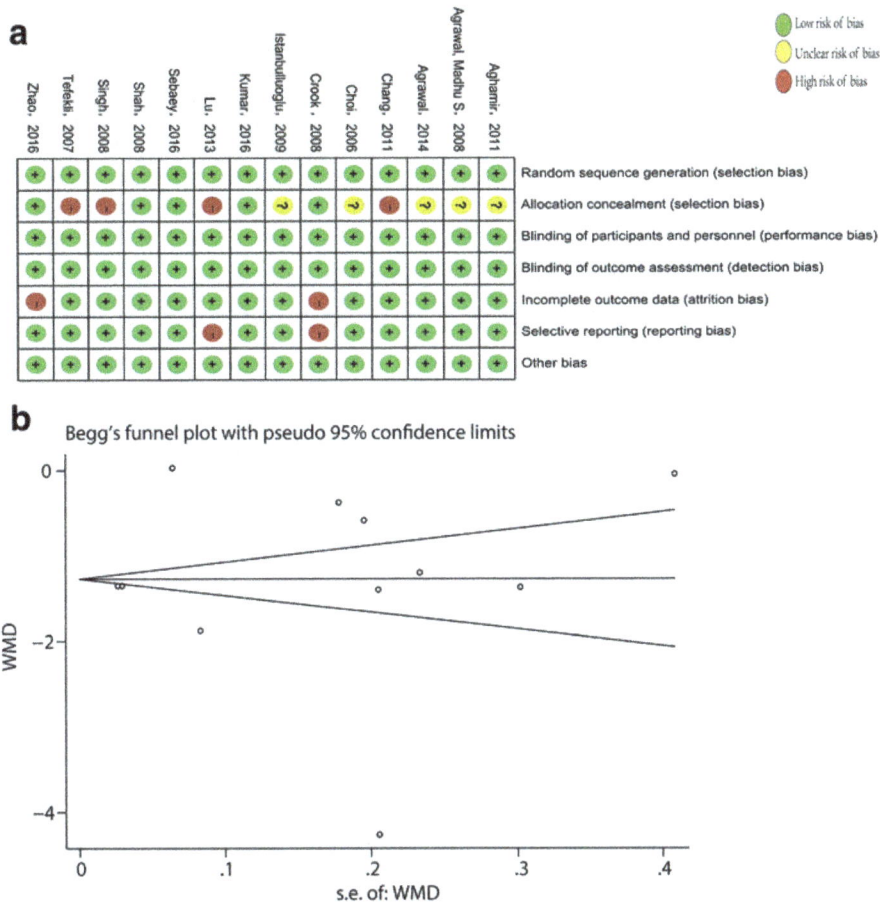

Fig. 2 (**a**) Risk of bias for each included study. (**b**) Begg's funnel plot of the hospital stay. WMD = weighted mean difference

the two groups ($P > 0.05$). Another 13 studies reported postoperative hemoglobin drop. Because the SD was not reported, three trials [13, 16, 22] were excluded from the data combination. A meta-analysis was performed for the other ten studies [12, 14, 15, 17–21, 23, 24], using a fixed effect model. The pooled results revealed no significant statistical differences between the tubeless group and standard PCNL group (WMD, –0.02 g/dL; 95% CI, –0.04 to 0.01; $P = 0.172$; $I^2 = 41.5\%$) (Fig. 5A).

Postoperative analgesia requirements
The study by Agrawal, Madhus et al. [15] showed the mean (SD) postoperative analgesic requirements (meperidine) in the first 24 h postoperatively was 81.7 (24.5) mg in the tubeless PCNL group and 126.5 (33.3) mg in the standard group. There was no significant statistical difference between the two groups ($P < 0.01$). Chang et al. [19] reported the postoperative analgesic requirements of both ketorolac and buprenorphine; the mean (SD) ketorolac dosage was 63.38 (15.22) mg in the tubeless PCNL group and 75.56 (16.44) mg in the standard PCNL group; and the dosage of buprenorphine was 0.09

(0.16) mg and 0.24 (0.76) mg in tubeless PCNL group and standard PCNL group, respectively. Ketorolac requirements favored the tubeless group ($P < 0.001$), but not the buprenorphine dosage ($P = 0.09$). The average tramadol dose required for analgesia postoperatively in Agrawal's study [21] was 81.3 (24.3) mg in the tubeless PCNL group and in the standard group, respectively; differences in doses were statistically significant ($P < 0.001$). As Kumar et al. [24] reported, cases in the tubeless group consumed significantly lower mean (SD) amounts of rescue analgesics (paracetamol), 1.48 (0.50) g in the tubeless group vs. 4.09 (1.11) g in the standard group ($P < 0.05$). A meta-analysis was also performed of the other five studies [11, 12, 14, 18, 23], using SMD for statistical analysis. These studies were divided into two subgroups according to the analgesic requirements (morphine or diclofenac sodium). The pooled result for the overall effect indicated the analgesic requirements in the tubeless PCNL group were significantly reduced (SMD, –1.09 mg; 95% CI, –1.35 to –0.84; $P < 0.001$; $I^2 = 46.8\%$) (Fig. 5B). In subgroup analysis, the results

Table 3 Begg's test for various factors

Factors	No. of studies	P value[a]	95% CI
Stone-free rate	11	0.956	[−0.711, 0 .675]
Operative time	9	0.385	[−3.073, 1.344]
Hospital stay	11	0.874	[−8.048, 9.303]
Return to normal activity	7	0.24	[−17.820, 5.653]
Postoperative hemoglobin drop	10	0.694	[−1.720, 1.202]
Postoperative analgesia equivalents	5	0.747	[−9.673, 12.096]
Postoperative pain scores	10	0.011	[1.664, 9.500]
Blood transfusion	7	0.545	[−2.640, 4.426]
Fever	7	0.627	[−1.311, 1.972]
Urine leakage	7	0.487	[−4.716, 2.585]

CI Confidence interval;
[a]P < 0.05 was considered statistically significant

for each subgroup ["morphine" subgroup [11, 18] (SMD, −1.01 mg; 95% CI, −1.45 to −0.58; P < 0.001; I^2 = 60.7%) and "diclofenac sodium" subgroup [12, 14, 23] (SMD, −1.13 mg; 95% CI, −1.45 to −0.82; P < 0.001; I^2 = 58.1%) (Fig. 5B)], were consistent with the overall results.

Postoperative pain scores

Seven studies [11, 13–15, 19, 21, 24] reported postoperative pain scores estimated using the visual analog scale (VAS). Analyzing these studies revealed that the tubeless PCNL group had statistically significant lower postoperative pain scores (WMD, −16.55 mm; 95% CI, −21.60 to

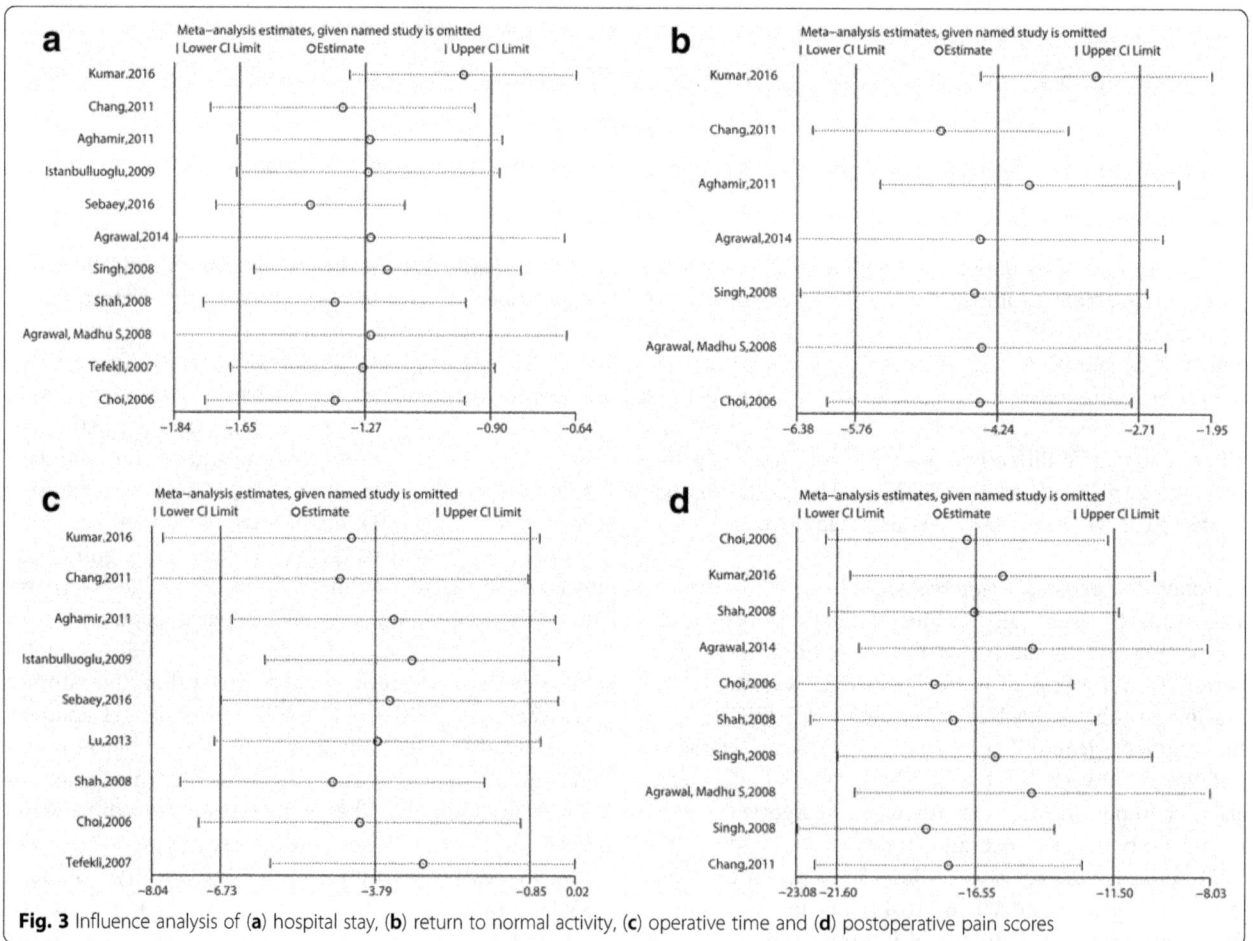

Fig. 3 Influence analysis of (**a**) hospital stay, (**b**) return to normal activity, (**c**) operative time and (**d**) postoperative pain scores

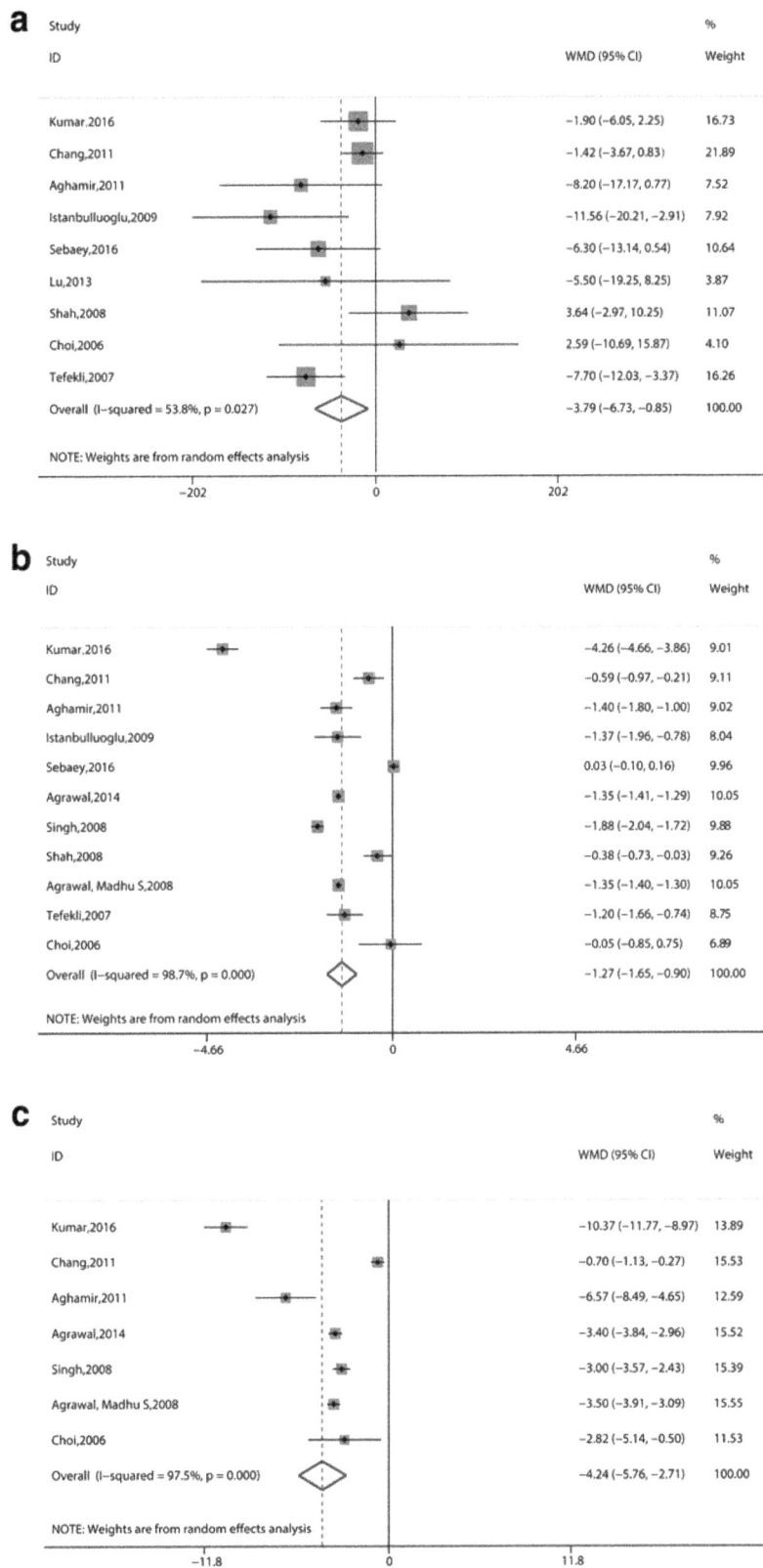

Fig. 4 Forest plots and meta-analysis of (**a**) operative time, (**b**) hospital stay, (**c**) return to normal activity. WMD = weighted mean difference, CI = confidence interval

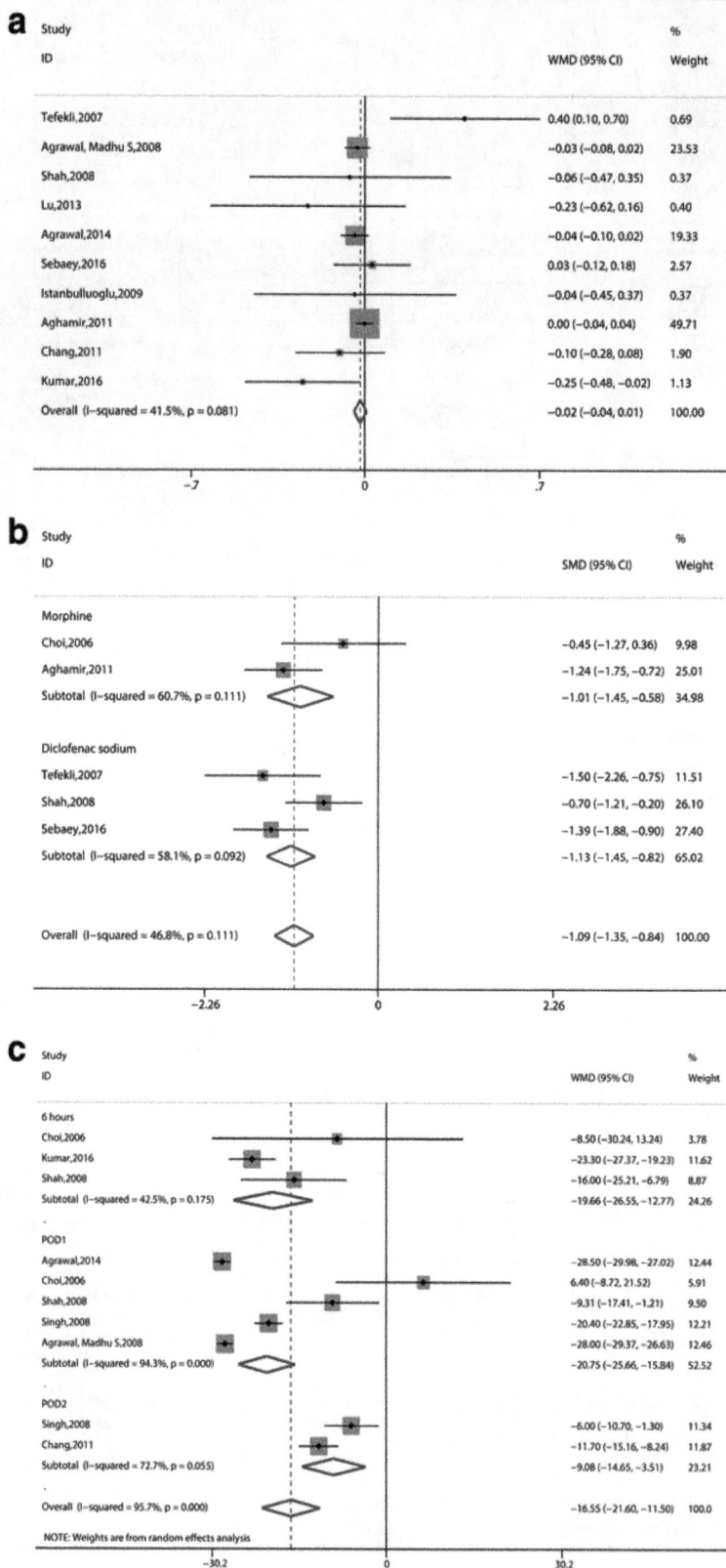

Fig. 5 Forest plots and meta-analysis of (**a**) postoperative hemoglobin drop, (**b**) postoperative analgesia requirements, (**c**) postoperative pain scores. WMD = weighted mean difference, SMD = standardized mean difference, CI = confidence interval, POD = postoperative day

−11.50; P < 0.001; I^2 = 95.7%) (Fig. 5C). Moreover, the results of the subgroup analysis for the "6 h" subgroup [11, 14, 24] (WMD, −19.66 mm; 95% CI, −26.55 to −12.77; P < 0.001; I^2 = 42.5%), "POD1" subgroup [11, 13–15, 21] (WMD, −20.75 mm; 95% CI, −25.66 to −15.84; P < 0.001; I^2 = 94.3%) and the "POD2" subgroup [13, 19] (WMD, −9.08 mm; 95% CI, −14.65 to −3.51; P = 0.001; I^2 = 72.7%) (Fig. 5C), indicated the same tendency.

Stone-free rate

Eleven studies [12–14, 16, 18–24] reported the stone-free rate. The pooled results of the overall data showed no significant statistical difference between the tubeless PCNL and the standard PCNL groups (RR, 1.01; 95% CI, 0.97 to 1.05; P = 0.776; I^2 = 0.0%) (Fig. 6A). The studies were divided into two subgroups according to the time when the stone-free rate was assessed. The pooled results of "the postoperative stone-free rate" subgroup, which included 11 studies [12–14, 16, 18–24], showed no significant difference between the two groups (RR, 1.01; 95% CI, 0.96 to 1.06; P = 0.703; I^2 = 0.0%) (Fig. 6A). "The 3rd-month stone-free rate" subgroup consisted of two studies [14, 19] with similar results (RR, 0.99; 95% CI, 0.93 to 1.06; P = 0.834; I^2 = 0.0%) (Fig. 6A).

Blood transfusion

The postoperative blood transfusion rate was measured in seven studies [11, 13, 14, 17, 18, 22, 24]. There was no significant statistical difference between the tubeless PCNL and the standard PCNL groups (RR, 0.79; 95% CI, 0.36 to 1.70; P = 0.538; I^2 = 0.0%) (Fig. 6B).

Fever

Postoperative fever rate (temperature more than 38 °C) was evaluated in seven studies [14, 15, 17, 20–22, 24]. The meta-analysis of these studies revealed no statistical difference between the tubeless PCNL and the standard PCNL group (RR, 1.05; 95% CI, 0.57 to 1.93; P = 0.867; I^2 = 0.0%) (Fig. 6B).

Urine leakage

Postoperative urine leakage was reported in seven studies [14, 15, 17, 19–21, 24]; a meta-analysis including these studies was performed using RR for effect size. Patients who underwent tubeless PCNL, rather than standard PCNL, were associated with a lower risk of postoperative urine leakage (RR, 0.30; 95% CI, 0.15 to 0.59; P = 0.001; I^2 = 41.2%) (Fig. 6B).

Readmission

Several studies [12, 15, 24] mentioned the readmission rate, but in two of these studies, postoperative issues did not require readmission [12, 15]. Only Kumar et al. [24]

reported that the standard PCNL group had a relatively higher rate of readmission, however the difference was not statistically significant between the two groups (7.1% vs. 1.8%; P = 0.21).

Sensitivity analysis

The results of the sensitivity analysis for partial and total tubeless PCNL are presented in Table 4. When the studies of partial tubeless PCNL [11–15, 20–23] were included, most of the outcomes such as hospital stay, return to activities, stone-free rate, postoperative hemoglobin drop, postoperative pain scores, blood transfusion, fever, urine leakage were constant. Though there was no significant difference in operative time between the two groups, it showed a similar tendency across studies. When only the studies of total tubeless PCNL [16–19, 24] were analyzed, only urine leakage was no longer detectable in the sensitivity analysis, the other outcomes remained consistent. Moreover, Ferakis and Stavropoulos [30] have reported that mini-PCNL is usually related to less morbidity than the standard method. A mini-PCNL is defined as a PCNL performed with a sheath diameter ≤ 22F [31]. This mini procedure was used in only two of the included studies [20, 23]. Thus, we performed a sensitivity analysis excluding the mini-PCNL studies. The results show that all outcomes remained consistent (Table 5).

Discussion

Percutaneous nephrolithotomy is now the major surgical treatment for patients with renal and upper ureteral stones [32, 33]. Using a nephrostomy tube at the end of the PCNL procedure was intended to be an integral part of the procedure [34]; however, it may also cause some significant postoperative discomfort. Therefore, tubeless PCNL has gained widespread popularity in recent years. Patients who were free from nephrostomy tube could be considered as tubeless PCNL.

In this meta-analysis, data from 1148 patients who underwent PCNL from 14 RCTs [11–24] were analyzed to update the effectiveness and safety of tubeless PNCL. Our main findings showed that tubeless PCNL was associated with significantly shorter operative time, shorter hospital stay, and shorter time to return to normal activities. Moreover, lower postoperative pain scores and reduced analgesia requirement were observed in the tubeless PCNL group. There was no significant statistical difference in the postoperative hemoglobin drop or the stone-free rate between the two groups. Concerning the main complications of PCNL, tubeless PCNL could significantly reduce urine leakage. However, no statistically significant difference was found in postoperative fever rate and blood transfusion rate.

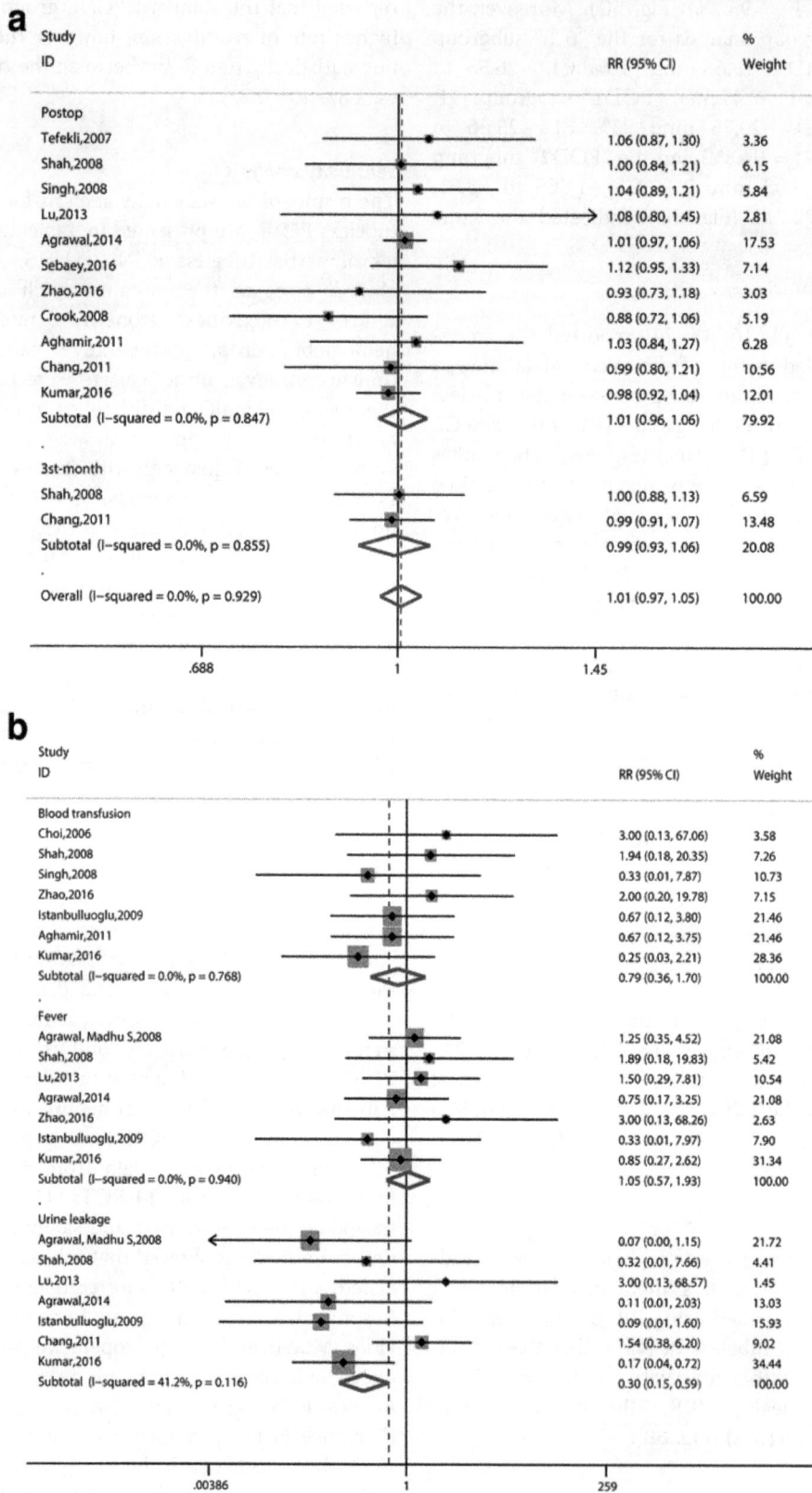

Fig. 6 Forest plots of (**a**) stone-free rate, (**b**) blood transfusion, fever and urine leakage. RR = relative risk, CI = confidence interval

Table 4 Results of sensitivity analysis for partial and total tubeless PCNL

Items	No. ofstudies	Reference of studies	Sample size TB/SD	Tests forheterogeneity I^2	P^a	Analysis model	Test for overalleffect Z	P^a	RR/WMD/SMD 95% CI	Favor
Analysis of partial tubeless studies										
Stone-free rate	7	[12, 20–23]	234/234	0%	0.830	Fixed	1.22	0.222	1.033[0.980,1.089]	TB
Operative time	5	[11, 12, 14, 20, 23]	118/118	57%	0.054	Random	1.20	0.229[b]	−3.253[−8.547,2.041]	TB
Hospital stay	7	[11–13, 21, 23]	316/316	99%	<0.0001	Random	4.52	<0.0001	−0.931[−1.335,-0.528]	TB
Return to normal activity	4	[11, 13, 15, 21]	226/226	0%	0.528	Fixed	24.76	<0.0001	−3.346[−3.610,-3.081]	TB
Postoperative hemoglobin drop	6	[12, 14, 15, 20, 21, 23]	290/290	48%	0.088	Fixed	1.43	0.152	−0.026[−0.063,0.010]	TB
Postoperative analgesic requirements	6	[11, 12, 14, 15, 21, 23]	286/286	65%	0.013	Random	7.33	<0.0001	−1.262[−1.600,-0.925]	TB
Postoperative pain scores	5	[11, 13–15, 21]	259/258	94%	<0.0001	Random	8.28	<0.0001	−20.750[−25.661,-15.839]	TB
Blood transfusion	4	[11, 13, 14, 22]	90/89	0%	0.761	Fixed	0.63	0.528	1.487[0.434,5.088]	SD
Fever	5	[14, 15, 20–22]	250/248	0%	0.920	Fixed	0.59	0.556	1.253[0.592,2.650]	SD
Urine leakage	4	[14, 15, 20, 21]	233/232	18%	0.303	Fixed	2.45	0.014	0.213[0.062,0.736]	TB
Analysis of total tubeless studies										
Stone-free rate	4	[16, 18, 19, 24]	184/180	0%	0.650	Fixed	0.58	0.565	0.976[0.900,1.059]	SD
Operative time	4	[17, 24]	204/200	55%	0.082	Random	2.00	0.045	−3.844[−7.609,-0.078]	TB
Hospital stay	4	[17, 24]	204/200	98%	<0.0001	Random	2.20	0.028	−1.907[−3.606,-0.207]	TB
Return to normal activity	3	[18, 19, 24]	159/155	99%	<0.0001	Random	1.70	0.090	−5.855[−12.618,0.909]	TB
Postoperative hemoglobin drop	4	[17, 24]	204/200	44%	0.147	Fixed	0.53	0.597	−0.009[−0.043,0.025]	TB
Postoperative analgesic requirements	3	[18, 19, 24]	159/155	97%	<0.0001	Random	1.86	0.062	−1.502[−3.081,0.077]	TB
Postoperative pain scores	2	[19, 24]	124/120	95%	<0.0001	Random	3.01	0.003	−17.448[−28.816,-6.081]	TB
Blood transfusion	3	[17, 18, 24]	136/137	0%	0.746	Fixed	1.29	0.198	0.503[0.176,1.432]	TB
Fever	2	[17, 24]	101/102	0%	0.585	Fixed	0.55	0.583	0.745[0.260,2.133]	TB
Urine leakage	3	[17, 19, 24]	169/165	68%	0.046	Fixed	1.14	0.254[c]	0.351[0.058,2.122]	TB

TB Tubeless percutaneous nephrolithotomy, *SD* Standard percutaneous nephrolithotomy, *RR* relative risk, *WMD* Weighted mean difference, *SMD* Standard mean difference, *CI* Confidence interval

[a]$P < 0.05$ was considered statistically significant

[b]Originally significant before studies using total tubeless percutaneous nephrolithotomy were excluded

[c]Originally significant before studies using partial tubeless percutaneous nephrolithotomy were excluded

The mean operative time was significantly shorter in the tubeless PCNL group than in the standard PCNL group in our analysis. However, in the review by Jiawu Wang et al. [8], there was no statistically significant difference in operative time between the two groups. We considered that these differences in operative times might have been attributed to the study selection. Each study may have calculated operative time using different criteria, and several studies did not provide a clear definition of the operative time involved. Furthermore, patient characteristics and surgeon's experience were likely the main factors influencing operative time.

The results of this meta-analysis indicated that the hospital stay and the time to return to normal activity were significantly reduced in the tubeless PCNL group.

Possible reasons could be attributed to less pain and the procedure did not involve the nephrostomy tube. The use of nephrostomy tubes in the standard PCNL group could have resulted in more postoperative discomfort, as well as requiring an additional procedure for tube removal, which means the prolongation of hospital stay and of time to return to normal activity. Hospital stay plays an important role in the evaluation of tubeless PCNL. Shorter hospital stay and shorter time to return to normal activity could decrease the costs of treatment and improve quality of health-care, which are indicated as advantages of the tubeless procedure.

Tubeless PCNL has been shown to be associated with decreased postoperative pain and analgesic requirements, differences that were statistically significant.

Table 5 Results of sensitivity analysis for standard PCNL

Items	No. of studies	Reference of studies	Sample size TB/SD	Tests for heterogeneity I²	Tests for heterogeneity Pᵃ	Analysis model	Test for overall effect Z	Test for overall effect Pᵃ	RR/WMD/SMD 95% CI	Favor
Stone-free rate	10	[12, 18, 19, 21, 22, 24]	463/459	0%	0.910	Fixed	0.32	0.747	0.992 [0.946,1.041]	SD
Operative time	7	[11, 12, 14, 17–19, 24]	266/262	62.8%	0.013	Random	1.98	0.048	−3.436 [−6.837,-0.036]	TB
Hospital stay	10	[11–15, 17–19, 21, 24]	480/476	96.9%	<0.0001	Random	10.02	<0.0001	−1.435 [−1.716,-1.154]	TB
Return to normal activity	7	[11, 13, 15, 18, 19, 21, 24]	385/381	97.5%	<0.0001	Random	5.44	<0.0001	−4.235 [−5.761,-2.709]	TB
Postoperative hemoglobin drop	8	[12, 14, 15, 17–19, 21, 24]	438/434	49.7%	0.053	Fixed	1.37	0.169	−0.018 [−0.043,0.008]	TB
Postoperative analgesic requirements	8	[11, 12, 14, 15, 18, 19, 21, 24]	405/401	91.4%	<0.0001	Random	4.79	<0.0001	−1.234 [−1.739,-0.729]	TB
Postoperative pain scores	7	[11, 13–15, 19, 21, 24]	383/378	94.9%	<0.0001	Random	6.35	<0.0001	−15.787 [−20.660,-10.913]	TB
Blood transfusion	7	[11, 13, 14, 17, 18, 22, 24]	226/226	0%	0.768	Fixed	0.62	0.538	0.785 [0.364,1.696]	TB
Fever	6	[14, 15, 17, 21, 22, 24]	333/333	0%	0.906	Fixed	<0.001	0.999	1.001 [0.521,1.922]	SD
Urine leakage	6	[14, 15, 17, 19, 21, 24]	386/381	40.4%	0.136	Fixed	3.64	<0.0001	0.259[0.125,0.537]	TB

TB Tubeless percutaneous nephrolithotomy, *SD* Standard percutaneous nephrolithotomy, *RR* Relative risk; *WMD* weighted mean difference, *SMD* standard mean difference, *CI* confidence interval
ᵃP < 0.05 was considered statistically significant

Drainage-tube related pain is one of the most common urologic complaints in the standard PCNL patient [35]. Multiple studies have demonstrated significant morbidity associated with indwelling nephrostomy tubes following PCNL, namely increased postoperative discomfort with significant analgesic requirements [14–19, 24, 36]. Thus, by performing tubeless PCNL for selected patients, we can achieve significantly improved patient pain profiles and the restrict usage of analgesic.

We found that the mean postoperative hemoglobin drop was lower in the tubeless PCNL group, but no statistical difference was found between the two groups. Patients with no noticeable hemorrhage during the operation were selected to undergo the tubeless procedure in our study. The main factors influencing the postoperative hemoglobin drop could be postoperative hemorrhage and the use of a nephrostomy tube. In the study by Shoma et al. [37], placement of a nephrostomy tube did not decrease the postoperative hemoglobin drop nor the development of perinephric hematoma. Furthermore, several investigators [14, 15, 17–21, 23] reported there was no significant difference between the two groups. The change in hemoglobin level may not be related to the use of a nephrostomy tube.

In our meta-analysis, there was no significant difference between the two groups in the stone-free rate; which is also similar to results of previous reviews [7, 9] and other published studies [11–24, 38]. The nephrostomy tube was placed at the end of the procedure in the standard group without affecting the stone-free rate. The incidence of stone clearance may be associated with the stone characteristics and renal anatomy in selected patients [24]. In addition, we found the vast majority of the included studies [12–14, 16, 18–22, 24] could not achieve a stone clearance of 100%. Although there were strict inclusion criteria, four studies [13, 18, 21, 22] in our review still reported the requirement of a second PCNL to treat the residual stone. It is sometimes difficult to exclude the existence of residual stones at the completion of the procedure. In some patients, performing a new puncture tract may sometimes be unavoidable [39]. This could represent a potential limitation of the tubeless procedure. However, flexible ureteroscopy has become a viable option for the treatment of renal stones in recent years due to its high stone-free rate and low morbidity [40]. Thus, it may be considered as a more suitable alternative to manage the residual stone.

The standard approach to PCNL includes placement of a nephrostomy tube designed to aid in hemostasis and drain the pelvicalyceal system [37]. However, our meta-analysis indicated that the tubeless PCNL did result in any increase in related complications. There was no significant difference in postoperative fever and blood transfusion between the two groups. Moreover, tubeless PCNL could significantly diminish urine leakage in comparison to the standard PCNL group. In our review, standard PCNL was not superior in terms of postoperative complications. Of course, this may be due to the fact that the study consisted of strictly selected patients with no complete or partial staghorn calculi, no congenital urinary tract anomalies, no noticeable hemorrhage during the operation, and no major collecting-system injury. In addition, many innovative techniques have been used recently to prevent postoperative bleeding and urinary leakage in the absence of an indwelling nephrostomy tube [41]. Santosh Kumar et al. [24] occluded the access tract with a 'Santosh-PGI hemostatic seal' following the stone clearance in the tubeless group and Shah et al. [42] instilled a fibrin sealant and gelatin matrix hemostatic sealant in the percutaneous tract after the completion of PCNL. Of course, the use of sealants remains controversial. Whether or not sealants can decrease bleeding and urinary extravasation deserves further exploration [43]. Nonetheless, tubeless PCNL may still result in fewer complications in appropriately selected patients when compared to PCNL performed with the presence of nephrostomy tube.

Though we have described many advantages of tubeless PCNL, it still has some limitations. One important issue pertinent to partial tubeless PCNL is the complication of the indwelling ureteral stent. Limb and Bellman [44] have reported that a subset of young men was unable to tolerate the internal Double-J stent. An additional drawback of tubeless PCNL is that it may interfere with a subsequent routine second-look procedure required to clear the residual stone fragments. In the study of Singh et al. [13], three patients had missed residual stones (invisible on initial postoperative fluoroscopy) that become apparent later. Last but not the least, tubeless PCNL may only be suitable for carefully selected patients.

Patients with ureteric obstruction, significant bleeding during the surgery, major collecting-system injury, or abnormal renal function may require a nephrostomy tube to aid in hemostasis and to drain the pelvicalyceal system. Patients without the above conditions were included in the study. We excluded those patients who underwent bilateral PCNL simultaneously. Though a small series of patients treated with simultaneous bilateral tubeless PNL have been reported [45, 46], and a timely drainage of the kidneys to prevent renal function damage should be considered. Furthermore, patients with staghorn stones, congenital urinary tract anomalies, serious urinary infection, solitary functioning kidneys, or kidneys with prior open surgery were also excluded from the study. Patients with staghorn stones always required subsequent surgery, and removing percutaneous access by the tubeless procedure may have necessitated a repeat of the PNL [43]. Patients with congenital urinary tract anomalies, serious urinary infection, and solitary functioning kidneys also need timely renal drainage which means they were unfit for tubeless PCNL. Finally, since prior open renal surgery might cause ureteral damage, we did not consider these patients in our study.

Some potential limitations of our meta-analysis should be considered. Firstly, we did not define the specific size of the stone as inclusion criteria due to the lack standards in some studies, however all patients included in the studies were suited to PCNL. Secondly, we did not analyze other potential complications, except for those mentioned above, such as pleural effusion, postoperative urinary tract infection, and septicemia. Due to the lack of adequate relevant data, these complications could not be included in our meta-analysis. Thirdly, the studies did not unify the category and specifications of postoperative analgesia, which may have led to a potential bias. We hope that uniform treatment standards will be discussed and defined in the future. Fourthly, due to the lack of sufficient description in some studies or in the limitations in the design and implementation of the included studies, the assessment of article quality could not be performed. This may have resulted in a potential bias. Finally, the pooled results relative to operative time, hospital stay, postoperative pain scores, and the time to return to normal activities showed significant heterogeneity. Thus, subgroup analysis, influence analysis, and sensitivity analysis were all performed to reduce heterogeneity, but these analyses did not significantly alter the results. Consequently, statistical heterogeneity may have influenced the conclusions. Lastly, the Begg's test of postoperative pain scores indicated that there might have been a publication bias for the included studies.

Conclusions

In conclusion, this updated meta-analysis showed that tubeless PCNL may be an effective and safe procedure for selected patients, resulting in significantly shorter hospital stay and shorter time to return to normal activity. Moreover, lower postoperative pain scores, reduced analgesia requirement, and urine leakage were also observed in tubeless PCNL without increasing other complications. We consider tubeless PCNL an acceptable and safe management option with experience and careful patient selection. Of course, larger high quality multi-center long-term RCTs are required to confirm the outcomes of our meta-analysis in the future.

Abbreviations
BMI: Body mass Index; CI: Confidence interval; PCNL: Percutaneous nephrolithotomy; POD: Postoperative day; RCTs: Randomized controlled trials; RR: Relative risk; SD: Standard deviation; SMD: Standardized mean difference; UTI: Urinary tract infection; VAS: Visual analog scale; WMD: Weighted mean difference

Acknowledgements
Not applicable.

Funding
No funding was obtained for this study.

Authors' contributions
Study concept and design: XY, SGW, QW and HLH. Acquisition of data: XY, QW, YDG and BLQ. Analysis and interpretation of data: XY, QW, BLQ, YDG and JQZ. Drafting of the manuscript: XY, SGW, JQZ and YCL. Critical revision of the manuscript for important intellectual content: XY, YCL and SGW. Study supervision: XY and SGW. All authors read and approved the final manuscript.

Competing interests
The authors declare that they have no competing interests.

Author details
[1]Department of Urology, Tongji Hospital, Tongji Medical College, Huazhong University of Science and Technology, No.1095 Jiefang Avenue, Wuhan, China. [2]Reproductive medicine center, Tongji Hospital, Tongji Medical College, Huazhong University of Science and Technology, Wuhan, China.

References
1. Türk C, Neisius A, Petrik A, et al. Guidelines on urolithiasis. EAU. 2017. Available at: http://uroweb.org/guideline/urolithiasis/. Accessed 15 April 2017.
2. Geraghty R, Jones P, Somani BK, et al. Worldwide trends of urinary stone disease treatment over the last two decades: a systematic review. J Endourol. 2017;31:547–56.
3. Ganpule AP, Vijayakumar M, Malpani A, et al. Percutaneous nephrolithotomy (PCNL) a critical review. Int J Surg. 2016;36:660–4.
4. Tirtayasa PMW, Yuri P, Birowo P, et al. Safety of tubeless or totally tubeless drainage and nephrostomy tube as a drainage following percutaneous nephrolithotomy: A comprehensive review. Asian J Surg. 2016;doi: https://doi.org/10.1016/j.asjsur.2016.03.003.
5. Bellman GC, Davidoff R, Candela J, et al. Tubeless percutaneous renal surgery. J Urol. 1997;157:1578–82.
6. Song G, Guo X, Niu G, et al. Advantages of tubeless mini-percutaneous nephrolithotomy in the treatment of preschool children under 3 years old. J Pediatr Surg. 2015;50:655–8.
7. Yuan H, Zheng S, Liu L, et al. The efficacy and safety of tubeless percutaneous nephrolithotomy: a systematic review and meta-analysis. Urol Res. 2011;39:401–10.
8. Wang J, Zhao C, Zhang C, et al. Tubeless vs standard percutaneous nephrolithotomy: a meta-analysis. BJU Int. 2012;109:918–24.

9. Zhong Q, Zheng C, Mo J, et al. Total tubeless versus standard percutaneous nephrolithotomy: a meta-analysis. J Endourol. 2013;27:420–6.

10. Mandhani A, Goyal R, Vijjan V, et al. Tubeless percutaneous nephrolithotomy – should a stent be an integral part? J Urol. 2007;178:921–4.

11. Choi M, Brusky J, Weaver J, et al. Randomized trial comparing modified tubeless percutaneous nephrolithotomy with tailed stent with percutaneous nephrostomy with small-bore tube. J Endourol. 2006;20(10):766-70.

12. Tefekli A, Altunrende F, Tepeler K, et al. Tubeless percutaneous nephrolithotomy in selected patients: a prospective randomized comparison. Int Urol Nephrol. 2007;39:57–63.

13. Singh I, Singh A, Mittal G. Tubeless percutaneous nephrolithotomy: is it really less morbid? J Endourol. 2008;22:427–34.

14. Shah HN, Sodha HS, Khandkar AA, et al. A randomized trial evaluating type of nephrostomy drainage after percutaneous nephrolithotomy: small bore v tubeless. J Endourol. 2008;22:1433–9.

15. Agrawal MS, Agrawal M, Gupta A, et al. A randomized comparison of tubeless and standard percutaneous nephrolithotomy. J Endourol. 2008;22:439–42.

16. Crook TJ, Lockyer CR, Keoghane SR, et al. A randomized controlled trial of nephrostomy placement versus tubeless percutaneous nephrolithotomy. J Urol. 2008;180:612–4.

17. Istanbulluoglu MO, Ozturk B, Gonen M, et al. Effectiveness of totally tubeless percutaneous nephrolithotomy in selected patients: a prospective randomized study. Int Urol Nephrol. 2009;41:541–5.

18. Aghamir SMK, Modaresi SS, Aloosh M, et al. Totally tubeless percutaneous nephrolithotomy for upper pole renal stone using subcostal access. J Endourol. 2011;25:583–6.

19. Chang CH, Wang CJ, Huang SW. Totally tubeless percutaneous nephrolithotomy: a prospective randomized controlled study. Urol Res. 2011;39:459–65.

20. Lu Y, Ping JG, Zhao XJ, et al. Randomized prospective trial of tubeless versus conventional minimally invasive percutaneous nephrolithotomy. World J Urol. 2013;31:1303–7.

21. Agrawal MS, Sharma M, Agarwal K. Tubeless percutaneous Nephrolithotomy using Antegrade tether: a randomized study. J Endourol. 2014;28:644–8.

22. Zhao PT, Hoenig DM, Smith AD, et al. A randomized controlled comparison of nephrostomy drainage vs ureteral stent following percutaneous nephrolithotomy using the Wisconsin stone QOL. J Endourol. 2016;30:1275–84.

23. Sebaey A, Khalil MM, Soliman T, et al. Standard versus tubeless mini-percutaneous nephrolithotomy: a randomised controlled trial. Arab journal of urology. 2016;14:18–23.

24. Kumar S, Singh S, Singh P, et al. Day care PNL using 'Santosh-PGI hemostatic seal' versus standard PNL: a randomized controlled study. Cent European J Urol. 2016;69:190–7.

25. Moher D, Liberati A, Tetzlaff J. Preferred reporting items for systematic reviews and meta-analyses: the PRISMA statement. BMJ. 2009; https://doi.org/10.1136/bmj.b2535.

26. Huskisson EC. Measurement of pain. Lancet. 1974;2:1127–31.

27. Phillips B, Ball C, Sackett D, et al. Oxford Centre for Evidence-Based Medicine Levels of Evidence. CEBM. 2017. http://www.cebm.net/ocebm-levels-of-evidence/. Accessed 15 Apr 2017.

28. Higgins JPT, Green S. Cochrane handbook for systematic reviews of interventions Version 5.1.0 [updated June 2017]. The Cocharane Collaboration 2017. http://handbook.cochrane.org. Accessed 15 Apr 2017.

29. Hozo SP, Djulbegovic B, Hozo I, et al. Estimating the mean and variance from the median, range, and the size of a sample. BMC Med Res Methodol. 2005; https://doi.org/10.1186/1471-2288-5-13.

30. Ferakis N, Stavropoulos M. Mini percutaneous nephrolithotomy in the treatment of renal and upper ureteral stones: lessons learned from a review of the literature. Urology annals. 2015;7:141–8.

31. Schilling D, Husch T, Bader M, et al. Nomenclature in PCNL or the tower of babel: a proposal for a uniform terminology. World J Urol. 2015 Nov;33(11):1905–7. https://doi.org/10.1007/s00345-015-1506-7.

32. Segura JW, Patterson DE, LeRoy AJ, et al. Percutaneous removal of kidney stones: review of 1,000 cases. J Urol. 1985;134:1077–81.

33. Skolarikos A, Alivizatos G, de la Rosette JJMC. Percutaneous nephrolithotomy and its legacy. Eur Urol. 2005; 47:22–28.

34. Maheshwari PN, Andankar MG, Bansal M. Nephrostomy tube after percutaneous nephrolithotomy: large-bore or pigtail catheter? J Endourol. 2000;14:735–7. 737-8

35. Abbott JE, Deem SG, Mosley N, et al. Are we fearful of tubeless percutaneous nephrolithotomy? Assessing the need for tube drainage following percutaneous nephrolithotomy. Urology annals. 2016;8:70–5.

36. Pietrow PK, Auge BK, Lallas CD, et al. Pain after percutaneous nephrolithotomy: impact of nephrostomy tube size. J Endourol. 2003;17(6):411–4.

37. Shoma AM, Elshal AM. Nephrostomy tube placement after percutaneous nephrolithotomy: critical evaluation through a prospective randomized study. Urology. 2012;79:771–6.

38. Ni S, Qiyin C, Tao W, et al. Tubeless percutaneous nephrolithotomy is associated with less pain and shorter hospitalization compared with standard or small bore drainage: a meta-analysis of randomized controlled trials. Urology. 2011;77:1293–8.

39. Kara C, Resorlu B, Bayindir M, et al. A randomized comparison of totally tubeless and standard percutaneous nephrolithotomy in elderly patients. Urology. 2010;76:289–93.

40. Proietti S, Knoll T, Giusti G. Contemporary ureteroscopic management of renal stones. Int J Surg. 2016;36:681–7.

41. de Cogain MR, Krambeck AE. Advances in tubeless percutaneous nephrolithotomy and patient selection: an update. Current urology reports. 2013;14:130–7.

42. Shah HN, Hegde S, Shah JN, et al. A prospective, randomized trial evaluating the safety and efficacy of fibrin sealant in tubeless percutaneous nephrolithotomy. J Urol. 2006;176:2488–92.

43. Zilberman DE, Lipkin ME, de la Rosette JJ, et al. Tubeless percutaneous nephrolithotomy–the new standard of care? J Urol. 2010;184:1261–6.

44. Limb J, Bellman GC. Tubeless percutaneous renal surgery: review of first 112 patients. Urology. 2002;59:527–31.

45. Istanbulluoglu MO, Ozturk B, Cicek T, et al. Bilateral simultaneous totally tubeless percutaneous nephrolithotomy: preliminary report of six cases. J Endourol. 2009;23(8):1255–7.

46. Bagrodia A, Raman JD, Bensalah K, et al. Synchronous bilateral percutaneous nephrostolithotomy: analysis of clinical outcomes, cost and surgeon reimbursement. J Urol. 2009;181(1):149–53.

8

Effects of increasing the PSA cutoff to perform additional biomarker tests before prostate biopsy

Tobias Nordström[1,2]⊙, Jan Adolfsson[3,4], Henrik Grönberg[1] and Martin Eklund[1*]

Abstract

Background: Multi-step testing might enhance performance of the prostate cancer diagnostic pipeline. Using PSA >1 ng/ml for first-line risk stratification and the Stockholm 3 Model (S3M) blood-test >10% risk of Gleason Score > 7 prostate cancer to inform biopsy decisions has been suggested. We aimed to determine the effects of changing the PSA cutoff to perform reflex testing with S3M and the subsequent S3M cutoff to recommend prostate biopsy while maintaining the sensitivity to detect Gleason Score ≥ 7 prostate cancer.

Methods: We used data from the prospective, population-based, paired, diagnostic Stockholm 3 (STHLM3) study with participants invited by date of birth from the Swedish Population Register during 2012–2014. All participants underwent testing with PSA and S3M (a combination of plasma protein biomarkers [PSA, free PSA, intact PSA, hK2, MSMB, MIC1], genetic polymorphisms, and clinical variables [age, family, history, previous prostate biopsy, prostate exam]). Of 47,688 men in the STHLM3 main study, we used data from 3133 men with S3M >10% and prostate biopsy data. Logistic regression models were used to calculate prostate cancer detection rates and proportion saved biopsies.

Results: 44.2%, 62.5% and 67.9% of the participants had PSA <1, <1.5 and <1.7 ng/ml, respectively. Increasing the PSA cut-off for additional work-up from 1 ng/ml to 1.5 ng/ml would thus save 18.3% of the performed tests, 4.9% of the biopsies and 1.3% (10/765) of Gleason Grade ≥ 7 cancers would be un-detected. By lowering the S3M cutoff to recommend biopsy, sensitivity to high-grade prostate cancer can be restored, to the cost of increasing the number of performed biopsies modestly.

Conclusion: The sensitivity to detect prostate cancer can be maintained when using different PSA cutoffs to perform additional testing. Biomarker cut-offs have implications on number of tests and prostate biopsies performed. A PSA cutoff of 1.5 ng/ml to perform additional testing such as the S3M test might be considered.

Keywords: Prostate cancer, Prostate neoplasm, Prostate-specific antigen (PSA), Biomarker, Stockholm3, STHLM3

Background

Recently, Crawford and colleagues proposed an approach of using PSA 1.5 ng/ml as first-line testing before using biomarker-based tests to inform prostate biopsy decisions [1]. Such a multi-step work-up is an attractive approach for improving prostate cancer diagnostics. Men with PSA below the population median carries a low risk to develop metastatic or lethal disease also during long follow-up [2]. Since testing with PSA has high availability and low cost, base-line PSA testing is a attractive for efficient first-line risk stratification [2].

For second-line testing, the S3M (Stockholm3 Model) blood-test has been developed, including data on proteins, a genetic score and clinical information (age, digital rectal examination, prostate volume, and previous biopsy) [3]. Compared with both organized PSA-screening and current prostate cancer testing (without organized screening but with high rates of PSA testing),

* Correspondence: martin.eklund@ki.se
[1]Department of Medical Epidemiology and Biostatistics, Karolinska Institutet, S-171 77 Stockholm, Sweden
Full list of author information is available at the end of the article

the STHLM3 studies have shown that use of the S3M test may decrease both the number of prostate biopsies and over-diagnosis, while maintaining sensitivity to high-grade disease [3, 4]. This was done using PSA >1 ng/ml as cutoff for performing the S3M blood-test and a risk of high-grade disease exceeding that of PSA = 3 ng/ml to indicate recommendation for prostate biopsies.

With the approach suggested by Crawford et al. [1], two thirds of men would be identified as having a very low risk of developing high-grade disease. Compared with a lower PSA cutoff, using 1.5 ng/ml would decrease the number of performed biomarker tests. However, while performing the biomarker test for fewer men, it would also yield a smaller pool of men in which to identify prostate cancer cases, potentially affecting overall sensitivity.

It is unknown how changing the PSA cut-off for performing a reflex test affects the overall diagnostic sensitivity, the number of performed biopsies, and number of performed biomarker tests. We therefore illustrate such effects for the first-line test PSA and the second-line biomarker test S3M.

Methods

STHLM3 (ISRCTN84445406) is a prospective and population-based prostate cancer diagnostic study conducted 2012–2014 including men between 50 and 69 years of age [3]. The S3M test is a blood test based on a model including a combination of plasma protein biomarkers (PSA, free PSA, intact PSA, hK2, MSMB, MIC1), genetic polymorphisms (232 SNPs), and clinical variables (age, family, history, previous prostate biopsy, prostate exam). The test gives a prediction on the individual risk of finding Gleason Score ≥ 7 on prostate biopsies, where ≥10% risk was considered increased risk in the main study. The 10% risk cutoff was choosen because it represent equal sensitivity to detect Gleason Score ≥ 7 cancer as PSA = 3 ng/

ml, used in major screening studies [5]. The exact cut-off used can be chosen to fit different individuals and healthcare systems [6]. As for September 2017, the S3M test is clinically availiable for analysis at Karolinska University Laboratory, Stockholm, Sweden.

Of 47,688 participants in the STHLM3 study, 26,458 men had a PSA ≥ 1 ng/ml and underwent further testing with S3M. By design, a prostate biopsy was recommended to men with ≥10% risk of high-grade prostate cancer as predicted by PSA (≥3 ng/ml) or the S3M test. Gleason Score ≥ 7 (ISUP ≥2) defined high-grade cancer. 65.0% of participants with high risk followed the recommendation to undergo prostate biopsy during the main study period. For this analysis we included 3133 men in the STHLM3 validation cohort with biopsy data and an S3M test ≥10%.

We calculated detection rates and proportion saved biopsies when S3M was used as a reflex test after a range of a priori choosen PSA cutoff levels, keeping overall sensitivity fixed at the same level as PSA ≥ 3 (or, equivalently, S3M ≥ 10% as a reflex test in men with PSA ≥ 1). Data on men with less than 10% risk of Gleason Score ≥ 7 prostate cancer was thus incomplete. To calculate results for this group of men, we imputed case status of each non-biopsied man using Bernoulli experiments with the risk prediction from the S3M as parameter [7].

Results

44.2%, 62.5% and 67.9% of the participants in the population-based STHLM3 study had PSA <1, <1.5 and <1.7 ng/ml, respectively. Solely increasing the cut-off for additional work-up from 1 ng/ml to 1.5 ng/ml would thus save 18.3% of the performed tests, 4.8% of the biopsies and only 1.3% (10/765) of Gleason Grade ≥ 7 cancers would be un-detected (Table 1). Participant characteristics in men with PSA ≥ 3 or S3M ≥ 10% risk of Gleason Score ≥ 7 cancer and thus undergoing a prostate biopsy are described in Table 2.

Table 1 Prevalence of prostate cancer different PSA ranges for men with S3 M ≥ 10% risk of Gleason Score ≥ 7 cancer. Number of men with respective finding among 47,688 men in the STHLM3 study of which 3133 had a S3 M test >10% and a subsequent prostate biopsy

PSA ng/ml	Proportion of men by PSA in STHLM3 [3] % (n)	Men with high risk of PCa (S3 M > 10%) % (n)	Gleason Score (GS) n (%)			
			3 + 3	3 + 4	4 + 3	≥4 + 4
0–0.9	21,230 (44.2)	0 (0)	N/A	N/A	N/A	N/A
1–1.4	8777 (18.3)	100 (3.2)	24 (3.1)	5 (1.1)	2 (2.0)	0 (0)
1.5–1.6	2593 (5.4)	54 (1.7)	17 (2.2)	3 (0.6)	0 (0.0)	0 (0)
1.7–1.9	2993 (6.2)	105 (3.4)	35 (4.5)	10 (2.1)	0 (0.0)	1 (0.7)
2.0–2.9	5906 (12.3)	394 (12.6)	96 (12.4)	67 (14.2)	18 (11.5)	7 (5.0)
3.0–3.9	2721 (5.7)	817 (26.1)	218 (28.2)	110 (23.3)	34 (21.7)	25 (17.9)
>4.0	3808 (7.9)	1663 (53.0)	382 (49.5)	277 (58.7)	103 (65.6)	107 (76.4)
Total	47,688 (100)	3133 (100)	772 (100)	472 (100)	157 (100)	140 (100)

Table 2 Cohort description. Characteristics of 3133 men in the STHLM3 study [3] with S3 M test indicating ≥10% risk of prostate cancer

Variable	
Participants, n	3133
Age, years (mean, SD)	63.4, 5.0
PSA, ng/ml (median, IQR)	6.1, 2.9
S3 M test, % risk Gleson Score ≥ 7 cancer (median, IQR)	0.20, 0.17
Biopsy findings (n, %)	
Benign	1578, 50.4
Gleason Score 6 (ISUP 1)	772, 24.6
Gleason Score 3 + 4 (ISUP 2)	472, 15.1
Gleason Score 4 + 3 (ISUP 3)	157, 5.0
Gleason Score ≥ 4 + 4 (ISUP ≥4)	140, 1.8

To infer the mortality benefit of early detection of prostate cancer reported in ERSPC, the sensitivity to detect high-grade disease needs to be at least as high as when performing systematic prostate biopsies with a PSA cut-off of 3 ng/ml, being the threshold primarily used for biopsy in ERSPC [5]. To adjust for the slightly decreased cancer detection when increasing the first-line PSA threshold from 1 to 1.5 ng/ml, the S3M cutoff to recommend biopsy can be tuned, as previously illustrated [7]. Figure 1 illustrates how the PSA cutoff to perform the S3M test and the S3M cutoff to recommend biopsy are inter-related to maintain sensitivity to high-grade disease. For example, the total number of biopsies would increase slightly by 4% if increasing the cutoff for performing the S3M test from PSA 1.0 ng/ml to 1.5 ng/ml while maintaining sensitivity to high-grade prostate cancer (Fig. 1). A small number of Glason Score ≥ 4 + 3 were detected in low PSA ranges (Table 1). If choosing

PSA 2 ng/ml for threshold to perform S3 M testing, only 1.0% (3/197) of Gleason Score ≥ 4 + 3 cancers would be undetected, but missing also 3.8% (18/472) of Gleason Score 3 + 4 cancers. Availiable number of higher-grade cases were to small in low PSA ranges for additional analyses such as in Fig. 1 on this endpoint.

Discussion

With a possibly increasing complexity of the diagnostic chain including a multi-step approach with PSA, additional biomarker-based algorithms, and imaging before deciding to recommend further work-up, several cut-offs need to be adjusted to optimize performance. Here, we illustrate the effects of simultaneously tuning both the PSA cut-off for performing the reflex test S3M and the S3M cutoff for recommending a prostate biopsy. Using this approach, the sensitivity to detect high-grade disease can be maintained, while the number of prostate biopsies is slightly affected.

From a health-economical point of view, it is efficient to maximize the use of cheap tools such as PSA early in the diagnostic chain, with the more expensive and specialized tests used downstream. Further, as many men with low risk of high-grade disease as possible should be identified early in the process, without being subjected to additional tests or extended workup. Thus, it is interesting both from the perspective of an individual and from the healthcare system to explore how an increased cut-off to perform e.g. the S3M test might be done without compromising the overall diagnostic performance.

This analysis was based on prospective, population-based data from the STHLM3 study. It illustrates the relationship between two sequential diagnostic tests when maintaining sensitivity to detect high-grade

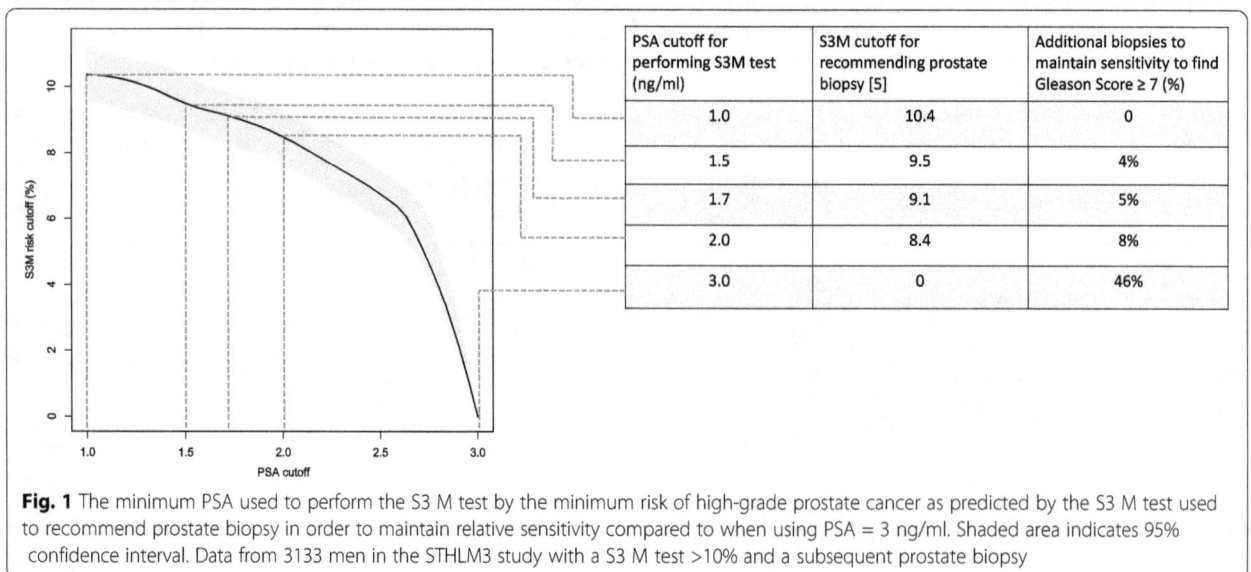

PSA cutoff for performing S3M test (ng/ml)	S3M cutoff for recommending prostate biopsy [5]	Additional biopsies to maintain sensitivity to find Gleason Score ≥ 7 (%)
1.0	10.4	0
1.5	9.5	4%
1.7	9.1	5%
2.0	8.4	8%
3.0	0	46%

Fig. 1 The minimum PSA used to perform the S3 M test by the minimum risk of high-grade prostate cancer as predicted by the S3 M test used to recommend prostate biopsy in order to maintain relative sensitivity compared to when using PSA = 3 ng/ml. Shaded area indicates 95% confidence interval. Data from 3133 men in the STHLM3 study with a S3 M test >10% and a subsequent prostate biopsy

disease. The detection rates in low PSA intervals are well comparable with previously presented data [8] and the internal validity of these data is high. While extrapolation outside the STHLM3 context is hard, corresponding analyses regarding other suggested reflex tests are warranted. Limitations of this work include lack of external validation, lack of true disease prevalence while men with <10% risk of Gleason Score ≥ 7 cancer as predicted by both PSA and S3M did not undergo prostate biopsy, and lack of long-term follow-up.

Conclusion

We conclude that the sensitivity to detect prostate cancer can be maintained while avoiding a substantial proportion of reflex tests and biopsies by carefully choosing the PSA cutoff to perform additional testing. For instance, a PSA cutoff of 1.5 ng/ml to perform additional biomarker tests such as the S3 M test might be considered.

Abbreviations
5-ARI: 5-alfa reductase inhibithor; ERSPC: European Randomized Study of Screening for Prostate Cancer; PSA: prostate-specific antigen; S3 M: stockholm3 model; STHLM3: Stockholm3 study

Acknowledgements
We thank all study participants, the STHLM3 core management group, STHLM3 outpatient urologists, KI Biobank, Karolinska University Hospital Laboratory, Unilabs AB Stockholm, and Histocenter Gothenburg for dedicated work with all aspects of the STHLM3 study.

Funding
The main funder of the STHLM3 study is the Stockholm County Council (Stockholms Läns Landsting) who is the main healthcare provider in Stockholm. Martin Eklund is supported by the Swedish Research Council for Health, Working Life and Welfare, the Swedish Research Council, and the Swedish Cancer Society. The funding sources had no role in the study design; the collection, analysis, and interpretation of data; in the writing of the report; or in the decision to submit the paper for publication.

Authors' contributions
HG is principal investigator for the STHLM3 study. TN, HG and ME designed the study. TN and ME performed statistical analyses and drafted the manuscript. TN, HG, JA and ME interpreted study results and finalized the manuscript. All authors read and approved the final manuscript.

Competing interests
TN and JA declare nor conflict of interest. HG has five prostate cancer diagnostic-related patents pending, has patent applications licensed to Thermo-Fisher Scientific, and might receive royalties from sales related to these patents. ME is named on four of these five patent applications. Karolinska Institutet collaborates with Thermo-Fisher Scientific in developing the technology for STHLM3.

Author details
[1]Department of Medical Epidemiology and Biostatistics, Karolinska Institutet, S-171 77 Stockholm, Sweden. [2]Department of Clinical Sciences at Danderyd Hospital, Karolinska Institutet, S-182 88 Stockholm, Sweden. [3]Department of Clinical Science, Intervention and Technology, Karolinska Institutet, Stockholm, Sweden. [4]Swedish Agency for Health Technology Assessment and Assessment of Social Services, Stockholm, Sweden.

References
1. Crawford ED, Rosenberg MT, Partin AW, Cooperberg MR, Maccini M, Loeb S, et al. An approach using PSA levels of 1.5 ng/mL as the cutoff for prostate cancer screening in primary care. Urology. 2016;96:116–20.
2. Vickers AJ, Cronin AM, Bjork T, Manjer J, Nilsson PM, Dahlin A, et al. Prostate specific antigen concentration at age 60 and death or metastasis from prostate cancer: case-control study. BMJ. 2010 ed. 2010;341:c4521.
3. Grönberg H, Adolfsson J, Aly M, Nordström T, Wiklund P, Brandberg Y, et al. Prostate cancer screening in men aged 50-69 years (STHLM3): a prospective population-based diagnostic study. Lancet Oncol. 2015;16:1667–76.
4. Eklund M, Nordström T, Aly M, Adolfsson J, Wiklund P, Brandberg Y, et al. The Stockholm-3 (STHLM3) Model can Improve Prostate Cancer Diagnostics in Men Aged 50–69 yr Compared with Current Prostate Cancer Testing. European Urology Focus [Internet]. 2016. Available from: http://www.eu-focus.europeanurology.com/article/S2405-4569(16)30156-0/fulltext.
5. Schröder FH, Hugosson J, Roobol MJ, Tammela TLJ, Zappa M, Nelen V, et al. Screening and prostate cancer mortality: results of the European randomised study of screening for prostate cancer (ERSPC) at 13 years of follow-up. Lancet. 2014;384:2027–35.
6. Nordström T, Grönberg H, Adolfsson J, Aly M, Eklund M. Balancing Overdiagnosis and early detection of prostate cancer using the Stockholm-3 model. European Urology Focus. 2016;
7. Nordström T, Grönberg H, Adolfsson J, Aly M, Eklund M. Balancing Overdiagnosis and Early Detection of Prostate Cancer using the Stockholm-3 Model. Catto J, editor. European Urology Focus. 2016.
8. Thompson IM, Pauler DK, Goodman PJ, Tangen CM, Lucia MS, Parnes HL, et al. Prevalence of prostate cancer among men with a prostate-specific antigen level. N. Engl. J. Med. 2004 ed. 2004;350:2239–46.

9

The R.I.R.S. scoring system: An innovative scoring system for predicting stone-free rate following retrograde intrarenal surgery

Yinglong Xiao[1†], Deng Li[2†], Lei Chen[2], Yaoting Xu[3], Dingguo Zhang[4], Yi Shao[1,2*] and Jun Lu[1*]

Abstract

Background: To establish and internally validate an innovative R.I.R.S. scoring system that allows urologists to preoperatively estimate the stone-free rate (SFR) after retrograde intrarenal surgery (RIRS).

Methods: This study included 382 eligible samples from a total 573 patients who underwent RIRS from January 2014 to December 2016. Four reproducible factors in the R.I.R.S. scoring system, including renal stone density, inferior pole stone, renal infundibular length and stone burden, were measured based on preoperative computed tomography of urography to evaluate the possibility of stone clearance after RIRS.

Results: The median cumulative diameter of the stones was 14 mm, and the interquartile range was 10 to 21. The SFR on postoperative day 1 in the present cohort was 61.5% (235 of 382), and the final SFR after 1 month was 73.6% (281 of 382). We established an innovative scoring system to evaluate SFR after RIRS using four preoperative characteristics. The range of the R.I.R.S. scoring system was 4 to 10. The overall score showed a great significance of stone-free status ($p < 0.001$). The area under the receiver operating characteristic curve of the R.I.R.S. scoring system was 0.904.

Conclusions: The R.I.R.S. scoring system is associated with SFR after RIRS. This innovative scoring system can preoperatively assess treatment success after intrarenal surgery and can be used for preoperative surgical arrangement and comparisons of outcomes among different centers and within a center over time.

Keywords: Urolithiasis, Stone surgery, Anatomy, Classification, Prognosis

Background

Urolithiasis is one of the most common diseases in urology. It has a prevalence rate of 5.8% in China, of which the most common form is kidney stones [1]. Treatments such as extracorporeal shock wave lithotripsy (SWL), ureteroscopic lithotripsy, retrograde intrarenal surgery (RIRS) and percutaneous nephrolithotomy (PNL) are first-line interventional therapies for urolithiasis according to the European Association of Urology (EAU) guidelines [2]. RIRS, however, has recently become the preferred choice in the management of renal calculi (smaller than 20 mm). Several studies have reported RIRS to be a safe technique, and it is associated with minimal and minor complications for intrarenal stones [3, 4].

As a string of scoring systems have been established for evaluating stone-free rate (SFR) and complications, PNL can be more easily predicted than ever before; [5] yet few criteria remain to preoperatively assess the SFR after RIRS due to a relatively short period of popularization as a first-line treatment for renal stones based on guidelines of the EAU. The Resorlu-Unsal stone score (RUSS) reported by Resorlu et al. can effectively estimate the SFR, and the modified Seoul National University Renal Stone Complexity score (S-ReSC) proposed by Jung et al. can predict the SFR after RIRS on the basis of the affected site without stone size and numbers, [6, 7] however neither of these scoring systems can predict the outcomes of the procedure universally, simply and specifically [8]. In this study, the primary aim was to develop an innovative scoring system and to

---

* Correspondence: drshaoyi@163.com; 842320@163.com
†Equal contributors
[1]Department of Urology, Shanghai General Hospital of Nanjing Medical University, No.100, Haining Road, Hongkou District, Shanghai 200080, China
Full list of author information is available at the end of the article

validate this system with regard to its capacity. This could estimate the SFR preoperatively, minimize complications, and provide a quantification of stone characteristics and patient outcomes between different centers.

Methods

R.I.R.S. scoring system

All components of the R.I.R.S. scoring system were obtained by computed tomography urography (CTU), which enabled a confidently reproducible prediction of the stone characteristics [9]. Renal calculus density was defined as an attenuation coefficient of 1 to 2 points as determined by ≤1000 Hu or >1000 Hu. The renal infundibulopelvic angle (RIPA) of the inferior pole stone was defined as the inner angle of the intersection of ureteropelvic axis and the axis of the lower renal calyx. This was separately scored from 1 to 3 points as determined by a non-inferior pole stone or inferior pole stone with RIPA >30° or ≤30°. RIL, the distance from most distal point at bottom stone-containing calix to midpoint of lip of renal pelvis [10] was assigned 2 points and was determined by whether the infundibulopelvic length was more than 25 mm; otherwise, 1 point was recorded. Stone burden, which we described as the cumulative stone diameter (CSD), was obtained by perioperative CTU. We assigned 1 to 3 points for stone burden according to CSD ≤10 mm, >10 mm and ≤20 mm, and >20 mm, respectively. The cumulative stone diameter on CTU was determined using digital calipers (PACS Software Program System) [11].

A summary of this scoring system ranging from a minimum of 4 to a maximum of 10 points is shown in Table 1. A score of 4 points indicates the simplest calculus, and a score of 10 indicates the most complex situation (Fig. 1).

Patients and procedures

All recruited patients underwent RIRS at the Department of Urology in Shanghai General Hospital from January 2014 to December 2016. All participating patients had CTU scans before the surgery to obtain clinical factors. Patients with no available preoperative CTU images, pelviureteric mass, multi-stage procedure and musculoskeletal or renal malformation were excluded.

Although the most suitable indication of RIRS is a stone size of less than 20 mm according to the EAU guidelines, several studies have reported favorable results after multi-stage RIRS with lower morbidities [12, 13]. Therefore, we attempted RIRS for larger stones (>20 mm) based on both patient and physician preferences. Postoperative day 1 (POD 1) and postoperative month 1 (POM1) kidney-ureter-bladder (KUB) film were required to estimate surgical outcomes. Additionally, non-contrasted computed tomography (NCCT) was likely to be required if the KUB film at POM1 showed any high-densities, or radiolucent stones in the case of intraoperative findings. A stone-free (SF) status was regarded as no detectable stone on KUB, and fragments of less than 2 mm were also considered negligible stones [14].

Preoperative single-dose antibiotic prophylaxis was used for all patients, however sensitive antibiotics were used for positive urine culture patients until negative [2]. All patients were performed on with a ureteral access sheath (UAS, COOK Medical, USA), which would equally facilitate stone extraction and reduce the intrarenal pressure [15]. A flexible ureteroscope (Olympus type V, Japan) was then advanced through the UAS. The stones were fragmented by holmium: YAG laser lithotripsy, and fragments were removed by a stone extractor (COOK Medical, USA) [16]. If the operation time exceeded 90 min, the procedure was stopped to minimize morbidities. Postoperative double-J stent catheterization was performed and removed at approximately POM1. All procedures were performed under general anesthesia in the lithotomy position by one experienced urologist (Jun Lu).

This study was accepted by the Ethics Review Board of Shanghai General Hospital. All patients were required to provide written informed consent for their data to be used for research purposes.

Data and statistical analysis

Demographics of the patients, variables of stones and the collecting system, and clinical data were recorded retrospectively. Continuous variables were expressed as the mean ± SD or median (Q3-Q1; interquartile range), and categorical data were presented by n (%). The continuous variables were analyzed using Student's t or

Table 1 Summary of R.I.R.S. scoring system

	Score		
	1	2	3
Renal stone density (Hu)	≤1000	>1000	
Inferior pole stone	non-inferior	inferior with RIPA > 30°	inferior with RIPA ≤ 30°
RIL (mm)	≤25	>25	
Stone burden (mm)	≤10	>10 and ≤20	>20

Range = 4~10 points

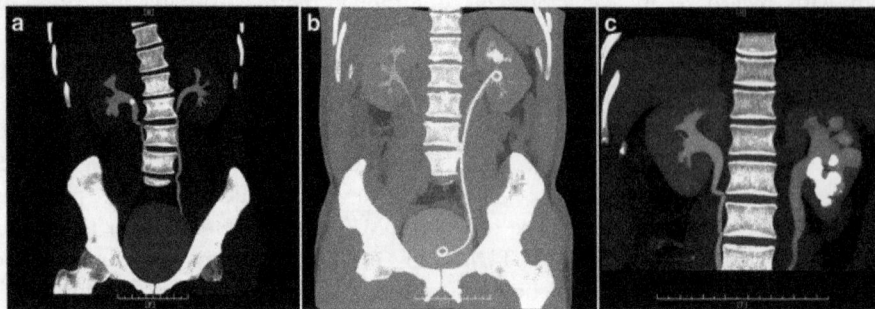

Fig. 1 The demonstration of the simplest calculus to the most complicated renal stone presented by computed tomography of urography. **a** The R.I.R.S. score was calculated as 4, the simplest calculus. **b** The R.I.R.S. score was calculated as 7. **c** The R.I.R.S. score was calculated as 10, the most complex situation

Mann-Whitney U tests depending on Kruskal-Wallis tests, and categorical data were analyzed by chi-square. The cut-off points of each continuous variable were subjectively set based on Youden's index, previous literature reviews and clinical practice experience. The multivariate logistic regression models were used to assess the significance of SF status and each score component. Bootstrapping (1000 resamples) was used to internally validate for the R.I.R.S. scoring system. The correlation of the present scoring system with the duration of procedure and hospitalization was tested using correlation analysis. The predictive ability of the R.I.R.S. scoring system was evaluated by the area under the receiver operating characteristic (AUROC) curve. Statistical significance was set at $p < 0.05$. The statistical analysis was performed using SPSS 23.0 (IBM, USA) and presented with GraphPad Prism 6.0 (GraphPad Software, USA).

Results

Of the 573 patients who underwent RIRS from January 2014 to November 2016, 382 eligible samples were included. The mean renal stone density was 1067.76 ± 336.93 Hu (range 272 to 1899). There were 145 (38.0%) patients who presented with inferior pole stones, and 32 cases were defined as narrow RIPA (≤30°) among those patients. The mean RIL was 23.55 ± 7.53 (range 9 to 63). The median CSD was 14 mm, and the interquartile range was 10 to 21. Other patient demographics and stone characteristics were compared between the SF group and non-SF group and are shown in Table 2 and Table 3.

The SFR on POD1 in the present cohort was 61.5% (235 of 382), and the POM1 outcome following RIRS was 73.6% (281 of 382). The SF group and non-SF group were similar with regard to age, hypertension, diabetes, BMI, history of renal surgery, UAS, relocation, laterality and urine culture in univariate analysis; however, gender ($p = 0.017$), diabetes (0 = 0.030), duration of procedure ($p < 0.001$), hospitalization (p < 0.001), complications (p

= 0.008), RIPA ($p = 0.003$), inferior pole stone ($p < 0.001$), RIL (p < 0.001), renal infundibular width (RIW, $p = 0.036$), renal stone density ($p < 0.001$), numbers of stone (p < 0.001) and stone burden (p < 0.001) showed to be statistically significant. Among these potential variables, the points of renal stone density ($p = 0.001$), inferior pole stone with narrow RIPA (p < 0.001), RIL ($p = 0.003$) and stone burden ($p < 0.001$) were regarded as independent factors in multivariate logistic regression. The R.I.R.S. score of the residual stone group was greater than that of the SF group (8.21 ± 1.22 vs 5.81 ± 1.24). Using bootstrapping (1000 resamples), the R.I.R.S. scoring system correlated with the SF status ($p < 0.001$). Furthermore, a greater R.I.R.S. score was associated with spontaneous clearance (p < 0.001), and correlated with a longer duration of procedure (p < 0.001, correlation coefficient = 0.415). However, the correlation between the R.I.R.S. score and hospitalization did not seem relevant in the present cohort ($p = 0.009$, correlation coefficient = 0.141). The AUROC curve of the R.I.R.S. scoring system for SF status prediction yielded 0.828 in POD1, but 0.904 in POM1 (Fig. 2).

Discussion

Since the invention of the flexible ureteroscope in the 1970s, advancements in endourological treatments of stones have become increasingly promising. However, because of some limitations, [17] RIRS was not recommended as a first-line treatment for renal calculi until 2013 according to the EAU guidelines. An applicable classification must be established to evaluate RIRS due to its relatively short period of use in clinical practice. In the past few years, a series of scoring systems have been established to estimate the SFR after the procedure, [6, 7, 18] but none of these systems have been effectively and conveniently embraced in clinical practice. Resorlu et al. first reported a scoring system called RUSS to preoperatively classify the probability of SF status [6]. Although RUSS is an uncomplicated and independent

Table 2 Demographics of patients and clinical data

	No. of patients	SF	Non-SF	P value
No. of patients (%)	382	281 (73.6%)	101 (26.4%)	
Gender				0.017*
Male	256 (67.0%)	198 (77.3%)	58 (22.7%)	
Female	126 (33.0%)	83 (65.9%)	43 (34.1%)	
Age (yo)	51.93 ± 12.32	52.14 ± 12.19	51.37 ± 12.74	0.590[a]
Hypertention				0.069
Yes	120 (31.4%)	81 (67.5%)	39 (32.5%)	
No	262 (68.6%)	200 (76.3%)	62 (23.7%)	
Diabetes mellitus				0.030*
Yes	36 (9.4%)	21 (57.3%)	15 (41.7%)	
No	346 (90.6%)	260 (75.1%)	86 (24.9%)	
BMI (kg/m2)	21.68 (23.79–19.1; 4.69)	21.57 (23.63–19.13; 4.50)	22.07 (24.29–19.08; 5.21)	0.406[b]
History of surgery				0.064
SWL	13 (3.4%)	11 (84.6%)	2 (15.4%)	
URL or RIRS	36 (9.4%)	22 (61.1%)	14 (38.9%)	
PNL	29 (7.6%)	16 (55.2%)	13 (44.8%)	
Laparoscopic ureterolithotomy	15 (3.9%)	13 (86.7%)	2 (13.3%)	
Pyuloplasty	3 (0.8%)	1 (33.3%)	2 (66.7%)	
Open surgery	3 (0.8%)	2 (66.7%)	1 (33.3%)	
No	294 (77.0%)	223 (75.9%)	71 (24.1%)	
UAS				0.927
Yes	373 (97.6%)	275 (73.7%)	98 (26.3%)	
No	9 (2.4%)	6 (66.7%)	3 (33.3%)	
Relocation				0.317
In situ	346 (90.6%)	252 (72.8%)	94 (27.2%)	
Ex situ	36 (9.4%)	29 (80.6%)	7 (19.4%)	
Duration of procedure (min)	50 (60–40; 20)	50 (60–40; 20)	60 (85–50; 35)	<0.001[b]*
Hospitalization (days)	5 (7–4; 3)	5 (6–3; 3)	6 (7–4; 3)	<0.001[b]*
Complications				0.008*
Yes	27 (7.1%)	14 (51.9%)	13 (48.1%)	
No	335 (92.9%)	267 (75.2%)	88 (24.8%)	

*Statistical significance was set at $P < 0.05$
UAS: Ureteral Access Sheath
[a] Student's t test, [b] Mann-Whitney U test

predictive scoring system for the SFR, the four-point scoring system might not prognosticate the SFR effectively and comprehensively when considering a complicated scenario in clinical practice [8]. Subsequently, Jung et al. established a modified S-ReSC score, which is based on stone sites without stone burden and numbers [7]. Along with improvements to the technique and experiences, urologists have more choices to manage larger renal stones (≥20 mm), and the stone burden is always considered an indispensable indicator for the SFR [12, 19]. Ito et al. recently performed a nomogram for the SFR after RIRS, but one of the limitations of their study

was in the high point range (0–25), which might be time-consuming for physicians [18]. In this study, we aimed to develop and internally validate a novel scoring system for predicting SFR following retrograde intrarenal surgery.

Considering the relation between stone composition and renal calculus density were often reported, meanwhile the maximum renal calculus density measured by Hounsfield Units on CT scans were related to fragmentation efficiency and operative time which would represent stone fragility [20, 21]. We used renal calculus density as the preoperative prediction of outcomes

Table 3 Characteristics of stones

	No. of patients	SF	Non-SF	P value
No. of patients (%)	382	281 (73.6%)	101 (26.4%)	
Laterality				0.370
Left	201 (52.6%)	144 (71.6%)	57 (28.4%)	
Right	181 (47.4%)	137 (75.7%)	44 (24.3%)	
RIPA (°)	47.91 ± 19.05	52.84 ± 18.51	43.50 ± 18.56	0.003[a]*
Inferior pole stone				<0.001*
Yes	145 (38.0%)	69 (47.6%)	76 (52.4%)	
No	237 (62.0%)	212 (89.5%)	25 (10.5%)	
RIL (mm)	23.55 ± 7.53	22.17 ± 7.02	27.40 ± 7.61	<0.001[a] *
RIW (mm)	10 (13–8; 5)	10 (12–7; 5)	11 (14–8; 6)	0.036[b]*
Stone burden (mm)	14 (21–10; 11)	12 (17–9; 8)	25 (29–18; 11)	<0.001[b]*
Numbers of stone				<0.001*
Single	233 (61.0%)	200 (85.8%)	33 (32.7%)	
Multiple	149 (39.0%)	81 (54.4%)	68 (45.6%)	
Renal stone density (Hu)	1067.76 ± 336.93	1022.59 ± 342.97	1193.43 ± 285.44	<0.001[a]*
Urine Culture				0.264
Positive	45 (11.8%)	30 (66.7%)	15 (33.3%)	
Negative	337 (88.2%)	251 (74.5%)	86 (25.5%)	

RIPA renal infundibulopelvic angle, *RIL* renal infundibulopelvic length, *RIW* renal infundibular width
*Statistical significance was set at $P < 0.05$
[a]Student's t test, [b] Mann-Whitney U test

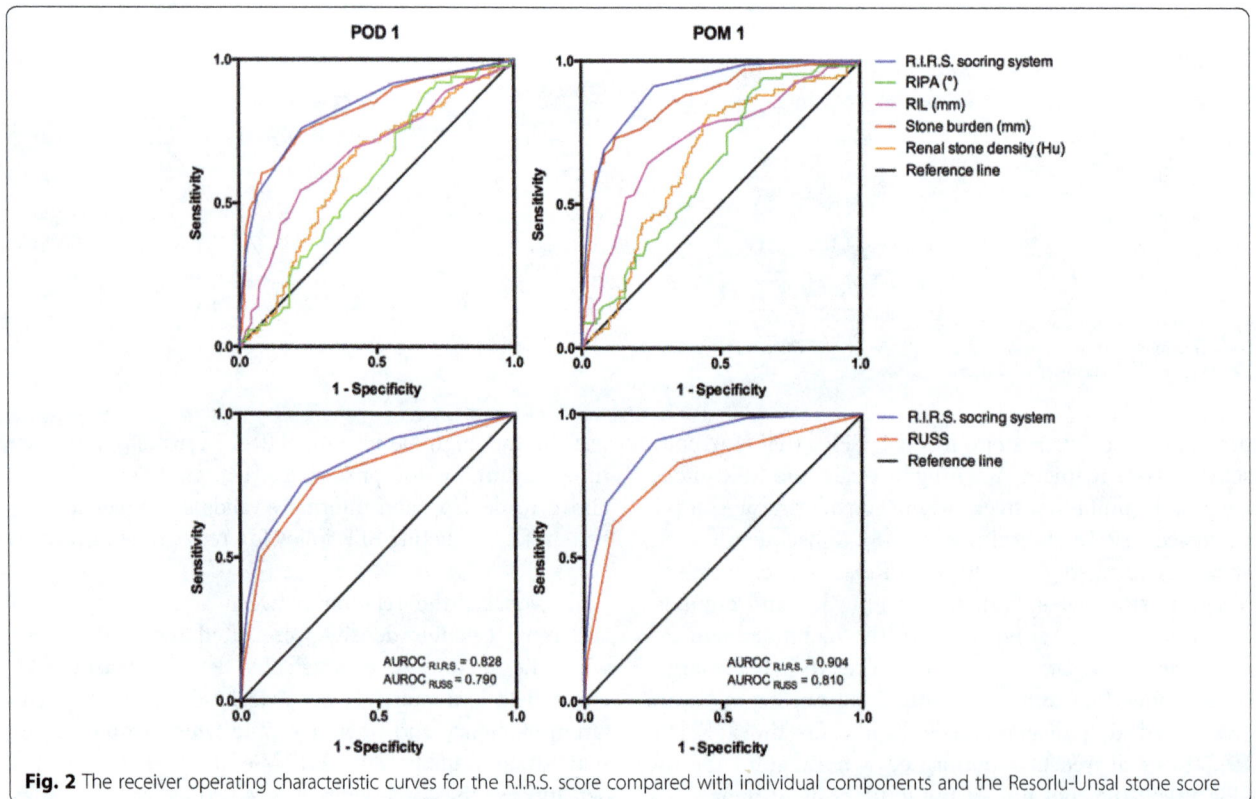

Fig. 2 The receiver operating characteristic curves for the R.I.R.S. score compared with individual components and the Resorlu-Unsal stone score

which enabled us to consult with patients, choose the suitable indications and avoid morbidities. We set 1000 Hu of attenuation coefficient as a cut-off point in this study, which was demonstrated to be appropriate for predicting the SF status in a multivariate logistic regression analysis and ROC curve.

Despite the rapid development of a flexible ureteroscope over the past decades, the management of lower pole stones remains a challenge for urologists. Ito et al. retrospectively validated the presence of lower pole calculi and stone size to be independent predictive factors of SF status after RIRS [22, 23]. Subsequently, Jessen et al. reported that a limited RIPA negatively influenced RIRS [24]. We revealed that a narrower RIPA and an increasing stone burden were independent factors in this cohort. These findings support those two variables as critical parameters for predicting outcomes of the procedure.

Inoue et al. retrospectively reviewed that a longer RIL, narrower RIPA and wider RIW would be unpropitious factors. Furthermore, only RIPA <30° was an independent factor for the probability of stone clearance in the multivariate analysis [25]. Resorlu et al. reported that the RIL was longer in the residual stone group compared with the SF group, but this finding was not significant retrospectively [26]. Jessen et al. reported that a negative influence would emerge by a greater RIL for RIRS [24]. In the present study, we discovered that a longer RIL was robustly correlated with SF status in both univariate and multivariate analysis, which was similar to previous literature.

In terms of the reasoning for endoscopic procedures, the stone burden is an independent prognostic factor for the SF status after RIRS, among other characteristics. Ito et al. initially found that the stone area had a relatively lower clinical reliability, while the CSD denoted by KUB films, and, in particular, stone volume described by NCCT is meaningful and impartial predictors of the SF status after RIRS [22]. Considering the inconvenience of calculating stone volume using NCCT by an additional algorithm, the CSD is the most regularly used parameter of stone size in clinical practice [13, 19, 27]. It was further concluded that the CSD obtained would validly and easily estimate the SFR preoperatively [28].

We developed a novel R.I.R.S. scoring system, comprising renal stone density, inferior pole stone, RIL and stone burden. The significance of each factor was defined through statistical analysis to determine the likely SF status after RIRS. Despite nearly overlapping curves with stone burden in POD1, the R.I.R.S. scoring system was found to be strongly prognostic of the final SF status in POM1, which was better than any other variable alone (Fig. 2). These findings supported that, in addition to stone burden, an adverse anatomical condition affects the postoperative spontaneous clearance as well. Moreover, a review of available studies of RIRS demonstrated

that operative time was affected by both attenuation co-efficients and stone burden, which in turn may affect the complications rate, especially fever and urosepsis [4, 20, 21]. Similar to these findings, the R.I.R.S. score is also correlated with operative time. We believe that it will help urologists to have more appropriate indications of procedure, predict the need for additional sessions of RIRS, and prevent surgical complications. The score was calculated as 4–5 (mild) for 115 (30.1%) patients, 6–8 (moderate) for 211 (55.2%) patients and 9–10 (severe) for 56 (14.7%) patients in this cohort (Fig. 3). The SFR values were 99.1%, 75.4% and 14.3%, respectively. With the intricacy of every procedure and case, the benefits of the R.I.R.S. scoring system appear to be supported by these perioperative observations. All parameters of the scoring system can be easily obtained from regular preoperative testing and do not require any additional software. Moreover, all the variables can provide information about the individual case. To our knowledge, this is the first report of a comprehensive scoring system for predicting SFR after RIRS, which was based on a large cohort of patients. The R.I.R.S. scoring system can favorably predict the outcomes of RIRS, especially the SFR of nephrolithiasis, which could facilitate not only clinical decision making but also patient counseling.

The primary limitations of our study include the retrospective design and analysis of a single center. Another possible study limitation was our exclusion criteria, which included musculoskeletal and renal malformation. These cases were excluded since they were low incidence and do not reflect the typical experience, but affect the outcomes. In addition, since not all patients underwent NCCT for follow-up, the evaluation between preoperative and postoperative imaging may involve a certain degree of bias. Because of these restrictions, the confidence level and bias could not be compared with a prospective and multi-center research study.

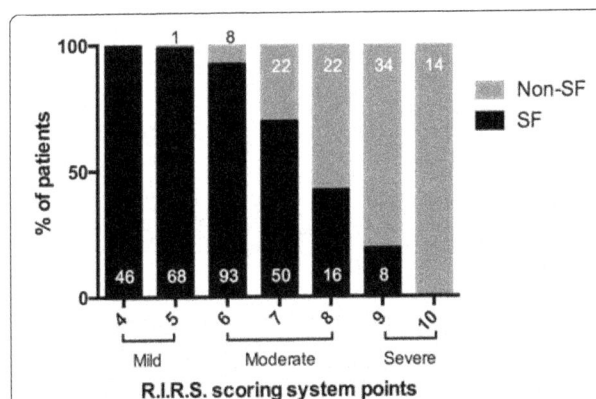

Fig. 3 The percentage and number of stone-free and non-stone-free groups stratified by mild, moderate and severe cases

Conclusions

The R.I.R.S. scoring system is associated with SFR after RIRS. This innovative scoring system can be used to pre-operatively assess treatment success after intrarenal surgery and can be used for preoperative surgical arrangement and comparison of outcomes among different centers and within a center over time.

Abbreviations

CSD: Cumulative stone diameter; CTU: Computed tomography of urography; RIL: Renal infundibular length; RIPA: Renal infundibulopelvic length; RIRS: Retrograde intrarenal surgery; RUSS: Resorlu-Unsal stone score; SFR: Stone-free rate

Acknowledgements

The authors appreciate all our participants for their gracious contribution in this study.

Funding

This study is supported by the Appropriate Health Technology Project of Shanghai Hospital Development Center (SHDC12016226).

Authors' contribution

YX and DL contributed equally to this work. YX drafted the paper and DL was responsible for radiological evaluation. LC, YX, DZ conducted the data collection and analysis. The corresponding authors, YS and JL, designed the study. All authors read and approved the final manuscript.

Competing interests

The authors declare that they have no competing interests.

Author details

[1]Department of Urology, Shanghai General Hospital of Nanjing Medical University, No.100, Haining Road, Hongkou District, Shanghai 200080, China. [2]Department of Urology, Shanghai Jiao Tong University School of Medicine, Shanghai General Hospital, No.100, Haining Road, Hongkou District, Shanghai 200080, China. [3]Department of Urology, Branch of Shanghai General Hospital, No. 1878, Middle Sichuan Road, Hongkou District, Shanghai 200081, China. [4]Department of Urology, Shanghai Pudong New Area People's Hospital, No. 490, South Chuanhuan road, Shanghai Pudong New Area, Shanghai 201200, China.

References

1. Zeng G, Mai Z, Xia S, Wang Z, Zhang K, Wang L, Long Y, Ma J, Li Y, Wan SP, et al. Prevalence of kidney stones in China: an ultrasonography based cross-sectional study. BJU Int. 2017;120(1):109–16.
2. Turk C, Petrik A, Sarica K, Seitz C, Skolarikos A, Straub M, Knoll T, Guidelines EAU. On interventional treatment for Urolithiasis. Eur Urol. 2016;69(3):475–82.
3. Hyams ES, Monga M, Pearle MS, Antonelli JA, Semins MJ, Assimos DG, Lingeman JE, Pais VM, Preminger GM, Lipkin ME, et al. A prospective, multi-institutional study of flexible Ureteroscopy for proximal ureteral stones smaller than 2 cm. J Urol. 2015;193(1):165–9.
4. Skolarikos A, Gross AJ, Krebs A, Unal D, Bercowsky E, Eltahawy E, Somani B, de la Rosette J. Outcomes of flexible Ureterorenoscopy for solitary renal stones in the CROES URS global study. J Urol. 2015;194(1):137–43.
5. WJ W, Okeke Z. Current clinical scoring systems of percutaneous nephrolithotomy outcomes. Nat Rev Urol. 2017;14(8):459–469.
6. Resorlu B, Unsal A, Gulec H, Oztuna D. A new scoring system for predicting stone-free rate after retrograde intrarenal surgery: the "resorlu-unsal stone score". Urology. 2012;80(3):512–8.
7. Jung JW, Lee BK, Park YH, Lee S, Jeong SJ, Lee SE, Jeong CW. Modified Seoul National University renal stone complexity score for retrograde intrarenal surgery. Urolithiasis. 2014;42(4):335–40.
8. Erbin A, Tepeler A, Buldu I, Ozdemir H, Tosun M, Binbay M. External comparison of recent predictive Nomograms for stone-free rate using retrograde flexible Ureteroscopy with laser lithotripsy. J Endourol. 2016;30(11):1180–4.
9. Thiruchelvam N, Mostafid H, Ubhayakar G. Planning percutaneous nephrolithotomy using multidetector computed tomography urography, multiplanar reconstruction and three-dimensional reformatting. BJU Int. 2005;95(9):1280–4.
10. Elbahnasy AM, Clayman RV, Shalhav AL, Hoenig DM, Chandhoke P, Lingeman JE, Denstedt JD, Kahn R, Assimos DG, Nakada SY. Lower-pole caliceal stone clearance after shockwave lithotripsy, percutaneous nephrolithotomy, and flexible ureteroscopy: impact of radiographic spatial anatomy. J Endourol. 1998;12(2):113–9.
11. Eisner BH, Kambadakone A, Monga M, Anderson JK, Thoreson AA, Lee H, Dretler SP, Sahani DV. Computerized tomography magnified bone windows are superior to standard soft tissue windows for accurate measurement of stone size: an in vitro and clinical study. J Urol. 2009;181(4):1710–5.
12. Akman T, Binbay M, Ozgor F, Ugurlu M, Tekinarslan E, Kezer C, Aslan R, Muslumanoglu AY. Comparison of percutaneous nephrolithotomy and retrograde flexible nephrolithotripsy for the management of 2-4 cm stones: a matched-pair analysis. BJU Int. 2012;109(9):1384–9.
13. Breda A, Angerri O. Retrograde intrarenal surgery for kidney stones larger than 2.5 cm. Curr Opin Urol. 2014;24(2):179–83.
14. Ghani KR, Wolf JSJ. What is the stone-free rate following flexible ureteroscopy for kidney stones? Nat Rev Urol. 2015;12(5):281–8.
15. Traxer O, Thomas A. Prospective evaluation and classification of ureteral wall injuries resulting from insertion of a ureteral access sheath during retrograde intrarenal surgery. J Urol. 2013;189(2):580–4.
16. Schatloff O, Lindner U, Ramon J, Winkler HZ. Randomized trial of stone fragment active retrieval versus spontaneous passage during holmium laser lithotripsy for ureteral stones. J Urol. 2010;183(3):1031–5.
17. Cindolo L, Castellan P, Scoffone CM, Cracco CM, Celia A, Paccaduscio A, Schips L, Proietti S, Breda A, Giusti G. Mortality and flexible ureteroscopy: analysis of six cases. World J Urol. 2016;34(3):305–10.
18. Ito H, Sakamaki K, Kawahara T, Terao H, Yasuda K, Kuroda S, Yao M, Kubota Y, Matsuzaki J. Development and internal validation of a nomogram for predicting stone-free status after flexible ureteroscopy for renal stones. BJU Int. 2015;115(3):446–51.
19. Breda A, Ogunyemi O, Leppert JT, Lam JS, Schulam PG. Flexible ureteroscopy and laser lithotripsy for single intrarenal stones 2 cm or greater–is this the new frontier? J Urol. 2008;179(3):981–4.
20. Ito H, Kawahara T, Terao H, Ogawa T, Yao M, Kubota Y, Matsuzaki J. Predictive value of attenuation coefficients measured as Hounsfield units on noncontrast computed tomography during flexible ureteroscopy with holmium laser lithotripsy: a single-center experience. J Endourol. 2012;26(9):1125–30.
21. Knoll T, Jessen JP, Honeck P, Wendt-Nordahl G. Flexible ureterorenoscopy versus miniaturized PNL for solitary renal calculi of 10-30 mm size. World J Urol. 2011;29(6):755–9.
22. Ito H, Kawahara T, Terao H, Ogawa T, Yao M, Kubota Y, Matsuzaki J. The most reliable preoperative assessment of renal stone burden as a predictor of stone-free status after flexible ureteroscopy with holmium laser lithotripsy: a single-center experience. Urology. 2012;80(3):524–8.
23. Ito H, Kuroda S, Kawahara T, Makiyama K, Yao M, Matsuzaki J. Preoperative factors predicting spontaneous clearance of residual stone fragments after flexible ureteroscopy. Int J Urol. 2015;22(4):372–7.
24. Jessen JP, Honeck P, Knoll T, Wendt-Nordahl G. Flexible ureterorenoscopy for lower pole stones: influence of the collecting system's anatomy. J Endourol. 2014;28(2):146–51.
25. Inoue T, Murota T, Okada S, Hamamoto S, Muguruma K, Kinoshita H, Matsuda T, Group SS. Influence of Pelvicaliceal anatomy on stone clearance after flexible Ureteroscopy and holmium laser lithotripsy for large renal stones. J Endourol. 2015;29(9):998–1005.
26. Resorlu B, Oguz U, Resorlu EB, Oztuna D, Unsal A. The impact of pelvicaliceal anatomy on the success of retrograde intrarenal surgery in patients with lower pole renal stones. Urology. 2012;79(1):61–6.
27. Turk C, Petrik A, Sarica K, Seitz C, Skolarikos A, Straub M, Knoll T, Guidelines EAU. On diagnosis and conservative Management of Urolithiasis. Eur Urol. 2016;69(3):468–74.

10

Should manual detorsion be a routine part of treatment in testicular torsion?

Arif Demirbas[1]*, Demirhan Orsan Demir[1], Erim Ersoy[1], Mucahit Kabar[1], Serkan Ozcan[1], Mehmet Ali Karagoz[1], Ozgecan Demirbas[2] and Omer Gokhan Doluoglu[1]

Abstract

Background: It was aimed to investigate the efficiency and reliability of the manual detorsion (MD) procedure in patients diagnosed with testicular torsion (TT).

Methods: A retrospective analysis was made of the data of 57 patients diagnosed with TT, comprising 20 patients with successful MD (Group I), 28 patients who underwent emergency orchiopexy (Group II), and 9 patients applied with orchiectomy (Group III). The groups were compared in respect of age, and duration of pain. The success rate of MD, the time of testicular fixation (TF), any problems encountered in follow-up, and follow-up times were analyzed in Group I. Data were analyzed with P-P pilot, Mann-Whitney U, Kruskal Wallis and Chi-square tests. A value of $p < 0.05$ was considered statistically significant.

Results: MD was successful and detorsion could be achieved in 20 of 26 patients. The groups were similar in respect of age ($p = 0.217$). The median duration of pain was 3 (1–8), 4 (1–72), and 48 (12–144) hours in Groups I, II, and III, respectively, and determined as similar in Groups I and II ($p = 0.257$), although a statistically significant difference was determined between the 3 groups ($p < 0.001$). TF was applied to Group I after median 10 (0–45) days, and no parenchymal disorder was determined in the median follow-up period of 21.5 (2–40) months.

Conclusion: MD that can be easily and immediately performed after the diagnosis of TT decreases ischemia time. This seems to be an efficient and reliable procedure when applied together with elective orchiopexy, as a part of the treatment.

Keywords: Testicular torsion, Manual detorsion, Orchiopexy, Orchiectomy

Background

Testicular (spermatic cord) torsion (TT), which was first described by Hunter, is an emergency urological diagnosis that results in ischemic organ injury in the affected testis, and requires urgent diagnosis and treatment [1, 2]. Cold weather, activation of the cremasteric reflex, trauma, undescended testis, and fast enlargement of testis during puberty are the known risk factors in susceptible individuals. It shows a bimodal distribution, and peaks in the neonatal period and puberty. Prevalence has been reported as 8.6/ 100,000 between the ages of 10 and 19 years in the United States [1–4].

With the exception of neonates, patients usually present with unilateral severe pain that has been present for a few hours [5, 6]. Pain is rarely mild, and it radiates to the inguinal region and abdomen. The most frequent physical examination findings are testicular tenderness and loss of the cremasteric reflex [1, 7]. An abnormal position of the testis is more common than other causes for acute scrotal pain [8]. Doppler ultrasonography (USG), scintigraphy, dynamic magnetic resonance (MR), and high-resolution USG are the diagnostic imaging modalities [3].

The most important factors for testicular salvage before it atrophies are known to be the duration between the onset of symptoms and detorsion, and the degree of the torsion [9, 10]. Emergency surgery after the diagnosis aims to shorten the duration of ischemia [1, 2, 11]. Manual detorsion (MD), as described by Nash, has been

* Correspondence: demirbas-arif@hotmail.com
[1]Department of Urology, Ankara Training and Research Hospital, 06340, Sukriye, Altındağ Ankara, Turkey
Full list of author information is available at the end of the article

suggested before surgery to return blood flow faster, and some authors have indicated it as an alternative to surgery [1, 12, 13].

In this study, it was aimed to investigate the efficiency of MD, whether it could be a routine part of treatment or an alternative to surgery in patients with TT due to time saved by the application, and the reliability of elective orchiopexy rather than emergency orchiopexy in the light of information provided in literature.

Methods

A retrospective analysis was made of a total of 57 patients admitted to our outpatient clinic or Emergency Department between 2011 and 2015 with acute scrotal pain, and who were diagnosed with TT based on physical examination findings and decreased or absent testicular blood flow on Doppler USG. The approval of the Local Ethics Committee was obtained before starting the study. The MD procedure was applied by three urologists in our clinic, and it was not performed by other urologists. Group I comprised 20 patients with successful MD, Group II comprised 28 patients who underwent emergency orchiopexy or orchiopexy after failure of MD, and Group III comprised 9 patients that had emergency scrotal exploration and orchiectomy. The patients in Group I had bilateral testicular fixation (TF) under elective conditions after MD, and the patients in Group II had bilateral TF during emergency orchiopexy.

The groups were compared in respect of age, and the time from onset of scrotal pain to admission to hospital (duration of pain). In Group I, the time of elective TF performed after MD and the number of the patients with a successful MD procedure were determined. In addition, the follow-up period, and the presence of testicular atrophy findings on Doppler USG were analyzed in Group I. The patients that had orchiopexy and orchiectomy (Groups II and III) were analyzed in respect of the time from onset of pain to the start of surgery in order to determine the gain in ischemia duration with MD compared to emergency scrotal exploration.

MD was performed without using any anesthesia technique to preserve the feeling of pain, in consideration of retorsion risk in the affected testis. The affected testis was rotated laterally for detorsion. However, when lateral rotation was not successful due to lateral TT, then medial rotation was applied [14]. The success of MD was defined as the immediate relief of symptoms and improvement of the physical examination findings, and the success was confirmed by normal testicular arterial and venous blood flow on Doppler USG, which was performed immediately after MD.

Patients in Group I and Group II were followed up with monthly physical examinations for the first 6 months after diagnosis and Doppler USG was applied

at 3-month intervals. Subsequent follow-up was physical examinations at 6-month intervals.

The study was conducted in accordance with the principles of Declaration of Helsinki 2008.

Statistical analysis

The statistical analysis of data was performed using SPSS version 15.0 (SPSS Inc., Chicago, IL, United States) statistics software. Conformity to normal distribution of the data was analyzed with histogram and P-P pilot test. The Mann-Whitney U and Kruskal Wallis tests were used to compare continuous variables that did not show normal distribution. The Chi-square test was used to compare categorical variables. A value of $p < 0.05$ was considered statistically significant.

Results

MD was performed in 26 patients diagnosed with TT. Successful MD was recorded in 20 (76%) patients, and 6 (24%) patients had emergency orchiopexy due to failure of MD. The ages of the patients were similar in all 3 groups ($p = 0.217$). The median duration of pain was 3 (1–8) hours in Group I, 4 (1–72) hours in Group II, and 48 (12–144) hours in Group III, with a significant difference determined between the groups ($p < 0.001$) (Table 1). The comparison of Groups I and II where testicular salvage could be achieved revealed that those groups were similar in respect of duration of pain ($p = 0.257$) (Table 2).

TF was performed under elective conditions at median 10 (0–45) days after MD in 18 of 20 patients. The other 2 patients, aged 45 and 36 years, respectively, were followed up without TF, as they did not accept the procedure. In the follow-up of these 2 patients, no painful episodes developed and no pathological findings were determined on physical examination or on Doppler USG. During the median follow-up period of 21.5 (2–40) months, none of the patients in Group I had atrophy or parenchymal disorders on physical examination or Doppler USG after MD and TF. No painful episode developed in any patient in the period up to elective orchiopexy. In the 6 patients applied with emergency orchiopexy due to unsuccessful MD, no testicular atrophy or other pathological findings were encountered. The median ischemia durations between diagnosis and scrotal

Table 1 The symptoms on admission in patients diagnosed with testicular torsion

	Group I n = 20	Group II n = 28	Group III n = 9	p
Age	17.5	19.5	20	= 0.217
Duration of pain (hours, min-max)	3, 1–8	4, 1–72	48, 12–144	<0.001

Table 2 Comparison of duration of pain in the groups that had testicular salvage

	Group I n = 20	Group II n = 28	p
Duration of pain (hours, min-max)	3, 1–8	4, 1–72	= 0.257

exploration were 90 (20–240) and 80 (45–180) minutes in Groups II and III, respectively (p = 0.636) (Table 3).

Discussion

TT is regarded as a race against time, and the histological changes of testicular injury appear in hours, and even in minutes [1–3]. It has been reported that irreversible ischemic changes occur 4–6 h after ischemic scrotum, and that 80% of patients need orchiectomy due to necrosis after 24 h if the testis is not detorsioned [3, 14, 15]. Studies have also shown that the duration between onset of symptoms and treatment caused disturbances in semen quality through autoimmune mechanisms [16].

Emergency scrotal exploration has been recommended as the standard treatment method for derotation of the rotated spermatic cord, and restoration of testicular blood flow [1–3]. However, minutes and even hours may be needed to prepare for this emergency procedure. Our five-year experience showed there was a significant time loss between diagnosis and treatment (80–90 min, Table 3) and this was reflected in the ischemia time.

MD was first described in 1893. It was performed to restore blood flow and give rapid pain relief. The efficiency of the procedure has been investgated by various authors [17–20]. Catolica [18] published the largest series with 34 patients, and reported that MD was successful in all patients, TF was performed under elective conditions in 6 patients, and the duration between urological consultation and surgery was between 1 h and 2 months in the 34 patients included in the study. The author also reported that retorsion was not evident in any of the patients, the ischemic testis was saved, and an emergency procedure became an elective procedure. A study from the Netherlands reported MD in 17 patients, 14 of which were successful, orchiopexy was performed electively (waiting time was mean 12 h, ranging from 2 h to 3 months), retorsion was not seen in any of the patients, and none of the patients had testicular atrophy after a mean follow-up period of 22 months. The procedure failed in 3 patients, and excessive scrotal edema and pain were considered to be responsible for this since

no anesthesia was used to be able to determine "sudden relief of pain" that was used as the success criterion [20]. In a study by Sessions et al. [14], residual torsion was determined during orchiopexy in 17/53 (38%) patients who had been applied with manual detorsion and it was concluded that orchiopexy should not be delayed. However, as there are no studies of high level evidence on this subject in literature, whether orchiopexy should be applied electively or not following manual detorsion does not come under the heading of a recommendation.

In the current series of 26 patients, MD was successful in 20 (76%) patients at the time of diagnosis, and it was determined that testicular salvage was achieved after long term follow-up (median: 21.5 months). Attempting MD and success after the procedure made a significant timesaving compared to orchiopexy in respect of testicular ischaemia time (median: 90 min). In the development of testicular damage, as it is known that every minute is valuable, the median ischaemia-free time of 90 mins gained with MD, suggests that it is important in the treatment of TT [1–3]. Elective TF and the absence of any retorsion in this waiting period can be considered to show the safety of MD. However, even if it is wanted to apply TF immediately after MD, it can be considered necessary to apply it at the time of MD diagnosis. Even after diagnosis, the time of transporting the patient to the operating room and preoperative preparation means 'a period with ischaemia'. A comparison was made of the patients that had MD and those with emergency orchiopexy (Group II) in order to determine the effect of the duration of torsion on the success of MD and no effect was observed.

Conclusion

MD is a non-invasive procedure, may be applied as soon as the diagnosis is made, decreases the duration of ischemia when compared to emergency scrotal exploration, and the long-termresults of this study have shown that it is safe when applied together with elective orchiopexy. MD is a simple procedure that may be performed safely with little to no delay in definite scrotal exploration and orchiopexy, which remains the gold standard.

Abbreviations
MD: Manual detorsion; TF: Testicular fixation; TT: Testicular torsion

Table 3 The time between diagnosis and scrotal exploration in patients that had orchiopexy or orchiectomy

	Group II n = 28	Group III n = 9	p
The time between diagnosis and exploration (minutes, min-max)	90, 20–240	80, 45–180	0.636

Acknowledgements
None.

Funding
None

Authors' contributions

Study concept and design: AD, DOD and OD Acquisition of data: MAK, MK, SO and AD Analysis and interpretation of data: OGD and EE Drafting of the manuscript: EE Critical revision of the manuscript for important intellectual content: EE Statistical analysis: OGD and O.D Administrative, technical, and material support: MAK, MK, SO and AD Study supervision: AD and DOD. All authors read and approved the final manuscript.

Competing interests

The authors declare that they have no competing interests.

Author details

[1]Department of Urology, Ankara Training and Research Hospital, 06340, Sukriye, Altındağ Ankara, Turkey. [2]Department of Pediatrics, Ankara Dr. Sami Ulus Women Health, Children's Training and Research Hospital, 06340 Ankara, Turkey.

References

1. Kapoor S. Testicular torsion: a race against time. Int J Clin Pract. 2008;62:821–7.
2. Barthold JS. Abnormalities of the testes and scrotum and their surgical management. In: Wein AJ, editor. Campbell-Walsh urology. 10th ed. Philadelphia, Pa: Saunders Elsevier; 2011. p. 3587–92.
3. Tekgül S, Doğan HS, Erdem E, et al. Guidelines on pediatric urology. European Association of Urology. 2015:13–5.
4. Cunningham RF. Familial occurrence of testicular torsion. JAMA. 1960;174:1330–1.
5. McAndrew HF, Pemberton R, Kikiros CS, et al. The incidence and investigation of acute scrotal problems in children. Pediatr Surg Int. 2002;18:435–7.
6. Sauvat F, Hennequin S, Slimane MAA, et al. Age for testicular torsion? Arch Pediatr. 2002;9:1226–9.
7. Kadish HA, Bolte RG. A retrospective review of pediatric patients with epididymitis, testicular torsion, and torsion of testicular appendages. Pediatrics. 1998;102:73–6.
8. Makela E, Lahdes-Vasama T, Rajakorpi H, et al. A 19-year review of paediatric patients with acute scrotum. Scan J Surg. 2007;96:62–6.
9. Visser AJ, Heyns CF. Testicular function after torsion of the spermatic cord. BJU Int. 2003;92:200–3.
10. Tryfonas G, Violaki A, Tsikopoulos G, et al. Late postoperative results in males treated for testicular torsion during childhood. J Pediatr Surg. 1994;29:553–6.
11. Murphy FL, Fletcher L, Pease P. Early scrotal exploration in all cases is the investigation and intervention of choice in the acute paediatric scrotum. Pediatr Surg Int. 2006;22:413–6.
12. Nash WG. Acute torsion of the spermatic cord: reduction: immediate relief. Br Med J. 1893;1:742.
13. Lee LM, Wright JE, McLoughlin MG. Testicular torsion in the adult. J Urol. 1983;130:93–4.
14. Sessions AE, Rabinowitz R, Hulbert WC, et al. Testicular torsion: direction, degree, duration and disinformation. J Urol. 2003;169:663–5.
15. Anderson JB, Williamson RC. Testicular torsion in Bristol: a 25-year review. Br J Surg. 1988;75:988–92.
16. Anderson JB, Williamson RC. Fertility after torsion of the spermatic cord. BJU Int. 1990;65:225–30.
17. Kiesling VJ, Schroeder DE, Pauljev P, et al. Spermatic cord block and manual reduction: primary treatment for spermatic cord torsion. J Urol. 1984;132:921–3.
18. Catolica EV. Preoperative manual detorsion of the torsed spermatic cord. J Urol. 1985;133:803–5.
19. Vordermark JS. Testicular torsion: management with ultrasonic Doppler flow detector. Urology. 1984;14:41–2.
20. Cornel EB, Karthaus HFM. Manual derotation of the twisted spermatic cord. BJU Int. 1999;83:672–4.

11

Qualitative insights into how men with low-risk prostate cancer choosing active surveillance negotiate stress and uncertainty

Emily M. Mader[1], Hsin H. Li[1,2], Kathleen D. Lyons[4], Christopher P. Morley[1,2,3], Margaret K. Formica[2*], Scott D. Perrapato[5], Brian H. Irwin[5], John D. Seigne[6], Elias S. Hyams[6], Terry Mosher[4], Mark T. Hegel[4,7] and Telisa M. Stewart[2]

Abstract

Background: Active surveillance is a management strategy for men diagnosed with early-stage, low-risk prostate cancer in which their cancer is monitored and treatment is delayed. This study investigated the primary coping mechanisms for men following the active surveillance treatment plan, with a specific focus on how these men interact with their social network as they negotiate the stress and uncertainty of their diagnosis and treatment approach.

Methods: Thematic analysis of semi-structured interviews at two academic institutions located in the northeastern US. Participants include 15 men diagnosed with low-risk prostate cancer following active surveillance.

Results: The decision to follow active surveillance reflects the desire to avoid potentially life-altering side effects associated with active treatment options. Men on active surveillance cope with their prostate cancer diagnosis by both maintaining a sense of control over their daily lives, as well as relying on the support provided them by their social networks and the medical community. Social networks support men on active surveillance by encouraging lifestyle changes and serving as a resource to discuss and ease cancer-related stress.

Conclusions: Support systems for men with low-risk prostate cancer do not always interface directly with the medical community. Spousal and social support play important roles in helping men understand and accept their prostate cancer diagnosis and chosen care plan. It may be beneficial to highlight the role of social support in interventions targeting the psychosocial health of men on active surveillance.

Keywords: Active surveillance, Prostatic neoplasm, Qualitative research, Coping behavior

Background

The introduction of the prostate-specific antigen (PSA) blood test has increased detection of prostate cancer in the US, and most men are now diagnosed with localized, early stage and low-risk tumors (PSA < 10 ng/mL, clinical staging T1-T2a, and Gleason score ≤6) [1–3]. Expectant management strategies, including active surveillance (AS), are now being increasingly recommended

to low-risk prostate cancer patients in an effort to avoid unnecessary treatment and its associated risks [1].

AS is a process of closely monitoring men with low-risk prostate cancer through PSA blood tests, digital rectal exams (DREs), ultrasounds, and prostate biopsies, with the goal of averting active treatment unless disease progression is detected or the patient chooses treatment [4, 5]. The small volume of research evaluating the psychosocial health and coping mechanisms of men following AS indicates that a lack of social support, illness uncertainty and anxiety are predictive factors in reduced quality of life among men with low-risk prostate cancer, and the psychosocial burden of living with

* Correspondence: FormicaM@upstate.edu
[2]Department of Public Health and Preventive Medicine, SUNY Upstate Medical University, 766 Irving Ave., Rm. 2262, Syracuse, NY 13210, USA
Full list of author information is available at the end of the article

prostate cancer affects adherence to AS and disease outcomes [6–8]. In addition, a recent study found that men who have low levels of coping confidence and high levels of treatment concern had higher intrusive thoughts about their cancer [9], underscoring the value of a better understanding of the coping strategies employed by men on active surveillance. Our research presented in this article investigates the primary coping mechanisms for men who have chosen to follow AS, with a specific focus on how these men interact with their social network as they negotiate the stress and uncertainty of their diagnosis and treatment approach.

Methods

This project is an extension of a prior qualitative study grounded in self-regulation theory investigating the decision-making process for low-risk prostate cancer patients [10, 11]; the initial data collection procedures are described in detail elsewhere [12]. Briefly, patient and provider semi-structured interviews were conducted at two academic institutions in the northeastern US. Patient inclusion criteria was based on patient age of 18 years or older, diagnosis of T1 or T2 prostate cancer within the past year, PSA value ≤10, Gleason Score ≤ 6, adequate fluency in English, and consent to participate. Interviews were conducted via telephone at the participants' convenience, and were transcribed by professional transcriptionists; transcriptions were proofread by an interviewer for assurance of quality and accuracy. The study was reviewed and approved by the institutional review boards (IRB) at Geisel School of Medicine at Dartmouth College, University of Vermont, and SUNY Upstate Medical University.

In the current study, only those transcripts from interviews with patients following AS were analyzed, as we were particularly focused on the coping and uncertainty management strategies of men who had chosen this treatment approach. Transcript data were analyzed following an immersion/crystallization process. Immersion and crystallization is a cyclical process of organizing and connecting data involving repeated readings of the data (immersion) followed by periods of reflection wherein themes and patterns are developed (crystallization); this process continues until meaningful patterns emerge from the data that can be well articulated and substantiated [13, 14]. Following this process, two authors (EMM and HHL) independently conducted initial coding of the transcripts, followed by a joint review and consolidation of the code list. Finalized codes and identified themes were then reviewed by the wider research team for confirmation. All transcript analysis was managed using ATLAS.ti, software version 7.

Results

Fifteen men following AS were interviewed; all men were white, non-Hispanic, with a mean age of 65 years. The majority of the men interviewed were married (73.3%), with a college or graduate degree (66.7%), and were evenly split between working full time or retired. Details on respondent demographics can be found in Table 1.

Three overarching themes emerged from our analysis of the interview transcripts. First, the choice to follow AS is related to how men cope with the anxieties experienced over the diagnosis and treatment of prostate cancer. Second, the reliance men place on individuals in their social networks during the decision-making process

Table 1 Summary of patient demographic characteristics

Patient characteristic	Mean (SD)
Age	65 (6.45)
	Count (%)
Race/Ethnicity	
White	15 (100)
Non-Hispanic	15 (100)
Marital Status	
Never Married	3 (20)
Married	11 (73.3)
Divorced	1 (6.7)
Employment	
Full Time	7 (46.7)
Retired	7 (46.7)
Declined to answer	1 (6.7)
Annual Income	
Less than $40,000	3 (20)
$40,000 or more	9 (60)
Declined to answer	3 (20)
Education	
High school graduate/GED[a]	2 (13.3)
Some college/technical school	2 (13.3)
College graduate	7 (46.7)
Graduate degree	3 (20)
Declined to answer	1 (6.7)
Household	
Living with spouse	11 (73.3)
Living alone	4 (26.7)
Insurance	
Private	7 (46.7)
Medicare	1 (6.7)
Medicaid	1 (6.7)
Medicare + Private	6 (40)

[a]*GED* general educational development test

extends to the period following the decision, in which they adjust and learn to cope with their untreated cancer. Lastly, the trust men place in their providers and the medical community has a strong impact on their ability to follow AS while effectively managing uncertainty and anxiety. Figure 1 provides an overview of these themes.

Selection of AS as part of coping

Ten participants described the risks associated with active treatment options as an area of significant concern. These men perceived urinary incontinence and erectile dysfunction as concrete and imminent risks, which would have a larger impact on their day-to-day lives than their current prostate cancer diagnosis. The potential of experiencing these side effects generated concern for several of the individuals interviewed.

Additionally, several men discussed the negative impact erectile dysfunction would have on the health of their personal relationships with spouses and partners:

"I certainly let him know that my wife and I, we're very close and active sexually, and very much in love with each other. So, he went through all of the potential outcomes of the surgery, none of which are very enticing to me." [pt 13]

Participants viewed AS as a viable treatment option that would appropriately manage their cancer while avoiding the risk of negative side effects. Several men also expressed relief in the diagnosis of a non-aggressive cancer, stating that since their cancer was "controllable and treatable" they were able to take a "less emotional attitude" about treatment choices. These participants

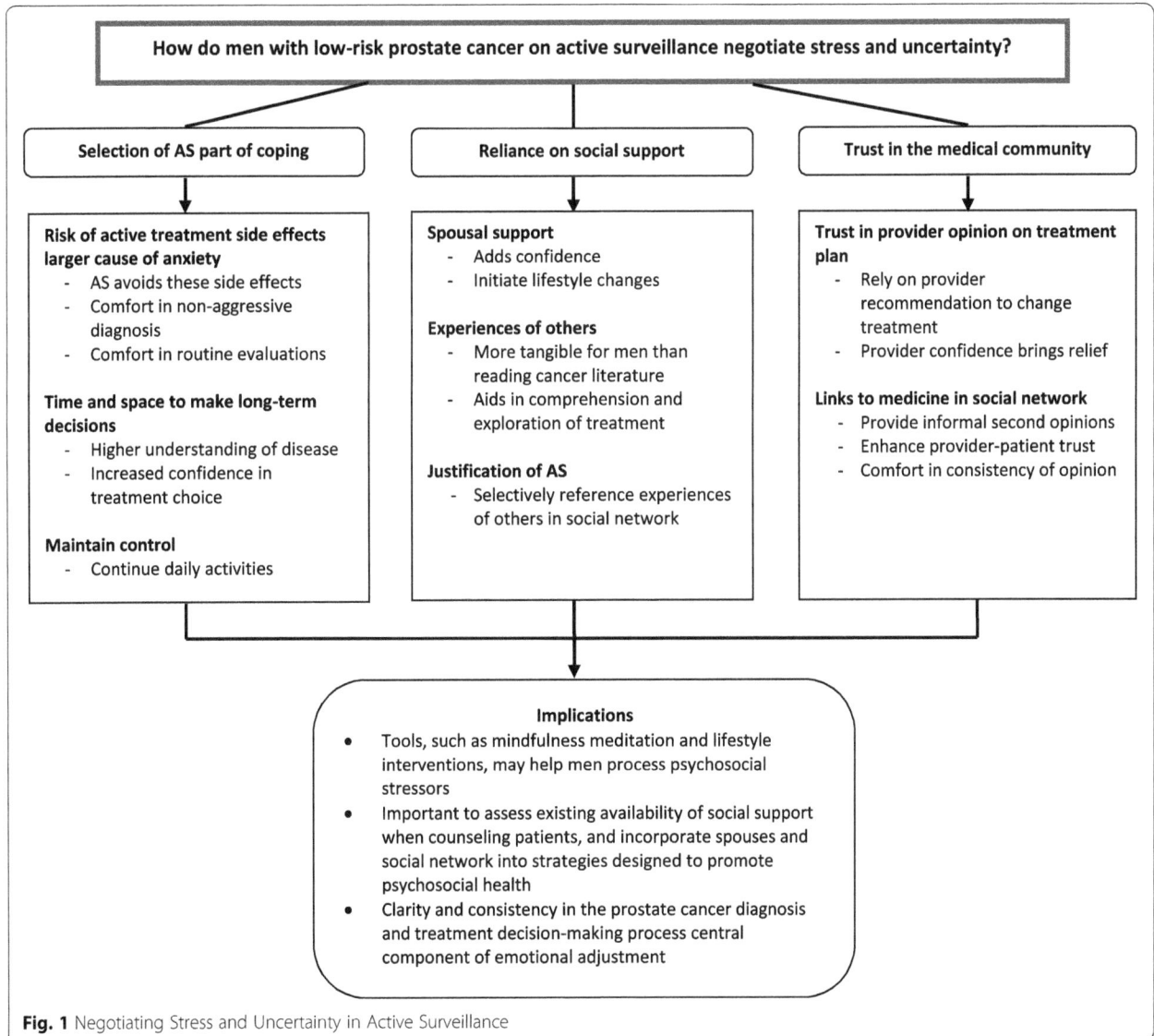

Fig. 1 Negotiating Stress and Uncertainty in Active Surveillance

were reassured by the ability to follow routine evaluations to track the progression of their cancer:

> "We're going to deal with it in that I'm gonna have
> another biopsy this fall because it'll be a year. That's
> the way the active surveillance is set up...I just, I'd
> rather do it this way. I'd rather be goin' up there and
> checkin' in and havin' a blood test than goin' to the
> hospital for radiation or do this. If it's not necessary,
> it's a waste of money and time." [pt 02]

It is important to note that the choice to follow AS did
not eliminate all anxieties regarding the cancer diagnosis.
Two participants felt increased worry in the period leading
up to their next PSA test or biopsy. However, it appears
that the anxiety felt prior to these regular checkups was
less than that experienced when contemplating life with
side effects from active treatment, and several men indicated feeling a sense of relief and reassurance after receiving benign test results:

> "So, it's seems like we are doing the right thing, and it
> gives me a little more peace of mind each three
> months when I go back in, well, we're on the right
> track here."[pt 01]

Some participants reported that following the AS
plan allowed them valuable time to contemplate the
need for future prostate cancer treatment, and what
their preferred treatment choice would be. This con-
templation period allowed men to reach a higher level
of understanding of their disease, as well as a higher
degree of confidence in their ability to make the right
decision for themselves:

> "In one way, it's a relief because it can postpone any
> potential confrontation with, 'Okay, doggone it. Now
> I've really got to make a decision for surgery or ignore
> the damn thing.' So it's been comforting." [pt 13]

Several men also reported that following the AS treatment plan allowed them to continue living their lives as
normal. These individuals valued this capability, and felt
that many of their daily activities would face interference
through more active treatment interventions:

> "I had thought that the radiation treatment would be
> like you go like a couple of times, and you don't. You
> go many times, almost every day for, like, a long
> time." [pt 15]

The ability to continue routine activities allowed them
to maintain a sense of control in a scenario with a large
degree of uncertainty, and this control over daily life

decreased the anxiety some men experienced over their
diagnosis:

> "They tell you, 'You have prostate cancer,' but, at the
> same time, 'We're monitoring it,' and I'm kinda going
> on like, just, ah, normal living. And so I don't - I don't
> think about it that much." [pt 03]

Comments from three men also suggest that the diagnosis of prostate cancer sparked a desire to "enjoy the
rest of" their lives, and following AS was viewed as a
window in time to be healthy and functional without
treatment regimens and side effects.

Reliance on social support
Ten of the men on AS expressed a strong sense of
reliance on their spouses not only during the treatment
decision-making process, but also during the period
thereafter in which they adjusted to life on AS. Spouses
were viewed as partners in this process, and their
support brought added confidence to many of the
participants:

> "We say it's a joint effort – we are in this together.
> And, you know, figure out what is the best decision
> for us." [pt 02]

> "But ya gotta have a good outlook. And I've got
> probably one of the most positive women that I've ever
> met in my life for a wife, which is a big help." [pt 02]

Several participants mentioned that their spouses initiated lifestyle changes that they felt could potentially
reduce the impact or slow the progression of prostate
cancer. Similar to the maintenance of routine activities,
these changes in habits were a way in which men could
maintain a sense of control over and cope with their
diagnosis:

> "She packs my lunch in the morning and makes
> sure I have all the right stuff, and a lot of fruits
> and vegetables, and none of the sweets I loved
> having (*laughing*) ...went on with the tea, only have
> minimal beef from the beef industry and a lot of
> fruits and vegetables, and trying to get an alkaline
> diet rather than an acidic diet. So that's what I
> tried to do to counteract this." [pt 01]

Participant responses also indicate that talking to
and reflecting upon the experiences of individuals
who had previously been diagnosed with prostate cancer is an important component of the decision to go
on and stay on AS. Several participants described a
process wherein after reviewing the medical literature

offered by physicians, they sought out individuals within their social networks who had previous encounters with prostate cancer to learn about their experiences with treatment:

"Well, I've contacted several people, family and different relationships. Why you, you learn from them who has had it, and yes, I have contacted probably, oh, probably half a dozen different individuals." [pt 01]

The majority of participants spoke with men who had undergone active treatment for prostate cancer, with only three speaking with individuals following AS. Most men spoke with family members and friends, but one individual specifically attended a prostate cancer support group meeting. Communication within the social network seemed to provide more tangible information to the participants compared to information they learned through reviewing medical literature; hearing about others' experiences and opinions allowed the participants to contextualize the potential risks and outcomes of active treatment to their own lives.

Several participants referenced stories shared by friends or family members who had negative outcomes from active treatment as evidence to support their choice to follow AS:

"I was gonna say one of the factors that weighed a little into my decision was my friend who had this, and, you know, he felt like overreacted after. He said, 'You know I just want to get rid of it,' and like a year later he told me he regretted that decision, you know, having it removed. He should have waited – that maybe because he's having a lot of side effects, I don't know." [pt 05]

Additionally, two participants referenced stories from family members who also chose not to seek active treatment for cancer; these family members lived longer than expected and died from causes other than cancer:

"And my father had prostate cancer. His, they claimed, had spread and were really pretty pessimistic. But he was older. And he decided not to do anything. And he lived – I don't know – something like seven or eight years and died of a heart attack." [pt 07]

By referencing these stories from their social networks, the participants were able to justify their own choice to follow AS by providing evidence that a) a slow-moving cancer would not be the ultimate cause of death, and b) active treatment would have a larger, negative impact on quality of life than the prostate cancer itself.

Trust in the medical community

Six men directly referenced conversations with friends or family members who were linked to the medical community, mostly through occupation. The advice received from these individuals was particularly emphasized, as their connection to the medical community added weight and legitimacy to their opinions over that of other members of the participants' social networks. For some men, the advice gained from these individuals was viewed as an informal second opinion:

"Being a professor...and having a number of students who were – they're both MD students and PhD students – I talked to them about it and...the basic conclusion that I got from them was I would be insane to go through radiation treatment with a Gleason index, you know, so extremely low, with just one sample." [pt 15]

Furthermore, the decision to follow AS was strengthened for participants when the second opinions obtained from specialists, or the opinions they heard from their friends or family members within the medical community, were concordant with the recommendations received by their providers. This consistency increased the trust participants held with their own providers, and brought a sense of relief and confidence that they made an appropriate decision in following AS:

"I had been doing some processing and it was reassuring to hear him say the same thing as the first doctor." [pt V01]

Seven participants also mentioned trust in their provider as they discussed their rationalization of the choice to follow AS. Several men took comfort in the notion that their providers would be able to recognize changes in their disease and make responsive recommendations to change treatment plans if or when necessary:

"I put a lot of faith in them. I have a lot of trust in them. They're very good at what they're doing." [pt 9]

"I really would wait for the physician to say, you know, it's time to take it out, take the prostate out." [pt 06]

Discussion

Much of the approach that men on AS take to negotiating the anxiety and uncertainty of their low-risk prostate cancer stems from the identification of their cancer as an indolent – or not life-threatening – disease with an extended time line of progression. Several studies evaluating the treatment decision-making process for men with low-risk prostate cancer generally conclude that men choosing aggressive interventions, such as surgery or radiation, do so from a strong desire to eradicate or cure a disease they view as life threatening, especially if they have a longer life expectancy at the age of diagnosis; conversely, men choosing AS tend to not view their prostate cancer as an immediate health threat [15–20]. The first theme developed in our analysis builds on this understanding of why men choose AS: the men in our sample did not view their prostate cancer as a direct threat to their well-being, but rather considered the potential side effects of aggressive treatment as threats. In this manner, the anxiety men on AS experience can stem in great part from prostate cancer treatment. The first approach to combat treatment-related anxiety for the individuals in our sample was to avoid the negative outcomes and risks associated with active treatment, and following AS was an agreeable method by which they could do this while ensuring their disease was not neglected.

The statements made by men in our sample also highlight the importance of maintaining control in coping with the unease of untreated cancer. For some men within our sample, this control took the form of maintaining routine activities without interruption, while for others it took the form of altering dietary and exercise habits. If men on AS characterize their prostate cancer as a slow-moving, non-threatening disease, any interruption to daily life would indicate that the cancer is not indolent and trigger a re-assessment of their illness representation. Additionally, adopting changes in diet and exercise are tangible actions that men perceive as beneficial to their disease state, and bring a sense of assurance to an otherwise uncertain scenario [21].

Concordant with prior investigations, our findings indicate that some men on AS may experience increased anxiety prior to routine follow-up procedures [6, 22]. Despite these initial anxieties, several of the men in our sample reported feeling reassured by the findings of their follow-up testing, which reaffirmed the suitability of AS. In fact, recent evidence indicates that routine testing plays an important role in the psychological health of men on AS by mollifying fears associated with disease progression. Thus, testing is an important component of anxiety management [22]. The time line of the AS protocol also afforded men the opportunity to become more familiar with all prostate cancer treatment options by extending the timeframe during which they could gather and digest information. Some men in our sample were concerned over the potential need to select an active treatment in the future due to disease progression. Following AS allowed these individuals the time necessary to reach a comfortable familiarity with available active treatment options and reduced their current anxiety over future changes. This finding complements that of qualitative research conducted by Volk et al. among men with localized prostate cancer, which concluded that the ability to slow the decision-making process allowed men on AS to gain a better understanding of the AS approach to cancer treatment and overcome the prevailing heuristic for immediate and aggressive treatment [19].

Existing literature focused on the role of social support during the diagnosis and decision-making process for prostate cancer treatment indicates that men seek opinions from their spouses and social connections as they make their treatment decisions [6, 17, 19, 23]. Comments from the men in our sample reflect this influence of social support, and particularly highlight the role of personal experiences with prostate cancer shared from within men's social networks in the decision-making process. It appears that these anecdotal stories may be more informative or salient for men compared to information gathered from the general literature, or, at times, even from medical professionals.

The results of our study further indicate that this reliance on the social network does not end once the treatment decision has been made; rather, men continue to rely upon spousal support as they make adjustments to life with untreated cancer, and continue to justify their treatment choice by learning from and referencing the experiences of others. The intersection between feedback from social connections and feedback from the medical community is also a significant component of the confidence men have in their decision to follow AS. Concordance between the opinions obtained from men's providers and those received from individuals within their social networks further legitimized AS as a valid treatment option for men in our sample, especially when those social connections had ties to the medical community.

Clinical implications

Providers may not always be aware of the psychosocial issues men with low-risk prostate cancer on AS experience. However, there are tools or potential interventions providers can share with their patients to help them process psychosocial stressors associated with their cancer diagnosis and management, including instruction in mindfulness meditation, cognitive-behavioral stress management, and diet and exercise lifestyle interventions [24–26]. A study of one such lifestyle intervention conducted in California, US, found that men felt the program supported feelings of optimism, hope and well-being [27]. Several men in our sample reported making similar lifestyle changes independently, indicating that the topics addressed in these interventions are salient among AS patients and present a viable avenue through which their psychosocial health can be supported.

Spouses and family members often act as health advocates, sources of emotional support, and facilitate patient-provider communication among men with prostate cancer [28–30]. Spouses of prostate cancer patients can frequently experience issues related to emotional wellness, balancing their health needs with those of the patient, and lack of communication [28]. Therefore, it may be important for providers to offer support resources to men's spouses and families as well. Engaging spouses and families in support services not only addresses their individual anxieties related to the prostate cancer diagnosis, but educate these individuals on AS management and enable them to adopt supportive roles for the prostate cancer patient [31].

Clarity in the diagnosis and treatment decision-making process is a central, salient component of emotional adjustment for men with low-risk prostate cancer [32]. Men who receive corroborating information from both their social network and from within the medical community may have less confusion and anxiety over their treatment decision, and increased trust in provider recommendations [33]. It is important for providers to acknowledge the role outside opinion – whether gathered internally or externally from the medical community – has on men's perceptions of prostate cancer.

Limitations

This study was conducted with a small convenience sample at academic institutions with multidisciplinary cancer centers. The multidisciplinary centers allow patients to receive timely feedback from providers in multiple specialties, often in the same day, prior to making treatment decisions. This study site likely influenced the degree to which the experiences of the men in our sample are generalizable to those of men receiving treatment outside a multidisciplinary setting. Additionally, the participants in our study were largely homogenous in demographic characteristics, and our findings may not generalize to men from other demographic groups and settings.

Some men in our sample may have been following AS for longer periods than others. It is possible that men with more months on AS were able to use that time to gain a more in-depth understanding of their disease and security in their treatment decision compared to other men in the sample. Additionally, the variability in time since treatment decision among men in our sample may have introduced recall bias in the content of the interviews. Future investigations targeting specific subgroups of prostate cancer patients may yield insight into variations in coping strategies among men based on time since diagnosis.

Finally, the research question described in this report emerged from a prior analysis originally targeting the decision-making process for men diagnosed with low-risk prostate cancer. As such, the interview transcripts analyzed in this project were originally constructed to elicit responses regarding that subject area, rather than directly focusing on coping and the role of men's social networks in managing stress and anxiety.

Conclusions

The decision to follow AS in many ways reflects the need to maintain control, as this treatment choice avoids more aggressive treatment options. Men on AS manage their prostate cancer-related anxiety by both maintaining a sense of control over their daily lives, as well as relying on the support provided them by their social networks and the medical community. Social networks, and more specifically spouses, support men on AS by encouraging lifestyle changes and serving as a resource to discuss and ease cancer-related stress. Men who are able to maintain a sense of trust and connection to their providers experience less worry and anxiety over their untreated prostate cancer.

It is important to recognize that these coping mechanisms or approaches to life on AS are not independent from one another, but rather collectively influence the patient's perception of his illness. Education and support services offered to patients should incorporate their friends and family members. Furthermore, physicians may be better prepared to address areas of confusion, contradiction and anxiety for their patients on AS by identifying the availability of social support and acknowledging the feedback obtained from within their patients' social networks regarding prostate cancer.

Abbreviations

AS: Active surveillance; DRE: Digital rectal exam; IRB: Institutional review board; PSA: Prostate-specific antigen; US: United States

Funding

The study was funded by the Norris Cotton Cancer Center Prouty Research Program and its Dartmouth/UMass/UVM Collaborative Research Grant Award Program. This project was also partially supported by the Health Resources and Services Administration (HRSA) of the U.S. Department of Health and Human Services (HHS) under grant D54HP23297, "Administrative Academic Units," (Christopher P. Morley, PI/PD. This information or content and conclusions are those of the authors and should not be construed as the official position or policy of, nor should any endorsements be inferred by HRSA, HHS or the U.S. Government. Kathleen D. Lyons, ScD is supported by a Mentored Research Scholar Grant in Applied and Clinical Research (MRSG 12-113-01 – CPPB) from the American Cancer Society.

Authors' contributions

KDL, MTH, SDP, BHI, JDS, ESH, and TM participated in project conception, design and coordination. TMS, MKF, and CPM participated in project design and coordination. KDL and TM conducted participant interviews. EMM and

HHL conducted qualitative analyses and drafted the manuscript. TMS, MKF,and KDL helped draft and/or revise the manuscript. All authors read and approved the final manuscript.

Competing interests
The authors declare that they have no competing interests.

Author details
[1]Department of Family Medicine, SUNY Upstate Medical University, 475 Irving Ave., Suite 200, Syracuse, NY 13210, USA. [2]Department of Public Health and Preventive Medicine, SUNY Upstate Medical University, 766 Irving Ave., Rm. 2262, Syracuse, NY 13210, USA. [3]Department of Psychiatry and Behavioral Sciences, SUNY Upstate Medical University, 750 E Adams St., Syracuse, NY 13210, USA. [4]Department of Psychiatry, Geisel School of Medicine at Dartmouth, Dartmouth-Hitchcock Medical Center, 1 Medical Center Dr., Lebanon, NH 03756, USA. [5]Division of Urology, Department of Surgery, University of Vermont College of Medicine, Fletcher House 301, 111 Colchester Ave., Burlington, VT 05401, USA. [6]Urology Section, Geisel School of Medicine at Dartmouth College, Dartmouth-Hitchcock Medical Center, 1 Medical Center Dr., Lebanon, NH 03756, USA. [7]Cancer Control Program, Norris Cotton Cancer Center, Dartmouth-Hitchcock Medical Center, 1 Medical Center Dr., Lebanon, NH 03756, USA.

References
1. Filson C, Marks L, Litwin M. Expectant management for men with early stage prostate cancer. CA Cancer J Clin. 2015;65:264–82.
2. Mohler JL, Kantoff PW, Armstrong AJ, Bahnson RR, Cohen M, D'Amico AV, et al. Prostate cancer, version 2.2014. J Natl Compr Canc Netw. 2014;12:686–718.
3. Thompson I, Thrasher JB, Aus G, Burnett AL, Canby-Hagino ED, Cookson MS, et al. Prostate cancer: guideline for the management of clinically localized prostate cancer 2007 update. J Urol. 2007;177(6):2106–31.
4. Hayes JH, Ollendorf DA, Pearson SD, Barry MJ, Kantoff PW, Stewart ST, et al. Active surveillance compared with initial treatment for men with low-risk prostate cancer: a decision analysis. JAMA. 2010;304:2373–80.
5. American Cancer Society. Expectant management, watchful waiting, and active surveillance for prostate cancer [Internet]. Prostate Cancer. 2015 [cited 2015 May 13]. Available from: http://www.cancer.org/cancer/prostatecancer/detailedguide/prostate-cancer-treating-watchful-waiting.
6. Bellardita L, Rancati T, Alvisi MF, Villani D, Magnani T, Marenghi C, et al. Predictors of health-related quality of life and adjustment to prostate cancer during active surveillance. Eur Urol. 2013;64:30–6.
7. Kazer MW, Psutka SP, Latini DM, Bailey DE. Psychosocial aspects of active surveillance. Curr Opin Urol. 2013;23:273–7.
8. Parker PA, Davis JW, Latini DM, Baum G, Wang X, Ward JF, et al. Relationship between illness uncertainty, anxiety, fear of progression and quality of life in men with favourable-risk prostate cancer undergoing active surveillance. BJU Int. 2016;117(3):469–77.
9. Yanez B, Bustillo NE, Antoni MH, Lechner SC, Dahn J, Kava B, et al. The importance of perceived stress management skills for patients with prostate cancer in active surveillance. J Behav Med [Internet]. Springer US; 2015 [cited 2016 Aug 26];38:214–23. Available from: http://link.springer.com/10.1007/s10865-014-9594-1.
10. Leventhal H, Diefenbach M, Leventhal EA. Illness cognition: using common sense to understand treatment adherence and affect cognition interactions. Cogn Ther Res. 1992;16:143–63.
11. Leventhal H. Findings and theory in the study of fear communications. Adv Exp Soc Psychol. 1970;5:119–86.
12. Lyons KD, Li HH, Mader EM, Stewart TM, Morley CP, Formica MK, et al. Cognitive and affective representations of active surveillance as a treatment option for low-risk prostate cancer. Am J Mens Health [Internet]. 2016 [cited 2016 Aug 26]; Available from: http://www.ncbi.nlm.nih.gov/pubmed/27365211.
13. Meadows LM, Verdi AJ, Crabtree BF. Keeping up appearances: using qualitative research to enhance knowledge of dental practice. J Dent Educ. 2003;67:981 90.

14. Borkan J. Immersion/Crystallization. In: Crabtree BF, Miller WL, editors. Doing Qual. Res. 2nd ed. Thousand Oaks: SAGE Publications; 1999. p. 179–94.
15. Penson DF. Factors influencing patients' acceptance and adherence to active surveillance. J Natl Cancer Inst Monogr. 2012;2012:207–12.
16. Davison BJ, Goldenberg SL. Patient acceptance of active surveillance as a treatment option for low-risk prostate cancer. BJU Int [Internet]. 2011 [cited 2015 Apr 2];108:1787–93. Available from: http://www.ncbi.nlm.nih.gov/pubmed/21507187.
17. Gorin MA, Soloway CT, Eldefrawy A, Soloway MS. Factors that influence patient enrollment in active surveillance for low-risk prostate cancer. Urology. 2011;77:588–91.
18. van den Bergh RCN, van Vugt HA, Korfage IJ, Steyerberg EW, Roobol MJ, Schröder FH, et al. Disease insight and treatment perception of men on active surveillance for early prostate cancer. BJU Int. 2010;105:322–8.
19. Volk RJ, McFall SL, Cantor SB, Byrd TL, Le Y-CL, Kuban DA, et al. "It's not like you just had a heart attack": decision-making about active surveillance by men with localized prostate cancer. Psychooncology. 2014;23:467–72.
20. Davison BJ, Oliffe JL, Pickles T, Mroz L. Factors influencing men undertaking active surveillance for the management of low-risk prostate cancer. Oncol Nurs Forum. 2009;36:89–96.
21. Oliffe JL, Davison BJ, Pickles T, Mroz L. The self-management of uncertainty among men undertaking active surveillance for low-risk prostate cancer. Qual Health Res. 2009;19:432–43.
22. Simpson P. Does active surveillance lead to anxiety and stress? Br J Nurs. 2014;23 Suppl 1:S4–12.
23. Chapple A, Ziebland S, Herxheimer A, McPherson A, Shepperd S, Miller R. Is "watchful waiting" a real choice for men with prostate cancer? A qualitative study. BJU Int. 2002;90:257–64.
24. Pickles T, Ruether D, Weir L, Carlson L, Jakulj F, SCRN Communication Team. Psychosocial barriers to active surveillance for the management of early prostate cancer and a strategy for increased acceptance. BJU Int. 2007;100:544–51.
25. Rossen S, Hansen-Nord NS, Kayser L, Borre M, Larsen RG, Trichopoulou A, et al. The impact of husbands' prostate cancer diagnosis and participation in a behavioral lifestyle intervention on spouses' lives and relationships with their partners. Cancer Nurs. 2015. doi:10.1097/NCC.0000000000000259.
26. Victorson D, Hankin V, Burns J, Weiland R, Maletich C, Sufrin N, et al. Feasibility, acceptability and preliminary psychological benefits of mindfulness meditation training in a sample of men diagnosed with prostate cancer on active surveillance: results from a randomized controlled pilot trial. Psychooncology. 2016. doi:10.1002/pon.4135.
27. Kronenwetter C, Weidner G, Pettengill E, Marlin R, Crutchfield L, McCormac P, et al. A qualitative analysis of interviews of men with early stage prostate cancer: the Prostate Cancer Lifestyle Trial. Cancer Nurs. 2005;28:99–107.
28. Hawes SM, Malcarne VL, Ko CM, Sadler GR, Banthia R, Sherman SA, et al. Identifying problems faced by spouses and partners of patients with prostate cancer. Oncol Nurs Forum. 2006;33:807–14.
29. Voerman B, Visser A, Fischer M, Garssen B, VanAndel G, Bensing J. Determinants of participation in social support groups for prostate cancer patients. Psychooncology. 2007;16:1092–9.
30. Maliski SL, Heilemann MV, McCorkle R. From "death sentence" to "good cancer": couples' transformation of a prostate cancer diagnosis. Nurs Res. 2002;51:391–7.
31. Bottorff JL, Oliffe JL, Halpin M, Phillips M, McLean G, Mroz L. Women and prostate cancer support groups: the gender connect? Soc Sci Med. 2008;66:1217–27.
32. Traeger L, Penedo FJ, Gonzalez JS, Dahn JR, Lechner SC, Schneiderman N, et al. Illness perceptions and emotional well-being in men treated for localized prostate cancer. J Psychosom Res. 2009;67:389–97.
33. Underwood W, Orom H, Poch M, West BT, Lantz PM, Chang SS, et al. Multiple physician recommendations for prostate cancer treatment: a Pandora's box for patients? Can J Urol. 2010;17:5346–54.

12

Artificial urinary sphincter implantation: an important component of complex surgery for urinary tract reconstruction in patients with refractory urinary incontinence

Fan Zhang[1,2] and Limin Liao[1,2]* ⓘ

Abstract

Background: We review our outcomes and experience of artificial urinary sphincter implantation for patients with refractory urinary incontinence from different causes.

Methods: Between April 2002 and May 2017, a total of 32 patients (median age, 40.8 years) with urinary incontinence had undergone artificial urinary sphincter placement during urinary tract reconstruction. Eighteen patients (56.3%) were urethral injuries associated urinary incontinence, 9 (28.1%) had neurogenic urinary incontinence and 5 (15.6%) were post-prostatectomy incontinence. Necessary surgeries were conducted before artificial urinary sphincter placement as staged procedures, including urethral strictures incision, sphincterotomy, and augmentation cystoplasty.

Results: The mean follow-up time was 39 months. At the latest visit, 25 patients (78.1%) maintained the original artificial urinary sphincter. Four patients (12.5%) had artificial urinary sphincter revisions. Explantations were performed in three patients. Twenty-four patients were socially continent, leading to the overall success rate as 75%. The complication rate was 28.1%; including infections ($n = 4$), erosions ($n = 4$), and mechanical failure ($n = 1$). The impact of urinary incontinence on the quality of life measured by the visual analogue scale dropped from 7.0 ± 1.2 to 2.2 ± 1.5 ($P < 0.001$).

Conclusions: The primary sources for artificial urinary sphincter implantation in our center are unique, and the procedure is an effective treatment as a part of urinary tract reconstruction in complicated urinary incontinence cases with complex etiology.

Keywords: Artificial urinary sphincter, Urinary tract reconstruction, Refractory urinary incontinence, Outcomes

Background

Artificial urinary sphincter (AUS) implantation is a well-established treatment for refractory stress urinary incontinence (SUI) resulting from intrinsic sphincter deficiency (ISD) [1]. It is versatile and effective in a wide range of situations, including post-prostatectomy incontinence (PPI) or other urethral surgery-related incontinence, traumatic urethral disruption as a result of a prior pelvic fracture, radical pelvic surgery, neurogenic causes, and as a salvage procedure after other treatments have failed [2, 3].

AUS placement is primarily performed in men with post-radical prostatectomy (RP) incontinence [4]; there is scant published data for other etiologies [1–3, 5]. Interestingly, the majority priority cases for AUS implantation in our institute have been incontinence secondary to urethral injuries and neurogenic cases. A series of urinary tract reconstruction (UTR) might be needed combining AUS placement and other additional procedures in complex cases [3]. The type of injury, possibility of a previous failed repair, relatively restricted surgical access, or urethral stricture, together with inherent detrusor-sphincter dysfunction, make UTR more complicated [6]. Thus, the quality and choice of management modalities should be tailored to the unique needs of each individual. The purpose of this study was to

---

* Correspondence: lmliao@263.net
[1]Department of Urology, China Rehabilitation Research Center, Beijing 100068, China
[2]Department of Urology, Capital Medical University, Beijing, China

present our experience of AUS implantation as a part of UTR for patients with complex and refractory urinary incontinence (UI).

Methods

Subjects

With the approval of the Ethics Committee of the China Rehabilitation Research Center, we reviewed 32 patients (31 males and 1 female) who underwent AUS placement (AMS 800; American Medical Systems, Minnetonka, MN, USA) for the treatment of UI secondary to different causes (April 2002 to May 2017). Written informed consent for participation was obtained from all participants in the study. All participants were adults and the mean age was 40.78 ± 16.58 years. Eighteen patients (56.3%) had pelvic fracture-associated urethral injuries (PFUI) (car accident or fall down) that were initially treated elsewhere and presented to us 8 months to 30 years after the injury with intractable incontinence, nine of whom developed urethral stricture after the Bank's method and had recurrent contractures after initial management; two underwent male slings surgeries but had recurrent incontinence. Nine patients (28.1%) had neurogenic bladder (NB) dysfunction (meningomyelocele, 5; spinal cord injury, 4) and 5 (15.6%) underwent prostatectomies (Table 1). The consent to publish these information (age and detailed medical history) was obtained from all participants.

The pre-implantation evaluation comprised a clinical interview, surgical history, analysis of voiding diaries (time and voided volumes, pad changes, and UI episodes), physical examination, urinalysis, and urine culture. More invasive testing included urethrography and video-urodynamic assessment. Cystourethroscopy was required to verify urethral integrity, bladder neck patency, and vesicourethral anastomotic strictures. Ultrasound was routinely used to assess the upper urinary tract (UUT) and post-void residual urine. The UUT was also evaluated by magnetic resonance urography (MRU).

Surgical technique

According to patients' individual condition, the following operations were conducted before AUS placement, including two strictures incision, three sphincterotomies, and five urethral dilations in urethral injuries associated UI patients due to the refractory urethral stricture post Bank's method; four patients with neurogenic UI underwent sphincterotomies or urethral dilations out of detrusor sphincter dyssynergia (DSD), 3 subsequently had augmentation cystoplasties. A urethral stricture was incised in one PPI patient. These surgeries were performed 3–6 months prior to AUS implantation as staged procedures in the series of UTR (Table 2).

Table 1 Clinic characteristics of the patients treated with an artificial urinary sphincter ($n = 32$)

Characteristics	Value
Number of patients	32
Age (yrs)	40.78 ± 16.58
Mean follow-up time (yrs)	3.3 ± 0.7
Type UI	
PFUI	18 (56.3%)
NB	9 (28.1%)
TURP	3 (9.4%)
RP	2 (6.2%)
Number of previous surgeries for UI	
0–1	10 (31.3%)
2	5 (15.6%)
3	5 (15.6%)
≥ 4	12 (37.5%)
Cuff size	
4 cm	21 (65.6%)
4.5 cm	10 (31.3%)
8 cm	1 (3.1%)*
Operative approach	
transperineal	16 (50%)
trans-scrotal	15 (46.9%)
trans-retropubic	1 (3.1%)
transcorporal (intracavernous)	1*

Values are presented as the mean (±standard deviation) or number (%)
PFUI pelvic fracture-associated urethral injuries, NB neurogenic bladder, TURP transurethral resection of the prostate, RP radical prostatectomy. *8 cm cuff was implanted on the female case. *One transperineal case had a transcorporal approach implantation when revised

AUS implantation was performed as the standard procedure [2. 3]. Sixteen patients (50%) had the transperineal approach (two incisions) and 15 (46.9%) had the advanced trans-scrotal approach (one incision); based on individual local skin conditions. The female case had a trans-retropubic approach. Intravenous antibiotics (ceftriaxone and vancomycin) were given within 12 h prior to AUS surgery. Under general or spinal anesthesia, all patients were placed in the lithotomy position and the perineum was generously prepped with an alcohol and Betadine solution. Then, a Foley catheter with 8F–16F was inserted into the bladder. The AUS cuffs were placed at the bulbar urethra for the male cases and the bladder neck for the female case. The pump and balloon were implanted in the scrotum or labium majus and abdomen, respectively. The balloon pressure was 61–70 cm H_2O in all cases. The indwelling catheter remained in situ for the first 24 h, then switched to an external urine collection device before system activation (4–6 weeks postoperatively). Antibiotic prophylaxis was maintained 3 days post-operatively, followed by 2 weeks of oral ciprofloxacin. The length of hospital stay ranged from 5 to 7 weeks, including 1 week of preoperative evaluation and 4–6 weeks post-operative

Artificial urinary sphincter implantation: an important component of complex surgery for urinary tract...

83

Table 2 Patient operative history and treatment measures before AUS implantation

Number of patients (N = 32)		Etiology	Previous procedures (Times)	Least treatment to AUS interval (Yrs)	Our treatment before AUS	Complications	Management
1		PFUI	Upl,Spl,USD,USI	21	USD	none	none
2		PFUI	Upl,RV	0.5	cystoscopy*	none	none
3		NB	spondylolysis	none	cystoscopy	dysuria	revision
4		NB	Cty	3	Sty + AC	infection, erosion	explantation
5	1st time	NB	Cty	1	Sty	RI	revision explantation
	2nd time		AUS(RI)	0.5	cuff removal	infection	
6		PFUI	Upl,Spl,USD,USI	2	Sty	RI, erosion	explantation
7	1st time	PFUI	Upl,USI(2),MS	10	USD	erosion, infection	revision
	2nd time		AUS (erosion)	3	Cuff removal	Transcorporal implantations	none
8		PFUI	Upl,USD,USI	0.7	USD	none	none
9		NB	spondylolysis	13	USD,AC	none	none
10		PPI	TURP,USD	2	cystoscopy	none	none
11		NB	Spondylolysis	20	cystoscopy	none	none
12		PFUI	Upl,Spl,USI(2)	20	USD	none	none
13		PFUI	Upl,Spl,USD	1	USI	none	none
14		PPI	TURP,Upl,USI(2)	20	USI	none	none
15		PFUI	Upl,Spl,USI	3	Sty	none	none
16		PFUI	Upl,USI(2),US,MS	14	USI	none	none
17		PFUI	Upl,USI(2),Cty	1	USD	none	none
18		NB	Upl,Spl,USD	9	USD + AC	none	none
19	1st time	PFUI	Upl,USI	10	cystoscopy	fluid leakage	revision
	2nd time		AUS(mechanical failure)	one month	device removal	none	none
20		PFUI	Upl,Spl,USD,USI(2)	30	Sty	none	none
21		PFUI	Upl,USD,USI	18	cystoscopy	none	none
22		PPI	RP	3	cystoscopy	none	none
23		PPI	TURP,USD	3	cystoscopy	none	none
24		PFUI	USD,USI	11	cystoscopy	none	none
25		NB	Upl,USI(2),US,USD	36	cystoscopy	none	none
26		PFUI	Upl	2	cystoscopy	none	none
27		NB	USD	1	cystoscopy	none	none
28		PFUI	Upl,USD(2),USI,Spl	10	cystoscopy	none	none
29		PFUI	Upl,Spl,USI(2)	2	cystoscopy	none	none
30		NB	USD	2	Sty	none	none
31		PFUI	Upl	1	cystoscopy	none	none
32		PPI	RP	1	cystoscopy	none	none

Cystoscopy was routinely performed to identify the severity of urethra strictures. If the stricture was asymptomatic or not progressive within at least 12 months, and if the post-void residual volume (< 50 ml) and Qmax were acceptable, then the AUS device was implanted with the maintenance of the current stricture. *PFUI* pelvic fracture-associated urethral injuries, *NB* neurogenic bladder, *PPI* post-prostatectomy incontinence, *Upl* urethroplasty, *Sty* sphincterotomy, *Spl* sphincteroplasty, *Cty* cystostomy, *RV* reconstruction of the vagina, *RI* recurrent incontinence, *USD* urethral stricture dilation, *USI* urethral stricture incision, *AC* augmentation cystoplasty, *MS* male sling, *TURP* transurethral resection of the prostate, *RP* radical prostatectomy, *US* urethral stent

in-patient time for patients from remote area. The local patients usually discharge from hospital 1 week after operation and visit out-patient clinic for system activation.

Assessment

All patients were assessed after AUS activation, followed by visits at 6 and 12 months, and by telephone interviews annually, or more frequently if needed.

The continence outcomes were assessed according to daily pad use. The impact of the UI in the patient's quality of life (QoL) was evaluated with a visual analogue scale (VAS). Specifically, the patients indicated on a numeric scale the impact of UI on QoL. Numbers 1–10 represented mild-to-severe impact on QoL. Efficacy and safety results were conducted on the following end points: infection/erosion rates; explantation rate (defined as complete removal of the whole device); and dry rate (defined as the proportion of patients wearing no pads). Patients were considered to have surgical success if they were socially continent (one pad per day or less). Failure was defined as that caused by any reason, such as mechanical failure, surgical revision, or removal.

Statistical analysis

Differences in durability according to different criteria were analyzed using the Student t-test. P-values <0.05 were considered significant. SPSS (version 17; SPSS, Inc., Chicago, IL, USA) was used for all analyses.

Results

All AUS procedures were performed successfully. The devices were activated in 31 cases at 1-month after surgery; patient 4 had device explantation because of an immediate infection due to scrotal skin erosion. At the time of adjustment, patient 3 had acute urinary retention and patient 5 had refractory incontinence (RI), both underwent cuff revision. The other early post-operative complications included two cases of transient perineal pain and one case of scrotal hematoma, all of which were managed conservatively. For initial evaluation, the success rate was 90.6% (29/32), 93.5% (29/31) patients had social continence including 80.6% (25/31) completely dry.

At 6-month follow-up, patient 5 had device explantation due to urethral atrophy induced RI and chronic infection; patient 19 had device revision due to balloon perforation. The success rate with original device was 90.3% (28/31); the success rate with revision was 96.8% (30/31). At 12-month follow-up, the success rate was maintained.

At 24-month follow-up, patient 6 had device explantation due to urethral erosion and chronic infection, leading to success rate 96.7% (29/30).

At 36-month follow-up, patient 7 had transcorporal single device (cuff) revision due to urethral erosion. Three cases had favorable outcomes in the first 2 years and then experienced descending efficacy due to recurrent incontinence (RI) (patient 2. 7 and 20), leading to success rate 89.7% (26/29).

The mean follow-up time was 39 months. At the latest follow-up, 25 patients maintained the original AUS. Four patients had AUS revisions. Explantations were performed in three patients. Twenty-four patients were socially continent, leading to the overall success rate as 75% (24/32), and 15 out of the 24 patients were completely dry 46.9% (15/32). The success rates were 77.8% (14/18), 66.7% (6/9) and 80% (4/5) in PFUI cases, NB cases and PPI cases, respectively. The daily pad count dropped from 3.6 ± 1.5 to 1.2 ± 0.2 pads per day (P <0.001; Table 3). The impact of UI on the QoL measured by the VAS dropped from 7.0 ± 1.2 to 2.2 ± 1.5 (P <0.001). Patients had preserved UUT

Table 3 Functional outcomes of pad use in patients with AUS device during post-operative period

Interval (months)	pad use ($n = 29$)[a]			
	none	1 pad	2–3 pads	> 4 pads
< 24	8	6	1	0
24–48	4	2	2	0
>48	3	1	1	1

At the end of the follow-up period, 24 patients were shown to be socially continent and 15 patients were completely dry. The daily pad count dropped from 3.6 ± 1.5 to 1.2 ± 0.2 pads per day (P <0.001). [a]Explantations were performed in three patients

function in the series of UTR; a typical case is shown in Fig. 1.

Discussion

AUS implantation has been the standard treatment for refractory SUI in males caused by sphincter deficiency. The quantity and level of evidence is 2b, as per the European Association of Urology guidelines [7]. Most information is gained from older case series after RP [8]. In the present study, the primary patients' source is urethral injuries associated UI with complex treatment experiences, which was quite different from previous literature [1–9]. Our success rate (75%) was comparable to the recent critical systematic review (61% and 100%) [9]. Despite known complications, the patient satisfaction rates remained favorable. There were several notable findings from the current study that merit further discussion.

The mechanism of urethral injuries associated UI may be related to the original trauma or as a complication of transpubic surgery and damage to the associated nerves or sphincter. A previous study indicated that the development of incontinence could be related to the trauma itself, rather than the method of initial management [10]. In our series, the majority of patients had undergone at least two urethral surgeries with recurrent incontinence. In our opinion, the subsequent urethral repair procedures, especially improper incision of urethral stricture, may contribute to the development of UI.

The use of AUS for urethral injuries associated UI has been limited because of functional urethral length, surrounding fibrosis, urethral strictures, and distorted anatomy of the pelvis. Scarring caused by previous urethral surgical procedures may lead to more difficult dissection. A decrease in functional urethral length may potentially reduce the efficacy of AUS surgery. Therefore, it is essential to confirm the status of the urethra and identify concomitant anastomotic strictures before AUS placement. If an anastomotic stricture is refractory or progressive, it is necessary to treat the stricture first. We prefer excising strictures narrower than 20-Fr, despite transient worsening of incontinence, and ensure an adequate recurrence-free period. The length of the period depends on individual conditions. If the stricture is

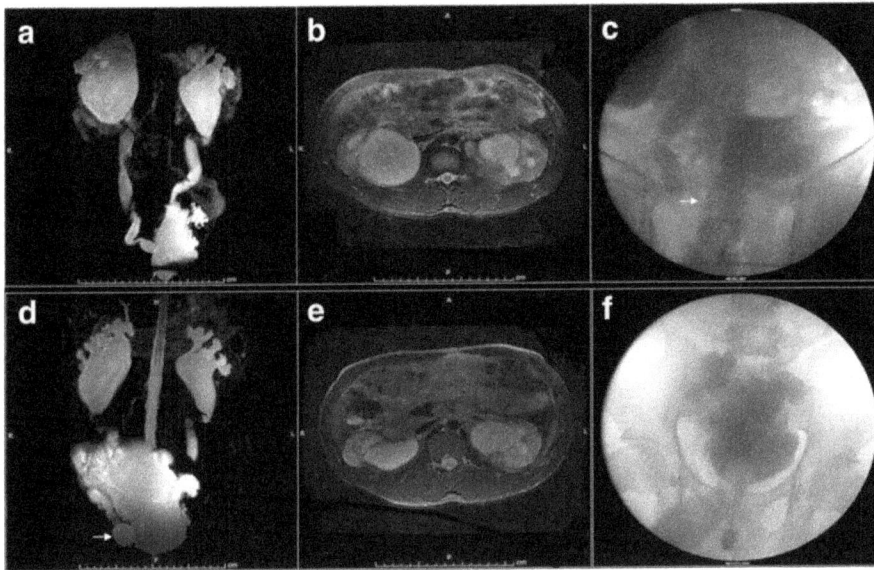

Fig. 1 Magnetic resonance urography and cystogram assessment before and after AUS implantation. Hydronephrosis (**a,b**) and vesicoureteral reflux (**c** represented by the white arrows) were presented before operation. Upper urinary dilation was ameliorated after augmentation cystoplasty and AUS surgery (**d** the white arrows represent the pressure regulating balloons, **e**) and reflux was cured (**f**) in 6-month follow up

asymptomatic or not progressive for at least 12 months and patients have acceptable post-void residual volumes (<50 ml), we suggest implanting the AUS device with maintenance of the current stricture, since aggressive excision may worsen a stable urethra.

NB dysfunction with UI secondary to ISD is also an indication for AUS implantation [3]. NB patients may suffer from low bladder outlet resistance, and the AUS can offer such patients the possibility of spontaneous voiding. In the present study, two NB patients had cuffs easily and effectively placed. Four patients with detrusor overactivity and DSD had sphincterotomy or urethral stricture dilations, three of whom subsequently had augmentation cystoplasty before AUS implantation. Only one patient with pre-existing renal insufficiency and urethral stricture had an immediate infection and erosion after AUS implantation, and this patient ultimately had an AUS explantation. One NB patient had hydronephrosis and high pressure vesicoureteral reflux. We performed augmentation cystoplasty and concomitant ureteral reimplantation before AUS implantation. The patient had UUT function preserved with appropriate manipulation of the device (Fig. 1). AUS implantation is usually coupled with specific complications in NB patients, leading to higher re-operative rate than non-neurogenic patients. We recommend performing a staged procedure, confirming stable UUT function and no urethral stricture recurrence at least 6-month before AUS implantation, especially in complex reconstruction cases.

It has been reported that 30%–40% of patients who undergo prostatectomies complain of persistent PPI [11]. Approximately 2%–5% of patients with PPI exhibit persistent incontinence for at least 1 year postoperatively, despite conservative therapy attempts [12]. The incidence of PPI cases remains high despite advances in surgical technologies and techniques [13]. The minor percentage of PPI cases in our report may reflect the relatively small number of RP performed in China compared to the United States, and a difference of referral pattern to our center. Based on our experience, some patients with PPI may undergo improvement of continence status to an acceptable extent over time; other patients prefer seeking treatment if the status worsens. A recent study concluded that preserving membranous urethral length, depth of the urethrovesical junction, and nerve were related to the recovery time and level of urinary continence after RP [14]. Petroski. et al. [15] reported that UI can improve for up to 24 months after RP and early radiotherapy (RT) may interfere with or prolong return to continence. UI was more common in the early RT group and UI rates gradually improved over 3 years post-RT. In the same study, only 12 patients (26%) had an AUS placed. The process of PPI improvement should be considered when making a decision in terms of AUS placement for such patients.

The relatively higher rates of complications in the initial few patients (up to patient 7) may be a reflection of the learning curve needed to perfect the surgical techniques [16]. Previous urethral damage (failed surgical procedures and urethral atrophy) can potentially result in technical difficulties and/or reduce the efficacy of AUS surgery [17]. Most patients presenting with an AUS infection will have underlying cuff erosion [18]. In the present study, infection currently developed in approximately 12.5% of our patients. Cuff erosion occurred early post-operatively (patient 4) due to infection and later after convalescence (patients 5, 6, and 7) due to urethral damage secondary to cuff pressure and improper catheterization. Patient 5 had a revision, but ultimately experienced explantation due to infection. Patient 7 had recurrent SUI related to erosion and infection 36 months after the initial implantation. The previous cuff was removed with the remainder of the device sealed in vivo and transcorporal implantation was performed 6 months later. A recent study showed urethral repair at the time of explantation for cuff erosion appears to prevent stricture development, thus facilitating successful replacement [19]. We prefer a staged procedure allowing a period for healing after explantation, since infection and erosion often coexist. An aggressive repair may worsen urethra condition.

The transcorporal approach has been described as salvage surgical technique in patients with a damaged or frail urethra [17]. Noticeably, the transcorporal-implanted patient experienced descending efficacy due to the refractory UI. An imaging study showed urethral atrophy at the 6-year visit. Urethral atrophy is a common cause of recurrence UI during follow-up with a functioning AUS [13]. Urethral atrophy may result secondary to chronic compression of the urethra and urethral tissue hypoxia.

In our series, two patients (7 and 16) had previous male sling surgery, but with unsatisfactory outcomes; they finally received AUS implantation. Although there is insufficient long-term efficacy data on the male sling, most patients with moderate incontinence would choose a male sling and cite the primary reason being a motivation to avoid a mechanical device [20]. The sling may be preferable as an initial procedure because an AUS can be attempted after sling failure [21]. Generally, it is accepted that a convenient male sling could be an option for mild-to-moderate SUI, while AUS remains the gold standard treatment for severe SUI cases.

A potential weakness of this study was the relatively small sample, leading to a lack of power to detect subtle associations. The relatively higher rates of complications and differences in the frequency of causes may be attributable to the variety of etiologies for UI, complex conditions and combination surgeries. It is noteworthy that long-term follow-up and UUT monitoring is essential in special populations.

Conclusion

The surgical management for complex UTR in UI cases including both neurogenic and non-neurogenic etiologies can be difficult. The present study indicated that AUS is a key procedure of UTR. The modalities of management must tailor to the unique needs of each individual. Appropriate patient counseling and adherence to surgical principles are vital for the success of surgery.

Abbreviations

AUS: Artificial urinary sphincter; DSD: Detrusor sphincter dyssynergia; ISD: Intrinsic sphincter deficiency; MRU: Magnetic resonance urography; NB: Neurogenic bladder; PFUI: Pelvic fracture-associated urethral injuries; PPI: Post-prostatectomy incontinence; QoL: Quality of life; RI: Recurrent incontinence; RP: Post-radical prostatectomy; RT: Radio therapy; SUI: Stress urinary incontinence; UI: Urinary incontinence; UTR: Urinary tract reconstruction; UUT: Upper urinary tract; VAS: Visual analogue scale

Acknowledgments

Not applicable.

Funding

This work was partially supported by the Natural Science Foundation of China (No. 81270847).

Authors' contributions

FZ collected data and drafted the manuscript. LML contributed to surgeries, the conception and design of the study, analysis interpretation of data, and helped to draft and revised the manuscript. Both authors read and approved the final manuscript.

Authors' information

Fan Zhang, MD & PhD is an urologist in the department of urology of China Rehabilitation Research Center (CRRC). Limin Liao, MD & PhD, is chairman of the department of urology of CRRC, and a professor of urology and vice-chairman of urologic department of Capital Medical University in Beijing. His main interests are neurourology, urodynamics and incontinence. He is a committee member of the neurourology promotion committee of the international continence society (ICS), and was chairman of 42nd ICS annual meeting in Beijing.

Competing interests

The authors declare that they have no competing interests.

References

1. Léon P, Chartier-Kastler E, Rouprêt M, Ambrogi V, Mozer P, Phé V. Long-term functional outcomes after artificial urinary sphincter (AMS 800®) implantation in men with stress urinary incontinence. BJU Int. 2015;115(6):951–7.
2. Kim SP, Sarmast Z, Daignault S, Faerber GJ, McGuire EJ, Latini JM. Long-term durability and functional outcomes among patients with artificial urinary sphincters: a 10-year retrospective review from the University of Michigan. J Urol. 2008;179(5):1912–6.
3. Lai HH, Hsu EI, Teh BS, Butler EB, Boone TB. 13 years of experience with artificial urinary sphincter implantation at Baylor College of Medicine. J Urol. 2007;177(3):1021–5.
4. Lee R, Te AE, Kaplan SA, Sandhu JS. Temporal trends in adoption of and indications for the artificial urinary sphincter. J Urol. 2009 Jun;181(6):2622–7.
5. Wang R, McGuire EJ, He C, Faerber GJ, Latini JM. Long-term outcomes after primary failures of artificial urinary sphincter implantation. Urology. 2012; 79(4):922–8.
6. Mundy AR, Andrich DE. Pelvic fracture-related injuries of the bladder neck and prostate: their nature, cause and management. BJU Int. 2010;105(9):1302–8.

Artificial urinary sphincter implantation: an important component of complex surgery for urinary tract...

87

7. Lucas MG, Bosch RJ, Burkhard FC, et al. EAU guidelines on surgical treatment of urinary incontinence. Eur Urol. 2012;62:1118–29.

8. Herschorn S, Brushini H, Comiter C, et al. Surgical treatment of urinary incontinence in men. Neurourol Urodyn. 2010;29:179–90.

9. Van der Aa F, Drake MJ, Kasyan GR, et al. The artificial urinary sphincter after a quarter of a century: a critical systematic review of its use in male non-neurogenic incontinence. Eur Urol. 2013;63(4):681–9.

10. Koraitim MM. Effect of early realignment on length and delayed repair of postpelvic fracture urethral injury. Urology. 2012;79(4):912–5.

11. Herschorn S, Bruschini H, Comiter C, et al. Committee of the International Consultation on I. Surgical treatment of stress incontinence in men. Neurourol Urodyn. 2010;29:179–90.

12. Bauer RM, Bastian PJ, Gozzi C, et al. Postprostatectomy incontinence: all about diagnosis and management. Eur Urol. 2009;55:322–3.

13. Chung E, Cartmill R. Diagnostic challenges in the evaluation of persistent or recurrent urinary incontinence after artificial urinary sphincter (AUS) implantation in patients after prostatectomy. BJU Int. 2013;112(Suppl 2):32–5.

14. Haga N, Ogawa S, Yabe M, et al. Association between postoperative pelvic anatomic features on magnetic resonance imaging and lower tract urinary symptoms after radical prostatectomy. Urology. 2014;84(3):642–9.

15. Petroski RA, Warlick WB, Herring J, et al. External beam radiation therapy after radical prostatectomy: efficacy and impact on urinary continence. Prostate Cancer Prostatic Dis. 2004;7:170–7.

16. Lai HH, Boone TB. The surgical learning curve of artificial urinary sphincter implantation: implications on prosthetic training and referral. J Urol. 2013; 189:1437–43.

17. Wiedemann L, Cornu JN, Haab E, et al. Transcorporal artificial urinary sphincter implantation as a salvage surgical procedure for challenging cases of male stress urinary incontinence: surgical technique and functional outcomes in a contemporary series. BJU Int. 2013;112(8):1163–8.

18. Rozanski AT, Tausch TJ, Ramirez D, Simhan J, Scott JF, Morey AF. Immediate urethral repair during explantation prevents stricture formation after artificial urinary sphincter cuff erosion. J Urol. 2014;192(2):442–6.

19. Brant WO, Erickson BA, Elliott SP, et al. Risk factors for erosion of artificial urinary sphincters: a multicenter prospective study. Urology. 2014;84(4):934–9.

20. Kumar A, Litt ER, Ballert KN, Nitti VW. Artificial urinary sphincter versus male sling for post-prostatectomy incontinence—what do patient's choose? J Urol. 2009;181:1231–5.

21. Sturm RM, Guralnick ML, Stone AR, Bales GT, Dangle PP, O'Connor RC. Comparison of clinical outcomes between "ideal" and "nonideal" transobturator male sling patients for treatment of post prostatectomy incontinence. Urology. 2014;83(5):1186–8.

13

The EEF1A2 gene expression as risk predictor in localized prostate cancer

Thomas Stefan Worst[1,2*], Frank Waldbillig[1], Abdallah Abdelhadi[1], Cleo-Aron Weis[2], Maria Gottschalt[2], Annette Steidler[1], Jost von Hardenberg[1], Maurice Stephan Michel[1] and Philipp Erben[1]

Abstract

Background: Besides clinical stage and Gleason score, risk-stratification of prostate cancer in the pretherapeutic setting mainly relies on the serum PSA level. Yet, this is associated with many uncertainties. With regard to therapy decision-making, additional markers are needed to allow an exact risk prediction. *Eukaryotic translation elongation factor 1 alpha 2* (EEF1A2) was previously suggested as driver of tumor progression and potential biomarker. In the present study its functional and prognostic relevance in prostate cancer was investigated.

Methods: EEF1A2 expression was analyzed in two cohorts of patients ($n = 40$ and $n = 59$) with localized PCa. Additionally data from two large expression dataset (MSKCC, Cell, 2010 with $n = 131$ localized, $n = 19$ metastatic PCa and TCGA provisional data, $n = 499$) of PCa patients were reanalyzed. The expression of EEF1A2 was correlated with histopathology features and biochemical recurrence (BCR). To evaluate the influence of EEF1A2 on proliferation and migration of metastatic PC3 cells, siRNA interference was used. Statistical significance was tested with t-test, Mann-Whitney-test, Pearson correlation and log-rank test.

Results: qRT-PCR revealed EEF1A2 to be significantly overexpressed in PCa tissue, with an increase according to tumor stage in one cohort ($p = 0.0443$). In silico analyses in the MSKCC cohort confirmed the overexpression of EEF1A2 in localized PCa with high Gleason score ($p = 0.0142$) and in metastatic lesions ($p = 0.0038$). Patients with EEF1A2 overexpression had a significantly shorter BCR-free survival ($p = 0.0028$). EEF1A2 expression was not correlated with serum PSA levels. Similar results were seen in the TCGA cohort, where EEF1A2 overexpression only occurred in tumors with Gleason 7 or higher. Patients with elevated EEF1A2 expression had a significantly shorter BCR-free survival ($p = 0.043$). EEF1A2 knockdown significantly impaired the migration, but not the proliferation of metastatic PC3 cells.

Conclusion: The overexpression of EEF1A2 is a frequent event in localized PCa and is associated with histopathology features and a shorter biochemical recurrence-free survival. Due to its independence from serum PSA levels, EEF1A2 could serve as valuable biomarker in risk-stratification of localized PCa.

Keywords: EEF1A2, Prostate cancer, Risk stratification, Biomarker, Expression, Outcome prediction

Background

In industrialized countries prostate cancer (PCa) is the cancer entity with the highest incidence in men. Though most tumors can be cured in early stages or are insignificant, without need for any treatment at all, around the world over 250,000 patients die from PCa per year [1]. Due to an increasing awareness, PCa screening has become more frequent throughout the last decades. Besides digital rectal exam, prostate specific antigen (PSA) is the current number one screening tool for PCa. But its value is debated controversially [2], due to limited PCa specificity and imprecise prediction of PCa aggressiveness [3]. Mixed models implementing PSA level, biopsy Gleason grade and clinical stage are typically utilized to estimate the individual risk for aggressive PCa with rapid progression along with early metastasization and – together with patient age and risk factors – lead to therapy decision in

* Correspondence: Thomas.Worst@medma.uni-heidelberg.de
[1]Department of Urology, University Medical Centre Mannheim, University of Heidelberg, Theodor-Kutzer-Ufer 1-3, 68167 Mannheim, Germany
[2]Institute of Pathology, University Medical Centre Mannheim, University of Heidelberg, Theodor-Kutzer-Ufer 1-3, 68167 Mannheim, Germany

order to avoid overtreatment by treating only relevant carcinomas [4].

Since these estimations are still imprecise, further markers, either blood- or urine-based or derived from biopsy tissue samples, are needed to specify the individual patient's risk and to facilitate therapy decision-making. Yet, PCa markers intensively studied during the last decade (e.g. genetic markers like the fusion gene TMPRSS2:ERG, circulating tumor cells or urine PCA3 test) are not used in clinical routine [3, 5, 6].

EEF1A2 (*eukaryotic translation elongation factor 1 alpha 2*) is part of a complex that enzymatically delivers aminoacyl tRNAs to the ribosome and is mainly expressed in brain, heart and skeletal muscles [7]. In general it is reported to favor oncogenesis by stimulating the phospholipid signaling and the Akt-dependent cell migration [8]. Besides its role in cancer, EEF1A2 mutations are associated with characteristic facial features, intellectual disability, autistic behavior and epilepsy [9].

There is also evidence, that EEF1A2 expression is predictive for patient outcome in various epithelial cancer entities [10–12]. In PCa one study found the more ubiquitously expressed isoform EEF1A1 to be overexpressed in peri-metastatic osteoblasts in PCa bone metastasis, compared to normal osteoblasts [13]. Another study found an overexpression of EEF1A2 in PCa tissue compared to matched benign tissue in a small preliminary cohort [14]. In the same study the authors could show an overexpression of EEF1A2 to inhibit apoptosis in metastatic PCa cells. Therefore they claimed EEF1A2 to be a hallmark for PCa progression. The impact of EEF1A2 expression – both on the mRNA and on the protein level – on clinical outcome has not been investigated, yet.

To validate recent findings about EEF1A2 overexpression in PCa on the mRNA level, sensitive qRT-PCR techniques were used on two independent cohorts of patients with localized PCa. Subsequent in silico analysis of RNA expression datasets served for validation. To gain further insight into the biological function of EEF1A2 in PCa siRNA interference experiments were conducted in vitro.

Methods

Cohorts and patient samples

qRT-PCR was used to asses EEF1A2 RNA expression in a cDNA array (Origene, Rockville, MD, USA; $n = 40$ PCa patients and $n = 8$ benign control samples). Patient characteristics of this cohort are shown in Table 1.

To further correlate EEF1A2 expression with clinical follow up data, a cohort of 59 patients who underwent radical prostatectomy in the Department of Urology of the Mannheim Medical Center between 1998 and 2001 was analyzed. Patient data of this cohort is given in Table 2. Prostate tissue specimens from patients who underwent

Table 1 Patient characteristics of the cDNA Array purchased from Origene

Parameter	n
Patients with PCa	40 (mean age 62.8 ± 8.2)
T stage	
T1	–
T2	22
T3	12
T4	–
n/a	6
N stage	
N0	20
N1	2
Nx	18
Gleason score	
5	2
6	8
7a	14
7b	8
8	3
9	4
n.a.	1
Control patients	8 (64.0 ± 10.9)

cystoprostatecomy or transurethral resection of the prostate, with histologically proven tumor-free prostate, served as controls. All experiments conducted in this retrospective analysis were in accordance with the institutional ethics review board (ethics approval 2013-845R-MA).

RNA-extraction, cDNA-synthesis and qRT-PCR from patient samples

Sections of tumor-bearing or tumor-free FFPE prostate tissue specimens were stained with hematoxylin and eosin and reviewed by a trained pathologist. Areas with at least 70% of tumor or tumor-free areas from control patients were marked and macrodissected from subsequent unstained 10 μm sections. RNA was extracted using the XTRAKT FFPE kit (Stratifyer, Cologne, Germany), as recommended by the manufacturer. In brief 150 μl of lysis buffer were added to the tissue sample and incubated for 30 min at 80 °C while shaking. After cooling down to 65 °C 50 μl of proteinase K (Roche) were added and incubated for 30 min at 65 °C while shaking. Subsequently 800 μl of MagiX-RNA buffer and 40 μl of MagiX-RNA beads were added and incubated at room temperature for 15 min while shaking. The mixed samples were put on a magnetic rack and washed three times. Finally the RNA was eluted in 100 μl of elution buffer. RNA samples were stored at −80 °C.

Table 2 Patient characteristics of the cohort recruited in Mannheim

Parameter	n
Patients with PCa	59 (mean age 62.9 ± 6.9)
T stage	
T1	–
T2	23
T3	33
T4	3
N stage	
N1	5
N0	47
Nx	7
Gleason score	
3	1
4	0
5	10
6	15
7a	15
7b	4
8	5
9	3
10	2
n.a. due to prior antihormonal therapy	4
average serum PSA level	13.3 ng/ml (2.8–73.0 ng/ml)
Control patients	15 (mean age 67.2 ± 11.3)

To receive a greater yield of target specific transcripts and to reduce contamination with other amplified cDNA sequences, we used a multiplexed specific cDNA synthesis with equimolar pooling of transcript specific reverse PCR primers (primer sequences see below). Superscript III (Life technologies) was used as reverse transcriptase at 55 °C for 120 min, followed by an incubation at 70 °C for 15 min. cDNA was immediately used for qRT-PCR or stored at –20 °C.

In the cDNA array the expression of EEF1A2 was determined in relation to the housekeeping gene Calmodulin 2 (CALM2). Intron spanning primer pairs (CALM2: forward GAGCGAGCTGAGTGGTTGTG reverse AGTCAGTTG GTCAGCCATGCT amplicon length 72 nt; EEF1A2: forward GGACCATTGAGAAGTTCGAGA, reverse AGCAC CCAGGCATACTTGAA, amplicon length 70 nt) compatible with the Universal Probe library (Roche Diagnostics) were designed using the primer3 algorithm [15]. In brief 10 µl of TaqMan Fast Universal PCR Mastermix (Life technologies), 0.75 µl of forward and reverse primer each (300 nM) (MWG Eurofins, Ebersberg, Germany) 0.5 µl of PCR probe (200 nM) (Roche Diagnostics) and 6 µl of nuclease free H_2O were added to 2 µl of cDNA template each. Subsequently 40 cycles of amplification with 1 s of

95 °C and 20 s of 60 °C were conducted on a Step One Plus qRT-PCR cycler (Applied Biosystems, Waltham, MA, USA). To allow a higher input of cDNA, the volume of primers was halved for qRT-PCR analysis of the Mannheim cohort. RNA-expression was calculated with the $2^{(-\Delta\Delta cT)}$-method [16].

Datamining and in silico validation

From the online platform CBioPortal [17] RNA expression data (z-score normalized) of two datasets also comprising clinical follow-up were downloaded: The MSKCC dataset consists of 131 primary an 19 metastatic tumor samples *(Taylor* et al., *Cancer Cell, 2010)* [18]. The TCGA (The Cancer Genome Atlas) dataset includes expression data of 499 primary PCa samples. EEF1A2 RNA expression was stratified by tumor characteristics and correlated with BCR-free (biochemical recurrence) survival and serum PSA levels.

Cell culture, siRNA knockdown and knockdown validation

Human PC3 metastatic PCa cells were obtained from ATCC (Wesel, Germany) and grown under standard conditions in DMEM (Life Technologies, Carlsbad, CA, USA) supplemented with 10% FCS (Sigma Aldrich, St. Louis, LA, USA). siGENOME pooled and individual siRNAs against EEF1A2 (No 1 GTACAAGATTGGCGGCATT, No 2 TCAAGAAGATCGGCTACAA, No 3 CTACAAAT GCGGAGGTATT, No 4 ATGCGGAGGTATTGACAAA) were transfected using Dharmafect I transfection reagent (Dharmacon, Lafayette, CO, USA). Dharmacon nontargeting siRNA were used as negative control. Briefly cells were detached, harvested, spun down and diluted to the desired concentration. Meanwhile siRNAs were diluted to a target concentration of 30nMol in pure RPMI (Life Technologies) and incubated for 10 min at room temperature. Dharmafect I was diluted 1:1000 in RPMI. After 10 min diluted siRNA and transfection reagent were mixed 1:1 and again incubated at room temperature for 30 min. Hereafter cell suspension was added to the transfection mix 3:1 and incubated at 37 °C.

qRT-PCR was conducted to validate knockdown of EEF1A2. RNA-extraction was performed using the RNeasy Mini Kit (Qiagen, Hilden, Germany) as recommended by the manufacturer. cDNA-Synthesis was performed as described previously [19]: in brief 40 µl of diluted RNA were mixed with 4 µl of 5 mg/ml pdN6 random primers, 4 µl of 10 mM dNTP Mix, 16 µl of 5× M-MLV buffer, 8 µl of 0.1 M RNase inhibitor, 4 µl of 0.1 M DTT and 4 µl of M-MLV reverse transcriptase (all from Roche Diagnostics, Basel, Switzerland). After an incubation for 2 h at 37 °C and a deactivation step of 5 min at 65 °C, cDNA was directly used for qRT-PCR or stored at –20 °C. qRT-PCR analyses were performed using the same primers, reagents and PCR protocol as described for tissue sample analyses.

Proliferation assay

PC3 cells were seeded and transfected following the protocol described above in 96-well plates (4500 cells in 100 μl/well). After 24 h the supernatant was replaced by 100 μl of fresh growth medium (DMEM with 10% FCS). After further 24, 48 and 72 h of incubation 10 μl of MTT-reagent (Promega, Mannheim, Germany) were added to each well and incubated for 3 h at 37 °C. Absorption measurement at 570 nm was done with an Infinite M1000 Pro plate reader (Tecan, Männerdorf, Switzerland).

Scratch assay

Using the same transfection protocol, PC3 cells were seeded in 24-well plates (250,000 cells in 1 ml of DMEM with 10% FCS per well). The medium was changed 24 h after transfection. Again 24 h later a defined scratch was introduced in the center of the well with a sterile 200 μl pipette tip and the medium was changed again. The scratch was photographed at 10× magnification. Subsequent images were acquired after further 24, 48 and 72 h. The cell free space in the scratch area was calculated with the open source software *tscratch* (ETH Zürich, Switzerland) [20]. The free area 24, 48 and 72 h after scratch were normalized to the initial scratch size.

Statistics

Statistical calculations were performed using Prism 6 (Graphpad, La Jolla, USA). Mann-Whitney-Test was used for calculation of inter-group expression changes in patient cohorts analyzed with qRT-PCR and in silico data. Outcome correlations were done using the log-rank test. Correlations with the PSA serum level were performed using Pearson correlation. Parametric t-test was used for in vitro assays. *P*-values ≤0.05 were deemed significant.

Results

qRT-PCR analysis indicates EEF1A2 overexpression in PCa patients

To investigate the expression of EEF1A2 in PCa qRT-PCR expression analyses in a cDNA array of 40 patients with localized PCa were performed. Compared to benign tissue samples EEF1A2 was overexpressed 6.76-fold in T2 tumors ($p = 0.006$) and 16.6-fold in T3 tumors ($p = 0.0011$) (Fig. 1a). The expression was also significantly higher in T3 compared to T2 tumors ($p = 0.0443$). Similar results were seen after stratification for Gleason grade (Fig. 1b). Tumors with a Gleason score ≤ 7a had a 7.22-fold higher expression of EEF1A2 ($p = 0.0064$). In tumors with Gleason ≥7b a 15.09-fold higher expression was seen ($p = 0.0004$). Though EEF1A2 expression was higher in tumors with higher Gleason score, no significant difference was seen between tumors with Gleason score ≤ 7a and ≥7b ($p = 0.0541$).

Since the analyzed cDNA array did not provide clinical follow-up data, the expression of EEF1A2 was further evaluated in a cohort of 59 patients treated with radical prostatectomy in the Mannheim Medical Center. EEF1A2 was significantly overexpressed in these tumor samples (Fig. 2a). In T2 tumors EEF1A2 was 2.16-fold overexpressed compared to benign controls ($p = 0.0277$). In T3/4 tumors a 2.23-fold overexpression was observed ($p = 0.0325$). In this dataset no significant difference in expression was seen between T2 tumors and locally advanced tumors.

EEF1A2 expression did not correlate with the serum PSA level ($r = -0.02058$; $p = 0.8771$). Kaplan-Meier analysis revealed a slightly shorter recurrence-free survival of patients with high EEF1A2 expression (mean follow-up 67.5 months, ± 51.2 months, Fig. 2b). Yet, log-rank test showed this difference not to be significant ($p = 0.14$). Taken together, these results point to a potential relevance of EEF1A2 risk predictor in localized PCa.

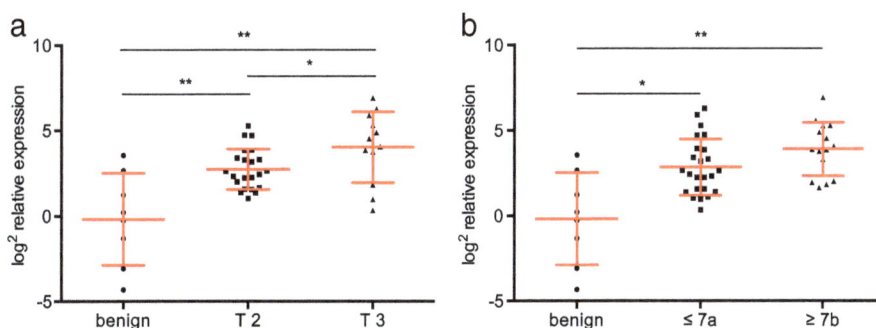

Fig. 1 qRT-PCR analysis in a panel of 40 PCa patients showed an overexpression of EEF1A2 in localized tumor samples. **a)** EEF1A2 expression was significantly dependent of tumor stage. **b)** The averages expression was higher in tumors with a Gleason score ≥ 7b, but this difference did not reach significance

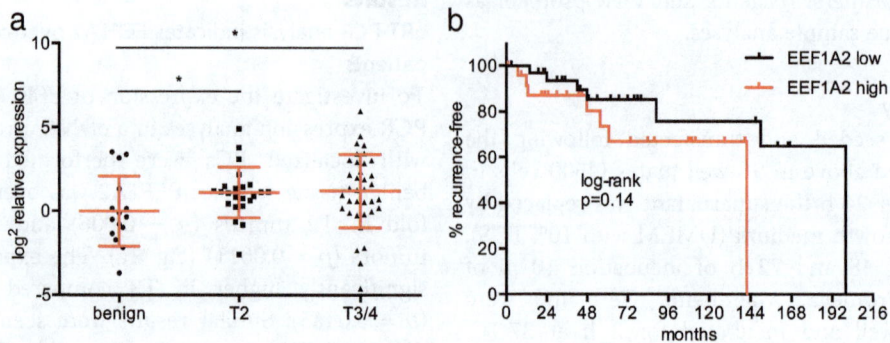

Fig. 2 a) In a cohort of 59 patients, undergoing radical prostatectomy EEF1A2 was overexpressed in PCa. There was no significant difference between tumor stages. **b**) Patients with high EEF1A2 expression in the primary tumor in tendency showed a shorter recurrence-free survival. Yet, log-rank test showed this difference not to be significant

In silico analyses reveal EEF1A2 as outcome predictor in localized PCa

To validate the expression of EEF1A2 in large cohorts of PCa patients, in silico analyses on the RNA expression microarray dataset by *Taylor* et al. *and on the RNA sequencing data of the TCGA cohort* were conducted. In the *Taylor* et al. dataset 16.8% of patients with localized PCa had a z-score ≥ 2, compared to benign controls (Fig. 3a). In metastatic tumor samples EEF1A2 overexpression was found in 52.6% of the patients. The highest expression was seen in PCa metastases ($p = 0.0038$ when compared with Gleason 6 localized tumors; Fig. 3b). Focusing on primary tumors, overexpression of EEF1A2 was a rare event in Gleason 6 tumors (2/41, 4.9%), and

rather seldom in Gleason 7 tumors (13/74, 17.6%). Among Gleason 8/9 tumors, 7 out of 15 (46.7%) had an EEF1A2 z-score > 2. In line with the qRT-PCR data presented here, this indicated a higher expression of EEF1A2 in more aggressive tumors ($p = 0.0142$ for Gleason 8/9 tumors vs. Gleason 6 tumors). Pearson correlation of EEF1A2 with the serum PSA levels at the time of surgery again showed no correlation ($r = 0.1590$; $p = 0.0708$).

Then EEF1A2 expression in primary tumors was correlated with patient outcome. Interestingly patients with an expression z-score of EEF1A2 ≥ 2 had a significantly shortened BCR-free survival compared to patients without EEF1A2 overexpression ($p = 0.0028$, mean follow-up 48.5 months, $\pm$ 29.6 months, Fig. 3c).

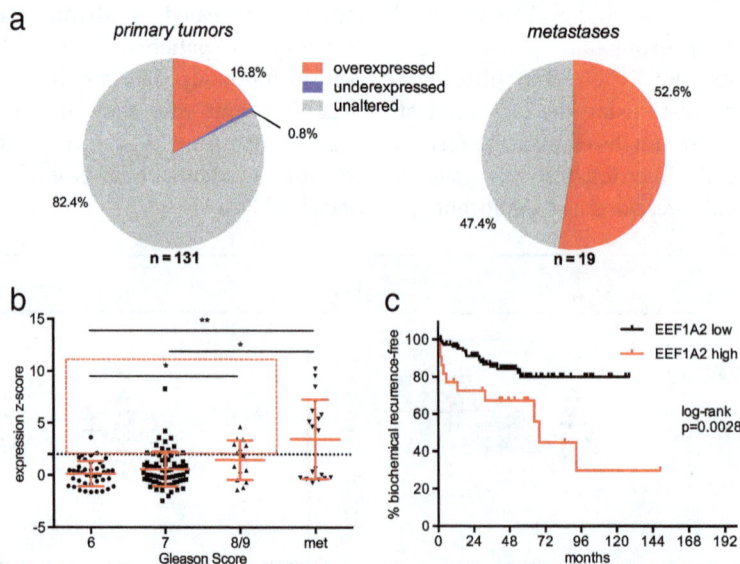

Fig. 3 In silico *validation of EEF1A2* **a**) Reanalysis of the microarray dataset by *Taylor* et al. revealed EEF1A2 to be overexpressed in 16.9% of localized PCA and in 52.6% of metastatic PCa (dashed line indicates an expression z-score of 2 compared to benign tissue). **b**) EEF1A2 overexpression was grade dependent in localized PCa and highest in metastases. **c**) Localized tumors with high EEF1A2 expression (indicated by a red square in **b**) had a significantly shorter biochemical recurrence-free survival

In the TCGA cohort (n = 499) there was no significant difference in the average expression of EEF1A2 according to the Gleason Score (Fig. 4a). Yet, only tumors with a Gleason Score of 7 or higher showed an overexpression of EEF1A2 (z-score $\geq$ 2). Tumors with an elevated EEF1A2 expression had a significantly shorter BCR-free survival (p = 0.043; Fig. 4b). The serum PSA levels of the patients in this cohort are not available and could therefore not be correlated with the EEF1A expression.

EEF1A2 is functionally involved in PCa migration but not in proliferation

To get a first insight into the function of EEF1A2 in PCa, transient transfection experiments were conducted in metastatic PC3 cells. qRT-PCR verified a strong knockdown effect for all used siRNAs (Fig. 5a). For further experiments siRNA No 3, which produced the strongest knockdown, was used.

In the MTT assay knockdown of EEF1A did not lead to a significant alteration of PC3 cell proliferation (Fig. 5b). By using scratch wound healing assay the influence of EEF1A2 knockdown on PC3 cell migration was studied. A significant reduction of migration in cells with EEF1A2 knockdown was observed (p = 0.035). After 24 h, 55.6% of the initial scratch area were covered by control-transfected cells, whereas only 44.7% were covered in EEF1A2-knockdown cells (Fig. 5c).

Discussion

The study aimed to determine the EEF1A2 expression in PCa tissue, to test for its potential relevance as risk predictor in localized PCa and to gain insight into its functional role of in PCa.

EEF1A2 was overexpressed in localized PCa with a stage-dependent increase in one of the two cohorts tested with qRT-PCR. In silico analyses of one *Taylor* et al. dataset confirmed the overexpression of EEF1A2 in aggressive localized PCa. The expression was dependent of the Gleason Score and patients with a high expression

in localized PCa had a significantly shorter BCR-free survival. In the TCGA dataset EEF1A2 overexpression only occurred in tumors with a Gleason Score of 7 or higher and again tumors with an elevated EEF1A2 expression had a significantly shorter BCR-free survival. qRT-PCR results also point to a potential association with recurrence-free survival. Though the cohorts analyzed with qRT-PCR were of limited patient number they are to date the largest series, in which EEF1A2 expression was profiled in PCa with a specific method. Furthermore this is the first study correlating clinical follow-up data with EEF1A2 expression in PCa.

Data on metastatic tumors has not been reported, yet. By reanalyzing existing microarray data, we revealed EEF1A2 to be overexpression in more than 50% of PCa metastases, underlining its association with an aggressive PCa phenotype.

Since EEF1A2 expression was not correlated with serum PSA levels it might provide additional value in PCa risk stratification of localized PCa as a tissue based marker, e.g. from prostate biopsy samples. In this setting qRT-PCR offers several advantages compared to conventional immunohistochemistry. qRT-PCR is more sensitive, allows a better quantification and therefore contributes to a better comparability between samples. Furthermore results are less observer-dependent. However, qRT-PCR does not give information about the expression pattern in the tissue.

The results of the present study are in accordance with results from the recent literature. *Scaggiante* et al. [21] deemed EEF1A2 as a marker for prostate cell transformation and a potential hallmark of cancer progression, since they found it overexpressed in metastatic PCa cell lines, compared with benign prostate cells. Additionally they found it to be overexpressed both in PCa tissue and peritumoral stroma in a small series of nine PCa patients.

Sun et al. [14] found a significantly higher RNA expression of EEF1A2 in 26 out of 30 primary PCa samples compared to matched control samples. Using the same

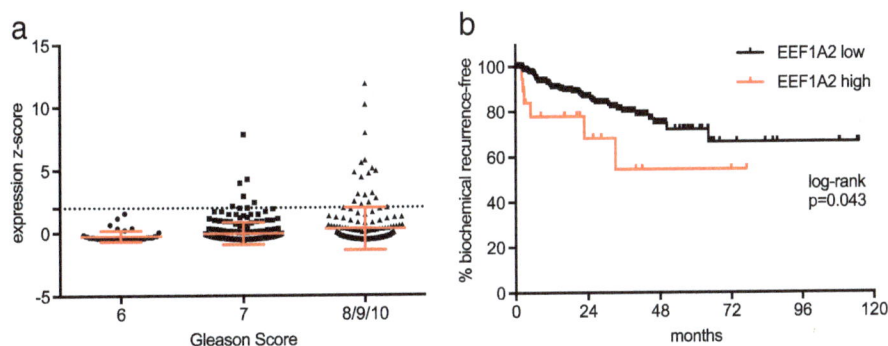

Fig. 4 a) EEF1A2 expression in the TCGA cohort (n = 499; dashed line indicated an expression z-score of 2). **b)** Tumors with an elevated EEF1A2 expression had a significantly shorter BCR-free survival

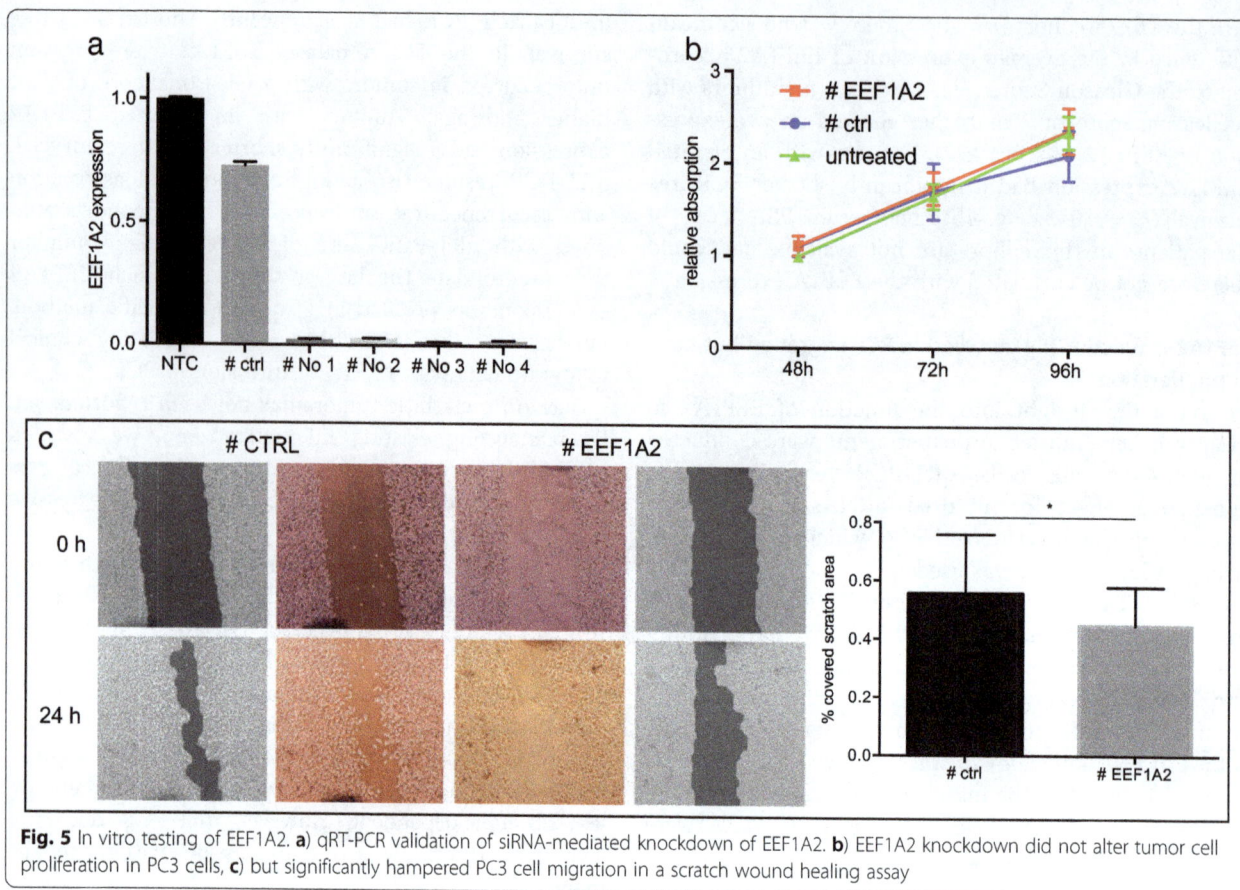

Fig. 5 In vitro testing of EEF1A2. **a)** qRT-PCR validation of siRNA-mediated knockdown of EEF1A2. **b)** EEF1A2 knockdown did not alter tumor cell proliferation in PC3 cells, **c)** but significantly hampered PC3 cell migration in a scratch wound healing assay

cohort they could validate these results on the protein level using immunohistochemistry. When they correlated their immunohistochemistry results with clinical features (age, PSA >/≤ 50 ng/ml, Gleason >/≤ 7, stages >/≤ T2), they did not find a significant correlation. Unfortunately they only performed these correlations on the protein level and did not further stratify their cohort. Additionally the number of patients in this study was comparably small. Therefore a correlation of EEF1A2 expression and the analyzed clinical features might have been missed. They also did not implement any follow-up data, making an outcome prediction impossible.

Reports on EEF1A2 expression in other tumor entities show differing results. Interestingly some studies attribute a higher expression of EEF1A2 with a poor prognosis, whilst others found it to be associated with a favorable outcome. In a large cohort of 438 primary breast cancer specimen, absence of EEF1A2 protein expression was a predictor of poor outcome [10]. EEF1A2 expression was not associated with other established prediction markers like HER-2 protein expression, tumor size, lymph node status, and estrogen receptor expression.

Controversially negative staining for EEF1A2 was a predictor for poor outcome in patients with non-small cell lung cancer [22]. In pancreatic ductal adenocarcinoma elevated expression of EEF1A2 was associated with nodal metastasis, perineural invasion and worse prognosis [11].

In vitro testing via siRNA-interference of EEF1A2 revealed a reduction of PC3 cell migration, indicating a potential tumor promoting function. Results on the impact of EEF1A2 on PCa cell migration have not been reported so far. The growth of PC3 cells was not altered. Interestingly another study showed a significant reduction of PCa cell growth and colony formation upon knockdown of EEF1A2 [14], which is partly controversial to the findings in the present study. Yet, differing results might be caused by different assay conditions like the growth media and siRNAs used.

A reduced growth of PCa cells upon EEF1A2 knockdown is in line with the proposed pro-oncogenic function of EEF1A2 in PCa. The same study also found an increase in apoptosis upon knockdown of EEF1A2, which had already been described in studies on other solid cancer entities [23, 24].

In pancreatic cancer EEF1A2 overexpression also resulted in an activation of AKT and led to an overexpression of the matrixmetallo-protease MMP9, which is a key player in extracellular matrix reorganization in context of cancer progression [12].

In hepatocellular carcinoma EEF1A2 was shown to inactivate P53 via an upstream activation of the PI3K/AKT/mTOR-pathway [25]. This gives rationale to a druggability of EEF1A2-dependent tumor growth in PCa with mTOR inhibitors, which are already in clinical use e.g. for metastatic renal cell carcinoma, breast cancer, neuroendocrine tumors and certain lymphomas [26, 27]. Actually, several early clinical trials using mTOR inhibitors in metastatic PCa are ongoing but merely show discouraging results [28–30]. A recent systematic review suggested reciprocal feedback mechanisms between PI3K and androgen receptor signaling to be causative for this and proposed a combinatorial targeted therapy of PI3K, mTOR and the androgen receptor [30].

Conclusion

qRT-PCR and in silico expression analyses confirm recent reports from smaller series about EEF1A2 overexpression in localized PCa. Furthermore this is the first study describing EEF1A2 expression to be stage- and grade dependent and EEF1A2 overexpression to be predictive for the outcome of patients with localized PCa. Since EEF1A2 expression is not correlated with serum PSA levels, it might serve as an additional biomarker for PCa risk stratification. Further prospective studies, investigating EEF1A2 expression e.g. in needle biopsy samples are needed to evaluate its value as prognostic biomarker. In vitro experiments give an outlook on the functional role of EEF1A2 in PCa.

Abbreviations

BCR: Biochemical recurrence; EEF1A2: Eukaryotic translation elongation factor 1 alpha 2; MSKCC: Memorial Sloan Kettering Cancer Center; PCa: Prostate cancer; qRT-PCR: Quantitative real-time PCR; TCGA: The Cancer Genome Atlas; TMPRSS2:ERG: Transmembrane protease, serine 2:ETS-related gene

Acknowledgements

None.

Funding

This work was supported by the foundation on cancer and scarlet research of the University of Heidelberg. T.S.W. was supported by a Ferdinand Eisenberger scholarship of the German Society of Urology.

Authors' contributions

TSW, FW, AA and AS processed and analyzed tissue samples. FW performed in vitro assays. TSW carried out in silico analyses. CAW and MG carried out pathologic review of tissue samples. TSW, JvH, MSM and PE planned the study and wrote the manuscript. All authors read and approved the final manuscript.

Competing interests

The authors declare that they have no competing interests.

References

1. Jemal A, Bray F, Center MM, Ferlay J, Ward E, Forman D. Global cancer statistics. CA Cancer J Clin. 2011;61:69–90.
2. Ilic D, Neuberger MM, Djulbegovic M, Dahm P. Screening for prostate cancer. Cochrane Database Syst Rev Online. 2013;1:CD004720.
3. Prensner JR, Rubin MA, Wei JT, Chinnaiyan AM. Beyond PSA: the next generation of prostate cancer biomarkers. Sci Transl Med. 2012;4:127rv3–3.
4. Heidenreich A, Bastian PJ, Bellmunt J, Bolla M, Joniau S, van der Kwast T, et al. EAU guidelines on prostate cancer. Part 1: screening, diagnosis, and local treatment with curative intent-update 2013. Eur Urol. 2014;65:124–37.
5. Choudhury AD, Eeles R, Freedland SJ, Isaacs WB, Pomerantz MM, Schalken JA, et al. The role of genetic markers in the management of prostate cancer. Eur Urol. 2012;62:577–87.
6. Armstrong AJ, Eisenberger MA, Halabi S, Oudard S, Nanus DM, Petrylak DP, et al. Biomarkers in the management and treatment of men with metastatic castration-resistant prostate cancer. Eur Urol. 2012;61:549–59.
7. Lee M-H, Surh Y-J. eEF1A2 as a putative oncogene. Ann N Y Acad Sci. 2009; 1171:87–93.
8. Abbas W, Kumar A, Herbein G. The eEF1A proteins: at the crossroads of Oncogenesis, apoptosis, and viral infections. Front Oncol. 2015;5:75.
9. Nakajima J, Okamoto N, Tohyama J, Kato M, Arai H, Funahashi O, et al. De novo EEF1A2 mutations in patients with characteristic facial features, intellectual disability, autistic behaviors and epilepsy. Clin Genet. 2015;87: 356–61.
10. Kulkarni G, Turbin DA, Amiri A, Jeganathan S, Andrade-Navarro MA, Wu TD, et al. Expression of protein elongation factor eEF1A2 predicts favorable outcome in breast cancer. Breast Cancer Res Treat. 2007;102:31–41.
11. Duanmin H, XC. eEF1A2 protein expression correlates with lymph node metastasis and decreased survival in pancreatic Ductal Adenocarcinoma. Hepato-Gastroenterology. 2012;60
12. Xu C, Hu D, Zhu Q. eEF1A2 promotes cell migration, invasion and metastasis in pancreatic cancer by upregulating MMP-9 expression through Akt activation. Clin Exp Metastasis. 2013;30:933–44.
13. Rehman I, Evans CA, Glen A, Cross SS, Eaton CL, Down J, et al. iTRAQ identification of candidate serum biomarkers associated with metastatic progression of human prostate cancer. PLoS One. 2012;7:e30885.
14. Sun Y, Du C, Wang B, Zhang Y, Liu X, Ren G. Up-regulation of eEF1A2 promotes proliferation and inhibits apoptosis in prostate cancer. Biochem Biophys Res Commun. 2014;450:1–6.
15. Untergasser A, Cutcutache I, Koressaar T, Ye J, Faircloth BC, Remm M, et al. Primer3–new capabilities and interfaces. Nucleic Acids Res. 2012;40:e115.
16. Livak KJ, Schmittgen TD. Analysis of relative gene expression data using real-time quantitative PCR and the 2−ΔΔCT method. Methods. 2001;25:402–8.
17. Cerami E, Gao J, Dogrusoz U, Gross BE, Sumer SO, Aksoy BA, et al. The cBio cancer genomics portal: an open platform for exploring multidimensional cancer genomics data. Cancer Discov. 2012;2:401–4.
18. Taylor BS, Schultz N, Hieronymus H, Gopalan A, Xiao Y, Carver BS, et al. Integrative genomic profiling of human prostate cancer. Cancer Cell. 2010; 18:11–22.
19. Worst TS, Meyer Y, Gottschalt M, Weis C-A, von Hardenberg J, Frank C, et al. RAB27A, RAB27B and VPS36 are downregulated in advanced prostate cancer and show functional relevance in prostate cancer cells. Int J Oncol. 2017;50:920–32.
20. Ashby WJ, Zijlstra A. Established and novel methods of interrogating two-dimensional cell migration. Integr Biol Quant Biosci Nano Macro. 2012;4: 1338–50.
21. Scaggiante B, Dapas B, Bonin S, Grassi M, Zennaro C, Farra R, et al. Dissecting the expression of EEF1A1/2 genes in human prostate cancer cells: the potential of EEF1A2 as a hallmark for prostate transformation and progression. Br J Cancer. 2012;106:166–73.
22. Kawamura M, Endo C, Sakurada A, Hoshi F, Notsuda H, Kondo T. The prognostic significance of eukaryotic elongation factor 1 alpha-2 in non-small cell lung cancer. Anticancer Res. 2014;34:651–8.
23. Anand N, Murthy S, Amann G, Wernick M, Porter LA, Cukier IH, et al. Protein elongation factor EEF1A2 is a putative oncogene in ovarian cancer. Nat Genet. 2002;31:301–5.
24. Migliaccio N, Martucci NM, Ruggiero I, Sanges C, Ohkubo S, Lamberti A, et al. Ser/Thr kinases and polyamines in the regulation of non-canonical functions of elongation factor 1A. Amino Acids. 2016;48:2339–52.
25. Pellegrino R, Calvisi DF, Neumann O, Kolluru V, Wesely J, Chen X, et al. EEF1A2 inactivates p53 by way of PI3K/AKT/mTOR-dependent stabilization of MDM4 in hepatocellular carcinoma. Hepatol Baltim Md. 2014;59:1886–99.

26. Voss MH, Molina AM, Motzer RJ. mTOR inhibitors in advanced renal cell carcinoma. Hematol Oncol Clin North Am. 2011;25:835–52.

27. Zhu AX, Abrams TA, Miksad R, Blaszkowsky LS, Meyerhardt JA, Zheng H, et al. Phase 1/2 study of everolimus in advanced hepatocellular carcinoma. Cancer. 2011;117:5094–102.

28. Armstrong AJ, Shen T, Halabi S, Kemeny G, Bitting RL, Kartcheske P, et al. A phase II trial of temsirolimus in men with castration-resistant metastatic prostate cancer. Clin Genitourin Cancer. 2013;11:397–406.

29. Emmenegger U, Booth CM, Berry S, Sridhar SS, Winquist E, Bandali N, et al. Temsirolimus maintenance therapy after Docetaxel induction in castration-resistant prostate cancer. Oncologist. 2015;20:1351–2.

30. Statz CM, Patterson SE, Mockus SM. mTOR Inhibitors in Castration-Resistant Prostate Cancer: A Systematic Review. Target Oncol. 2017;12:47-59.

14

Efficacy of commercialised extracorporeal shock wave lithotripsy service: a review of 589 renal stones

Tommy Kjærgaard Nielsen*⊙ and Jørgen Bjerggaard Jensen

Abstract

Background: Extracorporeal shockwave lithotripsy (ESWL) is the management of choice for renal stones 20 mm or smaller, with a stone clearance rate of up to 89%. The purpose of the present is to investigate the efficacy of a commercialised ESWL service, being performed as an outsourced treatment using a mobile lithotripsy system on an outpatient basis. Furthermore, the study aims to evaluate the risk of needing treatment with an internal ureteral double-J stent (JJ) after ESWL treatment.

Methods: During an eight-year period, 461 patients with a total of 589 renal stones were treated using a mobile lithotripsy system at a single Danish institution. A commercial company performed all treatments using a Storz Modulith SLK® system. Each stone was prospectively registered according to size, intra renal location and the presence of a JJ at the time of treatment. The number of required ESWL treatments and auxiliary procedures were retrospectively evaluated.

Results: The success rate after the initial ESWL procedure was 69%, which increased to an overall success rate of 93% after repeated treatment. A negative correlation was found between stone size and the overall success rate ($r = -0.2$, $p < 0.01$). The upper calyx was associated with a significantly better success rate, but otherwise intra renal stone location was not predictive for treatment success. A total of 17 patients (2.9%) required treatment with a JJ after the ESWL procedure. No significant difference was observed between the stone size or intra renal location and the risk of needing treatment with JJ after ESWL.

Conclusions: Commercialised ESWL treatment can achieve an overall success rate of more than 90% using a mobile lithotripsy system. As expected, an inverse relation between stone size and success rate was found. Patients who do not require treatment with a JJ prior to ESWL will only rarely need treatment with a JJ after ESWL, irrespective of stone size and intra renal stone location.

Keywords: Urinary calculi, Eswl, Lithotripsy, Mobile, Shockwave, Stones, Ureteral stent

Background

Extracorporeal shock wave lithotripsy (ESWL) was introduced in the 1980s and is still considered an effective and minimal invasive treatment of symptomatic as well as asymptomatic nephrolithiasis.

In most cases, treatment can be preformed on an outpatient basis with none or minimal anaesthesia. ESWL is a well-established management for nephrolithiasis and is the suggested first line treatment together with retrograde intrarenal surgery (RIRS) for stones smaller than 2 cm in the renal pelvis or upper/middle calyx, according to European Association of Urology (EAU) guidelines. However, it is still debated what the best practice is for patients with lower pole stones. The overall efficacy of ESWL for nephrolithiasis depends mainly on stone size, location, stone composition, patient habitus and performance of ESWL [1, 2]. Reports from high volume centres with static machines suggests stone clearance rates of 86–89%, 71–83%, 73–84% and 37–68% for stones in the renal pelvis, upper calyx, middle calyx and lower pole calyx, respectively [3–6].

* Correspondence: tomnie@rm.dk
Department of Urology, Hospitalsenheden Vest, Holstebro, Denmark

Outsourcing of EWSL procedures has routinely been used in Denmark where a static system was unavailable. Lithotripsy services were performed by dedicated technicians who visited hospitals periodically and provided treatments using a mobile lithotripsy system. However, such outsourcing of medical procedures may lack clinical ownership and inconsistencies, thus potentially risking inferior clinical results [7]. There are only a very limited number of studies that explores the efficacy of mobile lithotripter services being performed by commercial companies. And as health care services continuously are being outsourced to private operators it seems reasonable to investigate the efficacy of such treatment.

This study presents an assessment of the efficacy of such commercialised lithotripsy service in terms of stone free rate and auxiliary procedures. Furthermore, the study assesses the risk of having treatment with a JJ after the ESWL procedure due to complications associated with acute ureteral obstruction.

Methods

During an eight-year period a total of 461 patients (261 males and 200 females) with a mean age of 59 years (range 20–90 years) and with a total of 589 renal stones, underwent commercialised ESWL treatment at The Regional Hospital Holstebro, Denmark. All patients were prior to treatment radiographically diagnosed by noncontast computed tomography (CT).

Information regarding stone size (<5 mm, 5–10 mm, 10-20 mm and >20 mm) and intra renal stone location (upper calyx, middle calyx, lower calyx and renal pelvis), as well as treatment with JJ prior to ESWL was registered at the time of treatment. Treatment outcome and auxiliary procedures were retrospectively evaluated. Stone characteristics are summarized in Table 1.

All treatments were preformed on an outpatient basis by a commercial company (MLS Medical, Denmark) using a mobile lithotriptor system (Storz Modulith® SLK, Stortz Medical, Switzerland) featuring X-ray and ultrasound localization. Experienced technicians performed all treatment and were assisted by the responsible urologist. Treatment protocols followed producer recommendations: a) maximum 3500 impulses by 0,82 mJ/mm2 and later b) maximum 4000 impulses by 0,77 mJ/mm2. The amount of analgesia used was individualised and was at the discretion of the treating urologist. Post-

ESWL stone-expulsive treatment such as tamsulosin was not used.

Stone fragmentation was assessed two weeks after treatment using non-contrast CT and patients were considered stone free if CT confirmed stone clearance or the persistence of fragments smaller than 2 mm in maximum diameter. The treating policy towards ESWL was liberal, and there was no maximum fixed number of ESWL attempts as long as progress was observed. If there was no progress after two ESWL attempts auxiliary procedures was initiated.

The department had a restrictive policy towards the use of JJ in patients with nephrolithiasis. Thus, patients were not routinely treated with a JJ either prior to or after ESWL as a result of stone size or intra renal stone location. A JJ was only placed if the patient had hydronephrosis or was discomforted in such a degree that it could not be controlled with oral analgesics.

For statistical analysis of the data, chi-squared, Fischer's exact or Student's t-test were used as appropriate. In correlation analysis Pearson correlation coefficient were estimated. Statistical significance was evaluated based on a two-sided significance level of 0.05. Data analysis was performed using STATA v.14 software (StataCorp, LP, USA).

Results

A total of 408 stones (69%) were successfully treated with the initial ESWL procedure, which increased to 549 stones (93%) after repeated ESWL treatments (average number of treatments per stone = 1.4). A total of 40 stones (7%) did not respond to ESWL treatment and were treated with RIRS (n = 26) or percutaneous nephrolithotomy (PNL) (n = 14).

The mean number of ESWL sessions required for stones <5 mm, 5-10 mm, 10-20 mm and >20 mm were 1.1, 1.3, 1.6 and 1.4, respectively ($p < 0.01$). The overall ESWL success rates were 98%, 95%, 88%, and 75% respectively ($p < 0.05$). A correlation analysis between stone size and the overall ESWL success rate demonstrated a significant decrease in success rate as stone size increases (r = –0.2, $p < 0.01$). Treatment outcomes according to stone size are summarized in Table 2.

The mean number of ESWL sessions for stones in upper-, middle-, lower calyx and renal pelvis was 1.3, 1.2, 1.4 and 1.3 respectively ($p > 0.05$). The overall

Table 1 Distribution of intra renal stone location and stone size. Number of stones (%)

	Total	< 5 mm	5–10 mm	10–20 mm	>20 mm
Upper calyx, n (%)	77 (13)	23 (30)	46 (60)	8 (10)	0
Middle calyx, n (%)	76 (13)	21 (28)	47 (62)	8 (10)	0
Lower calyx, n (%)	257 (44)	46 (18)	147 (57)	59 (23)	5 (2)
Renal pelvis, n (%)	179 (30)	15 (9)	101 (56)	56 (31)	7 (4)

Table 2 Treatment outcome in relation to stone size

	< 5 mm n = 105 (18%)	5–10 mm n = 341 (58%)	10–20 mm n = 131 (22%)	> 20 mm n = 12 (2%)
Mean no of sessions (range)	1.1 (1–3)	1.3 (1–4)	1.6 (1–4)	1.4 (1–3)
Success after initial ESWL, n (%)	90 (86)	245 (72)	67 (51)	6 (50)
Accumulated success after 2nd ESWL, n (%)	102 (97)	303 (89)	99 (76)	8 (67)
Accumulated success after ≥3rd ESWL, n (%)	103 (98)	322 (95)	115 (88)	9 (75)
JJ present at ESWL, n (%)	5 (5)	29 (9)	20 (15)	2 (17)
Acute JJ placement after ESWL, n (%)	0	11 (3)	6 (5)	0

ESWL success rates were 99%, 95%, 93% and 91% respectively. With the exception of the upper calyx ($p < 0.05$), intra renal stone location did not prove to be predictive for ESWL efficacy ($p > 0.05$). Treatment outcomes according to intra renal stone location are summarized in Table 3.

The majority of patients (90.5%) did not have a JJ at the time of ESWL treatment. As expected, significantly more patients were treated with a JJ prior to ESWL when stones were located in the renal pelvis compared to other intra renal stone locations ($p = 0.05$). Table 4 provides the efficacy rates according the presence of a JJ. A total of 17 patients (2.9%) were treated with a JJ due to post-ESWL hydronephrosis, pain or steinstrasse. The median time from ESWL to treatment with a JJ were 31 days (95%CI±13). No significant difference was

Table 3 Treatment outcome according to intra renal stone location

	Upper Calyx n = 77 (13%)	Middle Calyx n = 76 (13%)	Lower Calyx n = 257 (44%)	Renal Pelvis n = 179 (30%)
Mean no of sessions (range)	1.3 (1–3)	1.2 (1–3)	1.4 (1–4)	1.3 (1–4)
Success after 1st ESWL, n (%)	53 (69)	59 (78)	171 (67)	124 (69)
Accumulated success after 2nd ESWL, n (%)	73 (95)	69 (91)	215 (84)	154 (86)
Accumulated success after ≥3rd ESWL, n (%)	76 (99)	72 (95)	238 (93)	163 (91)
JJ present at ESWL, n (%)	3 (4)	3 (4)	17 (7)	33 (18)
JJ placement after ESWL, n (%)	0	1 (1)	10 (4)	6 (3)

observed between either stone size or intra renal stone location and the risk of needing treatment with a JJ after ESWL ($p > 0.05$).

Discussion

The overall rate of stone clearance in this study was found to be in line with the reported stone free rate of centres with static machines. The overall stone free rate of 93% found in this study is significantly different from what was described in a recent study by Nafie et al., reporting a stone clearance rate of 49% [7]. In the study by Nafie it was speculated whether the low rate of stone clearance was due to a relative high proportion of patient with stones in the lower pole (43.3%). This is in significant contrast to a stone clearance of 93% for lower pole stones found in the present study, were 44% of the stones were located in the lower pole.

With regard to patient selection, information on the lower pole anatomy was not available and might have favoured stone clearance rates in this study but is unlikely to account for such large differences. Furthermore, the efficacy of ESWL is very dependent on the skills of the technician performing the treatment and in the present study treatments were carried out by a small team of very skilled and dedicated technicians [8]. In a previous multicentre study it was demonstrated that a transportable ESWL system had a high margin of safety with low complications rates and no apparent sacrifice of efficacy with regard to non-transportable systems [9].

Management of stones in the lower calyx using ESWL remains somewhat controversial. It has been reported that lower pole stones carry a lower success rate after ESWL monotherapy compared to stones in upper and middle calyx [1, 10]. However, a study with 246 cases of lower pole stones treated with EWSL concluded that stone size rather than lower pole anatomy was predictive of the efficacy [11]. Another study with nearly 600 renal stones fund no significant difference in stone clearance rate between stones located in the lower, middle and upper pole [12]. In the present study, no significant difference in ESWL success rate was observed between intra renal stone locations. Stones in the lower calyx were just as sensitive to ESWL as stones in other intra renal locations.

With a retreatment rate of 31%, the majority of stones required only a single treatment. However, the slightly higher retreatment rate found in this study compared to other series is consistent with the department's liberal policy towards ESWL. By performing a second treatment of the stones that was initially unsuccessfully treated, the overall stone free rate increased from 69% to 87%. Performing three or more ESWL attempts only increases the overall success rate slightly from 87% to 93%. Based on the finding in the present study, it seems reasonable

Table 4 Effect of JJ on stone clearance. Number of stones (%)

	Lower Calyx, n = 257		Renal Pelvis, n = 179		Stones 5–10 mm, n = 341		Stones 10–20 mm, n = 131	
	JJ not present n = 240	JJ present n = 17	JJ not present n = 146	JJ present n = 33	JJ not present n = 312	JJ present n = 29	JJ not present n = 111	JJ present n = 20
Succes after 1st ESWL	163 (68)	8 (47)	106 (73)	18 (55)	226 (72)	19 (66)	59 (53)	8 (40)
Accumulated succes after 2nd ESWL	202 (84)	13 (76)	128 (88)	26 (79)	278 (89)	25 (86)	85 (77)	14 (70)
Accumulated succes after ≥ 3rd ESWL	223 (93)	15 (88)	136 (93)	27 (82)	296 (95)	26 (90)	99 (89)	16 (80)

to offer a patient who was initially unsuccessful treated with ESWL at least one other attempt before considering invasive procedures.

The literature contains only little information on JJ-usage in relation to ESWL treatments and indications remains unclear and without consensus. The intention of a JJ is to prevent complications associated with ureteral obstruction as stone fragments is cleared trough the ureter. Conversely, the main drawbacks of JJ are bladder and kidney discomfort, risk of infections and calcification of the JJ. A survey among American urologists reported the JJ usage prior to ESWL to be 28% for 10 mm stones, 57% for 15 mm stones and 87% for 20 mm stones [13]. The results in the present study indicate a similar correlation between stone size and treatment with JJ prior to ESWL, though the results did not reach statistically significance. With respect to intra renal stone location, we found that significantly more patients with stones in the renal pelvis than elsewhere in the kidney were treated with JJ prior to ESWL. As expected, stones in the renal pelvis did give rise to to JJ-demanding obstruction more frequently than other intra renal locations. Previously, only a few studies have reported on JJ usage in relation to ESWL and concludes that treatment with a JJ prior to ESWL does not significantly influence stone free rates but generally results in more discomfort [14–17]. In the group of patients not treated with JJ prior to ESWL, we found that only 17 patients (3%) subsequently required treatment with an acute JJ because of complications associated with ureteral obstruction. Furthermore, we found association between stone size or intra renal stone location and the risk of needing treatment with JJ after the ESWL procedure.

The present study highlights the discrepancy in the efficacy of ESWL being reported in the literature, especially regarding mobile lithotripsy service. Although this study presents a large number of stones treated with EWSL the study is limited to being a single-centre design. Also, the retrospective design raises the issue of potential selection bias which are likely to have influenced the results of the present study. Further studies are warranted into the efficacy of mobile lithotripsy service, learning curve for ESWL technicians and commercialised health care services in general.

Conclusions

The initial success rate after one ESWL procedure was 69%, which increased to an overall success rate of 93% after repeated treatment. Apart from the upper calyx, intra renal stone location was not associated with treatment efficacy, whereas an inverse relation was found between stone size and treatment efficacy. Patients that did not require treatment with a JJ prior to ESWL had only a minimal risk of needing such treatment subsequently, thus prophylactic placement before or after ESWL cannot be recommended.

Abbreviations

CT: Computed tomography; EAU: European Association of Urology; ESWL: Extracorporeal shock wave lithotripsy; JJ: Internal ureteral double-J stent; PNL: Percutaneous nephrolithotomy; RIRS: Retrograde intrarenal surgery

Funding

Not applicable.

Authors' contributions

TN carried out the data collection, performed the statistical analysis and drafted the manuscript. JB participated in the study design, statistical analysis and coordination of the project. Both authors read and approved the final manuscript.

Competing interests

All authors declare that they have no competing interest.

References

1. Madaan S, Joyce AD. Limitations of extracorporeal shock wave lithotripsy. Curr Opin Urol. 2007;17:109–13.
2. Gerber R, Studer UE, Danuser H. Is newer always better? A comparative study of 3 lithotriptor generations. J Urol. 2005;173:2013–6.
3. Sahinkanat T, Ekerbicer H, Onal B, et al. Evaluation of the effects of relationships between main spatial lower pole calyceal anatomic factors on the success of shock-wave lithotripsy in patients with lower pole kidney stones. Urology. 2008;71:801–5.
4. Turna B, Ekren F, Nazli O, et al. Comparative results of shockwave lithotripsy for renal calculi in upper, middle, and lower calices. J Endourol. 2007;21:951–6.
5. Preminger GM. Management of lower pole renal calculi: shock wave lithotripsy versus percutaneous nephrolithotomy versus flexible ureteroscopy. Urol Res. 2006;34:108–11.
6. Albala DM, Assimos DG, Clayman RV, et al. Lower pole I: a prospective randomized trial of extracorporeal shock wave lithotripsy and percutaneous nephrostolithotomy for lower pole nephrolithiasis-initial results. J Urol. 2001;166:2072–80.

7. Nafie S, Dyer JE, Minhas JS, et al. Efficacy of a mobile lithotripsy service: a one-year review of 222 patients. Scand J Urol. 2014;48:324-7.

8. Nicholson A, Lee C, Ugarte R, et al. The Medstone fixed, mobile, and modular configurations: impact on efficacy. J Endourol. 2007;21(5):494-8.

9. Albala DM, Siddiqui KM, Fulmer B, et al. Extracorporeal shock wave lithotripsy with a transportable electrohydraulic lithotripter: experience with >300 patients. BJU Int. 2005;96:603-7.

10. Lingeman JE, Siegel YI, Steele B, et al. Management of lower pole nephrolithiasis: a critical analysis. J Urol. 1994;151:663-7.

11. Sorensen CM, Chandhoke PS. Is lower pole caliceal anatomy predictive of extracorporeal shock wave lithotripsy success for primary lower pole kidney stones? J Urol. 2002;168:2377-82.

12. Obek C, Onal B, Kantay K, et al. The efficacy of extracorporeal shock wave lithotripsy for isolated lower pole calculi compared with isolated middle and upper caliceal calculi. J Urol. 2001;166:2081-4.

13. Hollowell CM, Patel RV, Bales GT, Gerber GS. Internet and postal survey of endourologic practice patterns among American urologists. J Urol. 2000;163:1779-82.

14. Bierkens AF, Hendrikx AJ, Lemmens WA, Debruyne FM. Extracorporeal shock wave lithotripsy for large renal calculi: the role of ureteral stents. A randomized trial. Urol. 1991;145:699-702.

15. Chandhoke PS, Barqawi AZ, Wernecke C, Chee-Awai RA. A randomized outcomes trial of ureteral stents for extracorporeal shock wave lithotripsy of solitary kidney or proximal ureteral stones. J Urol. 2002;167:1981-3.

16. Musa AAK. Use of double-J stents prior to extracorporeal shock wave lithotripsy is not beneficial: results of a prospective randomized study. Int Urol Nephrol. 2007;40:19-22.

17. Pryor JL, Jenkins AD. Use of double-pigtail stents in extracorporeal shock wave lithotripsy. J Urol. 1990;143:475-8.

15

Role of calcifying nanoparticles in the development of testicular microlithiasis in vivo

Xia-cong Lin[1†], Xiang Gao[2†], Gen-sheng Lu[3], Bo Song[3] and Qing-hua Zhang[2*]

Abstract

Background: Calcifying nanoparticles (NPs) have been proven to be associated with a variety of pathological calcification and previously detected in semen samples from patients with testicular microlithiasis (TM). The present study was designed to test the hypothesis if human-derived NPs could invade the seminiferous tubules and induce TM phenotype.

Methods: The animals were divided into three groups. Normal saline (0.2 mL) was injected into the proximal right ductus deferens in group A as a control group. The experimental groups, B and C received *Escherichia coli* (10^6 cfu/mL, 0.2 mL) and human-derived NPs suspension (0.2 mL), respectively. Rats were euthanized in 2 batches at 2 and 4 weeks. Testicular pathology, ultrastructure and inflammatory mediators were assessed.

Results: Chronic inflammatory changes were observed at 2 weeks in both groups B and C. Moreover, the innermost layer of sperm cells were structurally impaired and a zone of concentrically layered collagen fibers around the human NPs body was formed in the lumen of the seminiferous tubule in group C only, in which TM phenotype of remarkable calcification surrounded by cellular debris within the seminiferous tubules was built at 4 weeks.

Conclusions: The results obtained from our study suggested a potential pathogenic effect of NPs in the development of calcification within the seminiferous tubules, which should be addressed in the future studies.

Keywords: Calcification, Calcifying nanoparticles, Inflammation, Testicular microlithiasis, seminiferous tubules

Background

Testicular microlithiasis (TM) is an uncommon condition of unknown etiology with multiple tiny calcifications present within the seminiferous tubules [1–3], which is associated with both malignant and benign conditions such as testicular neoplasms [4, 5]. So far no valid clinical or research approaches used to investigate the activity of TM in malignant conditions and infertility are available because of its unknown etiology. From clinical and laboratory studies, the existing evidence has confirmed that TM is formed by the intratubular deposits consisting of calcified central cores surrounded by multiple concentric layers of cellular debris, glycoprotein, and collagen within the seminiferous tubules [6]. However, possible

pathophysiological mechanisms leading to the formation of calcified central cores of TM are not yet fully understood. Recently, nano-sized bacteria-like organisms (nanobacteria) have been proven to be involved in the process of pathological calcifications and previously detected in semen samples from patients with testicular microlithiasis (TM) [6–10].

The terminology 'nanobacteria' referring to nano-sized bacteria-like organisms were first discovered in a cell culture and named by Kajander and Cifcioglu [7]. They were self-replicating, 0.1–0.5 μm in size, and had the capacity of forming calcium phosphate minerals under subsaturation levels of calcium and/or phosphate [8, 9]. Nanobacteria, as an emerging cause of pathological calcification, were therefore also called calcifying nanoparticles (NPs). Although there is insufficient proof that calcifying nanoparticles are living organisms, a great deal of evidence from previous studies has established a

* Correspondence: zhangqh1123@163.com
†Equal contributors
2Department of Obstetrics and Gynecology, Daping Hospital, Third Military Medical University, Chongqing 400038, People's Republic of China
Full list of author information is available at the end of the article

possible relationship between nanoparticles and pathological calcifications, such as aortic valve calcification, prostatic calculi, renal tubular calcification, and dental pulp stone [6–10]. This study was to test the hypothesis if human-derived NPs could invade the seminiferous tubules and induce TM phenotype.

Methods

Generation and preparation of human NPs

Referring to our previous research methods [10], nine patients with TM (multiple foci <3 mm in diameter in testicular parenchyma with sonography) were recruited and gave informed consent to participate in the investigation, which was approved by the local Institutional Review Board of our department. According to the culture techniques described by Kajander and Ciftçioğlu [7], after semen and urine samples were pretreated with oscillation, diluted, filtrated (using pinhole filter, 0.45 and 0.22 μm, Millex; Millipore Carrigtwohill, Cork, Ireland), and centrifuged, the samples were routinely cultured in flasks containing serum-free RPMI-1640 (GIBCO, Invitrogen, Carlsbad, CA, USA) medium at 37 °C (pH 7.4) in 5% CO2/95% air. After 5 weeks of inoculation, cultures were harvested by 30-min centrifugation at 20,000×g and resuspended in 10 ml PBS (pH 7.2) to prepare human NPs suspension under the same ionic condition in normal saline (1 McFarland U) for further experiments.

Rats infections with human NPs

All animal experiments were approved by the Institutional Animal Care and Use Committee. Sixty male Sprague Dawley rats (6 months old, 300–350 g) were divided into three groups: group A (control) with normal saline (0.2 mL) injected into the proximal right ductus deferens; group B receiving E. coli (10^6 cfu/mL, 0.2 mL); group C receiving human-derived NPs suspension (0.2 mL).

Sample collection

All rats were raised with the same conditions and were euthanized by asphyxiation with carbon dioxide (CO_2) followed by cervical dislocation in 2 batches(ten rats in each)at 2 and 4 weeks, respectively. By aseptic technique the testis and epididymis were harvested before the epididymis was completely removed.

Histological staining

Testis was fixed in 10% buffered formaldehyde for 24-48 h, and then embedded in paraffin. The paraffin blocks were cut into 3-μm thick pieces and then stained with hematoxylin and eosin.

Testis ultrastructural study

Referring to our previous research methods [11], for transmission electron microscopy (TEM), fresh testis tissue were cut into 1–2 μm pieces, fixed overnight in 2.5% glutaraldehyde, embedded on a membrane coated copper screen, and stained with 3% phosphotungstic acid for 1–2 min before being viewed on a Tecnai 10 transmission electron microscope (Philips, Eindhoven, The Netherlands) with an 80 kV working voltage.

For scanning electron microscopy (SEM), fresh testis tissues were cut into small blocks before being analyzed. Briefly, tissues were fixed for 1 h with 2.5% glutaraldehyde and dehydrated in an ethanol gradient, followed by cryodesiccation and metal plating. Samples were observed under a KYKY-EM3200 SEM (KYKY Technology Development, Beijing, People's Republic of China) using an accelerating voltage of 30 kV.

Statistical analysis

Statistical analysis was performed with the unpaired student t test or with a one-way analysis of variance with the Tukey post hoc test. Data were processed using the SPSS statistical software (version 16.0; SPSS, Inc., Chicago, IL, USA). Significance was accepted at a P value of less than 0.05.

Results

Human NPs, existing as white granular sediments in cultures, were isolated from semen samples of TM patients. Under TEM, the NPs displayed as crystalline spheroids with approximately 80–200 nm in size (Fig. 1).

Histopathological findings

The control group revealed normal histological features, which were characterized by regularly-organized distribution of cells in the seminiferous epithelium, including the outermost layer of spermatogonia and Sertoli cells,

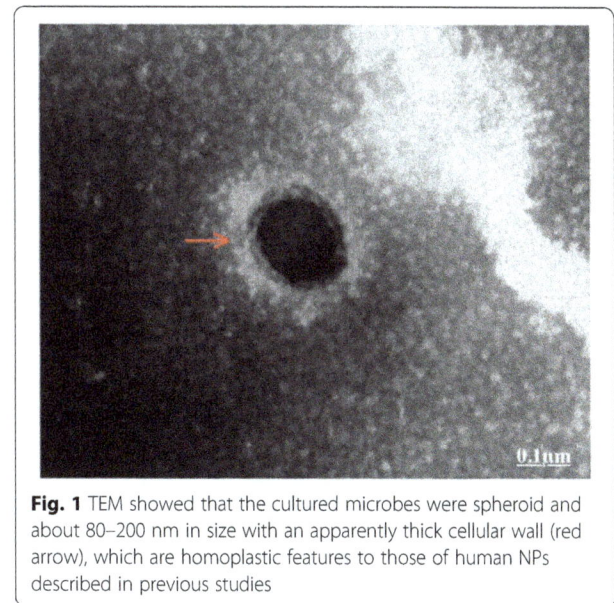

Fig. 1 TEM showed that the cultured microbes were spheroid and about 80–200 nm in size with an apparently thick cellular wall (red arrow), which are homoplastic features to those of human NPs described in previous studies

the middle layer of spermatocytes, and the innermost layer of sperm cells (Fig. 2a). At 2 weeks, significant leukocytic infiltration changes in the innermost layer of sperm cells were observed in groups B and C (Fig. 2b and c). In addition, the innermost layer of sperm cells were structurally impaired and a zone of concentrically layered collagen fibers around the human NPs body was formed in the lumen of the seminiferous tubule in group C (Fig. 2c). At 4 weeks, atrophy of seminiferous tubule was observed and a well-recognized form of intratesticular calcification surrounded by cellular debris within the seminiferous tubules following inflammatory disease resulting from NP infusion was formed in group C only (Fig. 2d), which indicated the establishment of a successfully reproduced model exhibiting the TM phenotype.

Ultrastructural observations

In the testis of control rats, a normal cell population was found typically localized in the seminiferous tubules while no morphological changes were discovered (Fig. 3a). In the testis at 2 weeks, consistent with the histological findings, many globoid or racket-shaped particles in cytoplasm were observed under TEM in group C (Fig. 3b and c). In addition, microcalcification surrounded by globoid human NPs within the seminiferous tubules increasingly occurred

in affected tubules in group C (Fig. 3c), which suggests that the formation of microcalcification is likely linked with NP exposure. At 4 weeks, microcalcification surrounded by cellular debris within the seminiferous tubules displayed characteristic features of testicular microlithiasis in group C only (Fig. 3d).

The SEM examination showed the interstitial tissue of control rats with an intricate three-dimensional network and each seminiferous tubule with large fenestrae and well spaced cells (Fig. 4a). Distinct globoid particles were observed between the interstitial tissue and the seminiferous tubules in the testis after 2 weeks in group C (Fig. 4b and c). In addition, the seminiferous tubules showed a compact, fibrous appearance with absence of fenestrae, but with a larger number of cellular debris, and microcalcification surrounded by globoid NPs within the seminiferous tubules were obviously visble in affected tubules in group C (Fig. 4c-d). At 4 weeks, the epithelium height significantly diminished and no spermatozoa in the lumen could be witnessed except microcalcification filled in the seminiferous tubule only in group C (Fig. 4e).

Discussion

The emergence of nanobacteria, which are nanometer-scale spherical particles capable of producing nucleate

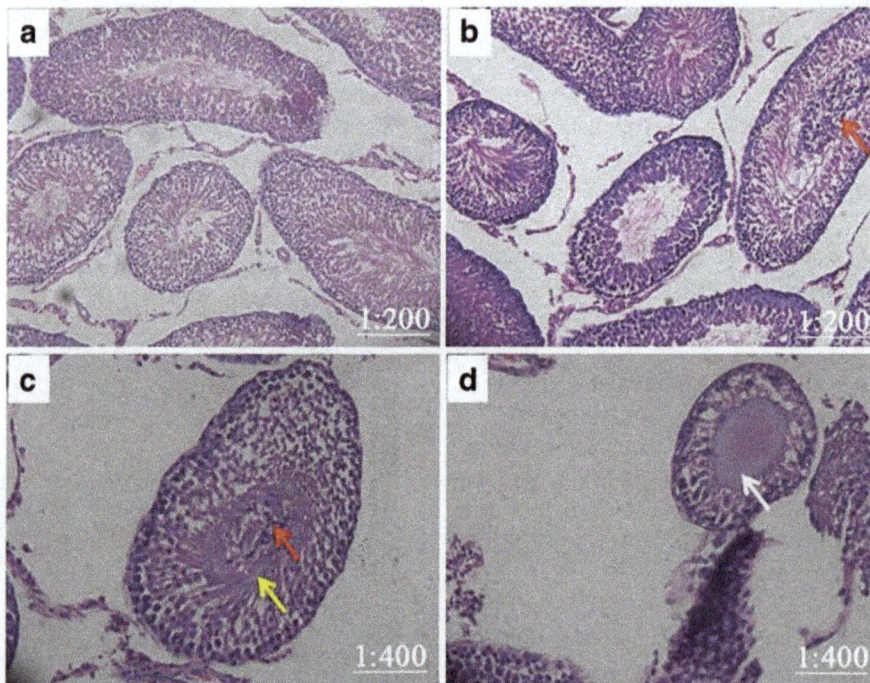

Fig. 2 Effect of *E. coli* and human NPs on testis histopathology. **a** The testes from control mice showed normal morphology and spermatogenesis. H&E, reduced from ×200. **b** and **c** At 2 weeks, significantly leukocytic infiltration changes in the innermost layer of sperm cells were noted in groups B and C (Fig. 2b and c; red arrows). In addition, the innermost layer of sperm cells were structurally impaired and a zone of concentrically layered collagen fibers around the human NPs body was formed in the lumen of the seminiferous tubule in group C (Fig. 2c; yellow arrow). H&E, reduced from ×400. **d** At 4 weeks after infusion, seminiferous tubule was atrophic and a well-recognised form of intratesticular calcification surrounded by cellular debris within the seminiferous tubules was observed in group C only (white arrow), indicating a model of TM phenotype successfully reproduced. H&E, reduced from ×400

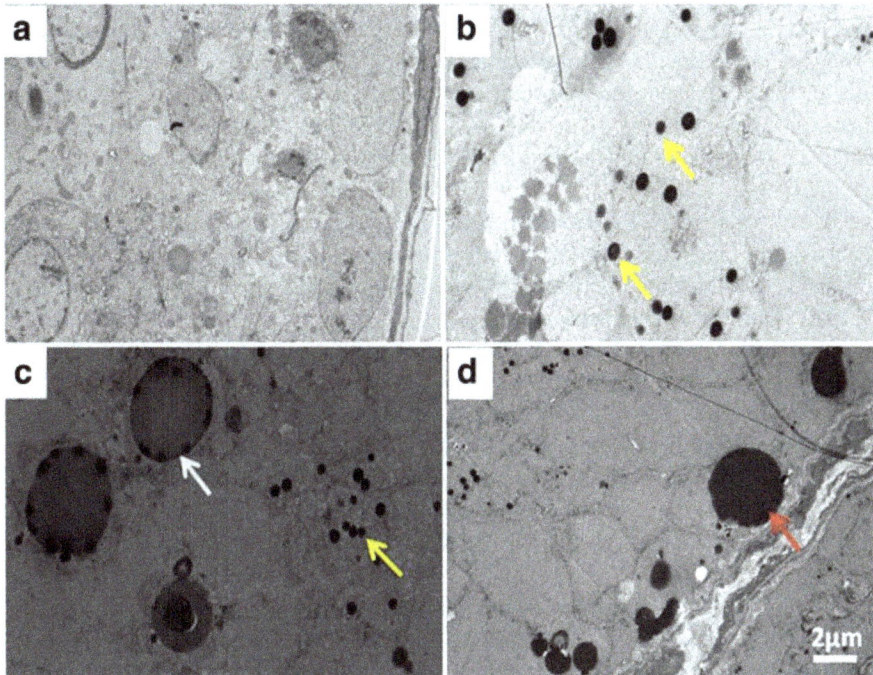

Fig. 3 Testis ultrastructural observations by TEM. **a** Normal cell population typically localized in the seminiferous tubules and no morphological changes were observed in the testis of control mice. **b** and **c** At 2 weeks, many globoid or racket-shaped particles in cytoplasm were observed under TEM in group B and C (yellow arrows). In addition, microcalcification surrounded by globoid human NPs within the seminiferous tubules increasingly occurred in affected tubules in group C (white arrows). **d** At four weeks, microcalcification surrounded by cellular debris within the seminiferous tubules displayed the characteristic features of testicular microlithiasis in group C only (Fig. 3d; red arrow)

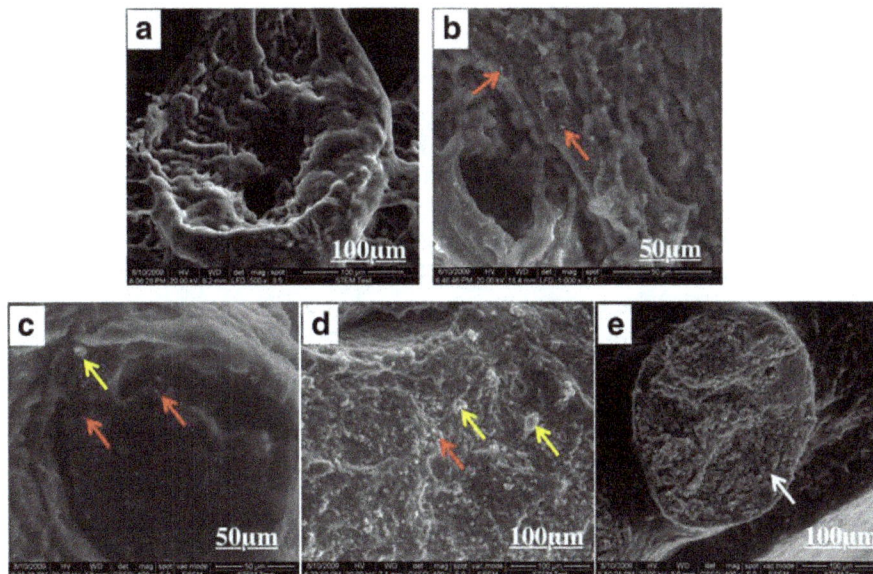

Fig. 4 Testis ultrastructural observations by SEM. **a** An intricate three-dimensional network and each seminiferous tubule with large fenestrae and well spaced cells were observed in the testis of control mice. **b-d** At 2 weeks, distinct globoid particles were observed between the interstitial tissue and the seminiferous tubules in the testis after 2 week in group C (Fig. 4b and c; red arrows). In addition, the seminiferous tubules showed a compact, fibrous appearance with absence of fenestrae, but with a larger number of cellular debris, and microcalcification surrounded by globoid NPs within the seminiferous tubules were obviously observed in affected tubules in group C (Fig. 4c-d; yellow arrow). **e** At 4 weeks, the epithelium height diminished and no spermatozoa in the lumen could be witnessed except microcalcification filled in the seminiferous tubule only in group C (Fig. 4e; white arrows)

hydroxyapatite, has spurred a major controversy in the field of microbiology [6, 7]. The absence of a fairly accurately sequenced genome for nanobacteria has led to various hypotheses of the characteristic and origin of nanobacteria. In this study, our cultured NPs successfully caused testicular inflammation, which suggested that they might be living entities.

Human NPs have been found mainly excreted from urinary tract and may flow back into seminiferous tubules, colonize there and cause testis infection [10, 12, 13]. To date, NPs have been found in periodontal diseases, urolithiasis, aortic valve calcification, human arthritic synovial fluid, and demonstrated to participate in the clinical pathological process of those diseases [10, 12, 13]. In a previous study, NPs were successfully cultured from 58.8% of semen samples of patients with TM [10]. Therefore, experimental studies on animal models focused on the uncovering of new connections between NPs and the etiopathogenesis of TM were needed.

To exclude the possibility of false positives of human NPs cultured from semen samples, three efforts were made in our study. Firstly, our experimental operations and testing instruments were conducted under strict aseptic conditions. Secondly, samples were cultured without fetal bovine serum, which usually contains inhibitors on apatite crystal formation, such as osteopontin, osteocalcin, and fetuin. Thirdly, the supernatants of human NPs cultures were filtered with a 0.22-μm minipore filter, which could effectively remove the common bacteria, mycoplasma, and fungi. In this study, human NPs were successfully cultured with serum-free RPMI-1640 from semen samples of patients with TM, which exhibited as spheroids with black coats and crystals around the bacterial body under TEM. All these results obtained from our experiments indicated that human NPs did reside in the testicular architecture of TM patients.

Furthermore, we injected the human NPs suspension into the male Sprague-Dawley rat proximal right ductus deferens, and pathological changes of the rats resulting from NP infection in the testis tissue were observed. Our investigation demonstrated that human NPs administration caused significant histopathological alterations in testis, manifested as leukocytic infiltration in the innermost layer of sperm cells at 2 weeks, structurally impaired sperm cells of the innermost layer and a zone of concentrically layered collagen fibers around the NP body formed in the lumen of the seminiferous tubules at 2 weeks, and a well-recognized form of intratesticular calcification surrounded by cellular debris within the seminiferous tubules at 4 weeks. However, no significant pathological changes were observed in the controls. Although significant leukocytic infiltration changes in the innermost layer of sperm cells were also observed in the groups receiving *E. coli* at 2 weeks, no intratesticular

calcification surrounded by cellular debris within the seminiferous tubules was observed after 4 weeks. Therefore, a model of TM phenotype was successfully reproduced in this study. Our results also confirmed that human NPs were the known agents of emerging infectious diseases and producing apatite, which agrees well with other reports [14, 15]. A possible calcification mechanism might be NP colonization in seminiferous tubules inducing an immune response, promoting inflammation development and further calcification.

Ultrasound (US) is an effective approach for monitoring formation of calcification, which can be seen as tiny bright echoes without acoustic shadow scattered throughout the testicular parenchyma. Unfortunately, we failed to find a suitable ultrasonic probe for rats. Instead we did testis ultrastructural study at different points. TEM and SEM illustrations showed that the pathological alterations and calcification in seminiferous tubules were not homogenous. Many globoid or racket-shaped particles in cytoplasm were only observed in the NP-instilled rats and were not present in any of the controls under TEM. Moreover, the fibrils and mineral deposits developed in seminiferous tubules had different sizes and morphology under SEM. These illustrations further proved that human NPs did participate in the formation of testicular microlithiasis.

The present study was a descriptive rather than mechanistic study. In our early experimental design, we intended to explore the formation mechanism of testicular microlithiasis by NPs, and thus chose *E. coli* as a control to uncover the differences in histopathological alterations. Unfortunately, we failed to observe any significant differences in terms of histological features. Further investigations on the differences of the leucocyte population by means of immunohistochemistry (IHC) between them may better define the character of NPs and their possible mechanistic role in TM pathogenesis. Therefore, more effort addressing this question is needed in our future work.

Conclusions

The results obtained from our study suggest a potential pathogenic effect of systemic inoculation of human-derived NPs to stimulate calcification within the seminiferous tubules.

Abbreviations
NPs: nanoparticles; SEM: scanning electron microscopy; TEM: transmission electron microscopy; TM: testicular microlithiasis

Acknowledgements
We thank Dr. Wei Liu and Dr. Peng Hui Chen for their technical and editorial assistance with this research project and manuscript preparation.

Funding
This study was supported by the National Natural Science Foundation in China (81,000,241 and 81,471,444).

Authors' contributions
Study conception and design: XC-Land QH-Z; Acquisition of data: XC-L, XG, GS-L, BS and QH-Z; Analysis and interpretation of data: XC-L,XG and QH-Z; Drafting of manuscript: XC-L,XG and QH-Z; Critical revision: BS. All authors read and approved the final manuscript.

Competing interests
The authors declare that they have no competing interests.

Author details
[1]Department of Urology, the 175th Hospital of PLA (Dongnan Affiliated Hospital of Xiamen University), Zhangzhou, Fujian 363000, People's Republic of China. [2]Department of Obstetrics and Gynecology, Daping Hospital, Third Military Medical University, Chongqing 400038, People's Republic of China. [3]Urological Research Institute of PLA, Southwest hospital, Third Military Medical University, Chongqing 400038, People's Republic of China.

References
1.   Maturen KE. Attributable risk calculations for testicular microlithiasisJ Clin Ultrasound. 2015;43(2):120–1.
2.   Xu C, Liu M, Zhang FF, et al. The association between testicular microlithiasis and semen parameters in Chinese adult men with fertility intention: experience of 226 cases. Urology. 2014;84(4):815–20.
3.   Ravichandran S, Smith R, Cornford PA, Fordham MV. Surveillance of testicular microlithiasis? Results of an UK based national questionnaire survey. BMC Urol. 2006;6:8.
4.   Richenberg J, Brejt N. Testicular microlithiasis: is there a need for surveillance in the absence of other risk factors? Eur Radiol. 2012;22(11):2540–6.
5.   Lee S, Choi HJ. Double Para-testicular Cellular Angiofibroma and Synchronous Testicular Microlithiasis. J Pathol Transl Med. 2016;50:75–7.
6.   Martel J, Peng HH, Young D, Wu CY, Young JD. Of nanobacteria, nanoparticles, biofilms and their role in health and disease: facts, fancy and future. Nanomedicine (Lond). 2014;9(4):483–99.
7.   Kajander EO, Ciftçioglu N. Nanobacteria: an alternative mechanism for pathogenic intra- and extracellular calcification and stone formation. Proc Natl Acad Sci U S A. 1998;95(14):8274–9.
8.   Hunter LW, Charlesworth JE, Yu S, Lieske JC, Miller VM. Calcifying nanoparticles promote mineralization in vascular smooth muscle cells: implications for atherosclerosis. Int J Nanomedicine. 2014;27:2689–98.
9.   Kutikhin AG, Brusina EB, Yuzhalin AE. The role of calcifying nanoparticles in biology and medicine. Int J Nanomedicine. 2012;7:339–50.
10. Zhang QH, Lu GS, Shen XC, et al. Nanobacteria may be linked to testicular microlithiasis in infertility. J Androl. 2010;31(2):121–5.
11. Xie QB, Lu GS, Song B, Zhang QH. Role of tiny nanoparticles in the development of interstitial cystitis in an animal model. Int J Clin Exp Pathol. 2017;10(1):250–7.
12. Ciftçioglu N, Björklund M, Kuorikoski K, et al. Nanobacteria: an infectious cause for kidney stone formation. Kidney Int. 1999;56(5):1893–8.
13. Hjelle JT, Miller-Hjelle MA, Poxton IR, et al. Endotoxin and nanobacteria in polycystic kidney disease. Kidney Int. 2000;57(6):2360–74.
14. Smith ER. Vascular Calcification in Uremia: New-Age Concepts about an Old-Age Problem. Methods Mol Biol. 2016;1397:175–208.
15. Hunter LW, Charlesworth JE, Yu S, Lieske JC, Miller VM. Calcifying nanoparticles promote mineralization in vascular smooth muscle cells: implications for atherosclerosis. Int J Nanomedicine. 2014;9:2689–98.

16

Prophylactic antibiotic use in pediatric patients undergoing urinary tract catheterization: a survey of members of the Society for Pediatric Urology

Alexander P. Glaser, Ilina Rosoklija, Emilie K. Johnson and Elizabeth B. Yerkes[*]

Abstract

Background: Current organizational guidelines regarding use of antibiotics during urinary tract catheterization are based on limited evidence and are not directly applicable to the pediatric urology population. We seek to improve understanding of this population by first evaluating current practices. This study aims to investigate practice patterns and attitudes of pediatric urologists regarding the use of antibiotics in the setting of urinary tract catheterization.

Methods: An online survey was sent to members of the Society for Pediatric Urology. Questionnaire sections included demographics, general questions about antibiotic use with catheterization, and specific clinical scenarios. Descriptive statistics were used, and chi-square analysis was performed to examine associations between demographics and specific responses.

Results: Of 448 pediatric urologists surveyed, 154 (34%) responded to the survey. A majority of surveyed urologists (78%) prescribe daily prophylactic antibiotics with a hypospadias stent in place, but extensive variation in use of antibiotics was reported with other catheters and tubes. Extensive variation in practice patterns was also reported for three case scenarios regarding antibiotic prophylaxis with catheterization. Urologists > 50 years of age and fellowship-trained urologists were more likely to prescribe antibiotics for hypospadias stents ($p = 0.02$, $p = 0.03$), but no other significant associations between demographic characteristics and antibiotic use were found.

Conclusions: There is substantial variation in practice patterns among surveyed pediatric urologists regarding prophylactic antibiotic use with urinary catheterization. This variation, combined with a lack of objective data and increasing pressure to decrease infectious complications and combat antibiotic resistance, highlights the need for development of management guidelines for this unique population.

Keywords: Urinary tract infection, Catheter-related infection, Antibiotic prophylaxis, Health care survey, Pediatrics

This manuscript was presented at the American Urological Association annual meeting in 2016 (MP55–15), and is published in abstract form [1].

Background

Catheter-associated urinary tract infections (CAUTIs) are the most common nosocomial infection in the United States and lead to increased cost of care as well as patient length-of-stay, morbidity, and mortality [2]. Recent national measures in the United States have sought to prevent and decrease the frequency of CAUTIs in the general population [3]. Furthermore, there has been increasing pressure from payers, including the Centers for Medicare & Medicaid Services, to decrease infectious complications by imposing financial penalties on hospitals that perform poorly with regard to hospital-acquired conditions.

Alongside pressure to decrease infectious complications there has been an increasing focus on the problems caused by antibiotic resistance [4]. According to the U.S.

* Correspondence: eyerkes@luriechildrens.org
Department of Surgery, Division of Urology, Ann and Robert H. Lurie Children's Hospital of Chicago, 225 E. Chicago Ave, Chicago, IL 60611, USA

Center for Disease Control and Prevention, each year over 2 million illnesses and over 20,000 deaths are directly attributable to antibiotic resistance [4]. Problematic resistance patterns have forced urologists to use broader-spectrum antibiotics on a routine basis [5]. Yet despite growing resistance patterns, antibiotic drug development has stymied and few new drugs are being developed [6–8]. Antibiotic stewardship has been proposed as a solution to promote use of optimal antibiotic regimens; however, due to a lack of evidence in the pediatric urology population, further research is needed to define appropriate and inappropriate antibiotic use [9, 10]. Current guidelines from the American Urological Association (AUA) and the European Association of Urology (EAU) recommend antibiotic prophylaxis with urinary tract catheter removal if bacteriuria and other risk factors (such as older age, smoking status, deficient nutritional status, immunosuppression, diabetes mellitus, and prolonged hospitalization) are present; however, these are based on limited evidence and are not directly applicable to the pediatric urology population [11–13]. Therefore, we sought to improve understanding of this unique population by first describing and measuring current practices. This study aimed to investigate current practice patterns and attitudes of pediatric urologists regarding the use of prophylactic antibiotics in patients undergoing urinary tract catheterization.

Methods

Survey and data collection

A 20-item online questionnaire regarding the use of prophylactic antibiotics with urinary catheterization was sent to 315 active and affiliate members of the Society for Pediatric Urology (SPU). The original request was sent via email in August, 2015 and two follow-up reminders were sent in September, 2015. Questionnaire sections included: (1) Demographics, (2) General questions about antibiotic use with urinary catheterization, and (3) Specific clinical scenarios (see Additional file 1). Study data were collected and managed using REDCap (Research Electronic Data Capture, http://project-redcap.org) electronic data capture tools hosted at Northwestern University [14]. This study received institutional review board approval (IRB #2015–462).

Statistical analysis

Descriptive statistics were used, and chi-square analysis was performed to examine associations between demographics and specific responses. Statistical comparisons were 2-sided with a type I error probability set at 0.05. Analysis was performed using SPSS Statistics (IBM, version 22).

Results

Respondent demographics

Of 448 members of the SPU surveyed, 154 (34%) responded to the survey (Table 1). SPU members from all AUA sections responded, ranging from 18% of all SPU members located in the New England section to 42% of all SPU members located in the North Central section. There was no statistically significant difference in response rates between sections ($p = 0.28$). The majority of respondents (91%) were fellowship-trained in pediatric urology or were currently in fellowship. Sixty-six percent of respondents practiced in an academic setting, while the remainder practiced in private practice or as a hospital employee.

Use of prophylactic antibiotics with urinary tract catheterization

The majority of respondents (78%) prescribe prophylactic antibiotics the entire time a hypospadias stent is in place (Fig. 1a). However, extensive variation in prescribing patterns was seen for prophylactic antibiotics with use of a Foley catheter, percutaneous nephrostomy tube (PCN), suprapubic tube (SPT), and internal double-J ureteral stent, with 30–50% of respondents prescribing no antibiotics for these tubes, and the remainder prescribing prophylactic antibiotics at least some of the time. The majority of respondents do not prescribe a dose of prophylactic antibiotics at the time of tube removal, with the exception of removal of a ureteral stent (Fig. 1b).

Use of urine cultures and culture data with urinary tract catheterization

The majority of respondents do not obtain urine cultures prior to removal of a hypospadias stent (90%), Foley catheter (75%), PCN (59%), SPT (69%), or internal double-J ureteral stent (67%) (Fig. 1c). If a urine culture is positive, 46% of respondents prescribe a 5–7 day course of antibiotics, while 25% prescribe 2–4 days of antibiotics, 6% prescribe 24 h of antibiotics, and 16% prescribe no antibiotics (Fig. 1d). If a urine culture is negative, 37% still prescribe 24 h or less of antibiotics, while 49% prescribe no antibiotics.

Use of prophylactic antibiotics with simple outpatient procedures

Sixty-one percent of respondents reported prescribing no prophylactic antibiotics for patients undergoing a voiding cystourethrogram, while the remainder (39%) prescribe prophylactic antibiotics at least some of the time (Fig. 2). Similar variation is seen for retrograde urethrogram and urodynamic studies.

Table 1 Respondent Demographics

Question	Responses, n (%)
Age (years)	
31–40	35 (23%)
41–50	42 (27%)
51–60	51 (33%)
> 60	25 (16%)
Gender	
Male	116 (75%)
Female	34 (22%)
Other	2 (1.3%)
Fellowship Trained	
Currently in fellowship	6 (4%)
Yes	134 (87%)
No	11 (7%)
Years in practice	
Currently in fellowship	6 (4%)
0–5	29 (19%)
6–10	23 (15%)
11–15	23 (15%)
16–20	21 (14%)
> 20	51 (33%)
Number of pediatric urologists in practice	
1–2	57 (37%)
3–4	51 (33%)
5–6	28 (18%)
7–10	15 (9.7%)
> 10	3 (1.9%)
Practice Setting	
Academic affiliation	102 (66%)
Hospital employee	17 (11%)
Private Practice	34 (22%)
Other	1 (0.6%)
AUA Section	
Mid Atlantic	16 (10%)
New England	6 (4%)
New York	9 (6%)
North Central	38 (25%)
Northeastern	9 (6%)
South Central	20 (13%)
Southeastern	24 (16%)
Western	29 (19%)
From another geographic location	3 (2%)

Use of antibiotics in clinical case scenarios

Substantial variation in practice patterns was reported for three case scenarios with indwelling catheters and no evidence of infection (Fig. 3). Full case descriptions are detailed in Fig. 3.

For an 8-year old male undergoing a direct visual internal urethrotomy and a subsequent indwelling catheter for 3 days, 66% of respondents prescribe antibiotics the entire time the catheter is in place, while 18% would prescribe antibiotics only at catheter removal, and 9% would prescribe no antibiotics.

For a 12-year old female being discharged from the hospital with a newly created continent catheterizable channel and an indwelling catheter through the channel for 2 weeks, 47% of respondents would prescribe antibiotics the entire time the catheter is in place, while 13% would prescribe antibiotics only at catheter removal, and 34% would prescribe no antibiotics.

Finally, for a 2-year old female with ureteropelvic junction obstruction and a PCN for 2 weeks, 32% of respondents prescribe antibiotics the entire time the PCN is in place, while 34% would prescribe antibiotics only at PCN removal, and 27% would prescribe no antibiotics.

Personal experience with infectious complications

Twenty-five percent of respondents reported having a patient with a serious complication (requiring an intensive care unit or an invasive procedure) or death related to a CAUTI. Thirty-one percent of these respondents reporting changing their practice based on this event, while 59% reported not changing their practice based on this event, and 10% reported being unsure if their practice changed based on this event.

Associations

Urologists > 50 years of age and fellowship-trained urologists were more likely to prescribe antibiotics > 50% of the time for hypospadias stents (95% vs. 82%, $p = 0.02$; 95% vs. 79%, $p = 0.03$). Respondents who reported changing practice patterns based on a serious complication or death related to CAUTI were more likely to prescribe antibiotics > 50% of the time with a ureteral double-J stent and for the entire time the catheter is in place for Case Scenario #2 (54% vs. 16%, $p = 0.04$; 60% vs 16%, $p = 0.02$). There was also a possible association noted for respondents who reported changing practice patterns based on an infectious complication to prescribe antibiotics > 50% of the time with a SPC, but this was not statistically significant (42% vs. 8%; $p = 0.06$). There was no difference in prescribing pattern based on gender, size of practice, practice setting, or AUA section.

Discussion

This survey of SPU members indicates that substantial variation exists in the use of prophylactic antibiotics in pediatric urology patients undergoing short-term urinary

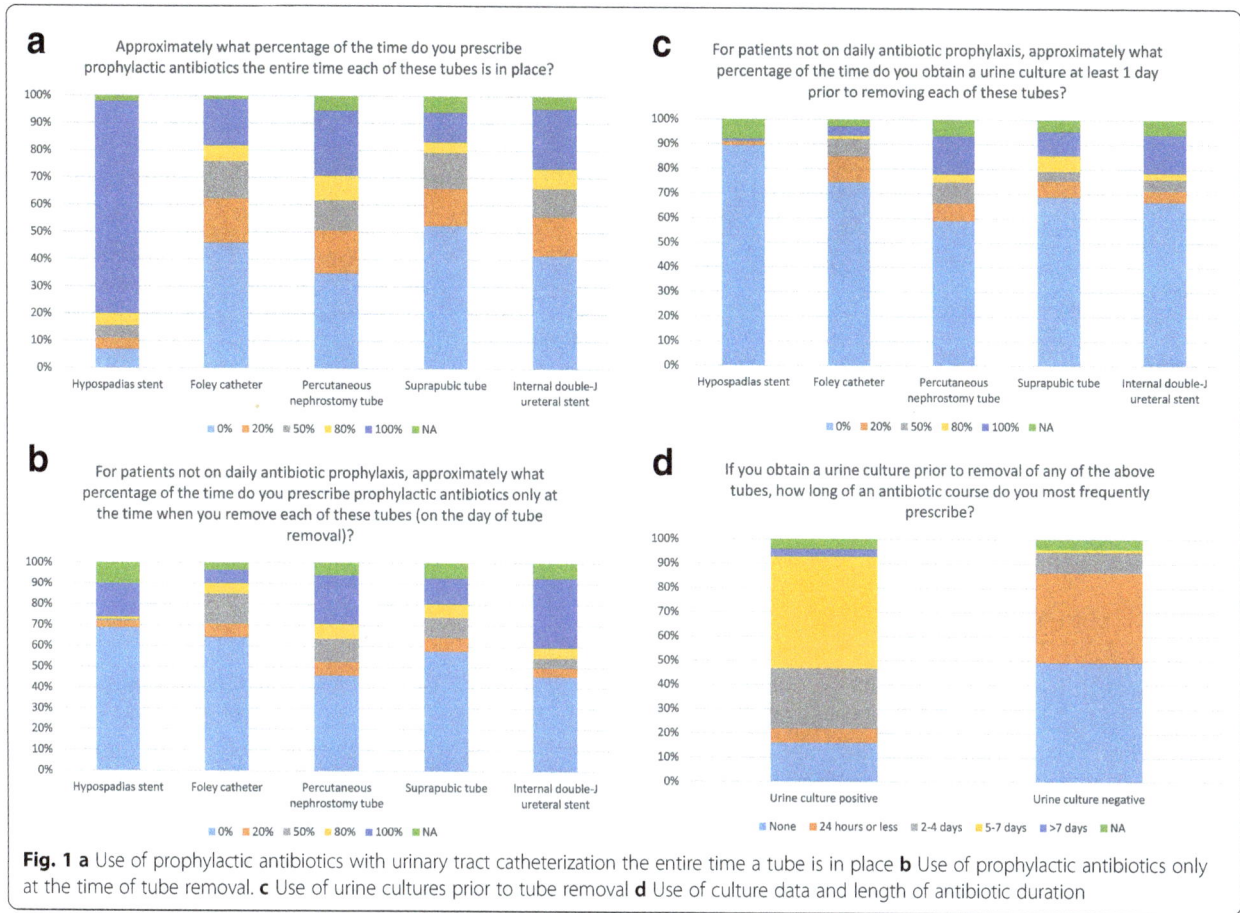

a Approximately what percentage of the time do you prescribe prophylactic antibiotics the entire time each of these tubes is in place?

b For patients not on daily antibiotic prophylaxis, approximately what percentage of the time do you prescribe prophylactic antibiotics only at the time when you remove each of these tubes (on the day of tube removal)?

c For patients not on daily antibiotic prophylaxis, approximately what percentage of the time do you obtain a urine culture at least 1 day prior to removing each of these tubes?

d If you obtain a urine culture prior to removal of any of the above tubes, how long of an antibiotic course do you most frequently prescribe?

Fig. 1 a Use of prophylactic antibiotics with urinary tract catheterization the entire time a tube is in place **b** Use of prophylactic antibiotics only at the time of tube removal. **c** Use of urine cultures prior to tube removal **d** Use of culture data and length of antibiotic duration

catheterization. Almost 80% of all survey respondents always prescribe with a hypospadias stent, but this was the only queried scenario with a clear consensus; extensive variation was seen in the remainder of scenarios and questions. For example, in Case Scenario #3, respondents were split with approximately 1/3 prescribing no antibiotics, 1/3 prescribing antibiotics at catheter removal only, and 1/3 prescribing antibiotics the entire time the catheter is in place. This variation speaks to the complexity of these patients, but also to the lack of evidence guiding antibiotic use.

Interestingly, in our study, respondents who reported changing their practice patterns based on an infectious complication were significantly more likely to prescribe antibiotics for internal double-J stents and for a newly created catheterizable channel ($p = 0.04$, $p = 0.02$). In addition, there was a possible association between respondents who changed their practice based on an infectious complication and more antibiotic use in patients with a SPC ($p = 0.06$). This suggests that the lack of evidence regarding antibiotic use in these populations may allow the availability bias of a prior adverse event to drive decision making.

The lack of consensus in antibiotic prescribing patterns in our study is similar to the survey of Wazait et al., who found that 60% of 237 healthcare professionals prescribe prophylactic antibiotics with urinary catheter removal for adult patients, while 40% did not use antibiotics [15]. Variation has also been reported for preoperative surgical antibiotic prophylaxis in a wide range of endoscopic, laparoscopic, and open surgical procedures in both the adult and pediatric populations [16–18]. While these studies examined preoperative surgical prophylaxis instead of antibiotic use with catheters, the similar variation in antibiotic use corroborates our findings.

In our study, urologists > 50 years of age and fellowship-trained urologists were more likely to prescribe antibiotics at least 50% of the time for hypospadias stents. Several studies have investigated the topic of antibiotic use with hypospadias stents, which may be why this was the only scenario with a clear consensus in our study, and especially for older urologists and fellowship-trained urologists, who may be more familiar with the literature. In 2004, Meir et al. reported a decreased risk of complicated UTI and a non-significant suggestion of a decreased rate of urethrocutanous fistula formation with antibiotic use while a hypospadias stent

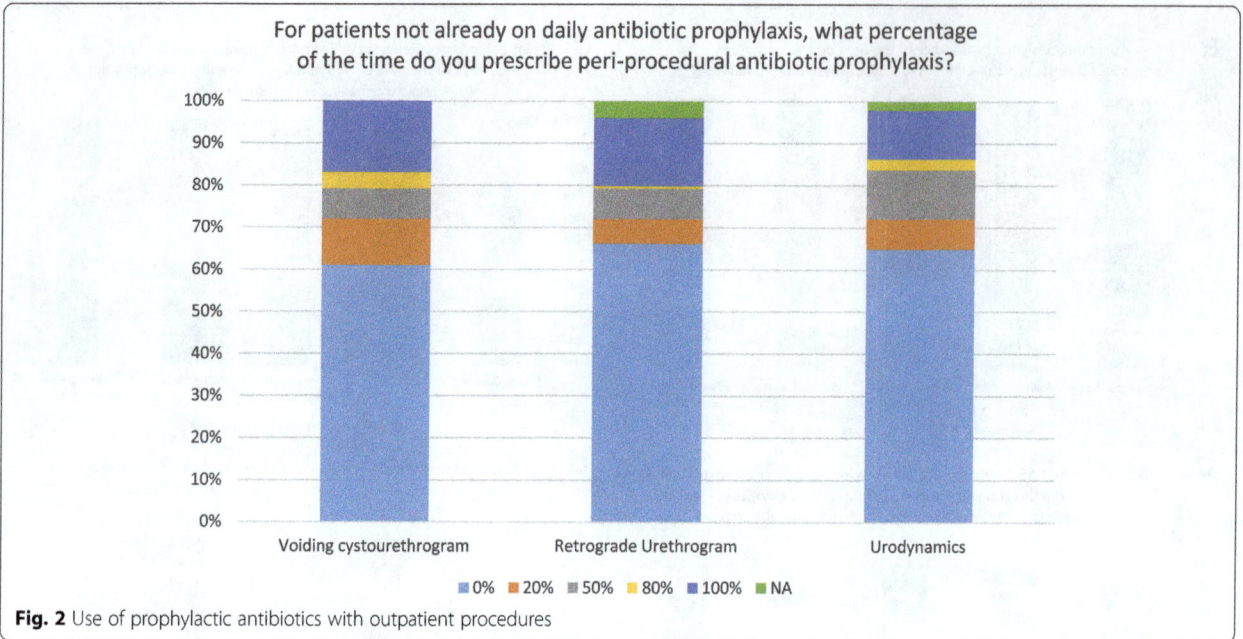

Fig. 2 Use of prophylactic antibiotics with outpatient procedures

is in place [19]. However, this result has not been replicated in other studies and the role of prophylactic antibiotics in hypospadias stents remains controversial [20, 21]. A multi-institutional randomized controlled trial is currently ongoing to investigate the role of antibiotics in this setting (PROPHY, clinicaltrials.gov identifier NCT02096159).

The relative lack of evidence guiding antibiotic use with catheterization in the pediatric population may explain the practice variation reported in our study. While there is some evidence that antibiotic use at the time of catheter removal can decrease symptomatic UTIs in adults [22, 23], these results are not consistently reported [24] and antibiotic use in this setting remains

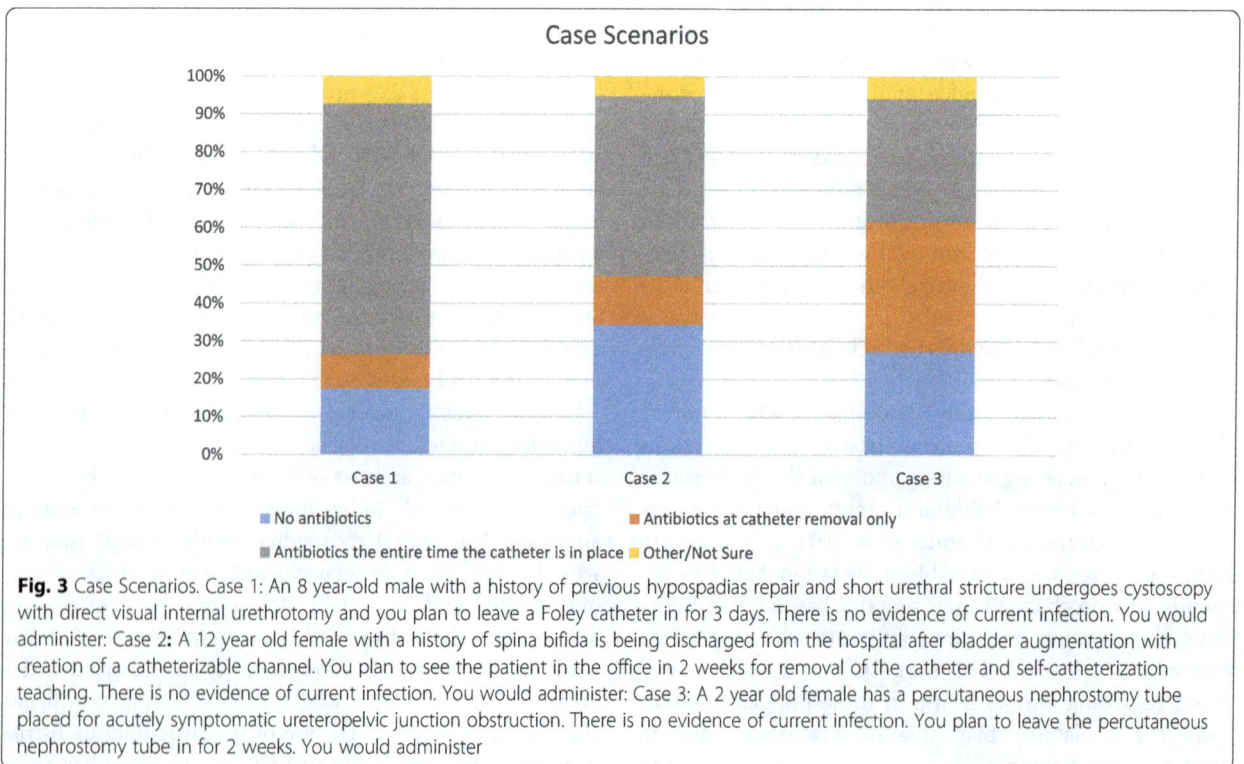

Fig. 3 Case Scenarios. Case 1: An 8 year-old male with a history of previous hypospadias repair and short urethral stricture undergoes cystoscopy with direct visual internal urethrotomy and you plan to leave a Foley catheter in for 3 days. There is no evidence of current infection. You would administer: Case 2: A 12 year old female with a history of spina bifida is being discharged from the hospital after bladder augmentation with creation of a catheterizable channel. You plan to see the patient in the office in 2 weeks for removal of the catheter and self-catheterization teaching. There is no evidence of current infection. You would administer: Case 3: A 2 year old female has a percutaneous nephrostomy tube placed for acutely symptomatic ureteropelvic junction obstruction. There is no evidence of current infection. You plan to leave the percutaneous nephrostomy tube in for 2 weeks. You would administer

controversial [25]. A recent Cochrane review of adult patients found limited evidence that prophylactic antibiotics reduce the incidence of bacteriuria, with even less evidence that this reduces febrile morbidity in those receiving antibiotic prophylaxis [26]. There is also limited evidence that antibiotics reduce bacteriuria for urodynamic studies in adults, but not enough evidence to suggest that antibiotics reduce symptomatic UTIs [27–29].

Variation in antibiotic use in our study may also be explained by a lack of specific management guidelines in this area. Organizational guidelines from the AUA, EAU, and others have limited applicability to the pediatric urology population, although they include the option to give antibiotics in complex scenarios. The AUA Best Practice Policy Statement on Urologic Surgery Antimicrobial Prophylaxis recommends antibiotic prophylaxis for removal of external urinary catheters and for urodynamics if risk factors such as urinary anatomic abnormalities, immunodeficiency, externalized catheters, colonized exogenous or endogenous material, and prolonged hospitalization are present [11]. Many pediatric urology patients will have one or more of these risk factors, yet in our survey many prescribers do not routinely give antibiotics in scenarios that include these risk factors, such as an externalized catheter. The AUA statement suggests that, for patients with risk factors, antimicrobial use at the time of catheter removal may be therapeutic in the setting of prolonged catheterization following a procedure, but the statement does not make a recommendation whether empiric antibiotics or culture-directed therapy is preferable in this setting. Evidence for this is primarily based on adult and post-prostatectomy literature and again may have limited applicability to the pediatric urology population [22, 30]. The EAU guideline on urological infections similarly states that when continuous drainage is in place after surgery, prolonged perioperative antibiotic prophylaxis is not routinely recommended; however, asymptomatic bacteriuria may be treated after removal of the catheter [12]. Finally, the United States Healthcare Infection Control Practices Advisory Committee, a division of the Centers for Disease Control and Prevention, also does not recommend routine antibiotics with short- and long-term catheterization, but does make a specific exception for patients with bacteriuria upon catheter removal following urologic surgery [3].

Although current guidelines include the option to give antibiotics in complex patients, there remains little guidance on which of these patients will actually benefit from antibiotic use. Our study shows that these patients are managed much differently by different practitioners – some with antibiotics, and some without. The risks of overuse of antibiotics are well-documented and include cost, unnecessary drug exposure, potential for allergic reactions, and antimicrobial resistance [2, 4]. Clinician-driven antibiotic stewardship has been proposed as the answer to reducing unnecessary antibiotic use [5, 9]. However, at this time, more directed evidence is needed to guide antibiotic use in pediatric urology. In this study, we approached this broad problem by first determining practice patterns. Next steps to establish effective stewardship include defining appropriate and inappropriate antibiotic use in this population and determining which patients will benefit the most.

Several limitations of this study should be acknowledged. First, only one-third of SPU members responded to our survey; however, this response rate is similar to other previous SPU surveys, and all sections of the AUA were represented in our sample [17, 31]. Also, it is unknown to us how many practicing pediatric urologists are not members of the SPU and were therefore not sent questionnaires; however, responders to our survey included academic, hospital-employed, and private-practice pediatric urologists. Antimicrobial resistance patterns may be different in different demographic areas, but we did not see a difference in prescribing patterns based on AUA section. Associations reported in this study are limited due to the lack of consensus for the majority of queried scenarios. Questions regarding specific antimicrobial agents were not asked. Also, in our study we cannot determine to what extent the reported responses correspond to actual clinical practice. However, we attempted to simulate the clinical environment in our survey by both asking general questions and using clinical scenarios. Finally, in this study we do not provide any information about what the best antimicrobial practice actually is, as this was not the study intent. Instead, this investigation was designed to define and measure current practice patterns as a first step in improving antimicrobial use for pediatric urology patients whose treatments require catheter use.

Conclusions

Our results indicate there is substantial variation in practice patterns among surveyed pediatric urologists regarding prophylactic antibiotic use with urinary catheterization and minor lower urinary tract procedures such as urodynamics, retrograde urethrogram, and voiding cystourethrogram. This lack of consensus in current management of these complex patients highlights the need for further research in this area and for the development of management guidelines for this unique population.

Abbreviations
AUA: American Urological Association; CAUTI: Catheter-associated urinary tract infection; EAU: European Association of Urology; PCN: Percutaneous nephrostomy tube; SPT: Suprapubic tube; SPU: Society for pediatric urology; UTI: Urinary tract infection

Acknowledgements
We would like to thank the Society for Pediatric Urology for assisting with distribution of this survey.

Funding

This research did not receive any specific grant from funding agencies in the public, commercial, or not-for-profit sectors.

Authors' contributions

All authors contributed to study conception and design. All authors have read and approve the final manuscript. IR contributed to acquisition of data. AG performed analysis and interpretation of data. AG, IR, and EJ contributed to drafting of manuscript.

Competing interests

The authors declare that they have no competing interests.

References

1. Glaser AP, Rosoklija I, Johnson E, Yerkes E. MP55-15 catheter-associated antibiotic use in pediatric urology: a survey of members of the Society for Pediatric Urology. J Urol. 2016;195(4):e741–2.

2. Hidron AI, Edwards JR, Patel J, Horan TC, Sievert DM, Pollock DA, Fridkin SK, National Healthcare Safety Network T, Participating National Healthcare Safety Network F. NHSN annual update: antimicrobial-resistant pathogens associated with healthcare-associated infections: annual summary of data reported to the National Healthcare Safety Network at the Centers for Disease Control and Prevention, 2006-2007. Infect Control Hosp Epidemiol. 2008;29(11):996–1011.

3. Gould CV, Umscheid CA, Agarwal RK, Kuntz G, Pegues DA, Healthcare Infection Control Practices Advisory C. Guideline for prevention of catheter-associated urinary tract infections 2009. Infect Control Hosp Epidemiol. 2010;31(4):319–26.

4. CDC: Antibiotic resistance threats in the United States. http://www.cdc.gov/drugresistance/pdf/ar-threats-2013-508.pdf 2013: [Accessed 2 July 2015].

5. Wagenlehner FM, Bartoletti R, Cek M, Grabe M, Kahlmeter G, Pickard R, Bjerklund-Johansen TE. Antibiotic stewardship: a call for action by the urologic community. Eur Urol. 2013;64(3):358–60.

6. Boucher HW, Talbot GH, Bradley JS, Edwards JE, Gilbert D, Rice LB, Scheld M, Spellberg B, Bartlett J. Bad bugs, no drugs: no ESKAPE! An update from the Infectious Diseases Society of America. Clinical infectious diseases : an official publication of the Infectious Diseases Society of America. 2009;48(1):1–12.

7. Bassetti M, Merelli M, Temperoni C, Astilean A. New antibiotics for bad bugs: where are we? Ann Clin Microbiol Antimicrob. 2013;12(22):1–15.

8. Boucher HW, Talbot GH, Benjamin DK Jr, Bradley J, Guidos RJ, Jones RN, Murray BE, Bonomo RA, Gilbert D, Infectious Diseases Society of A. 10 × '20 progress–development of new drugs active against gram-negative bacilli: an update from the Infectious Diseases Society of America. Clinical infectious diseases : an official publication of the Infectious Diseases Society of America. 2013;56(12):1685–94.

9. America SfHEo, America IDSo, Society PID. Policy statement on antimicrobial stewardship by the Society for Healthcare Epidemiology of America (SHEA), the Infectious Diseases Society of America (IDSA), and the Pediatric Infectious Diseases Society (PIDS). Infect Control Hosp Epidemiol. 2012;33(4):322–7.

10. Krieger JN. Prophylaxis in urology is no longer easy–should we use more or fewer antibiotics? J Urol. 2013;190(6):1972–3.

11. Wolf JS Jr, Bennett CJ, Dmochowski RR, Hollenbeck BK, Pearle MS, Schaeffer AJ, Urologic Surgery Antimicrobial Prophylaxis Best Practice Policy P. Best practice policy statement on urologic surgery antimicrobial prophylaxis. J Urol. 2008;179(4):1379–90.

12. Grabe M, Bartoletti R, Bjerklund-Johansen TE, Cek HM, Pickard RS, Tenke P, Wagenlehner F, Wullt B. Guidelines on urological infections. European Association of Urology. 2014:1–112. http://uroweb.org/guideline/urological-infections. Accessed 2 July 2015.

13. Bratzler DW, Dellinger EP, Olsen KM, Perl TM, Auwaerter PG, Bolon MK, Fish DN, Napolitano LM, Sawyer RG, Slain D, et al. Clinical practice guidelines for antimicrobial prophylaxis in surgery. Surg Infect. 2013;14(1):73–156.

14. Harris PA, Taylor R, Thielke R, Payne J, Gonzalez N, Conde JG. Research electronic data capture (REDCap)–a metadata-driven methodology and workflow process for providing translational research informatics support. J Biomed Inform. 2009;42(2):377–81.

15. Wazait HD, van der Meullen J, Patel HR, Brown CT, Gadgil S, Miller RA, Kelsey MC, Emberton M. Antibiotics on urethral catheter withdrawal: a hit and miss affair. J Hosp Infect. 2004;58(4):297–302.

16. Mossanen M, Calvert JK, Holt SK, James AC, Wright JL, Harper JD, Krieger JN, Gore JL. Overuse of antimicrobial prophylaxis in community practice urology. J Urol. 2015;193(2):543–7.

17. Hsieh MH, Wildenfels P, Gonzales ET Jr. Surgical antibiotic practices among pediatric urologists in the United States. J Pediatr Urol. 2011;7(2):192–7.

18. Cek M, Tandogdu Z, Naber K, Tenke P, Wagenlehner F, van Oostrum E, Kristensen B, Bjerklund Johansen TE, Global Prevalence Study of Infections in Urology I. Antibiotic prophylaxis in urology departments, 2005-2010. Eur Urol. 2013;63(2):386–94.

19. Meir DB, Livne PM. Is prophylactic antimicrobial treatment necessary after Hypospadias repair? J Urol. 2004;171(6):2621–2.

20. Baillargeon E, Duan K, Brzezinski A, Jednak R, El-Sherbiny M. The role of preoperative prophylactic antibiotics in hypospadias repair. Can Urol Assoc J. 2014;8(7–8):236–40.

21. Kanaroglou N, Wehbi E, Alotay A, Bagli DJ, Koyle MA, Lorenzo AJ, Farhat WA. Is there a role for prophylactic antibiotics after stented hypospadias repair? J Urol. 2013;190(4 Suppl):1535–9.

22. Marschall J, Carpenter CR, Fowler S, Trautner BW, Program CDCPE. Antibiotic prophylaxis for urinary tract infections after removal of urinary catheter: meta-analysis. BMJ. 2013;346:f3147.

23. Pfefferkorn U, Lea S, Moldenhauer J, Peterli R, von Flue M, Ackermann C. Antibiotic prophylaxis at urinary catheter removal prevents urinary tract infections: a prospective randomized trial. Ann Surg. 2009;249(4):573–5.

24. van Hees BC, Vijverberg PLM, Hoorntje LE, Wiltink EHH, Go PM, Tersmette M. Single-dose antibiotic prophylaxis for urinary catheter removal does not reduce the risk of urinary tract infection in surgical patients: a randomized double-blind placebo-controlled trial. Clin Microbiol Infect. 2011;17:1091–4.

25. Maki DG. ACP journal Club. Review: antibiotic prophylaxis on removal of urinary catheters reduces symptomatic urinary tract infections. Ann Intern Med. 2013;159(8):JC9.

26. Lusardi G, Lipp A, Shaw C. Antibiotic prophylaxis for short-term catheter bladder drainage in adults. Cochrane Database Syst Rev. 2013;7(7):CD005428.

27. Foon R, Toozs-Hobson P, Latthe P. Prophylactic antibiotics to reduce the risk of urinary tract infections after urodynamic studies. Cochrane Database Syst Rev. 2012;10(10):CD008224.

28. Lowder JL, Burrows LJ, Howden NL, Weber AM. Prophylactic antibiotics after urodynamics in women: a decision analysis. Int Urogynecol J Pelvic Floor Dysfunct. 2007;18(2):159–64.

29. Cundiff GW, McLennan MT, Bent AE. Randomized trial of antibiotic prophylaxis for combined urodynamics and cystourethroscopy. Obstet Gynecol. 1999;93(5 Pt 1):749–52.

30. Banks JA, McGuire BB, Loeb S, Shrestha S, Helfand BT, Catalona WJ. Bacteriuria and antibiotic resistance in catheter urine specimens following radical prostatectomy. Urol Oncol. 2013;31(7):1049–53.

31. Morganstern B, Ahmed H, Palmer LS. Pediatric Urologists' personal point-of-view of health related quality of life. Urology. 2016;88:179–82.

17

Intravescical prostatic protrusion is a predictor of alpha blockers response: results from an observational study

L. Topazio[1*], C. Perugia[1], C. De Nunzio[2], G. Gaziev[1], V. Iacovelli[1], D. Bianchi[1], G. Vespasiani[3] and E. Finazzi Agrò[3]

Abstract

Background: To investigate the efficacy of tamsulosin in patients with lower urinary tract symptoms (LUTS) and benign prostatic enlargement (BPE) with intravesical prostatic protrusion (IPP). Ultrasound measurement of the IPP has been previously described as an effective instrument for the evaluation of benign prostatic obstruction (BPO) and could help in clarifying the role of alpha-blockers in patients with (BPE).

Methods: Patients with BPE and LUTS were enrolled in this observational study. Intravesical prostatic protrusion was graded as grade 1 (< 5 ml), 2 (5 < IPP < 10 ml) and 3 (> 10 ml). Patients were treated with tamsulosin for twelve weeks. Evaluation was performed before and at the end of treatment by means of International Prostate Symptom Score (IPSS) and uroflowmetry. Patients were considered responders if a reduction of IPSS > 3 points was reported.

Results: One hundred forty-two patients were enrolled. Twelve patients were excluded because of incomplete data. Fifty patients showed an IPP grade 1 (group A), 52 a grade 2 (group B) and 28 a grade 3 (group C). Treatment success was obtained in 82%, 38,5% and 7,1% of patients respectively; these differences (group A vs B-C and group B vs C) were highly significant. The odd ratio to obtain a treatment success was of 59 and 8.1 in group A and group B respectively, in comparison to group C. After a multivariate regression, the relationship between IPP grade and treatment success remained significant. Improvement of uroflowmetry parameters has been reported in all the groups especially in patients with a low grade IPP (p value = 0,016 group A vs group B; p value = 0,005 group A vs group C). Prostate volume seems not to influence this relationship.

Conclusions: Intravesical prostatic protrusion has found to be significantly and inversely correlated with treatment success in patients with LUTS and BPE under alpha-blockers therapy. Alpha blockers odd ratio of success is 59 times higher in patients with a low grade IPP in comparison to patients with a high grade.

Keywords: LUTS, BPH, Alpha-blockers, Intravesical prostatic protrusion

Background

Benign prostatic hyperplasia (BPH) is found in over half of 60-year-old men and in almost all of 80-year-old men [1] and is the most frequent cause of bladder outlet obstruction (BOO) in males over the age of 50 who apply with lower urinary tract symptoms [2]. In this case, the term Benign Prostatic Obstruction (BPO) is currently used [3]. In BPO patients, medical therapy is the most commonly used [3] and provides relief in symptoms and alteration in disease progression [4]. However, long-term

dropout rates reach 30–43% [5] and not all patients benefit from the treatment. Therefore, it would be beneficial to identify patients that will not respond to medical treatment.

The evaluation of BPO is an important factor that can reflect the severity of disease and can aid in measuring the outcome of the treatment. Nowadays the standard practice investigation for BPO patients is composed of uroflowmetry and ultrasound (US) evaluation of the post-void residual urine (PVR) [3]. Unfortunately, such investigations have less possibility to clearly identify the degree of BOO in men affected by Benign prostatic enlargement (BPE) with respect to pressure-flow study

* Correspondence: lucatpz@hotmail.it
[1]School of Specialization in Urology, University "Tor Vergata", Rome, Italy
Full list of author information is available at the end of the article

(PFS) during invasive urodynamic investigation (UD) [6]. However, UD test before surgical BPO treatment is not always indicated in international guidelines because of the invasiveness and high costs of the method [3, 7].

In the last decade, several authors have tried to identify novel and less invasive parameters that could help the physician in evaluating the degree of BPO, thus predicting a treatment response. The most promising among them are bladder/detrusor wall thickness [8, 9], ultrasound-estimated bladder weight [10], non-invasive pressure-flow testing [11], prostatic urethral angle [12] and US measurement of the intravesical prostatic protrusion (IPP) [11, 13, 14].

US measurement of IPP was first described by Chia et al. in 2003 to correlate well with BPO (presence and severity) on urodynamic testing, with a PPV of 94% and a NPV of 79% [13]. The clinical significance of IPP can be explained by the fact that protrusion of the median lobe of the prostate into the bladder can cause a "ball valve" type of benign prostatic obstruction with incomplete opening and disruption of the funneling effect of the bladder neck [13, 15].

Further studies on this topic have shown that IPP may correlate with prostate volume, detrusor overactivity (DO), bladder compliance, detrusor pressure at maximum urinary flow, BOO index and PVR, and negatively correlates with Qmax [16]. Moreover, IPP also seems to predict successfully the outcome of a trial without catheter (TWOC) after acute urinary retention [17] and the success rate of TURP [18]. To date, however, few data have been reported in terms of the association between IPP and clinical outcomes in patients undergoing medical therapy. Studies investigating the relationship between IPP and alpha-blockers therapy outcomes [19, 20] have shown that it may be correlated to reduced efficacy of alpha blockers in patients with IPP and mild/moderate (< 40 ml) prostate volume (PV) [19, 20]. However, to our knowledge, no data are available on patients with PV ≥ 40 ml.

Aim of this study was to investigate the efficacy of an alpha-blocker (Tamsulosin) in patients with lower urinary tract symptoms (LUTS) and BPE with or without IPP.

Methods

This is an observational prospective study performed from January to December 2015 in the outpatient clinic of Tor Vergata University Hospital in Rome and reported following the STROBE statement.

We enrolled male patients between fifty and seventy-five years of age, affected by BPE defined as trans-rectal ultrasound (TRUS) estimated PV ≥ 30 ml, in whom tamsulosin had been prescribed for LUTS.

Exclusion criteria were:

- Prior urologic surgery;
- Patients affected by a urologic neoplasia, bladder calculus or any type of neurological abnormality;
- Prior treatment with alpha blockers and 5alpha reductase inhibitors;
- Absence of intravescical prostatic protusion.

All patients enrolled underwent a baseline evaluation by means of medical history, administration of the International Prostate Symptom Score and Quality of Life (IPSS/QoL) questionnaire, trans-rectal ultrasound of the prostate and uroflowmetry. All TRUS were performed by the same physician and at the standard bladder filling of 150 ml. Trans rectal ultrasound was performed in the midsagittal plane and IPP along with the prostatic volume were measured. IPP was identified according to the classification system used by Nose et al [21] and was defined by the distance from the tip of the prostate's protrusion into the vesical lumen to the bladder neck measured in millimetres. IPP estimated by TRUS was then graded as Grade 1 (if it was inferior to 5 mm), Grade 2 (if it was comprised between 5 and 10 mm) and Grade 3 (if it was superior to 10 mm). PV measurement was obtained during TRUS. All uroflowmetry were performed at the standard bladder filling of 250–300 ml as recommended by the guidelines for good urodynamic practices [22].

All patients enrolled were then treated with Tamsulosin (0,4 mg/day) for twelve weeks and re-evaluated after treatment by means of International Prostate Symptom Score and Quality of Life (IPSS/QoL) and uroflowmetry. Patients were considered responders (treatment success) if showing a reduction of IPSS > 3 points.

Statistical analysis

All data were classified in an Excel Database. All analyses were performed by means of the software STATA 13.0. Univariate logistic regression was used to evaluate relationships between each parameter (IPP grade, PV, IPSS, Qmax, PSA) and treatment success. A paired t test was used to evaluate change in time in uroflow parameters in each group separately. One way anova was used to compared these changes between the three groups. Bonferroni correction was applied in post hoc comparison. Univariable logistic regression was used to evaluate relationships between IPP grade and the treatment success. Odd Ratio (OR) and relative 95% confidence Interval (CI 95%) were reported. A stepwise logistic regression was applied considering as independent factor IPP grade, age PSA, PV and baseline value of Qmax IPSS and RPM. Adjusted OR (ORadj) and relative 95% confidence Interval (CI 95%) were reported. A p value < 0.05 was considered statistically significant.

Table 1 Baseline features of Patients

	Age, mean (DS)	Prostate volume, mean (DS)	Estimated IPP, mean (DS)	Pre-treatment Qmax, mean (DS)	Pre-treatment IPSS, mean (DS)	Pre-treatment PSA, mean (DS)
Group A	62 (8.9)	45.5 (16.9)	2.7 (0.8)	10.5 (2.9)	17.7 (3.9)	3.5 (2.5)
Group B	64 (9)	53.2 (21.2)	6.5 (1.3)	9.3 (1.5)	18 (4.1)	2 (1.4)
Group C	66 (8.6)	54.6 (13.1)	11.4 (1.1)	8.8 (2.3)	22.2 (5.1)	3.1 (1.7)

IPP Intravesical prostatic protrusion, *Qmax* Maximum flow at uroflowmetry, *IPSS* International prostatic symptoms score

Results

One hundred forty-two patients were enrolled. Twelve patients were excluded because of incomplete data. Of the remaining 130 patients, 50 (38.5%) showed an IPP grade 1 (group A), 52 (40%) an IPP grade 2 (group B) and 28 (21.5%) an IPP grade 3 (group C). Baseline features of patients are showed in Table 1. Treatment success, defined as post-treatment IPSS score reduction > 3 points, was obtained in 82%, 38,5% and 7,1% of patients respectively. The odd ratio to obtain a treatment success was of 59 (CI 95% 11.8–296) and 8.1 (CI95% 1.7–38) in group A and group B respectively, in comparison to group C (Table 2). Moreover, there is a positive improvement of uroflow parameters in each group (Table 3) with a better improvement after treatment in patients with a low grade IPP with respect to patients with a higher grade IPP (p value = 0,016 Group A vs Group B; p value = 0,005 Group A vs Group C).

After multivariate regression, the relationship between IPP grade and treatment success remained significant. Interestingly the multivariate regression shows that PV seems not influence this relationship and is not included in the final model (Table 4).

Discussion

IPP is a promising parameter, first described by Chia in 200, 313, that has shown a good correlation with the presence and severity of BPO on urodynamic testing. Further studies have found a strong correlation between IPP and DO, bladder compliance, detrusor pressure at maximum urinary flow, terminal dribbling, BOO index and PVR while a negative correlation was found between IPP and Qmax and/or alpha-blockers efficacy [16, 19, 20, 23]. Moreover a well-designed study from Luo GC et al. has shown that the presence of middle lobe is more obstructive than those of lateral lobes and could better correlate with BOO grade [24]. Data

coming from our study suggest that IPP is significantly and inversely correlated with treatment success in patients affected by BPE and with LUTS under alpha-blocker therapy. Alpha-blockers odd ratio of success is 59 times higher in patients with a low grade IPP in comparison to patients with a high grade IPP and 8 times higher with respect to patients with a moderate grade IPP. It is important to underline that the definition of success used in this study (a reduction of IPSS score > 3 points) is in line with previous and contemporary studies, considering this IPSS variation as clinically significant [25]. Interestingly even after multivariate regression with stepwise logistic regression IPP remains as independent predictive factors for alpha blockers treatment success.

Our data are similar to those in literature; Cumpanas et al. analyzed 183 patients with BPH (PV < 40 mL) treated with tamsulosin and found that approximately 40% of the patients in the high IPP group were treatment nonresponders and had significantly worse outcomes than patients in the low IPP group at 3 months [20]; even in a more recent paper Kalkanli et al. [26] showed that an increase in IPP was associated with a lower response level to medical treatment and indicated a significant negative correlation between IPP-Qmax and IPP-post treatmens IPSS. Similar data were also published by Hirayama et al [27] in Patients treated with Dutasteride 0.5 mg daily in which IPP was seen to be the strongest predictive factor for failure of medical therapy and conversion to surgical intervention with the optimal cutoff value of IPP of 8 mm. This value yielded a sensitivity of 91% and a specificity of 72%.

Interestingly our data show that PV seems not to influence the relationship between IPP and alpha-blockers success rate. This is, to our knowledge, one of the very first papers to investigate this relationship in Patients with PV higher than 40 ml and our results are similar to those already published by Wang et al. in 2015 [28] who showed a strong correlation between IPP and BPO and stated that IPP is superior to PV in predicting BPO in patients who present with LUTS.

Our result indicates that IPP helps to predict obstruction by BPH and therefore the progression of BPH (prostate adenoma) and response rate to alpha blockers therapy; therefore, IPP is useful in stratifying BPH patients with LUTS at initial evaluation, helping the urologist in

Table 2 Relationship between IPP grade and treatment success

	Responders	Not responders	OR	CI 95%	p
Group A	41 (65.1%)	9 (13.4%)	59	11.8–296	< 0.001
Group B	20 (31.7%)	32 (47.8%)	8.1	1.7–38	0.008
Group C	2 (3.2%)	26 (38.8%)	1		

OR Odd ratio, *CI* Confidence interval

Table 3 Pre post-treatment Qmax differences

	Pre-treatment Qmax, mean (SD)	Post-treatment Qmax, mean (SD)	Pre post-treatment Qmax differences, mean (SD)	pValue
Group A	10.5 (2.9)	14.1 (3.2)	3.6 (1.4)	< 0.001
Group B	9.3 (1.5)	11.7 (2.7)	2.4 (2.7)	< 0.001
Group C	8.8 (2.3)	10.8 (2.7)	2.0 (2.2)	< 0.001

Qmax Maximum flow at uroflowmetry

deciding which patient could benefit from medical therapy and avoiding lots of unuseful prescriptions for further cost-effective management.

It is interesting to observe that also Qmax showed a larger improvement in low or moderate IPP grade patients in comparison to severe IPP grade patients (p value = 0,016 Group A-B vs Group C). Furthermore, patients with a higher IPP grade showed lower pre-treatment Qmax, in comparison with patients with 1–2 IPP grade (p value = 0,029 Group A-B vs Group C). This finding seems to suggest that the degree of IPP could correlate with the degree of BPO, but the lack of an invasive urodynamic evaluation (pressure/flow study) do not allow us to draw conclusions on that point.

The study has several limitations; no RCT, no sample size calculation; non-invasive UD data. Besides we are conscious that EAU Guidelines on "Non neurogenic male LUTS" [3] suggest a combination therapy for patients with PV > 40 ml and therefore that the vast majority of patients in our study did not receive a Guideline conform therapy but the aim of this study was not to evaluate the efficacy of tamsulosin monotherapy in PV > 40 ml but to assess the efficacy of alpha-blockers in relationship to the IPP grade. Thus the results of this paper could reinforce the indication of a combination therapy in this patients' population. This study provides furthermore the information that IPP seems to be a negative prognosctic factor for success of Tamsulosin, independently by the prostate volume.

The strengths of the study are a proper statistical methodology and the use of a clinically meaningful primary outcome measure as modifications in IPSS score.

Table 4 Multivariate regression on treatment success

	ORadj	CI 95%		P value
IPP grade				
Grade 1	84.83	14.31	502.93	< 0.001
Grade 2	8.70	1.70	44.51	0.009
Grade 3	1			
Age	.95	.90	1.00	0.071
PSA	.74	.58	.94	0.014
PVR pre	.99	.97	.99	0.037

Stepwise regression. Initial model: IPP grade, PSA, PV, Qmax baseline, IPSS baseline, RPM baseline

Conclusions

IPP seems significantly and inversely correlated with treatment success in patients with LUTS and BPE under alpha-blockers and may be considered a useful tool to discriminate patients in whom medical treatment has higher (low grade IPP) or lower (high grade IPP) probability of success.

Abbreviations
BOO: Bladder outlet obstruction; BPE: Benign prostatic enlargement; BPH: Benign prostatic hyperplasia; BPO: Benign Prostatic Obstruction; CI: Confidence interval; DO: Detrusor overactivity; IPP: Intravesical prostatic protrusion; IPSS/QoL: International Prostate Symptom Score and Quality of Life; LUTS: Lower urinary tract symptoms; OR: Odd Ratio; PFS: Pressure-flow study; PV: Prostate volume; PVR: Post-void residual urine; TRUS: Trans-rectal ultrasound; TWOC: Trial without catheter; UD: Urodynamic investigation; US: Ultrasound

Acknowledgements
None

Funding
None

Authors' contributions
LT has participated in data analysis and interpretation and drafting the article; CP, VI and GG have participated in data collection; DB, CDN and VG have participated in critical revision of the article; EFA have participated in conception and design of the work. All authors have given final approval of the version to be published.

Competing interests
The authors declare that they have no competing interests

Author details
[1]School of Specialization in Urology, University "Tor Vergata", Rome, Italy. [2]Department of Urology, Sant'Andrea Hospital, University "La Sapienza", Rome, Italy. [3]Department of Experimental Medicine and Surgery, University "Tor Vergata", Rome, Italy.

References
1. Platz EA, Smit E, Curhan GC, Nyberg LM, Giovannucci E. Prevalence of and racial/ethnic variation in lower urinary tract symptoms and noncancer prostate surgery in U.S. men. Urology. 2002;59:877–83.
2. Martin SA, Haren MT, Marshall VR, et al. Prevalence and factors associated with uncomplicated storage and voiding lower urinary tract symptoms in community-dwelling Australian men. World J Urol. 2011;29:179–84.

3. EAU guidelines on Management of Non-Neurogenic Male Lower Urinary Tract Symptoms (LUTS), incl. Benign Prostatic Obstruction (BPO)S. Gravas (Chair), T. Bach, A. Bachmann, M. Drake, M. Gacci, C. Gratzke, S. Madersbacher, C. Mamoulakis, K.A.O. Tikkinen Guidelines Associates: M. Karavitakis, S. Malde, V. Sakkalis, R. Umbach. LIMITED UPDATE MARCH 2016.

4. Mc Connell JD, Roehrborn CG, Bautista OM, et al. The long-term effect of doxazosin, finasteride, a combination therapy on the clinical progression of benign prostatic hyperplasia. N Engl J Med. 2003;349:2387–98.

5. Lepor H. Long term efficacy and safety of terazosin in patients with benign prostatic hyperplasia. The terazosin research group. Urology. 1995;45:406–13.

6. Nitti VW, Kim Y, Combs AJ. Correlation of the AUA symptom index with urodynamics in patients with suspected benign prostatic hyperplasia. Neurourol Urodyn. 1994;13(5):521–7. discussion 527-9

7. van Venrooij GE, van Melick HH, Boon TA. Comparison of outcomes of transurethral prostate resection in urodynamically obstructed versus selected urodynamically unobstructed or equivocal men. Urology. 2003;62: 672–6.

8. Oelke M, et al. Diagnostic accuracy of noninvasive tests to evaluate bladder outlet obstruction in men: detrusor wall thickness, uroflowmetry, postvoid residual urine, and prostate volume. Eur Urol. 2007;52:827.

9. Blatt AH, et al. Ultrasound measurement of bladder wall thickness in the assessment of voiding dysfunction. J Urol. 2008;179:2275.

10. Kojima M, et al. Ultrasonic estimation of bladder weight as a measure of bladder hypertrophy in men with infravesical obstruction: a preliminary report. Urology. 1996;47:942.

11. Pel JJ, et al. Development of a non-invasive strategy to classify bladder outlet obstruction in male patients with LUTS. Neurourol Urodyn. 2002;21:117.

12. Park YJ, Bae KH, Jin BS, Jung HJ, Park JS. Is increased prostatic urethral angle related to lower urinary tract symptoms in males with benignprostatic hyperplasia/lower urinary tract symptoms? Korean J Urol. 2012 Jun;53(6): 410–3. doi:10.4111/kju.2012.53.6.410. Epub 2012 Jun 19.

13. Chia SJ, et al. Correlation of intravesical prostatic protrusion with bladder outlet obstruction. BJU Int. 2003;91:371–4.

14. Kessler TM, et al. Ultrasound assessment of detrusor thickness in men-can it predict bladder outlet obstruction and replace pressure flow study? J Urol. 2006;175:2170.

15. Zheng J, Pan J, Qin Y, Huang J, Luo Y, Gao X, Zhou X. Role for intravesical prostatic protrusion in lower urinary tract symptom: a fluid structural interaction analysis study. BMC Urol. 2015 Aug 19;15:86. doi:10.1186/s12894-015-0081-y.

16. Keqin Z, et al. Clinical significance of intravesical prostatic protrusion in patients with benign prostatic enlargement. Urology. 2007;70:1096.

17. Mariappan P, et al. Intravesical prostatic protrusion is better than prostate volume in predicting the outcome of trial without catheter in white men presenting with acute urinary retention: a prospective clinical study. J Urol. 2007;178:573.

18. Lee JW, Ryu JH, Yoo TK, Byun SS, Jeong YJ, Jung TY. Relationship between Intravesical prostatic protrusion and postoperative outcomes in patients with benign prostatic hyperplasia. Korean J Urol. 2012 Jul;53(7):478–482. doi:10.4111/kju.2012.53.7.478. Epub 2012 Jul 19.

19. Park HY, Lee JY, Park SY, Lee SW, Kim YT, Choi HY, Moon HS. Efficacy of alpha blocker treatment according to the degree of intravesical prostatic protrusion detected by transrectal ultrasonography in patients with benign prostatic hyperplasia. Korean J Urol 2012 Feb;53(2):92–97. doi:10.4111/kju.2012.53.2.92. Epub 2012 Feb 20.

20. Cumpanas AA, Botoca M, Minciu R, Bucuras V. Intravesical prostatic protrusion can be a predicting factor for the treatment outcome in patients with lower urinary tract symptoms due to benign prostatic obstruction treated with tamsulosin. Urology 2013 Apr; 81(4):859–863. doi:10.1016/j.urology.2012.12.007. Epub 2013 Jan 30.

21. Nose H, Foo KT, Lim KB, Yokoyama T, Ozawa H, Kumon H. Accuracy of two noninvasive methods of diagnosing bladder outlet obstruction using ultrasonography: intravesical prostatic protrusion and velocity-flow video urodynamics. Urology. 2005;65:493–7.

22. Werner Schafer,* Paul Abrams, Limin Liao, Anders Mattiasson, Francesco Pesce, Anders Spangberg, Arthur M. Sterling, Norman R. Zinner, and Philip van Kerrebroeck Good urodynamic practices: Uroflowmetry, filling Cystometry, and pressure-flow studies. Neurourol Urodyn 2002;21:261–274.

23. Kim JH, Shim JS, Choi H, Moon du G, Lee JG, Kim JJ, Bae JH, Park JY. Terminal dribbling in male patients with lower urinary tract symptoms: relationship with international prostate symptom score and with intravesical prostatic protrusion. BMC Urol. 2015 Aug 29;15:89. doi:10.1186/s12894-015-0082-x.

24. Luo GC, Foo KT, Kuo T, Tan G. Diagnosis of prostate adenoma and the relationship between the site of prostate adenoma and bladder outlet obstruction. Singap Med J. 2013 Sep;54(9):482–6.

25. Barry MJ, Williford WO, Chang Y. Benign prostatic hyperplasia specific health status measures in clinical research: how much change in the American urological association symptom index and the benign prostatic hyperplasia impact index is perceptible to patients? J Urol. 1995;154:1770–4.

26. Kalkanli A, Tandogdu Z, Aydin M, Karaca AS, Hazar AI, Balci MBC, Aydin M, Nuhoglu B. Intravesical prostatic protrusion:a potential marker of alpha-blocker treatment success in patients with benign prostatic enlargement. Urology. 2016;88:161–5.

27. Hirayama K, Masui K, Hamada A, Shichiri Y, Masuzawa N, Hamada S. Evaluation of Intravesical prostatic protrusion as a predictor of Dutasteride-resistant lower urinary TractSymptoms/benign prostatic enlargement with a high likelihood of surgical intervention. Urology. 2015;86:565–9.

28. Wang D, Huang H, Law YM, Foo KT. Relationships between prostatic volume and Intravesical prostatic protrusion on transabdominal ultrasound and benign prostatic obstruction in patients with lower urinary tract symptoms. Ann Acad Med Singap. 2015;44:60–5.

18

A pilot study in intraparenchymal therapy delivery in the prostate: a comparison of delivery with a porous needle vs standard needle

Martin L. Brady[1], King Scott Coffield[2,5]* ⓘD, Thomas J. Kuehl[3,6], Raghu Raghavan[1], V. O. Speights Jr[4,5], Belur Patel[2,5], Scott Wilson[7], Mike Wilson[7] and Rick M. Odland[7,8]

Abstract

Background: New biologic therapies directly injected into the prostate are in clinical trials for prostatic diseases. There is a need to understand distribution of injected therapies as a function of prostatic anatomy, physiology, and device design.

Methods: A needle with a porous length of customizable-length was tested and its performance compared with a standard needle. Injections of magnetic resonance contrast reagent were placed into ex-vivo human prostates after surgical excision in standard of care therapy for invasive bladder cancer patients. Magnetic resonance images were acquired using sequences to quantify volume delivered, distributed, and backflow.

Results: Magnetic resonance images analysis revealed heterogeneity distribution with injection into the specimens. There was low resistance to flow along ductal pathways and high resistance to flow into glandular nodules and smooth muscle/fibrous parenchyma. Data confirm previous studies showing injection loss via urethra backflow, urethra, and prostatic ducts. Tissue fraction of dose was significantly higher with porous needle compared with standard needle ($p = .03$). We found that a greater volume of distribution divided by the amount infused (Vd/Vi) increased by 80% with the porous needle, though no statistically significant association due to small sample size.

Conclusions: This study demonstrated that prostatic tissue is anatomically heterogenic and limits distribution of needle injection. There is greater distribution in the ex-vivo prostate using a porous needle. The complexity of intra prostatic flow pathways suggests preoperative imaging and pre-treatment planning will enhance therapy.

Keywords: Prostate, Porous Needle, Infusion, Imaging, Distribution

Background

Benign prostatic hyperplasia (BPH) and prostate cancer are two major diseases in men [1, 2]. Symptomatic BPH occurs in two-thirds of men by age 80. One in seven men has prostate cancer diagnosed; it is a common cause of cancer death in men later in life. Though low risk prostate cancer is more common, intermediate and high risk prostatic cancer remain morbidity and mortality risks for one in nine men between 50 and 80 years of age. Radical prostatectomy and external or implant radiation therapy (standard of care) are associated with serious side effects upon a man's quality of life. Common surgical and medical BPH therapies may fail or cause similar side effects. There is ample evidence of need for improved outcomes in both diseases.

Prostatic injection of biologicals to treat BPH and prostate cancer is a potential pathway to reduce serious side-effects of commonly used therapies. A major challenge for developing therapies based on prostatic injection is lack of predictable control of distribution of the

* Correspondence: King.Coffield@BSWHealth.org
[2]Department of Surgery, Division of Urology, Scott & White Medical Center, Temple, TX, USA
[5]Texas A&M Health Science Center College of Medicine, Temple, TX, USA
Full list of author information is available at the end of the article

injected agent into a specialized muscular organ that may have anatomic alteration of the prostatic ductal continuity, invasion and distortion of prostatic fibromuscular tissue, and ducts with intermediate and high risk prostatic adenocarcinoma. Prostatic adenoma enlargement also alters the glandular ductal drainage and prostatic fibromuscular tissue with compression and fibrous barriers rather than invasion. However, the impetus to develop minimally invasive therapies for benign and malignant disease has grown with recent advances in therapeutic related technologies of imaging, molecular innovation, and the interest of limiting the side effects of therapy for active and engaged patients. Intraprostatic injections have recently been explored, as these can be performed under local anesthesia. There has also been interest in development of two agents, Fexapotide triflutate (NX-1207) for symptomatic BPH and topsalysin (PRX-302) for BPH and organ confined prostatic cancer. Both have shown good safety profiles and early efficacy in phase II studies [3].

The goal of this study is to describe and define the distribution of liquid agents injected in ex-vivo prostates harvested at radical cystectomy. We aim to highlight a preliminary comparison of two different devices for infusion of fluid into prostate.

Methods
Devices and equipment
Institutional review board approval was obtained to undertake the tissue harvesting and injection of the prostates in this study. Inclusion criteria included 18 years of age, prior diagnosis of invasive bladder cancer, lack of prior bladder radiation, prostate radiation, bladder chemotherapy, prostate chemotherapy or prostate surgery, and the granting of IRB-approved tissue harvesting consent from each patient. We used a standard, control needle and a porous, investigation needle (Fig. 1) in this study, both 20 gauge MP35N alloy with a length of 20cm and plastic luer fitting on proximal end. The control needle was end port design with single bevel at the distal end. The distal end of the porous, investigational needle has a solid tri-bevel tip. The porous length

starts 3mm proximal to the tri-bevel tip point and was 1–2 cm long in this study. The porous length is a thermomechanical formed metallic structure designed to provide distribution along the entire porous length.

Sample preparation; device insertion and placement
Human prostates were harvested at radical cystoprostatectomy from 16 consented patients with muscle invasive transitional carcinoma. After bladder and seminal vesicles removal, the prostates were cooled in ice slush and transported to the research laboratory for processing. Prostate volumes were estimated using measurements of thickness, depth, and width, using the formula for an ellipsoid. Each prostate was positioned in a magnetic resonance (MR) compatible container encased in insulating foam, stabilized with the apex perpendicular to a brachytherapy guide template. The urethra was filled with insulating foam to permit localization without occlusion. The stabilized prostate was placed inside a body coil using a 3T Siemens Trios (Siemens, Enlagen, Germany) for imaging. High-resolution, serial axial sections were obtained with 1mm thick slices to plan the positioning of two devices for infusion. The pulse parameters for the FLASH acquisition were TR = 30 ms, and averaging acquisitions with TE from 2.2 to 23.2 msec. The voxels were isotropic and the resolution was 0.95 mm. Needle placement was performed by a single urological team (KSC, TJK) experienced with image guided prostate needle placement. The infusions targeted the mid transition zone of the prostate, since that is where it is easiest to envisage placing a needle traversing the peripheral and transition prostatic zones in a bilaterally symmetric manner. The insertion depth of the porous needle and standard needle was the same, about 20 mm, which was typically a few mm less than the dimension of the prostate along the trajectory of the catheter in the urethra. Each device was used to infuse from 1—1.5mL of modified Galbumin™ (gadolinium-labeled albumin; Biopal, Inc., Worcester, MA) (Additional files 1 and 2), using a duel channel syringe pump (Model KDS LEGATO 210, KD Scientific, Holliston, MA) during a 10-minute interval in all but four of the prostate

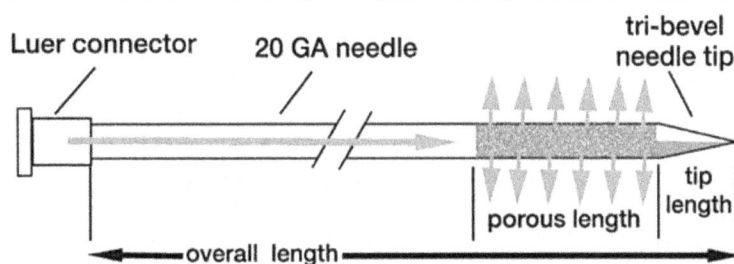

Fig. 1 Includes an appearance of a standard needle though the porous segment is readily visible with variable length. Study needle was 20 Ga with a tri-bevel tip for penetration ease and single lumen with standard luer-lok connector

specimens and during a 100-120 minute infusion in four to allow a more detailed evaluation of the distribution patterns. The infusion technique and times were selected to control pressure delivery into the prostates. The injected molecular agent was used to simulate molecular size of potential therapeutic agents. Serial dynamic images were obtained to document distribution through the gland in relation to anatomic landmarks and lesions. After each infusion, additional high-resolution images were obtained to determine quantitative distribution maps of infused contrast agent. The prostate was then removed from the container and immersed in formalin fixation. The prostate and urethra were processed for anatomic evaluation and sections were photographed and blocked for histologic examination.

Contrast agent infusions and imaging

Galbumin™ served as a surrogate for the proteins used in therapies for prostatic disease. This reagent was infused at a concentration of 25% of the supplied Galbumin™, diluted 1:3 with saline solution. The resulting concentration was 0.0845mmol/L. The infusate was prepared in a 10mL volumetric flask by adding full volume from two vials with 25mg/mL of Galbumin™ in each vial, along with 100μL of food coloring and filling with phosphate buffered saline. Four separate vials using Glowing Galbumin™-Fluorescein infusate from Biopal, Inc. were prepared and placed in small tubes located within the field of view of the prostate. The composition of these vials varied from 0—2.5mg/mL of Gd-conjugated albumin. The four vials, each holding about 300μL of the markers, were placed below the prostate in the container used in the MR scanner. The prostates were cooled and imaged with contrast injection within 6-8 hours from harvest. Imaging with sequencing was acquired before infusion and once after the infusion at either 10 minutes or 100-120 minutes (in four prostates) after initiation of infusion using T1 maps computed from pairs of 3D FLASH MR scans at flip angles of 6 and 34° using the variable nutation method [4, 5]. B1 field inhomogeneities were corrected using a method for measuring said angles [6]. We measured the concentration of MR reagents by the method described by Brady et al for in-vivo infusions [7]. Gadolinium concentration C was computed from the T1 maps using the equation $1/T1 = 1/T10 + R1C$, where relaxivity is denoted R1.

Line pressure measurements

The line pressures were measured using transducers placed between the infusion pump and 25ft of high pressure tubing. The tubing allows for instruments to be located outside of the 25 gauss line of the MR unit.

Data analysis

The volume of distribution V_d was estimated as the volume of the voxels containing a measureable concentration of gadolinium tracer and was used to compute the ratio V_d/V_i, where V_i is the volume of fluid infused. In calculating V_d, we applied a threshold to the concentration instead of applying a threshold to the T1-enhanced image of the contrast reagent. For Galbumin™, the threshold was 0.002mmol/L, or 4.8% of the infusate concentration (this was the minimum computable concentration). In the case of CellTrack™, the threshold was 0.8% of the infusate concentration. Thus, V_d is the total volume of all voxels that contain at least this concentration of reagent. Increasing or decreasing this threshold tended to decrease or increase V_d, respectively.

Comparison of the fraction of contrast delivered to prostate tissue with each needle type was tested with a two sided T test, corresponding to the conservative assumption that there is no a priori reason to favor the porous device delivering more or less infusate than the standard needle into a specialized muscular organ that was similar on both sides of injection.

Comparison of the ratio of volume of distribution to volume infused with each needle type was tested with two-sided T test, corresponding to the conservative assumption that there is no a priori reason to favor the porous device delivering more or less infusate than the standard needle into a specialized muscular organ that was similar on both sides of injection.

Results

Histopathological results

The histopathological analysis of each prostate was performed by a single pathologist utilizing the laboratory standard for prostate surgical specimens submitted with cystectomy for invasive transitional cell carcinoma. Final pathological reports revealed no incidental prostate cancer in the prostate specimens. There was a single transitional cell carcinoma focally extending into the proximal prostatic urethra without invasion into the prostatic stroma.

Backflow

Backflow is a well-known phenomenon due to the interaction of tissue elasticity with fluid flow [8]. However, there was essentially no measureable backflow beyond the proximal extent of the porous segment when the porous needle was used (Additional files 1 and 2). However, the standard needle did exhibit backflow (Fig. 2). Sometimes, there are other preferred pathways that prevent backflow reaching the prostatic capsule. Nevertheless, this remains a concern for needle infusions particularly at higher flow rates.

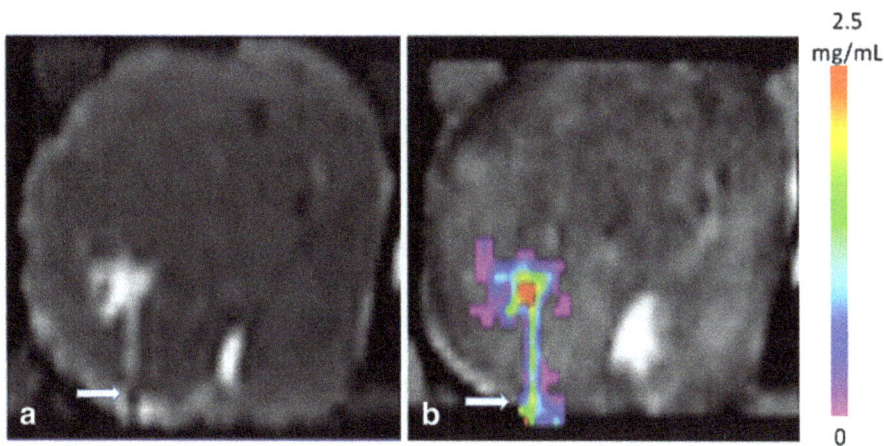

Fig 2 Image depicts standard needle infusate backflow (**a**) along the needle sides with concentration distribution (**b**) seen at highest in red and lowest in lavender. The Gadolinium distribution is seen in Fig. **a**. The concentration distribution is seen in Fig. **b**

Outflow

We use the word outflow in a very restricted sense to mean volume transmission of particle (tracer in this case) beyond the prostatic capsule or into the urethra before the prostate or the target zone (e.g. the peripheral zone of the prostate) is filled with infusate (Fig. 3). With little spread within the parenchyma, much of such outflow can be avoided if backflow is well contained. However, as shown in Tables 1 and 2, only a small fraction of the total infused amount of tracer stays within the prostate.

Preferred pathways

The ductal or directional pathways in the prostate seem also to lead to infusate loss to the outside as well as into the urethra (Fig. 4). The aim of a good delivery system is to reduce infusate loss and effective distribution to the targeted area.

Obstacles

Unlike preferred pathways, obstacles such as glandular or stromal nodules appear either highly resistant to fluid flow throughout their volume or are surrounded by a fibrous barrier preventing ingress or efflux. Figure 5 displays post-infusion images showing (top images from left to right) infused dye, T1-weighted MRI, and computed concentration in a single axial section. This figure shows a clear avoidance of a region in the prostate: it is likely enclosed by a relatively impermeable fibrous and/or muscle tissue barrier. In the few cases where the needle or porous catheter is inserted into such a nodule, flow within the nodule is limited. This may also be due to the nodule itself being of high resistance. We cannot sharply distinguish between these possibilities from the imaging data; though in T2 imaging (which would show water as high intensity), there tends to be a thin dark band

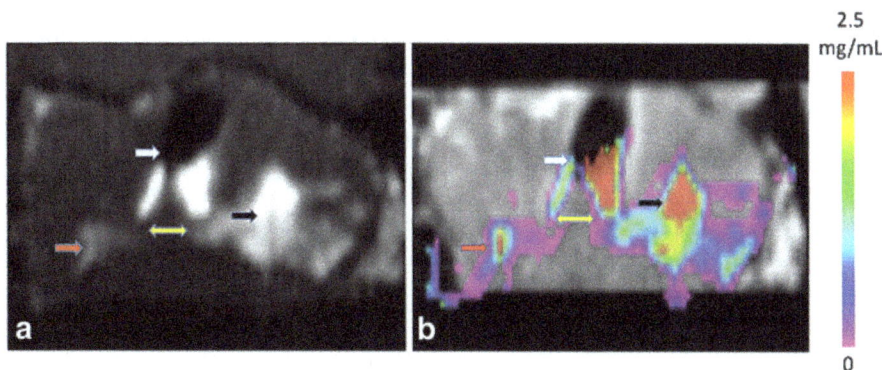

Fig. 3 Left (**a**): T1 Gadolinium injection image with standard needle (red arrow) and porous needle (black arrow) pointing to the linear needle image entering the prostate from lower edge of prostate. White arrow depicts infusate movement to the urethra. Yellow arrow depicts channels of infusate from the injection site to the urethra. Right (**b**): Gadolinium concentration map showing outflow moved from the injection site to urethra (dark oval upper center) and subcapsular region in both figures. Note larger porous needle infusate distribution and concentration (red) on right compared to standard needle on left

Table 1 Comparison of fraction of contrast delivered to prostate tissue

Device vs needle	Fraction in tissue (mean with SE)	N	p-value
Device 1cm length of porous segment	0.27 ± 0.12 (0.24 ± 0.14)	7 (8)	0.013 (0.05)
Device 2 cm length of porous segment	0.33 ± 0.24	5	0.035
Needle	0.10 ± 0.11	8	0.010 (0.02)

The numbers in parentheses use an infusion not included in calculating the other entry in the same element of the table (see text for further explanation). The p-values are two-sided, corresponding to the conservative assumption that there is no a priori reason to favor the porous device. The entry for the p-values compares the device in the row to the standard needle: the third row is a comparison where both porous devices are aggregated in the comparison

surrounding the nodule which would favor the hypothesis of an impermeable tissue barrier around the region.

Figure 5 also show excellent correspondence between the MR distribution of the contrast reagent and the visible distribution of the vegetable dye. In addition, a microscopic image of the portion of the tissue at the border of the nodule is shown at the bottom. An indication of why the infusion failed to penetrate is the fibromuscular capsule that surrounds the cystic nodule (as designated by the arrow).

Overall results

We summarize the simplest metrics from the infusions in Tables 1 and 2. These are the amount of tracer actually detected within the prostatic tissue compared with the total amount infused in Table 1 and the volume of distribution V_d calculated as discussed above relative to volume of infusion V_i in Table 2. The data presented in Additional files 1 and 2 were omitted in the computation of the statistics: (i) the infusions with Prohance™ which were done as preliminary experiments to refine the protocol; (ii) bolus infusions with the needle which were not continuous infusions; and (iii) one placement with the 2-cm porous needle which inadvertently missed the prostate entirely. Further, there was (iv) another placement with the 1cm porous device from which no infusate could be detected over the entire porous section. What we have done is to report the statistics separately with this one infusion witheld and then included.

We note that the distribution volumes are computed not by a threshold on the brightness of a contrast-enhanced image, as is customary, but on the computed concentration of the contrast agent itself (Table 2). Thus, they are somewhat more objectively measured than in the usual way, though varying this threshold will change the distribution volumes. However, the dose is not dependent on any arbitrary threshold (Table 1). The distribution volume with the porous versus the standard needle did not differ significantly between the 10 minute and the 100-120 minute infusion.

The porous needle was tested with injection on one side of the prostate and its performance compared with that of a standard needle injecting into the other side of prostate. The fraction of infused solution in the tissue was greater with the porous needle by almost 3-fold ($p = 0.03$) compared with standard needle. While the volume of distribution was greater with porous needle than the standard needle (80% higher), no statistically significant association could be determined with this small sample size. A Cohen's d was calculated to be .6 (medium to large) and .79 (large) for porous needle vs standard needle for all grouped 1 and 2cm porous needles and 2cm porous needle, respectively, indicating that this finding will be significantly different if this trend continues. A sample size to achieve a power >.80 and alpha error < .05 is estimated to be a total of 35 for each group, or roughly an additional 20 samples to achieve a p value < 0.05. For the 2cm porous needle, a total of 26 samples in each group would be needed.

Discussion

The purpose of a prostatic infusion is to deliver a planned dose to a planned targeted region. There are multiple pathways for flow of fluid carrying the agent that frustrate this goal, and therefore one needs a strategy to overcome these. Backflow does not seem to be an issue for the porous needle, and other strategies exist that can significantly limit backflow, though such approaches may create other procedural constraints. So, while backflow is an issue for standard needles at the high flow rates needed for clinical acceptability of the procedure, it does not appear a fundamental technological

Table 2 Comparison of ratio of Volume of distribution to Volume infused

Device vs needle	Vd/Vi	N	p-value
Device 1cm length of porous segment	1.32 ± 0.67 (1.17 ± 0.74)	7 (8)	0.211 (0.365)
Device 2 cm length of porous segment	1.46 ± 0.84	5	0.194
Needle	0.81 ± 0.81	7	0.116 (0.192)

The numbers in parentheses use an infusion not included in calculating the other entry in the same element of the table (see text for further explanation). The p-values are two-sided, corresponding to the conservative assumption that there is no a priori reason to favor the porous device. The entry for the p-values compares the device in the row to the standard needle: the third row is a comparison where both porous devices are aggregated in the comparison

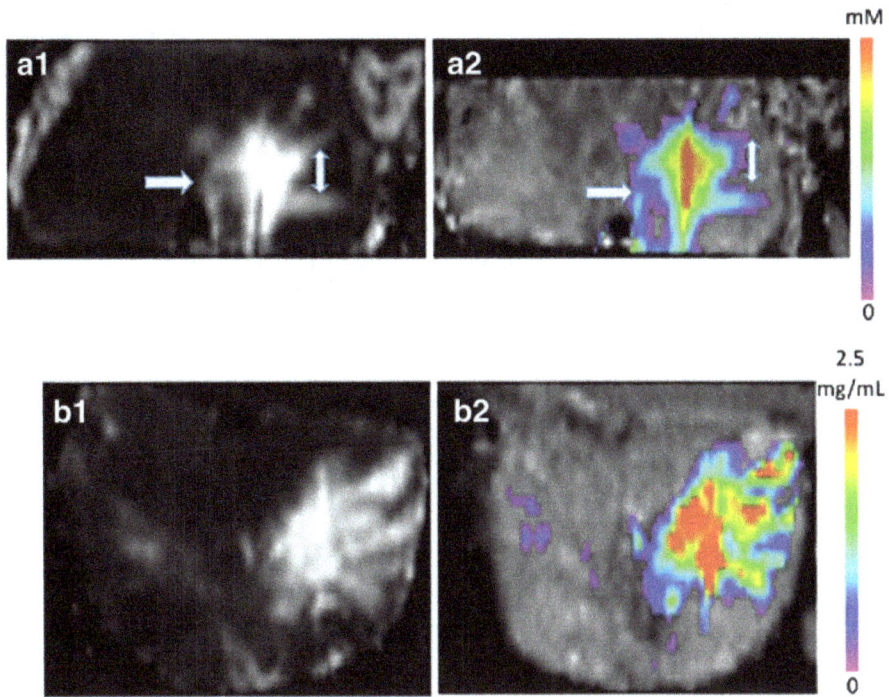

Fig. 4 Top (**a**) demonstrates T1 Gadolinium injection image with porous needle on left showing distribution of contrast along ductal or directional pathways in the prostate leading to infusate loss to the outside as well as into the urethra (lower mid image). Right image demonstrates Gadolinium concentration map with contrast concentration along ductal or directional pathways in the prostate with less high (red) concentration in center of infusate due to loss to urethra and subcapsular. Bottom (**b**) demonstrates T1 Gadolinium injection image with porous needle showing greater distribution on left and greater concentration (note red in center imageL) on the right with less ductal or directional preferred outflow loss of contrast.

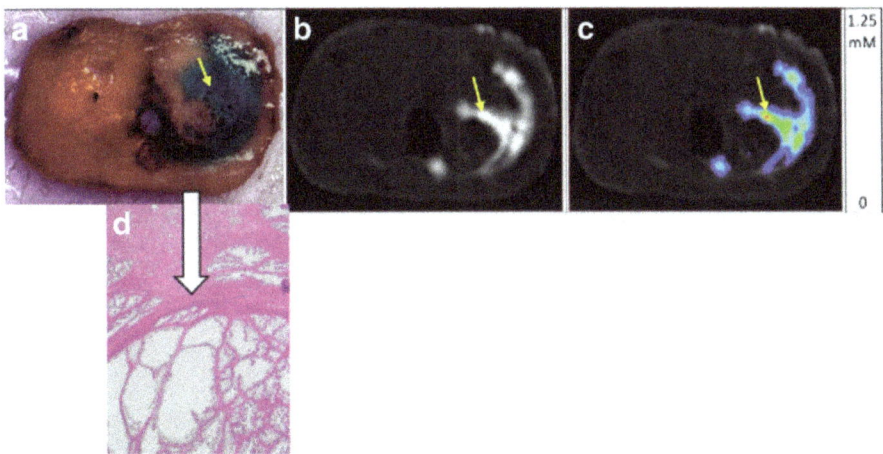

Fig. 5 Top (**a**) demonstrates T1 Gadolinium injection image with porous needle on left showing distribution of contrast along ductal or directional pathways in the prostate leading to infusate loss to the outside as well as into the urethra (lower mid image). Right image demonstrates Gadolinium concentration map with contrast concentration along ductal or directional pathways in the prostate with less high (red) concentration in center of infusate due to loss to urethra and subcapsular. Bottom (**b**) demonstrates T1 Gadolinium injection image with porous needle showing greater distribution on left and greater concentration (note red in center image L) on the right with less ductal or directional preferred outflow loss of contrast

problem for intraprostatic infusions. However, there is a multiplicity of preferred pathways that lead to the urethra, as well as to the boundary of the prostate. Such ductal losses certainly suggest the benefit of multiport needle(s), so that one misplaced port does not vitiate the entire infusion, or multiple infusions with multiple needles, as is more customary. However, these ductal losses are not eliminated with such precautions and must be tolerated. The goal of the procedure is to ensure adequate dosing of the target while accepting therapeutic agent loss within and beyond the prostate. This has implications for the allowed toxicity of any potential agent similar to considerations for systemically administered agents. Outflow, in the sense of volume transmission of agents reaching the capsule and beyond, is by itself not a major issue if the backflow and ductal losses can be constrained. Obstacles are an issue: they will need to be identified in the imaging and multiple needle trajectories may become necessary to ensure distribution into nodules, requiring infusion with therapeutic agent.

There are several limitations of ex-vivo studies, such as the lack of tissue perfusion and any other in-vivo infusion distribution contributing factors. The number of prostates infused is small as mentioned; a larger sample may define greater difference between the porous needle and the standard needle. Another key limitation is the impact of translation to clinical patient therapy delivery that will influence ability to place and stabilize the needles during infusion. Thus, while these ex-vivo results are instructive of prostatic injection distribution, clinical studies are required to obtain reliable representation as to the relative contribution of the different flow mechanisms identified in these ex-vivo intraprostatic injections. However, these ex-vivo and prior comparative results of porous and standard needles indicate the porous needles provide improved distribution with the prostate [9, 10], including one in-vivo study [11], all of which have shown porous needle superiority over standard needle injections.

The results also indicate a need for pre-operative imaging and planning for placement of needles. We can envisage a hierarchy of approaches for increasing complexity and precision. We can begin with the best pre-operative imaging to reveal the structures in the prostate that affect flow and offer guidelines for placement of needles, and of flow rates, that are likely to avoid failure of infusions. The surgeon then reviews this information when placing the needles. However, it has become increasingly acceptable clinically to offer MR-fused 3D ultrasound guidance in biopsies of the prostate. This same technology can be used for infusions, wherein a plan is created as an overlay and fused with the real time 3D ultrasound so that the surgeon has a plan as guidance or information directly in view.

Conclusions

This study demonstrated that prostatic tissue is anatomically heterogenic, which presents considerable challenge to achieving a desired distribution of injected agents, particularly from a standard needle. The complexity of flow pathways suggests that preoperative imaging and pre-infusion treatment planning to manage injectate distribution heterogeneity for consistent therapeutic results will be of potential value. The porous needle permitted greater fractional distribution of an injected complex agent compared to the standard needle. This approach to intraparenchymal therapy of prostate disease appears to warrant further investigation in the in vivo setting.

Abbreviation
Gad-HAS: Gadolinium chelate bound to human serum albumin

Acknowledgments
The studies reported in this paper were supported by research funds from the National Institutes of Health, the Institute of Diabetes and Digestive and Kidney Diseases (NIH/NIDDK), grant number DK085810. Rick Odland, Scott Wilson and Mike Wilson have a financial interest in Twin Star Medical, which owns the proprietary rights to the porous needle. We also thank Jilene Gendron for MRI technical support, and Michelle Reyes for laboratory technical support, both at the Scott and White Hospitals, Temple, Texas.

Funding
This study was funded by the National Institutes of Health, the Institute of Diabetes and Digestive and Kidney Diseases. Grant number: DK085810.

Authors' contributions
MLB: Protocol/project development, data collection or management, data analysis, manuscript writing/editing. KSC: Protocol/project development, data collection or management, data analysis, manuscript writing/editing. TJK: Protocol/project development, data collection or management, data analysis, manuscript writing/editing. RR: Protocol/project development, data analysis, manuscript writing/editing. VOS: Data collection or management, data analysis. BP: Data collection or management. SW: Protocol/project development, data collection or management. MW: Protocol/project development, data collection or management. RMO: Data Analysis, manuscript writing/editing. All authors read and approved the final manuscript.

Competing interests
RMO, SW, and MW have a financial interest in Twin Star Medical, which owns the proprietary rights to the porous needle.

Author details
[1]Therataxis, LLC, Baltimore, MD, USA. [2]Department of Surgery, Division of Urology, Scott & White Medical Center, Temple, TX, USA. [3]Department of Obstetrics & Gynecology, Scott & White Medical Center, Temple, TX, USA. [4]Department of Pathology, Scott & White Medical Center, Temple, TX, USA. [5]Texas A&M Health Science Center College of Medicine, Temple, TX, USA. [6]Departments of Obstetrics & Gynecology, Pediatrics, and Molecular & Cellular Medicine, Texas A&M Health Science Center College of Medicine, Temple, TX, USA. [7]Twin Star TDS, LLC, Lexington, KY, USA. [8]Department of Otolaryngology, Hennepin County Medical Center, University of Minnesota, Minneapolis, MN, USA.

References

1. Andersson KE. Intraprostatic injections for lower urinary tract symptoms treatment. Curr Opin Urol. 2015;25:12–8.
2. Gulley JL, Heery CR, Madan RA, et al. Phase I study of intraprostatic vaccine administration in men with locally recurrent or progressive prostate cancer. Cancer Immunol Immunother. 2013;62:1521–31.
3. Nair SM, Pimentel MA, Gilling PI. Evolving and investigational therapies for benign prostatic hyperplasia. Can J Urol. 2015;22(Suppl 1):82–7.
4. Brady M, Raghavan R, Chen Z, Broaddus W. Quantifying fluid infusions and tissue expansion in brain. IEEE Trans Biomed Eng. 2011;58:2228–37.
5. Deoni SCL, Peters TM, Rutt BK. Rapid combined T1 and T2 mapping using gradient recalled acquisition in the steady state. Magn Reson Med. 2003;49:515–26.
6. Deoni SCL, Peters TM, Rutt BK. Determination of optimal angles for variable nutation proton magnetic spin-lattice, T1, and spin-spin, T2, relaxation times measurement. Magn Reson Med. 2004;51:194–9.
7. Chowning SL, Susil RC, Krieger A, Fichtinger G, Whitcomb LL, Atalar E. A preliminary analysis and model of prostate injection distributions. Prostate. 2006;66:344–57.
8. Wang J, Qiu M, Constable RT. In vivo method for correcting transmit/receive nonuniformities with phased array coils. Magnc Reson Med. 2005;53:666–74.
9. Raghavan R, Mikaeilian S, Brady M, Chen ZJ. Fluid infusions from catheters into elastic tissue: I. Azimuthally symmetric backflow in homogeneous media. Phys Med Biol. 2010;55:281–304.
10. King BJ, Mann-Gow TK, Kida M, Plante MK, Perrapato SD, Zvara P. Intraprostatic ethanol diffusion: comparison of two injection methods using ex vivo human prostates. Prostate Cancer Prostatic Dis. 2015;18:237–41.
11. King BJ, Plante MK, Kida M, Mann-Gow TK, Odland R, Zvara P. Comparison of intraprostatic ethanol diffusion using a microporous hollow fiber catheter versus a standard needle. J Urol. 2012;187:1898–902.

19

Kidney stone formers have more renal parenchymal crystals than non-stone formers, particularly in the papilla region

Atsushi Okada* ⓘ, Shuzo Hamamoto, Kazumi Taguchi, Rei Unno, Teruaki Sugino, Ryosuke Ando, Kentaro Mizuno, Keiichi Tozawa, Kenjiro Kohri and Takahiro Yasui

Abstract

Background: We investigated the renoprotective ability of healthy people against kidney stone formation. To clarify intratubular crystal kinetics and processing in human kidneys, we performed a quantitative and morphological observation of nephrectomized renal parenchyma tissues.

Methods: Clinical data and pathological samples from 60 patients who underwent radical nephrectomy for renal cancer were collected from June 2004 to June 2010. The patients were retrospectively classified as stone formers (SFs; $n = 30$, kidney stones detected by preoperative computed tomography) and non-stone formers (NSFs; $n = 30$, no kidney stone history). The morphology of parenchymal intratubular crystals and kidney stone-related gene and protein expression levels were examined in noncancerous renal sections from both groups.

Results: SFs had a higher smoking rate ($P = 0.0097$); lower red blood cell, hemoglobin, and hematocrit values; and higher urinary red blood cell, white blood cell, and bacterial counts than NSFs. Scanning electron microscopy revealed calcium-containing crystal deposits and crystal attachment to the renal tubular lumen in both groups. Both groups demonstrated crystal transmigration from the tubular lumen to the interstitium. The crystal diffusion analysis indicated a significantly higher crystal existing ratio in the medulla and papilla of SFs and a significantly higher number of papillary crystal deposits in SFs than NSFs. The expression analysis indicated relatively high osteopontin and CD68, low superoxide dismutase, and significantly lower Tamm–Horsfall protein expression levels in SFs. Multivariate logistic regression analysis involving the above factors found the presence of renal papillary crystals as a significant independent factor related to SFs (odds ratio 5. 55, 95% confidence interval 1.08–37.18, $P = 0.0395$).

Conclusions: Regardless of stone formation, intratubular crystals in the renal parenchyma seem to transmigrate to the interstitium. SFs may have reduced ability to eliminate renal parenchymal crystals, particularly those in the papilla region, than NSFs with associated gene expression profiles.

Keywords: Kidney stones, Macrophages, Osteopontin, Oxidative stress, Tamm-Horsfall protein

Background

Since the introduction of extracorporeal shock-wave lithotripsy in 1980, [1] fewer opportunities for open surgery have led to fewer chances for pathological investigations of kidney stone formation (KSF) using human kidney parenchymal tissue. Therefore, studies of human KSF tend to focus on urinary inorganic concentrations [2, 3]

and epidemiological data, such as those investigating the relationship with diabetes [4] and metabolic syndrome [5]. Recent progress in endoscopic technology has directed attention to Randall's plaque [6]; interstitial apatite crystal deposits beginning at the basement membranes of the thin loops of Henle seem to be sites of calcium oxalate (CaOx) stone formation [7–9]. However, intraparenchymal events involving the kinetics of intratubular crystals have not been elucidated.

Previous basic studies using hyperoxaluric-animal and cell-culture models led to the detection of morphological

* Correspondence: a-okada@med.nagoya-cu.ac.jp
Department of Nephro-urology, Nagoya City University Graduate School of Medical Sciences, 1 Kawasumi, Mizuho-cho, Mizuho-ku, Nagoya, Aichi 467-8601, Japan

and genetic events in the renal parenchyma via the detection of stone matrix protein, [10] completion of the human genome project, and technological progress related to recombinant gene analysis [11–13]. In particular, the factors currently considered to affect calcium kidney stone formation are stone matrix proteins, cell injury caused by oxidative stress, monocyte/macrophage induction, and urinary stone inhibitors.

Osteopontin (OPN), the main component of stone matrix protein, is a glycoprotein present in human calcium-containing kidney stones [10] that may play an important role in crystal conversion to stones. OPN antisense-expressing cultured renal tubular cells demonstrate reduced aggregation of CaOx crystals and crystal-cell interactions [14] and OPN-knockout mice show reduced growth of renal crystals [12]. OPN is also involved in the formation of the organic layer of apatite plaque particles in the renal inner medulla of CaOx stone formers (SFs) [15]. Furthermore, renal tubular-cell injury caused by oxidative stress is essential for kidney stone formation [16]. Some studies have indicated that tubular-cell apoptosis caused by deviated free radicals and diminished superoxide dismutase (SOD) expression, [17] and collapsed organelles, including mitochondria and fragmented microvilli in the renal tubular lumen, lead to stone nidus formation [18]. We reported renal intratubular crystal elimination in a mouse model, increased expression of macrophage-related inflammatory genes in a DNA microarray analysis of stone-forming kidneys, [13] and phagocytosis of interstitial crystals by macrophages under transmission electron microscopy, [19] suggesting the kidney stone-preventive ability of macrophages by crystal processing. Moreover, Umekawa et al. [20] demonstrated that exposure to CaOx crystals promotes the expression of monocyte chemotactic protein-1 (MCP-1) and induces macrophage migration. Finally, Tamm–Horsfall protein (THP), a urinary inhibitor of stone formation, has been studied because THP-deficient mice demonstrate spontaneous calcium crystal formation [21].

The above experimental findings suggest that intratubular crystal formation involves several steps and that animal models may have the ability to eliminate the crystals. However, among the possible mechanisms of stone formation, these processes are thought to model Randall's plug due to hyperoxaluria or cystinuria rather than Randall's plaque. However, there is no definitive evidence to confirm this assumption. With the above in mind, we aimed to elucidate the intratubular crystal kinetics and processing in human kidneys using nephrectomized parenchymal tissues.

Methods
Patients
We obtained clinical data and pathological samples from 60 patients who underwent radical nephrectomy for stage I renal cell carcinoma (RCC) from June 2004 to June 2010. The Institutional Review Board of Nagoya City University Hospital approved the study design (Approval No. 551). The patients were retrospectively classified as SFs (30 patients with renal stones detected by preoperative computed tomography [CT]) and non-stone formers (NSFs; 30 age [± 1 year] - and sex-adjusted patients without renal stone and kidney disease history). In SFs, all stones were also detectable by abdominal X-ray and were presumed to be non-uric acid stones.

Clinical data analysis
We evaluated basic clinical and pathological data, comorbidities, and lifestyle factors. The preoperative laboratory data analyses included complete blood count, coagulability tests, and biochemical analyses. Using spot urine sampling, qualitative analysis of specific gravity, pH, protein, and glucose and flow cytometry-based quantitative analysis of urinary red blood cells (RBCs), white blood cells (WBCs), epithelial cells, and bacteria were conducted.

Aortic calcification index
Because of the similarity between atherosclerosis formation and kidney stone formation, [22] we calculated the aortic calcification index of both groups as the degree of calcification at the aortic arterial wall as follows: grade 0, none; grade 1, < 120 degrees of calcification; grade 2, ≥ 120 degrees but < 240 degrees of calcification; and grade 3, ≥ 240 degrees of calcification.

Detection and quantification of renal crystal deposits
Paraffin-embedded tissue blocks prepared from formalin-fixed excised kidneys were sliced to a 4-μm thickness and stained with hematoxylin and eosin (H&E). Crystal deposits in the normal renal parenchyma were detected by polarized light optical microphotography of the H&E-stained samples. The number of crystal deposits was quantified by counting the crystals per 100 visual fields (magnification, × 100) in noncancerous sections of the renal cortex, medulla, and papilla and as the existing ratio (number of kidneys with crystal deposits/whole kidneys). CaOx crystals were detected by Pizzolato staining [23].

Scanning electron microscopy (SEM) analysis
Dewaxed paraffin-embedded sections (4-μm thickness) were washed with a phosphoric acid buffer, re-fixed with 2.5% glutaraldehyde and subsequently with 2% osmium liquid, dehydrated in a 50–100% ethanol series, and embedded in epoxy resin. After sputtering a platinum filter on a stage, SEM specimens were prepared using electrical conduction. The crystal ultrastructure was then examined by SEM. The elemental spectra of the crystal deposits were determined by energy-dispersive X-ray spectroscopy (EDX).

Immunohistochemistry (IHC)

IHC for OPN, SOD, CD68 (a macrophage surface marker), and THP was performed using 4-µm-thick cross-sections. The tissues were autoclaved for antigen activation at 121 °C for 5 min, blocked with 0.5% hydrogen peroxide in methanol for 30 min, washed with 0.01 M phosphate-buffered saline (PBS), and treated with skimmed milk in PBS for 1 h at room temperature. They were then incubated overnight at 4 °C with the following polyclonal antibodies: rabbit anti-human OPN (Immuno-Biological Laboratories Co., Ltd., Gunma, Japan), rabbit anti-human CD68 (Santa Cruz Biotechnology, Santa Cruz, CA, USA), rabbit anti-human THP (Santa Cruz Biotechnology), and goat anti-human SOD (Santa Cruz Biotechnology). The reacted antibodies were detected using a Histofine simple stain kit for goat or rabbit immunoglobulin G (Nichirei Biosciences, Inc., Tokyo, Japan) according to the manufacturer's instructions.

Quantitative reverse transcription-polymerase chain reaction (qRT-PCR) analysis

Total RNA from noncancerous kidney sections was extracted using NucleoSpin FFPE RNA (Macherey-Nagel GmbH & Co., Düren, Germany) according to the manufacturer's instructions. All RNA samples were reverse-transcribed to complementary DNA with a High Capacity cDNA reverse transcription kit (Applied Biosystems, Life Technologies, Carlsbad, CA, USA). According to the annotation information of each gene, the TaqMan gene expression assay product, a 20× assay mix of forward and reverse primer sets, and TaqMan MGB probe (FAM dye labeled) with complementary sequences to each messenger RNA sequence were obtained. The qPCR was performed with the TaqMan Universal PCR master mix (404,437, Applied Biosystems) using the 7500 FAST real-time PCR system (Applied Biosystems). After denaturation at 95 °C for 10 min, PCR was initiated at 95 °C for 15 s and completed at 60 °C for 1 min. The reaction was repeated 45 times. The expression of each sample was determined as a ratio to the expression of the glyceraldehyde 3-phosphate dehydrogenase gene (GAPDH; internal control). TaqMan gene expression assay probe kits were used for the secreted phosphoprotein-1 gene (SPP1, encoding

OPN; Hs00959010_m1), SOD1 (Hs00533490_m1), CD68 (Hs00154355_m1), uromodulin gene (UMOD, encoding THP; Hs00358451_m1), and GAPDH (Hs03929097_g1).

Statistical analysis

We used the chi-square test using a 2 × 2 table to compare the comorbidities and lifestyle factors. The clinical and basic laboratory data were compared using Student's t-test. Furthermore, the pathological data, aortic calcification grades, urinalysis results, number of crystal deposits, and messenger RNA expression levels were analyzed using the Mann–Whitney U-test. The categorical pathological patient data, comorbidity data, and lifestyle factor data were assessed using the chi-square test. Repeated-measures analysis of variance (ANOVA) was used to compare the renal crystal distribution between the groups. Based on each analysis, the extracted factors were evaluated for their relationship with kidney stone formation using multivariate logistic regression analysis. In these analyses, a P-value < 0.05 was considered to indicate a statistically significant difference.

Results

Clinical findings

The groups were not significantly different in terms of clinical data. No significant sex difference was detected between the groups (Table 1). Both groups were predominantly composed of patients with clear-cell RCC. There were no significant differences in pathological diagnoses, grades, stages, and affected sides between the groups (Table 2). Comorbidities did not differ between the groups (Table 3). However, SFs had a significantly higher smoking rate than NSFs (P = 0.0097).

Although the RBC, hemoglobin, and hematocrit (Ht) values of SFs were within the normal limits, they were significantly lower than those of NSFs (P = 0.0290, 0.0360, and 0.0268, respectively; Table 4). The coagulation-related and blood biochemical data were not significantly different between the groups. Furthermore, no significant differences in urinalysis results were noted. However, SFs had significantly higher urinary RBC, WBC, and bacterial count values (P = 0.0343,

Table 1 Clinical patient data

Parameter	Total, mean (SD)		P-value*	Men, mean (SD)		P-value*	Women, mean (SD)		P-value*
	SFs	NSFs		SFs	NSFs		SFs	NSFs	
Age (years)	62.1 (10.6)	61.7 (10.9)	0.8856	62.7 (10.3)	63.0 (10.3)	0.9336	56.6 (13.3)	57.6 (12.2)	0.8856
Height (cm)	164.6 (7.4)	165.3 (6.7)	0.7016	166.1 (6.6)	166.7 (5.9)	0.7282	156.8 (6.6)	157.6 (5.2)	0.8366
Weight (kg)	62.2 (12.1)	66.0 (10.5)	0.1933	64.0 (11.7)	67.2 (9.6)	0.2902	53.2 (10.4)	59.8 (13.8)	0.4181
Body mass index (kg/m²)	22.9 (3.4)	24.0 (3.7)	0.2149	23.2 (3.4)	24.0 (3.0)	0.3587	21.6 (2.9)	24.2 (6.6)	0.4455
Abdominal circumference (cm)	77.7 (8.1)	80.4 (8.3)	0.2027	78.2 (8.1)	80.5 (8.1)	0.3260	74.9 (8.0)	79.8 (10.2)	0.4243

SD standard deviation, SFs stone formers, NSFs non-stone formers

*P < 0.05 indicates statistically significant differences by Student's t-test

Table 2 Pathological patient data

Parameter	Number of SFs (%)	Number of NSFs (%)	P-value*
Diagnosis			0.7879
Clear cell RCC	27 (90.0)	28 (93.3)	
Papillary RCC	1 (3.3)	1 (3.3)	
Chromophobe RCC	1 (3.3)	0 (0)	
Collecting duct carcinoma	1 (3.3)	1 (3.3)	
Grade			0.3529
1	8 (26.7)	9 (30.0)	
2	20 (66.7)	21 (70.0)	
3	2 (6.7)	0 (0)	
INF			0.5194
a	18 (64.3)	20 (69.0)	
b	10 (35.7)	8 (27.6)	
c	0	1 (3.4)	
pT			0.7249
1a	12 (40.0)	13 (43.3)	
1b	9 (30.0)	11 (36.7)	
2	2 (6.7)	1 (3.3)	
3a	2 (6.7)	3 (10.0)	
3b	5 (16.7)	2 (6.7)	
Side			0.0705
Right	12 (40.0)	19 (63.3)	
Left	18 (60.0)	11 (36.7)	

SFs stone formers, NSFs non-stone formers, RCC renal cell carcinoma
*P < 0.05 indicates statistically significant differences by the chi-square test

0.0117, and 0.0014, respectively); male patients had similar values for the above parameters ($P = 0.0108$, 0.0036, and 0.0010, respectively). Qualitative analysis of urinary protein and glucose levels did not yield significant differences between the groups (Table 5).

Table 3 Comparison of the comorbidities and lifestyle factors

Parameter	Number of SFs (%)	Number of NSFs (%)	P-value*
Comorbidity			
Hypertension	15 (50.0)	14 (46.7)	0.7961
Heart disease	4 (15.4)	3 (11.1)	0.6876
Cerebrovascular disease	0 (0.0)	2 (6.7)	0.1503
Diabetes	2 (6.7)	7 (23.3)	0.0706
Habituation			
Smoking	19 (63.3)	9 (30.0)	**0.0097**
Drinking	11 (36.7)	6 (20.0)	0.1520

SFs stone formers, NSFs non-stone formers
The bold number indicates a statistically significant difference (*P < 0.05) by the chi-square test for a 2 × 2 table

Aortic calcification rates
The aortic calcification rates of SFs and NSFs were 80.0 and 63.3%, respectively (Table 6). SFs tended to have an insignificantly higher incidence of aortic calcification ($P = 0.3032$); a similar tendency was observed in both sexes.

Morphology and composition of renal crystals
Polarized light optical microphotography revealed renal crystal deposits with birefringence in both groups (Fig. 1a). SEM demonstrated no significant difference in crystal morphology and crystal attachment to the tubular walls between the groups (Fig. 1b). EDX showed that the main component of the deposits was calcium-containing crystals (Fig. 1c).

Crystal transmigration
Pizzolato staining revealed renal intratubular CaOx crystals (Fig. 2). The cortex crystals existed in the tubular lumen and adapted to the tubular walls (Fig. 2a). In the medullary regions, crystal-attached tubular epithelial cells were abraded and crystal transmigration into the interstitium was observed (Fig. 2b). In the papillary region, almost all crystals were detected in the interstitium (Fig. 2c). These findings were the same in both groups.

Crystal distribution
In the renal cortex, the incidence ratios of SFs and NSFs were 48.1 and 40.7%, respectively ($P = 0.3190$; Fig. 3a). SFs had significantly higher incidence ratios in the medulla (40.9% vs. 23.1%, $P = 0.0064$) and papilla (55.6% vs. 30.8%, $P = 0.0004$). There were no significant differences in the number of crystal deposits (Fig. 3b) in the cortex (2.41 [0.63] vs. 1.44 [0.43], $P = 0.3833$) and medulla (1.84 [0.53] vs. 1.56 [0.63], $P = 0.4079$) between SFs and NSFs. However, SFs had a significantly higher number of papillary crystal deposits than NSFs (7.58 [2.42] vs. 2.75 [1.14], $P = 0.0235$). Furthermore, SFs had a significantly greater number of crystal deposits overall ($P = 0.0187$).

Kidney stone-related gene and protein expression levels
OPN was expressed at the apical side of the distal tubular cells (Fig. 4a). SOD expression was diffusely detected among the proximal tubular cells. CD68-positive cells were detected mainly at the interstitial area of the renal papilla and tubular lumen. THP expression was diffusely detected among the distal tubular cells. As shown in Fig. 4b, SFs had a relatively high expression level of *SPP1* ($P = 0.4959$) and relatively low expression levels of *SOD1* ($P = 0.0790$) and *CD68* ($P = 0.2764$). Finally, SFs had a significantly lower expression level of *UMOD* ($P = 0.0392$) than NSFs.

Table 4 Preoperative laboratory patient data

Parameter	Total, mean (SD)		P-value*	Men, mean (SD)		P-value*	Women, mean (SD)		P-value*
	SFs	NSFs		SFs	NSFs		SFs	NSFs	
WBC ($\times 10^3/\mu$L)	5.7 (1.4)	6.4 (1.8)	0.1172	5.9 (1.4)	6.7 (1.8)	0.0870	5.1 (0.9)	5.0 (1.2)	0.8366
Neutrophil (%)	62.1 (8.6)	62.4 (6.5)	0.8800	62.4 (8.9)	62.8 (6.0)	0.8742	59.3 (7.4)	61.1 (9.3)	0.8125
Eosinophil (%)	3.3 (3.3)	3.0 (2.3)	0.7481	3.6 (3.4)	3.1 (2.4)	0.5742	1.4 (0.80)	2.7 (1.9)	0.2588
Basophil (%)	0.4 (0.3)	0.5 (0.4)	0.3021	0.5 (0.3)	0.5 (0.4)	0.5532	0.2 (0.20)	0.5 (0.1)	0.0656
Monocyte (%)	5.2 (1.6)	5.5 (1.7)	0.5208	5.4 (1.4)	5.6 (1.2)	0.7515	3.6 (1.90)	4.9 (3.3)	0.5034
Lymphocyte (%)	27.6 (6.0)	28.7 (6.2)	0.5075	27.4 6.0)	28.3 (6.3)	0.6122	29.1 (6.9)	30.8 (5.1)	0.6899
RBC ($\times 10^6/\mu$L)	4.3 (0.6)	4.6 (0.6)	**0.0290**	4.3 (0.5)	4.7 (0.6)	0.0592	4.1 (0.40)	4.5 (0.3)	0.8366
Hemoglobin (g/dL)	13.0 (1.9)	14.0 (1.8)	**0.0360**	13.2 (1.8)	14.3 (1.7)	**0.0393**	11.8 (1.8)	12.4 (1.0)	0.4845
Hematocrit (%)	39.5 (4.7)	42.3 (4.8)	**0.0268**	40.1 (4.6)	43.2 (4.7)	**0.0248**	36.9 (4.4)	38.2 (2.7)	0.6088
Platelets ($\times 10^3/\mu$L)	216.0 (56.5)	211.7 (46.1)	0.7496	215.4 (61.9)	212.5 (46.4)	0.8554	218.9 (18.6)	207.4 (49.7)	0.6434
APTT (%)	97.1 (13.4)	96.3 (12.9)	0.8171	96.2 (12.1)	96.0 (13.7)	0.9551	101.4 (19.7)	97.9 (8.2)	0.7198
PT (%)	96.6 (13.2)	102.2 (14.5)	0.1611	86.1 (11.3)	102.7 (17.3)	0.1310	98.4 (21.8)	99.5 (12.8)	0.9303
PT/INR	1.04 (0.10)	1.01 (0.10)	0.2293	1.04 (0.09)	1.00 (0.11)	0.2641	1.04 (0.10)	1.01 (0.08)	0.6996
Fibrinogen (mg/dL)	327.8 (93.5)	319.6 (70.4)	0.7069	336.6 (98.2)	319.0 (74.1)	0.4818	285.4 (54.4)	322.8 (54.5)	0.3090
TP (g/dL)	7.3 (0.4)	7.33 (0.4)	0.6528	7.2 (0.4)	7.3 (0.5)	0.6805	7.5 (0.50)	7.6 (0.2)	0.8124
Albumin (g/dL)	4.3 (0.5)	4.33 (0.4)	0.9494	4.3 (0.60)	4.3 (0.4)	0.9010	4.6 (0.21)	4.4 (0.2)	0.3126
GOT (U/L)	20.8 (5.7)	23.3 (9.8)	0.2365	21.3 (5.9)	22.2 (8.0)	0.6390	18.4 (4.5)	28.6 (16.4)	0.2170
GPT (U/L)	20.9 (10.4)	26.2 (19.2)	0.1947	21.7 (10.3)	24.2 (11.6)	0.4303	16.8 (11.0)	36.0 (41.6)	0.3476
LDH (U/L)	198.1 (33.2)	185.8 (29.9)	0.1619	196.2 (34.9)	181.2 (24.6)	0.0975	212.3 (11.2)	213.5 (46.8)	0.9686
ALP (U/L)	233.6 (63.0)	241.3 (64.5)	0.6470	236.7 (57.9)	237.0 (62.2)	0.9828	219.0 (90.4)	262.4 (35.4)	0.4428
γ-GTP (U/L)	51.6 (63.2)	28.1 (10.2)	0.5916	60.5 (67.4)	29.0 (10.8)	0.1430	14.0 (0.1)	25.3 (0.1)	0.0771
Creatinine (mg/dL)	0.9 (0.2)	0.82 (0.2)	0.4937	0.9 (0.2)	0.9 (0.2)	0.4700	0.7 (0.2)	0.6 (0.0)	0.8480
Uric acid (mg/dL)	6.0 (1.7)	6.14 (1.6)	0.6891	6.1 (1.7)	6.5 (1.4)	0.4115	5.1 (1.3)	4.2 (1.2)	0.4009
BUN (mg/dL)	15.9 (4.9)	15.3 (3.3)	0.5500	15.9 (4.6)	15.5 (3.4)	0.7763	16.2 (6.6)	15.0 (2.6)	0.5092
Glucose (mg/dL)	122.5 (31.8)	129.2 (47.2)	0.5253	121.0 (33.4)	132.0 (49.6)	0.3690	130.0 (23.6)	115.4 (30.9)	0.4252
Calcium (mg/dL)	9.8 (0.3)	9.71 (0.4)	0.5741	9.8 (0.3)	9.7 (0.4)	0.3148	9.7 (0.3)	9.9 (0.1)	0.2483
e-GFR	71.4 (20.7)	74.9 (18.3)	0.4961	71.0 (20.8)	72.7 (14.0)	0.7287	73.4 (22.5)	85.2 (32.5)	0.5226
Urinary specific gravity	1.016 (0.006)	1.016 (0.006)	0.8782	1.016 (0.006)	1.016 (0.006)	0.9044	1.013 (0.006)	1.016 (0.009)	0.6434
Urinary pH	6.0 (0.7)	6.32 (0.8)	0.0899	5.9 (0.6)	6.3 (0.8)	0.0604	6.3 (1.2)	6.4 (0.8)	0.8783
Urinary RBC (/μL)	68.3 (37.8)	11.9 (5.5)	**0.0343**	80.1 (45.8)	5.7 (1.4)	**0.0108**	14.0 (9.1)	43.1 (30.9)	0.4647
Urinary WBC (/μL)	56.7 (38.7)	11.5 (7.4)	**0.0117**	54.5 (46.5)	3.6 (0.8)	**0.0036**	66.5 (40.5)	50.9 (43.4)	0.7540
Urinary epithelium (/μL)	4.0 (1.1)	2.66 (1.0)	0.1073	2.9 (1.0)	1.3 (0.2)	0.1428	9.4 (3.4)	9.7 (4.8)	0.6761
Urinary casts (/μL)	0.4 (0.1)	0.2 (0.1)	0.2339	0.5 (0.1)	0.1 (0.0)	0.1217	0.2 (0.2)	0.5 (0.4)	0.8345
Urinary bacteria ($\times 10^3/\mu$L)	5.4 (3.0)	1.12 (0.2)	**0.0014**	2.4 (0.6)	0.9 (0.1)	**0.0010**	19.2 (16.8)	2.3 (0.9)	0.4647
Urinary volume (L/day)	1.4 (0.5)	1.6 (0.6)	0.1511	1.4 (0.5)	1.6 (0.3)	0.3038	0.9 (0.4)	1.5 (0.7)	0.2225

SD standard deviation, *SFs* stone formers, *NSFs* non-stone formers, *WBC* white blood cell, *RBC* red blood cell, *APTT activated partial thromboplastin time*, *PT* prothrombin time, *PT/INR* prothrombin time international normalized ratio, *TP* total protein, *GOT* glutamic oxaloacetic transaminase, *GPT* glutamic pyruvic transaminase, *LDH lactate dehydrogenase*, *ALP* alkaline phosphatase, *γ-GTP* γ-glutamyl transpeptidase, *BUN blood urea nitrogen*, *e-GFR* estimated glomerular filtration rate
The bold numbers indicate statistically significant differences (*P < 0.05) by Student's *t*-test or the Mann–Whitney *U*-test

Multivariate analysis of the relationship between extracted factors and SFs

Multivariate logistic regression analysis was used to assess the relationship of the following factors with SFs: smoking habits, RBC, Ht, urinary RBC, urinary bacteria, existence of renal papillary crystals, and UMOD expression ratio. Continuous variables were adopted for analysis as two nominal scales with cut-off values set at the median values. The presence of renal papillary crystals was found to be a significant independent factor related to SFs (odds ratio 5.55, 95% confidence interval 1.08–37.18, P = 0.0395) (Table 7).

Table 5 Qualitative analysis of urinary protein and glucose

Parameter	Group	−, n (%)	±, n (%)	+, n (%)	++, n (%)	P-value*
Urinary protein	SFs	19 (63.3)	3 (19.0)	7 (23.3)	1 (3.33)	0.7007
	NSFs	20 (66.7)	5 (16.7)	4 (13.3)	1 (3.33)	
Urinary glucose	SFs	29 (96.7)	0 (0.0)	1 (3.3)	0 (0.0)	0.1785
	NSFs	23 (76.7)	1 (3.3)	3 (10.0)	3 (10.0)	

SFs stone formers, NSFs non-stone formers

*P < 0.05 indicates statistically significant differences by the Mann-Whitney U-test

Discussion

Kohri et al. [10] suggested that calcium kidney stone formation involves the expression of several stone matrix proteins, mainly OPN, in renal tubular cells, indicating that the phenomenon is inducible by both environmental and genetic factors [24]. However, their explanation has two major problems: (i) because kidney stone formation is asymptomatic, patients do not recognize its onset until colic pain occurs due to stone descent or chance detection by imaging studies; and (ii) due to the spread of extracorporeal shock wave lithotripsy, it has become difficult to extract tissues ethically from living kidneys, making it impossible to conduct detailed studies on kidney tissues, in contrast to the situation when open surgery was common. Due to the recent development of endoscopic instruments, morphological and pathological studies on Randall's plaque have become more common. We recently conducted a genome-wide study of plaque tissue, resulting in the confirmation of inflammatory cytokine expression, increased immune cell number, and cellular apoptosis in renal papilla stone tissue [25]. However, these findings were limited to the renal papilla tissue and represent only the change in expression levels after stone formation. To resolve these problems, we enrolled patients with asymptomatic stones detected contingently by preoperative CT for the diagnosis of renal tumors and investigated renal parenchyma integrally using pathological whole-kidney samples. Specifically, we analyzed the crystal morphology and transmigration in addition to kidney stone-related gene and protein expression.

Table 6 Analysis of aortic calcification grades

	Group	Grade 0, n (%)	Grade 1, n (%)	Grade 2, n (%)	Grade 3, n (%)	P-value*
Total	SFs	6 (20.0)	13 (43.3)	6 (20.0)	5 (16.7)	0.3032
	NSFs	11 (36.7)	10 (33.3)	4 (13.3)	5 (16.7)	
Men	SFs	5 (20.0)	11 (44.0)	5 (20.0)	4 (16.0)	0.4672
	NSFs	8 (32.0)	10 (40.0)	2 (8.0)	5 (20.0)	
Women	SFs	1 (20.0)	2 (40.0)	1 (20.0)	1 (20.0)	0.3808
	NSFs	3 (60.0)	0 (0.0)	2 (40.0)	0 (0.0)	

SFs stone formers, NSFs non-stone formers

*P < 0.05 indicates a statistically significant difference by the Mann–Whitney U-test

We found that SF group had a significantly higher smoking rate than NSFs. Słojewski et al. [26] did not detect significant correlations between smoking and kidney stone composition. Smoking is a significant, independent risk factor for atherosclerosis via the oxidative stress associated with mitochondrial damage [27]. Considering the similarity between kidney stone and atherosclerosis formation, [22] smoking might conceivably affect stone formation or crystal kinetics. The precise relationship between the risk of stone formation and smoking should be investigated in future studies.

SFs had significantly lower RBC, hemoglobin, and Ht values than NSFs. Renal ischemia via anemia could lead to renal tubular-cell injury, [28] implying that anemia might be involved in stone formation. However, patients with kidney stones have erythropoietin resistance caused by bone marrow oxalosis [29]. Furthermore, the increase in urine RBC, WBC, and bacterial counts may be the result of the erosion of the renal pelvic mucosa on Randall's plaque in patients with stones [30]. Unfortunately, we did not consider the existence of plaque in this study.

The notable findings of this study are as follows: (i) regardless of kidney stone history, intratubular crystal deposits were detectable in the renal parenchymal tissues; (ii) the crystals transmigrated from the tubular lumen to the papillary interstitium; and (iii) SFs had a significantly higher number of crystal deposits in the renal papilla. Bergsland et al. [31] noted that SFs, especially those with idiopathic hypercalciuria, have higher urinary calcium molarity than NSFs and that the difference becomes significant at night. CaOx supersaturation but not calcium phosphate supersaturation is higher in SFs than in NSFs, which could also explain CaOx stone formation on papillary Randal's plaques. CaOx crystal residues in the renal papilla could be another factor related to CaOx stone formation. Furthermore, Vervaet et al. [32] used hyperoxaluric rat model and human renal biopsy samples to indicate the gradual migration of intratubular crystals to the interstitium. In the hyperoxaluric mouse model we previously established, [11] intratubular crystal deposits were eliminated in about 6 days. The crystals were englobed and fragmented by macrophages and crystal deposits were undetectable in the renal papillary region at all time points. Boonla et al. [33] investigated MCP-1 and interleukin (IL)-6 messenger RNA expression in renal biopsy samples from SFs and extracted kidney samples from patients with renal cancer; they demonstrated relatively low MCP-1 and IL-6 expression levels in the cancerous samples compared to those in noncancerous tissues. In the present study, the significantly higher number of interstitial crystal deposits in

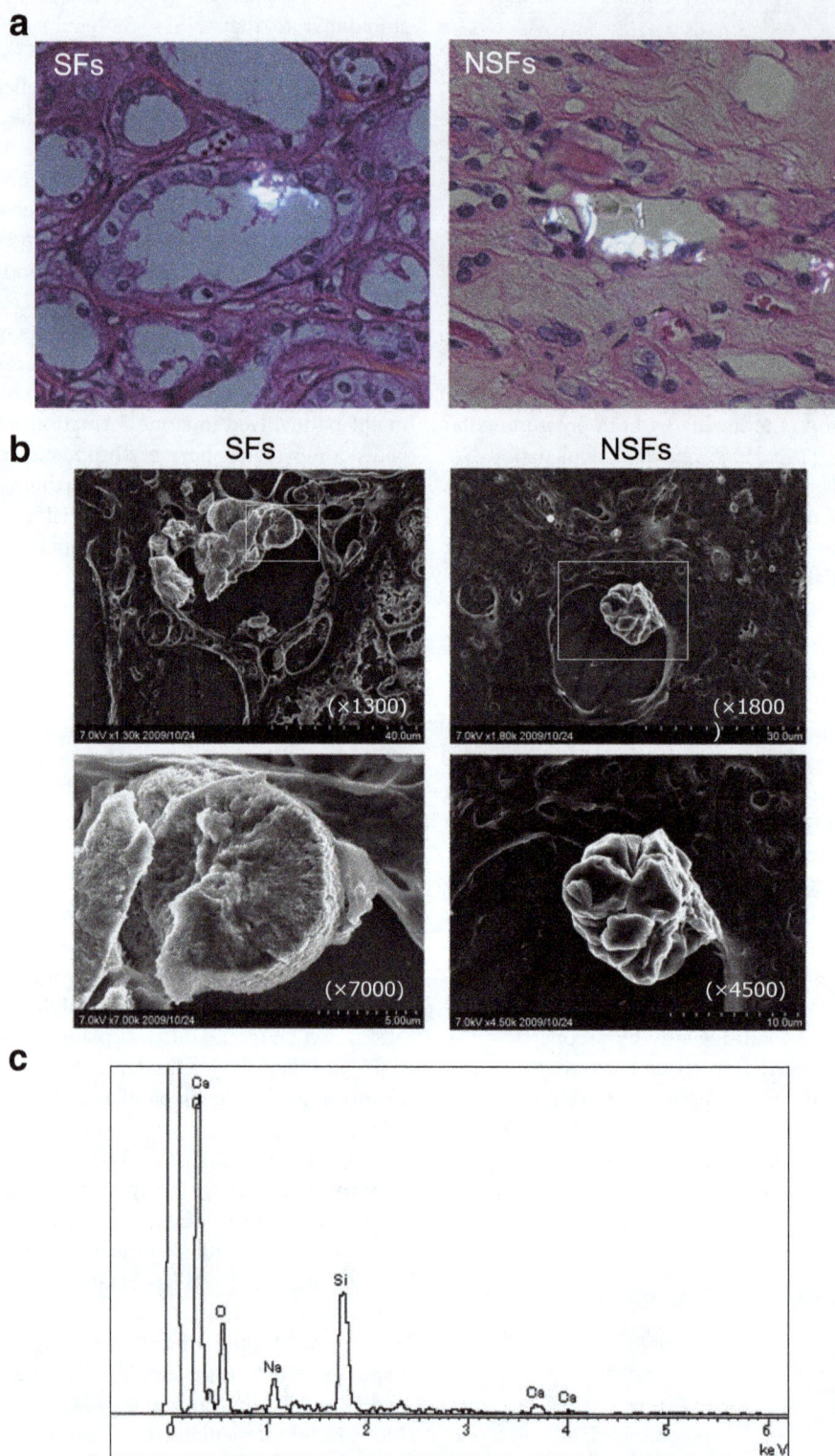

Fig. 1 Morphology and composition of renal tubular crystal deposits in stone formers (SFs) and non-stone formers (NSFs). **a** Crystal attachment to the tubular walls detected by polarized light optical microphotography of hematoxylin and eosin-stained renal cortex sections (magnification, × 800). **b** Crystal attachment to the tubular walls detected by scanning electron microscopy (SEM) of the crystal ultrastructure. **c** Energy-dispersive X-ray spectroscopy (EDX) of the mineral components on the surface of SEM-detected crystal deposits. The EDX spectrum shows calcium as the main component of the deposits

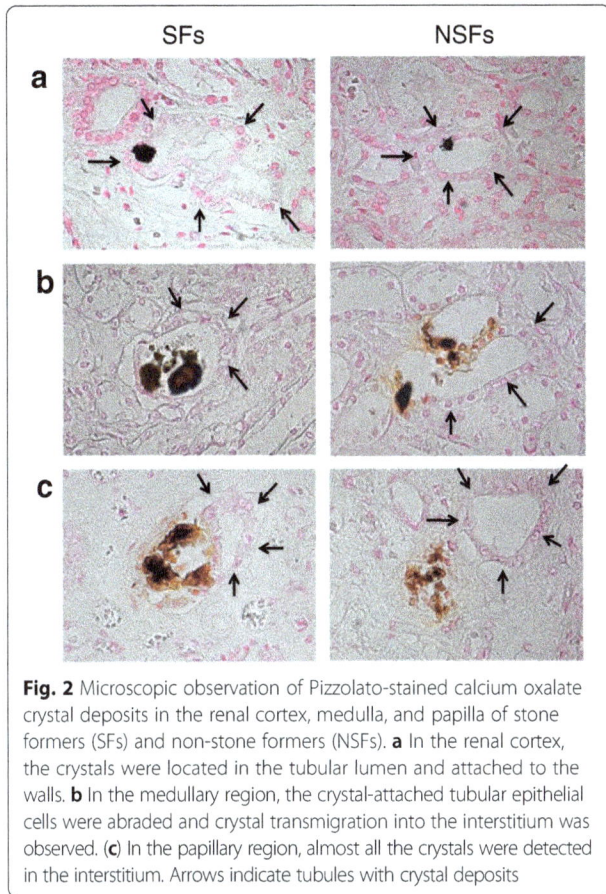

Fig. 2 Microscopic observation of Pizzolato-stained calcium oxalate crystal deposits in the renal cortex, medulla, and papilla of stone formers (SFs) and non-stone formers (NSFs). **a** In the renal cortex, the crystals were located in the tubular lumen and attached to the walls. **b** In the medullary region, the crystal-attached tubular epithelial cells were abraded and crystal transmigration into the interstitium was observed. (**c**) In the papillary region, almost all the crystals were detected in the interstitium. Arrows indicate tubules with crystal deposits

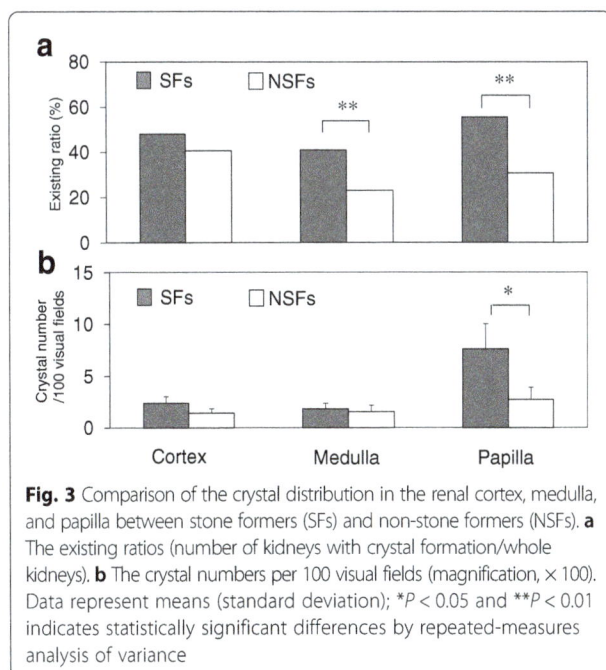

Fig. 3 Comparison of the crystal distribution in the renal cortex, medulla, and papilla between stone formers (SFs) and non-stone formers (NSFs). **a** The existing ratios (number of kidneys with crystal formation/whole kidneys). **b** The crystal numbers per 100 visual fields (magnification, × 100). Data represent means (standard deviation); *$P < 0.05$ and **$P < 0.01$ indicates statistically significant differences by repeated-measures analysis of variance

the papilla of SFs and relatively high *CD68* expression level in NSFs suggest some important roles of macrophages in kidney stone prevention. The OPN, SOD, and CD68 expression levels were similar to those indicated in previous basic studies: SFs had increased OPN expression in the renal tubular cells, tubular-cell injury by oxidative stress, and reduced migration of renal macrophages. In particular, the significantly lower THP expression level in SFs indicates that THP has a crucial role as a kidney stone-preventive factor in humans.

On the basis of our results, we hypothesize the phenomena of human renal intratubular crystal processing. First, crystal nidi are generated in the tubular lumen of the renal cortex because of a urinary supersaturated condition [2, 3]. Some oxidative stresses, such as anemia or smoking, and renal tubular-cell injuries cause collapse of mitochondria and microvilli with decreased SOD expression [16–18]. Consecutively, OPN expression increases and THP downregulation induces crystal-cell interaction and the adaptation of aggregated crystals to the tubular epithelium [26]. Thereafter, the tubular epithelium disintegrates via apoptosis and crystal clusters transmigrate to the renal interstitium via the regenerating epithelium [32]. Tubular-cell injury increases the expression of MCP-1 or various chemokines, in turn inducing monocytes, their transmigration to the renal interstitium, and their differentiation into macrophages [20]. The interstitial crystals can then be removed by macrophages.

These calcification processes, including epithelial-cell injury via oxidative stress, the participation of OPN via inflammation, macrophage activity with phagocytosis, and processing and conversion of foam cells into calcified tissue, are similar to the processes of atherosclerosis formation [34]. SFs tended to have higher levels of aortic calcification. These outcomes suggest a new approach to kidney stone formation involving similar biomolecular processes to those involved in metabolic syndrome that are not related to kidney stone disease because of hyperuricemia, decreased urinary pH, or hypocitraturia caused by metabolic syndrome [35–37].

Multivariate analysis indicated that the presence of renal papillary crystals was significantly and independently related to stone formation. This result represents all of the relationships discussed above. These findings suggest the possibility that the process of kidney stone formation depends on some renoprotective abilities related to the processing of crystals formed in the renal parenchyma, especially the renal papilla.

This study has some limitations that should be discussed. We could not clarify how cancer background,

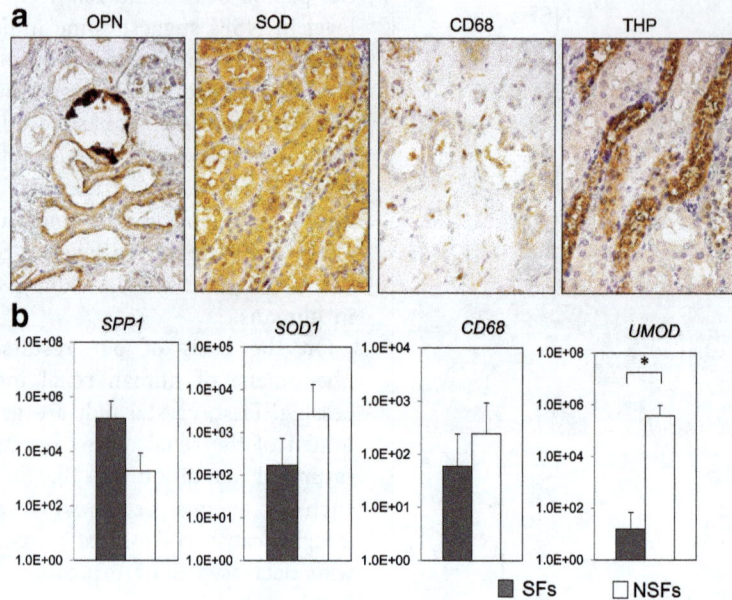

Fig. 4 Kidney stone-related gene and protein expressions in stone formers (SFs) and non-stone formers (NSFs). **a** Immunohistochemistry (magnification, × 100) for osteopontin (OPN), superoxide dismutase (SOD), CD68, and Tamm–Horsfall protein (THP). **b** mRNA expression levels of the secreted phosphoprotein-1 gene (SPP1), SOD1, CD68, and uromodulin gene (UMOD) detected by quantitative polymerase chain reaction (qPCR). The glyceraldehyde 3-phosphate dehydrogenase gene was used as the internal control. Data represent means (standard deviation). *$P < 0.05$ indicates statistically significant differences by the Mann-Whitney U-test

involving environmental and genetic factors, affected "true" kidney stone formation. Furthermore, because this study was conducted retrospectively, detailed analysis of stone component and urinary biochemistry could not be performed. Moreover, Randall's plaques were not detectable in the study sample.

Conclusions

We identified similar phenomena to those detected in previous basic studies, such as crystal-cell interactions, increased OPN expression, decreased SOD and THP expression, and macrophage involvement in the human renal parenchyma. The new findings of this study were crystal formation in patients without kidney stones, crystal transmigration to the papillary interstitium, and crystal processing at the renal papilla regardless of stone formation. SFs may have reduced ability to eliminate renal parenchymal crystals than NSFs (especially in the papilla region), with associated gene expression changes.

Table 7 Multivariate analysis for relationships between extracted factors and kidney stone formation

	OR (95% CI) For stone formers	P-value*
Smoking (+)	1.95 (0.40–9.92)	0.4037
RBC (≤ 4.6 × 10^6/μL)	0.30 (0.03–2.38)	0.2518
Ht (≤ 48%)	1.28 (0.17–12.01)	0.8135
Urinary RBC (≤ 4.3/μL)	1.52 (0.28–8.29)	0.6211
Urinary bacteria (≤ 0.99 × 10^3/μL)	4.46 (0.90–29.08)	0.0687
Renal papillary crystals (+)	5.55 (1.08–37.18)	0.0395
UMOD (existing ratio < 0.001)	4.15 (0.67–37.96)	0.1313

*$P < 0.05$ indicates a statistically significant difference. OR odds ratio, CI confidence interval, RBC red blood cell, Ht hematocrit, UMOD uromodulin

Abbreviations

CaOx: Calcium oxalate; CT: Computed tomography; EDX: Energy-dispersive X-ray spectroscopy; GAPDH: Glyceraldehyde 3-phosphate dehydrogenase; H&E: Hematoxylin and eosin; Ht: Hematocrit; IHC: Immunohistochemistry; IL-6: Interleukin-6; KSF: Kidney stone formation; MCP-1: Monocyte chemotactic protein-1; NSF: Non-stone former; OPN: Osteopontin; PBS: Phosphate-buffered saline; qRT-PCR: Quantitative reverse transcription-polymerase chain reaction; RBC: Red blood cell; RCC: Renal cell carcinoma; SEM: Scanning electron microscopy; SF: Stone former; SOD: Superoxide dismutase; SPP1: Secreted phosphoprotein-1; THP: Tamm–Horsfall protein; UMOD: Uromodulin; WBC: White blood cell

Acknowledgments

We thank N. Kasuga and M. Noda for administrative assistance.

Funding

This work was supported in part by Grants-in-Aid for Scientific Research from the Ministry of Education, Culture, Sports, Science, and Technology, Japan (grant Nos. 15H04976, 15 K10627, 16 K11054, 16 K15692, and 16 K20153) and research grants from the Aichi Kidney Foundation, Takeda Science Foundation, and Mitsui Life Social Welfare Foundation.

Authors' contributions

AO carried out the data collection, performed the statistical analysis, and drafted the manuscript. RU, TS, and KT performed sample staining and image analysis. RA, KM, TK participated in the study design and statistical analysis. KK and TY coordinated the project. All authors read and approved the final manuscript.

Competing interests

The authors declare that they have no competing interests.

References

1. Chaussy C, Brendel W, Schmiedt E. Extracorporeally induced destruction of kidney stones by shock waves. Lancet. 1980;2:1265–8.
2. Werness PG, Brown CM, Smith LH, Finlayson B. EQUIL2: a BASIC computer program for the calculation of urinary saturation. J Urol. 1985;134:1242–4.
3. Tiselius HG. An improved method for the routine biochemical evaluation of patients with recurrent calcium oxalate stone disease. Clin Chim Acta. 1982; 122:409–18.
4. Daudon M, Traxer O, Conort P, Lacour B, Jungers P. Type 2 diabetes increases the risk for uric acid stones. J Am Soc Nephrol. 2006;17:2026–33.
5. Taylor EN, Stampfer MJ, Curhan GC. Obesity, weight gain, and the risk of kidney stones. JAMA. 2005;293:455–62.
6. Randall A. The origin and growth of renal calculi. Ann Surg. 1937;105:1009–27.
7. Evan AP, Lingeman JE, Coe FL, Parks JH, Bledsoe SB, Shao Y, et al. Randall's plaque of patients with nephrolithiasis begins in basement membranes of thin loops of Henle. J Clin Invest. 2003;111:607–16.
8. Evan A, Lingeman J, Coe FL, Worcester E. Randall's plaque: pathogenesis and role in calcium oxalate nephrolithiasis. Kidney Int. 2006;69:1313–8.
9. Coe FL, Evan AP, Worcester EM, Lingeman JE. Three pathways for human kidney stone formation. Urol Res. 2010;38:147–60.
10. Kohri K, Suzuki Y, Yoshida K, Yamamoto K, Amasaki N, Yamate T, et al. Molecular cloning and sequencing of cDNA encoding urinary stone protein, which is identical to osteopontin. Biochem Biophys Res Commun. 1992;184:859–64.
11. Okada A, Nomura S, Higashibata Y, Hirose M, Gao B, Yoshimura, et al. Successful formation of calcium oxalate crystal deposition in mouse kidney by intraabdominal glyoxylate injection. Urol Res. 2007;35:89–99.
12. Okada A, Nomura S, Saeki Y, Higashibata Y, Hamamoto S, Hirose M, et al. Morphological conversion of calcium oxalate crystals into stones is regulated by osteopontin in mouse kidney. J Bone Miner Res. 2008;23:1629–37.
13. Okada A, Yasui T, Hamamoto S, Hirose M, Kubota Y, Itoh Y, et al. Genome-wide analysis of genes related to kidney stone formation and elimination in the calcium oxalate nephrolithiasis model mouse: detection of stone-preventive factors and involvement of macrophage activity. J Bone Miner Res. 2009;24:908–24.
14. Yasui T, Fujita K, Asai K, Kohri K. Osteopontin regulates adhesion of calcium oxalate crystals to renal epithelial cells. Int J Urol. 2002;9:100–8.
15. Evan AP, Coe FL, Rittling SR, Bledsoe SM, Shao Y, Lingeman JE, et al. Apatite plaque particles in inner medulla of kidneys of calcium oxalate stone formers: osteopontin localization. Kidney Int. 2005;68:145–54.
16. Itoh Y, Yasui T, Okada A, Tozawa K, Hayashi Y, Kohri K. Preventive effects of green tea on renal stone formation and the role of oxidative stress in nephrolithiasis. J Urol. 2005;173:271–5.
17. Hirose M, Tozawa K, Okada A, Hamamoto S, Shimizu H, Kubota Y, et al. Glyoxylate induces renal tubular cell injury and microstructural changes in experimental mouse. Urol Res. 2008;36:139–47.
18. Hirose M, Yasui T, Okada A, Hamamoto S, Shimizu H, Itoh Y, et al. Renal tubular epithelial cell injury and oxidative stress induce calcium oxalate crystal formation in mouse kidney. Int J Urol. 2010;17:83–92.
19. Okada A, Yasui T, Fujii Y, Niimi K, Hamamoto S, Hirose M, et al. Renal macrophage migration and crystal phagocytosis via inflammatory-related gene expression during kidney stone formation and elimination in mice; detection by association analysis of stone-related gene expression and microstructural observation. J Bone Miner Res. 2010;25:2701–11.
20. Umekawa T, Chegini N, Khan SR. Oxalate ions and calcium oxalate crystals stimulate MCP-1 expression by renal epithelial cells. Kidney Int. 2002;61:105–12.
21. Mo L, Huang HY, Zhu XH, Shapiro E, Hasty DL, Wu XR. Tamm-Horsfall protein is a critical renal defense factor protecting against calcium oxalate crystal formation. Kidney Int. 2004;66:1159–66.
22. Yasui T, Itoh Y, Bing G, Okada A, Tozawa K, Kohri K. Aortic calcification in urolithiasis patients. Scand J Urol Nephrol. 2007;41:419–21.
23. Pizzolato P. Histochemical recognition of calcium oxalate. J Histochem Cytochem. 1964;12:333–6.
24. Kohri K, Yasui T, Okada A, Hirose M, Hamamoto S, Fujii Y, et al. Biomolecular mechanism of urinary stone formation involving osteopontin. Urol Res. 2012;40:623–37.
25. Taguchi K, Hamamoto S, Okada A, Unno R, Kamisawa H, Naiki T, et al. Genome-wide gene expression profiling of Randall's plaques in calcium oxalate stone formers. J Am Soc Nephrol. 2017;28:333–47.
26. Słojewski M, Czerny B, Safranow K, Drozdzik M, Pawlik A, Jakubowska K, et al. Does smoking have any effect on urinary stone composition and the distribution of trace elements in urine and stones? Urol Res. 2009;37:317–22.
27. Puddu P, Puddu GM, Cravero E, De Pascalis S, Muscari A. The emerging role of cardiovascular risk factor-induced mitochondrial dysfunction in atherogenesis. J Biomed Sci. 2009;16:112.
28. Nemoto T, Yokota N, Keane WF, Rabb H. Recombinant erythropoietin rapidly treats anemia in ischemic acute renal failure. Kidney Int. 2001;59:246–51.
29. Sahin G, Acikalin MF, Yalcin AU. Erythropoietin resistance as a result of oxalosis in bone marrow. Clin Nephrol. 2005;63:402–4.
30. Ciftçioğlu N, Vejdani K, Lee O, Mathew G, Aho KM, Kajander EO, et al. Association between Randall's plaque and calcifying nanoparticles. Int J Nanomedicine. 2008;3:105–15.
31. Bergsland KJ, Coe FL, Gillen DL, Worcester EM. A test of the hypothesis that the collecting duct calcium-sensing receptor limits rise of urine calcium molarity in calcium kidney stone formers. Am J Physiol Renal Physiol. 2009; 297:F1017–23.
32. Vervaet BA, Verhulst A, Dauwe SE, De Broe ME, D'Haese PC. An active renal crystal clearance mechanism in rat and man. Kidney Int. 2009;75:41–51.
33. Boonla C, Hunapathed C, Bovornpadungkitti S, Poonpirome K, Tungsanga K, Sampatanukul P, et al. Messenger RNA expression of monocyte chemoattractant protein-1 and interleukin-6 in stone-containing kidneys. BJU Int. 2008;101:1170–7.
34. Scatena M, Liaw L, Giachelli CM. Osteopontin: a multifunctional molecule regulating chronic inflammation and vascular disease. Arterioscler Thromb Vasc Biol. 2007;27:2302–9.
35. Sakhaee K, Maalouf NM. Metabolic syndrome and uric acid nephrolithiasis. Semin Nephrol. 2008;28:174–80.
36. Cupisti A, Meola M, D'Alessandro C, Bernabini G, Pasquali E, Carpi A, et al. Insulin resistance and low urinary citrate excretion in calcium stone formers. Biomed Pharmacother. 2007;61:86–90.
37. Khan SR, Canales BK. Unified theory on the pathogenesis of Randall's plaques and plugs. Urolithiasis. 2015;43:109–23.

20

Hand-assisted living-donor nephrectomy: a retrospective comparison of two techniques

Jeannette D. Widmer[2*], Andrea Schlegel[1], Philipp Kron[1], Marc Schiesser[3], Jens G. Brockmann[4] and Markus K. Muller[1,2]

Abstract

Background: Living-donor nephrectomy (LDN) is challenging, as surgery is performed on healthy individuals. Minimally invasive techniques for LDN have become standard in most centers. Nevertheless, numerous techniques have been described with no consensus on which is the superior approach. Both hand-assisted retroperitoneoscopic (HARS) and hand-assisted laparoscopic (HALS) LDNs are performed at Zurich University Hospital. The aim of this study was to compare these two surgical techniques in terms of donor outcome and graft function.

Method: Retrospective single-center analysis of 60 consecutive LDNs (HARS $n = 30$; HALS $n = 30$) from June 2010 to May 2012, including a one-year follow-up of the recipients.

Results: There was no mortality in either group and little difference in the overall complication rates. Median warm ischemia time (WIT) was significantly shorter in the HARS group. The use of laxatives and the incidence of postoperative vomiting were significantly greater in the HALS group. There was no difference between right- and left-sided nephrectomies in terms of donor outcome and graft function.

Conclusions: Both techniques appear safe for both donors and donated organs. The HARS technique is associated with a shorter WIT and a reduced incidence of postoperative paralytic ileus. Therefore, we consider HARS LDN a valuable alternative to HALS LDN.

Background

For patients with end-stage renal disease, kidney transplantation is the only treatment to improve their survival, and it quickly enhances their quality of life [1, 2]. During the last several decades, living-donors have become the primary source of donor kidneys for transplantation [3]. As well as expanding the donor organ pool, living-donor kidneys allow preemptive transplantation, and surgery can be efficiently planned with both the donor and the recipient in optimum medical condition. Hence, the outcome of living-donor kidney transplantation is superior to transplantation of deceased donor kidneys in terms of improved long-term recipient survival, quality of life, early graft function and better graft survival [4–6]. However, living-donor nephrectomy

(LDN) remains a surgical challenge in terms of minimizing postoperative complications as it is performed on healthy individuals. Therefore, the most important goal is ensuring the safety and well-being of the voluntary donor [7–9]. The surgical technique must result in the least possible risk of morbidity without compromising the functional outcome of grafts.

The first laparoscopic donor nephrectomy was performed in 1995 by Kavoussi and Ratner [10] and became a well-established technique due to many advantages, including less postoperative pain, a shorter hospital stay and better cosmetics, when compared to open surgical approaches [11, 12]. In contrast, the prolonged warm ischemia time (WIT) has been highlighted as the major disadvantage [13, 14]. A compromise was found in the hand-assisted laparoscopic (HALS) donor nephrectomy technique, which was first described by Wolf et al. in 1998 [15]. This approach shortens the WIT compared to a purely laparoscopic nephrectomy. Further advantages

* Correspondence: jeannette.widmer@gmx.net
[2]Department of Surgery, Kantonsspital Frauenfeld, 8500 Frauenfeld, Switzerland
Full list of author information is available at the end of the article

include tactile feedback, easier and rapid control of bleeding by digital pressure and more rapid kidney recovery [16, 17]. Injuries to the bowel and/or other organs are more likely by a transperitoneal approach due to its nature of abdominal access [18]. In 2001, Wadström et al. combined the advantages of HALS nephrectomy and the retroperitoneoscopic approach favored by urologists and introduced the hand-assisted retroperitoneoscopic (HARS) LDN technique [19]. Direct access to the kidneys without entering the peritoneal cavity obviates bowel injury and is associated with shorter operating time, shorter WIT, less blood loss and a shorter length of hospital stay compared to HALS LDN [20, 21].

The aim of this study was to compare these two surgical techniques in terms of donor outcome and graft function.

Methods

Donors

All donors undergoing HARS or HALS LDNs at the University Hospital of Zurich between June 2010 and May 2012 and the corresponding recipients were identified. A preoperative work-up was carried out according to our standard donor protocol (conformable to the Amsterdam forum guidelines [22]). Indications and results were discussed by the donor kidney board, which is a panel of transplant surgeons, nephrologists, transplantation coordinators, and immunology and psychology experts who meet on a weekly basis. The decision of which donor kidney to retrieve was based first on functional investigations. In the case of functional differences of less than 3%, anatomical considerations guided surgical decision-making. The guiding principle was to leave the better, greater-functioning organ with the donor. The choice of surgical technique depended on the preference of the lead surgeon. All donors received standard postoperative analgesia plus on-demand medication. Donors were followed-up with in our surgical outpatient clinic at 3 months after surgery.

Surgical procedure

For both techniques, the donor was placed in the contralateral flank position with slight hip flexion, thereby extending the ipsilateral flank.

HARS technique: A Pfannenstiel incision was made to introduce the hand-port (GelPort™, Applied Medical Resources Corporation). The retroperitoneal space was created by blunt dissection. The introduction of the first trocar (camera) in the lateral upper abdomen was guided by the surgeon's hand, followed by insufflation of carbon dioxide up to 12 cm H_2O. One or two additional working trocars were placed under direct vision in the medial lower abdomen. Identification and dissection of the kidney, ureter and vascular structures were performed by

hand and with an endoscopic device (Harmonic Ultrasonic Shears, Ethicon). Following complete dissection of all structures, the ureter was clipped and transected distally, and the renal vein and artery were accurately exposed and then divided by a stapler device. The kidney was recovered through the open hand-port.

HALS technique: A periumbilical camera port was introduced into the abdominal cavity, followed by insufflation of carbon dioxide up to 15 cm H_2O. Two or three additional working trocars were placed in the lateral upper and lower abdomen under direct vision. Before clipping the ureter and dividing the renal vein and artery, the hand-port was introduced through a Pfannenstiel incision. After full mobilization, the kidney was extracted through the open hand-port.

Abdominal closure for both techniques was performed in a standard fashion. Drains were not routinely placed.

Recipients

All renal grafts were placed extraperitoneally into the iliac fossa. The immunosuppressive regimen was determined preoperatively depending on immunological and donor-specific risk stratification. Postoperative care was undertaken by the surgical lead. Recipients were followed-up regularly with by the Department of Nephrology at the University Hospital of Zurich.

Data collection

Demographic and clinical data were retrospectively obtained from the clinical information system, which maintains all patients' data electronically. The following parameters from donors and recipients were retrieved: preoperative renal retention parameters, BMI, blood group, and HLA status. Operative time (OT), WIT and organ site were noted. Kidney function (creatinine, GFR) before and after surgery were recorded for both donors and recipients. Delayed graft function (DGF) was defined as the use of dialysis in the first postoperative week [23]. In terms of postoperative parameters, the time to first bowel movement, laxative use, postoperative vomiting, use of analgesics and length of hospital stay were recorded. Complications were routinely ranked using the Clavien-Dindo classification, a five-grade therapy-based system in which higher grades reflect more severe complications [24]. In this study, the Comprehensive Complication Index (CCI), a new scale to better quantify postoperative morbidity, was also applied [25]. All complications arising from a single case and ranked by the Clavien-Dindo classification were summarized and expressed on a scale of 0 to 100. The calculation was made using the CCI® calculator (www.assessurgery.com). The CCI score allows quantification of all complications after a surgical procedure, while the Clavien-Dindo classification describes only the most severe complication. Donors were followed-up until 90 days after surgery.

Statistical analysis

Data analysis was performed using SPSS 21 (SPSS Inc., Chicago IL, USA). All data values presented are median values with an interquartile range (IQR) unless otherwise stated. A bivariate analysis was carried out comparing selected variables in the HALS and HARS cohorts. Differences in continuous variables between groups were tested for statistical significance using the Mann-Whitney U test. For comparison of proportions Fisher's exact tests was used. P values < 0.05 were considered statistically significant.

Availability of data and materials

The datasets used and/or analyzed during the current study are available from the corresponding author on reasonable request.

Results

Donor

Demographic and clinical data

A total of 60 live kidney donors were included in the study ($n = 30$ HARS, $n = 30$ HALS). The demographic and clinical characteristics of the kidney donors are summarized in Table 1. There was no relevant difference between the two groups.

Perioperative data

The median OT did not differ considerably between groups (Table 2). Conversion to laparotomy was never required. In the HARS group, 16 (53.3%) patients underwent right-sided donor nephrectomy, compared to 12 (40%) in the HALS group. There was no relevant difference between right- and left-sided nephrectomies within the two groups with regard to postoperative renal function. There was a trend for the OT to be shorter in both groups for right-sided nephrectomies, but these differences did not reach statistical significance (HARS: 132 min versus 145 min, $p = 0.15$; HALS: 140 min versus 180 min, $p = 0.06$).

Median WIT was significantly shorter in the HARS group than in the HALS group (120 s versus 150 s,

Table 2 Donors' intra- and postoperative data

	HARS ($n = 30$)	HALS ($n = 30$)	p-value
OT overall (min)	140 (34)	170 (47)	0.060
- OT right-sided (min)	132 (40)	140 (52)	0.315
- OT left-sided (min)	145 (75)	180 (28)	0.197
WIT (sec)	120 (49)	150 (16)	0.008
- WIT of right kidneys (sec)	120 (38)	150 (23)	0.208
- WIT of left kidneys (sec)	120 (60)	150 (4)	0.017
First bowel movement (d)	2.1 (0)	2.4 (1)	0.385
Use of laxatives	19 (63.3)	27 (90)	0.030
Vomiting [a]	4 (13.3)	7 (23.3)	0.506
- plus laxatives	1/4	7/7	0.010
Length of hospital stay (d)	6 (3)	6 (3)	0.062
Creatinine (umol/l)			
- Preoperative	69 (16)	69 (14)	0.646
- Postoperative	99 (28)	102 (26)	0.794
- Follow-up	104 (23)	100 (21)	0.556

OT operative time, *WIT* warm ischemia time
Values are median and IQR, frequencies are in absolute numbers and %
[a]vomiting after 24 h and 7 days postoperatively

$p = 0.008$). There was no relevant difference in WIT for left-sided compared to right-sided organ harvest for both surgical techniques.

The demand for postoperative analgesia was similar between groups. Median time to first bowel movement after surgery did not differ between the HARS and HALS groups. However, there was a significant difference in the use of laxatives: 19 (63.3%) donors in the HARS group received laxatives compared to 27 (90%) in the HALS group. In the HARS group, 4 (13.3%) patients experienced at least one episode of postoperative emesis (24 h - 7 days) compared to 7 (23.3%) in the HALS group. All HALS donors experiencing emesis required laxatives, while this was the case for only one donor in the HARS group.

It is institutional policy that donors can decide how long they would like to stay in the hospital following surgery, and their wishes are accommodated. However, the median length of hospital stay did not differ between the two groups. The median creatinine preoperatively, before discharge, and during 3 months of follow-up did not differ between the two groups.

Minor complications (grade 0–II)

Postoperative courses were uneventful in 22 (73.3%) donors in the HARS group and 18 (60%) in the HALS group (Table 3).

Two (6.6%) Grade I complications occurred in each group, including incisional pain, lumbago and shoulder ache. They all could be eased by either subcutaneous infiltration of local anesthetics or oral analgesia and

Table 1 Demographic and clinical characteristics of kidney donors

	HARS ($n = 30$)	HALS ($n = 30$)	p-value
Age (years)	56 (17)	50 (18)	0.268
Female	21 (70)	19 (63.3)	0.784
BMI (kg/m^2)	24.8 (4.4)	25.5 (3.8)	0.765
Art. hypertension	4 (13.3)	5 (16.6)	1.000
Right-sided donation	16 (53.3)	12 (40)	0.437

Values are median and IQR, frequencies are in absolute numbers and %

Table 3 Donor complications according to the Clavien-Dindo score and CCI within 90 days

	HARS (n = 30)	HALS (n = 30)	p-value
Clavien-Dindo Score			
Grade I	2 (6.6)	2 (6.6)	0.672
Grade II	3 (10)	6 (20)	
Grade IIIb	3 (10)	4 (13.3)	
None	22 (73.3)	18 (60)	
CCI			
Overall	6.16 (11.26)	10.36 (15.28)	0.245
Right-sided LDN	6.83 (12.25)	8.18 (11.97)	0.775
Left-sided LDN	5.39 (9.96)	11.70 (16.98)	0.307

Values are mean and SD, frequencies are in absolute numbers and %

physiotherapy. All Grade I complications corresponded to a CCI of 8.7 points.

Three (10%) Grade II complications occurred in the HARS group, including seroma, hematoma and a new onset of arterial hypertension. All complications required medical treatment with antibiotics combined with frequent wound hygiene or antihypertensive drugs and corresponded to a CCI of 20.9 points. Within the HALS group, six (20%) Grade II complications were observed, including newly diagnosed arterial hypertension, fever of unknown origin and wound seroma. All complications could be treated by drug therapy and corresponded to a CCI of 20.9 points except a donor with two postoperative complications (Grade I and Grade II), whose CCI totaled 22.6 points.

Major complications (grade III-V)
Three donors in the HARS group underwent surgical evacuation of subcutaneous hematoma in the area of the Pfannenstiel incision (Grade IIIb). The CCI was 33.7 points in all three cases. Four Grade IIIb complications occurred in the HALS group. Two subcutaneous hematomas required operative evacuation. One subcutaneous infection had to be treated surgically, followed by vacuum-assisted wound closure. One of those donors additionally underwent subcutaneous infiltration of local anesthetic (Grade I) due to persistent incisional pain. In that donor, the CCI was 34.8 points. The others corresponded to a CCI of 33.7 points. In addition, one donor underwent three surgical revisions (two subcutaneous evacuations of hematoma and one exploratory laparotomy) for a severe hemorrhage. During the exploratory laparotomy, laceration of the spleen and the small bowel mesentery was found. Treatment consisted of a splenectomy and mesenteric suture. The same donor developed a hypertensive crisis during postoperative monitoring in the ICU that required intravenous antihypertensive medication. The sum of complications in this donor

resulted in a CCI of 58.4 points. High-grade complications, i.e., single- or multi-organ failure (Grade IVa or IVb) as well as donor death (Grade V) did not occur in either group.

Recipients
Demographic and clinical data
The recipients' detailed preoperative characteristics are shown in Table 4. In the HARS group, 20 (66%) recipients underwent dialysis for a median of 8 months prior to transplantation; 14 had hemodialysis and 6 had peritoneal dialysis. In the HALS group, 23 (77%) recipients were dialyzed preoperatively for a median of 10 months, with 22 by hemodialysis and 1 by peritoneal dialysis.

Perioperative data
There were no relevant differences between the two groups in the median serum creatinine level and creatinine clearance before discharge and at 1 year after transplantation.

Survival and graft function
The recipients' one-year survival rate was 93.3% in the HARS group and 100% in the HALS group. The one-year graft survival rate was also comparable in both groups (90% versus 93.3%). In the HARS group, 29 recipients (96.6%) had an immediate or delayed onset of diuresis compared to all recipients (100%) in the HALS group (Table 4).

Table 4 Demographic and clinical characteristics of recipients' data

	HARS (n = 30)	HALS (n = 30)	p-value
BMI (kg/m^2)	23.9 (5.8)	25.6 (5.4)	0.174
Preoperative Dialysis	20 (3.3)	23 (76.6)	0.567
- Hemodialysis	14 (46.6)	22 (73.3)	
- Peritoneal Dialysis	6 (20)	1 (3.3)	
First Kidney-Tx	24 (80)	29 (96.6)	0.103
Retransplantation	6 (20)	1 (3.3)	0.103
AB0-Incompatibility	5 (16.6)	5 (16.6)	1.000
HLA			
- 0-2 mismatches	3	5	0.819
- 3-4 mismatches	12	15	0.604
- 5-6 mismatches	15	10	0.294
OT (min)	106 (39)	120 (20)	0.271
DGF/PNF	4	1	0.353
- PNF	1	0	
Creatinine (umol/l)			
- Before discharge	110 (47)	108 (41)	0.996
- After one year	118 (31)	115 (37)	0.605

Values are median and IQR, frequencies are in absolute numbers and %, *Tx* Transplantation, *DGF* delayed graft function, *PNF* primary non-function

The patient with primary non-function in the HARS group developed multiple complications, starting with an acute vascular rejection from the very beginning. In the further course a dehydrating diarrhea due to a pseudomembranous colitis occurred, followed by intestinal bleeding necessitating a hemicolectomy, and finally sepsis and multiple organ failure. The patient died 14 weeks after transplantation.

There were three cases of DGF in the HARS group and one in the HALS group. One of the DGF patients in the HARS group developed a subcutaneous hematoma postoperatively, which led to a hemodynamic instability and required two units of blood prior to the occurrence of diuresis. The second patient with DGF had a perforation of the cecum due to ischemic colitis, necessitating an ileocecal resection. The patient developed a burst abdomen postoperatively because of an abscess in the renal graft bed. The kidney, which worked perfectly before the ileoceacal resection, did not recover from this septic burst and was explanted 4 months after transplantation. The third recipient suffered from a very severe diarrhea postoperatively resulting in a metabolic derailment, which led to a temporary loss of kidney function. This recipient later developed necrotizing pancreatitis, resulting in permanent loss of graft function and the development of multiple organ failure 6 weeks after transplantation, and died. The DGF patient in the HALS group underwent immediate surgical revision due to bleeding from the venous anastomosis. Temporary hemodialysis was required, and the kidney did partially recover; the GFR was 21 ml/min at the one-year follow-up, but dialysis was not yet needed.

Discussion

There are two different approaches for hand-assisted donor nephrectomy: transabdominal and retroperitoneal. Evidence of the superiority of either technique is lacking. This analysis has shown equivalent donor outcomes after both techniques in terms of postoperative kidney function and complications. The overall WIT was significantly shorter for kidneys recovered by the retroperitoneal approach despite similar operating times for the two surgical techniques. There does, however, seem to be a trend for a shorter OT using the HARS approach. Laxatives were used significantly more often in the HALS group, and concurrent vomitus was observed in all of these patients, suggesting that the transabdominal technique has a greater effect on bowel function. Finally, both left and right nephrectomies appear to be safe and feasible with both surgical techniques.

The first LDN was performed in 1954 with an open approach [26], which remained the gold standard for more than 40 years. In 1995, a purely laparoscopic technique to procure kidneys from living-donors was pioneered [10]. Wolf et al. [15] described the HALS donor nephrectomy in 1998 for the first time, followed by Wadström et al. [19], who introduced the HARS nephrectomy 3 years later. Various advantages soon became obvious, such as the ability to use tactile feedback, easier and rapid control of bleeding by digital pressure, better exposure and dissection of structures, and more rapid kidney recovery [16]. Studies of HALS or HARS procedures describe superiority compared to purely laparoscopic nephrectomies with regard to OT and WIT [18]. Therefore, the laparoscopic approach with or without hand-assistance has become the gold standard at most kidney transplant centers [27].

Postoperative donor complication rates range from 0 to more than 40% in different reports, depending on how authors classify adverse events after a nephrectomy [20, 28–30]. Our analysis defined complications according to the Clavien-Dindo classification as well as to the CCI [24, 25]. The latter is a new scale to measure surgical morbidity and is not yet routinely used in clinical practice. Therefore, we were interested in its applicability to living kidney donors as well as in how it compares to the Clavien-Dindo classification. First, there were no mortalities or life-threatening complications except for one donor who required an emergency relaparotomy and splenectomy. There were no conversions from laparoscopic to open surgery. We found no relevant differences in graft survival and function between the two groups at the one-year follow-up. DGF occurred in three (10%) recipients transplanted with a kidney recovered by the retroperitoneal approach and in one (3.3%) patient with a kidney harvested by the transperitoneal approach. DGF as well as PNF (primary non-function, defined as permanent loss of allograft function starting immediately after transplantation) certainly are very important indicators for graft function and should not be neglected. In this regard the definition of DGF is crucial. We defined DGF as needed dialysis within the first week after transplantation [23]. In the literature, the frequency of DGF varies from 0 to 10% in living-donor transplantation, indicating that the presented results are within the expected range [28, 31, 32]. We hypothesized that the graft functions were delayed or not existing due to complications in the recipient. Either there was a hemodynamic instability postoperatively due to a subcutaneous bleeding, a sepsis because of a cecal perforation during the first week after transplant surgery, a severe diarrhea postoperatively which led to a metabolic derailment followed by a secondary anuria, an acute vascular rejection or a bleeding from the venous anastomosis. But still, contributing factors during the donor kidney harvesting cannot be totally ruled out. The overall donor complication rate according to the Clavien-Dindo classification during follow-up tended to be higher, though not significantly, in the HALS group for in-hospital minor adverse events. However, Dols et al. [21] reported in a randomized controlled trial an increased incidence for high-grade complications in HALS compared to HARS nephrectomy patients. On the other hand, Ruszat et al. [20] documented overall complication rates of 20% for the retroperitoneoscopic and 15% for the hand-assisted transabdominal approach. Interestingly, these complication rates were significantly lower than those for purely laparoscopic nephrectomies (42.9%). Analysis of the CCI of our donors showed higher scores in the HALS group compared to the HARS group, although these differences did not reach statistical significance. The CCI better represents the severity of adverse events than does the Clavien-Dindo Score. In our opinion, the new CCI scoring system is applicable and yields more information about overall complications following donor nephrectomy.

There was no relevant difference in the OT between the two techniques in our analysis, although there was a trend for a longer OT in the HALS group, mirroring other published results [21]. A key difference between the two techniques that may affect the OT is the timing of when the surgeon installs the hand-port and inserts his/her hand. In the HARS technique, hand assistance is part of the procedure from the very beginning, while in the HALS technique, hand assistance is only used for dissecting the vascular structures and for recovery of grafts. Whether this influences the recorded time of the operation remains speculative. OT is an important consideration, as there is sufficient evidence that both renal function and organ perfusion are compromised by the duration of pneumoperitoneum [33, 34]. The WIT was significantly shorter in our study for kidneys that were recovered by the retroperitoneal approach. Given the various definitions of WIT that exist, it is difficult to compare WITs across different studies. It has been previously reported that the WIT in the HARS technique is shorter than in the HALS technique [20, 35]. The differences in the WIT measured in our study did not translate into differences in delayed graft function, graft loss or renal function. This is consistent with previously published results [31].

Our study indicates for the first time that patients undergoing HALS procedures require significantly more laxatives compared to those undergoing HARS procedures. All of the donors in the HALS group who vomited after 24 h postoperatively required laxatives in contrast to only 25% in the HARS group. This is perhaps not surprising, but it confirms the hypothesis that patients undergoing transperitoneal nephrectomies are more frequently afflicted with a paralytic ileus. Still, other factors (e.g. OT) may have influenced these results. Matas et al. compared morbidity rates among open, hand-assisted laparoscopic

and pure laparoscopic nephrectomies [7]. Bowel obstruction also occurred significantly more often in the hand-assisted laparoscopic group then in the others. Other studies showed more serosa and splenic lesions in transperitoneal approaches [18].

There is repeated discussion concerning the preference for right or left donor nephrectomies. Most centers favor left kidneys for donation because of the longer renal vein, which makes implantation less demanding. On the other hand, some surgeons prefer the right kidney because it is easier to retrieve. A recent Meta-Analysis demonstrate a significant difference in terms of OT in favor of right-sided HALS nephrectomies [36]. In our study, there was a trend for a shorter OT in both groups for right-sided nephrectomies, although these differences did not reach statistical significance. A shorter OT for the right kidney can be expected due to the lower position of the right kidney and generally no adrenal, lumbar or genital veins draining into the right renal vein. There is also less need for colonic dissection and no risk of lacerating the spleen. Our OTs for right- and left-sided nephrectomies in both groups are shorter overall when compared to results of other similar studies [16, 37]. Eventually, the OT depends on the experience of the performing surgeon. The donor complication rates were comparable and did not show a relevant difference between right- and left-sided kidney donations.

An obvious limitation of our study is the small number of patients and, therefore, the low statistical power. The retrospective nature of the study is also a limitation. Only two surgeons carried out the donor procedures and patients were not randomized for the type of surgery performed. Hence, the procedures were always performed in the same way, and because both consultant surgeons were experienced, the results did not vary over time. The fact that the hand assistance in the two groups was at different time points during the procedure limits the direct comparison of the two groups. Recipient surgery in most of the cases was performed by just one of the two surgeons. Therefore, recipient surgery does not bias the presented results.

With respect to donor safety, surgeons should apply the surgical technique they are best trained in and feel most comfortable with. Future training of new surgeons should include various techniques to give them the confidence to use the best surgical approach to match individual circumstances and to be versatile enough to change procedures if research determines the superiority of one procedure. Furthermore, long-term follow-up is urgently needed because information about outcome (e.g., late complications caused by abdominal adhesions) over a longer time period in both groups is scarce.

Conclusion

There were no mortalities or intraoperative challenges leading to conversion in either donor group. In agreement with the current literature, it was demonstrated that HARS and HALS approaches for LDN are safe and feasible for renal graft recovery on either side. Neither of the two techniques provided clear evidence of superiority. And we found no relevant difference in graft function after 1 year postoperatively. However, given that the WIT is significantly shorter and the incidence of postoperative paralytic ileus is less frequent in the HARS group, we suggest that this technique might be preferred for living related kidney organ donors. Further advantages might be found for more complex patients, such as obese donors or donors with previous abdominal surgery.

Abbreviations

BMI: Body mass index; CCI: Comprehensive complication index; DGF: Delayed graft function; GFR: Glomerular filtration rate; HALS: Hand-assisted laparoscopic; HARS: Hand-assisted retroperitoneoscopic; LDN: Living-donor nephrectomy; OT: Operative time; WIT: Warm ischemia time

Authors' contributions

JW carried out the research design, wrote the paper, collected, analyzed and interpreted data. AS helped carrying out the research design, revised the paper critically, analyzed and interpreted data. PK collected and interpreted data. MS was one of the performing surgeons. JGB helped carrying out the research design, drafting the manuscript. He was one of the performing surgeons. MKM gave final approval of the version to be published, helped analyzing and interpreting data. All authors read and approved the final manuscript.

Competing interests

The authors declare that they have no competing interests.

Author details

[1]Division of Visceral and Transplantation Surgery, University Hospital, Zurich, Switzerland. [2]Department of Surgery, Kantonsspital Frauenfeld, 8500 Frauenfeld, Switzerland. [3]Department of Surgery, Kantonsspital St. Gallen, St. Gallen, Switzerland. [4]Department of Surgery, Kidney and Pancreas Transplantation, King Faisal Specialist Hospital, Riyadh, Kingdom of Saudi Arabia.

References

1. Reese PP, Shults J, Bloom RD, Mussell A, Harhay MN, Abt P, et al. Functional status, time to transplantation, and survival benefit of kidney transplantation among wait-listed candidates. Am J Kidney Dis Off J Natl Kidney Found. 2015;66(5):837–45.

2. Biancone L, Cozzi E, López-Fraga M, Nanni-Costa A. Long-term outcome of living kidney donation position paper of the European committee on organ transplantation (CD-P-TO), Council of Europe. Transpl Int Off J Eur Soc Organ Transplant. 2015.

3. Bundesamt für Gesundheit - Zahlen und Fakten [Internet]. [cited 2014 Aug 14]. Available from: https://www.bag.admin.ch/bag/de/home/service/zahlen-fakten/zahlen-fakten-zu-transplantationsmedizin/zahlen-fakten-zur-spende-und-transplantation-von-organen.html#925789694.

4. Hariharan S, Johnson CP, Bresnahan BA, Taranto SE, McIntosh MJ, Stablein D. Improved graft survival after renal transplantation in the United States, 1988 to 1996. N Engl J Med. 2000;342(9):605–12.

5. Branco F, Cavadas V, Rocha A, Vidinha J, Osório L, Martins L, et al. Living versus cadaveric-donor renal transplant recipients: a comparison on sexual function. Transplant Proc. 2013;45(3):1066–9.

6. Gozdowska J, Zatorski M, Torchalla P, Białek Ł, Bojanowska A, Tomaszek A, et al. Living-donor versus deceased-donor kidney transplantation: comparison of psychosocial consequences for recipients. Transplant Proc. 2016;48(5):1498–505.

7. Matas AJ, Bartlett ST, Leichtman AB, Delmonico FL. Morbidity and mortality after living kidney donation, 1999-2001: survey of United States transplant centers. Am J Transplant Off J Am Soc Transplant Am Soc Transpl Surg. 2003;3(7):830–4.

8. Morgan BR, Ibrahim HN. Long-term outcomes of kidney donors. Curr Opin Nephrol Hypertens. 2011;20(6):605–9.

9. Muzaale AD, Massie AB, Wang M-C, Montgomery RA, McBride MA, Wainright JL, et al. Risk of end-stage renal disease following live kidney donation. JAMA. 2014;311(6):579–86.

10. Ratner LE, Ciseck LJ, Moore RG, Cigarroa FG, Kaufman HS, Kavoussi LR. Laparoscopic live donor nephrectomy. Transplantation. 1995;60(9):1047–9.

11. Fonouni H, Mehrabi A, Golriz M, Zeier M, Müller-Stich BP, Schemmer P, et al. Comparison of the laparoscopic versus open live donor nephrectomy: an overview of surgical complications and outcome. Langenbeck's Arch Surg. 2014;399(5):543–51.

12. Nicholson ML, Elwell R, Kaushik M, Bagul A, Hosgood SA. Health-related quality of life after living donor nephrectomy: a randomized controlled trial of laparoscopic versus open nephrectomy. Transplantation. 2011;91(4):457–61.

13. Chin EH, Hazzan D, Edye M, Wisnivesky JP, Herron DM, Ames SA, et al. The first decade of a laparoscopic donor nephrectomy program: effect of surgeon and institution experience with 512 cases from 1996 to 2006. J Am Coll Surg. 2009;209(1):106–13.

14. Altinel M, Akinci S, Gunes ZE, Olcucuoglu E, Gonenc F, Yazicioglu AH. Open versus laparoscopic donor nephrectomy: perioperative parameters and graft functions. Transplant Proc. 2011;43(3):781–6.

15. Wolf JS, Tchetgen MB, Merion RM. Hand-assisted laparoscopic live donor nephrectomy. Urology. 1998;52(5):885–7.

16. Minnee RC, Bemelman F, Kox C, Surachno S, Ten Berge IJM, Bemelman WA, et al. Comparison of hand-assisted laparoscopic and open donor nephrectomy in living donors. Int J Urol Off J Jpn Urol Assoc. 2008;15(3):206–9.

17. Yuan H, Liu L, Zheng S, Yang L, Pu C, Wei Q, et al. The safety and efficacy of laparoscopic donor nephrectomy for renal transplantation: an updated meta-analysis. Transplant Proc. 2013;45(1):65–76.

18. Özdemir-van Brunschot DMD, Koning GG, van Laarhoven KCJHM, Ergün M, van Horne SBCE, Rovers MM, et al. A comparison of technique modifications in laparoscopic donor nephrectomy: a systematic review and meta-analysis. PLoS One. 2015;10(3):e0121131.

19. Wadström J, Lindström P. Hand-assisted retroperitoneoscopic living-donor nephrectomy: initial 10 cases. Transplantation. 2002;73(11):1839–40.

20. Ruszat R, Sulser T, Dickenmann M, Wolff T, Gürke L, Eugster T, et al. Retroperitoneoscopic donor nephrectomy: donor outcome and complication rate in comparison with three different techniques. World J Urol. 2006;24(1):113–7.

21. Dols LFC, Kok NFM, d'Ancona FCH, Klop KWJ, Tran TCK, Langenhuijsen JF, et al. Randomized controlled trial comparing hand-assisted Retroperitoneoscopic versus standard laparoscopic donor nephrectomy. Transplantation. 2013.

22. Delmonico FL, Dew MA. Living donor kidney transplantation in a global environment. Kidney Int. 2007;71(7):608–14.

23. Mallon DH, Summers DM, Bradley JA, Pettigrew GJ. Defining delayed graft function after renal transplantation: simplest is best. Transplantation. 2013; 96(10):885–9.

24. Clavien PA, Barkun J, de Oliveira ML, Vauthey JN, Dindo D, Schulick RD, et al. The Clavien-Dindo classification of surgical complications: five-year experience. Ann Surg. 2009;250(2):187–96.

25. Slankamenac K, Graf R, Barkun J, Puhan MA, Clavien P-A. The comprehensive complication index: a novel continuous scale to measure surgical morbidity. Ann Surg. 2013;258(1):1–7.

26. Murray JE, Tilney NL, Wilson RE. Renal transplantation: a twenty-five year experience. Ann Surg. 1976;184(5):565–73.

27. Klop KWJ, Dols LFC, Kok NFM, Weimar W, Ijzermans JNM. Attitudes among surgeons towards live-donor nephrectomy: a European update. Transplantation. 2012;94(3):263–8.

28. Baron PW, Ben-Youssef R, Ojogho ON, Kore A, Baldwin DD. Morbidity of 200 consecutive cases of hand-assisted laparoscopic living donor nephrectomies: a single-center experience. J Transp Secur. 2012;2012:121523.

29. Bachmann A, Wyler S, Wolff T, Gürke L, Steiger J, Kettelhack C, et al. Complications of retroperitoneoscopic living donor nephrectomy: single center experience after 164 cases. World J Urol. 2008;26(6):549 54.

30. Lentine KL, Lam NN, Axelrod D, Schnitzler MA, Garg AX, Xiao H, et al. Perioperative complications after living kidney donation: a National Study. Am J Transplant Off J Am Soc Transplant Am Soc Transpl Surg. 2016;16(6):1848–57.
31. Lucas SM, Liaw A, Mhapsekar R, Yelfimov D, Goggins WC, Powelson JA, et al. Comparison of donor, and early and late recipient outcomes following hand assisted and laparoscopic donor nephrectomy. J Urol. 2013;189(2):618–22.
32. Minnee RC, Bemelman WA, Donselaar-van der Pant KA, Booij J, ter Meulen S, ten Berge IJM, et al. Risk factors for delayed graft function after hand-assisted laparoscopic donor nephrectomy. Transplant Proc 201042(7):2422–2426.
33. Demyttenaere S, Feldman LS, Fried GM. Effect of pneumoperitoneum on renal perfusion and function: a systematic review. Surg Endosc. 2007;21(2):152–60.
34. Wever KE, Bruintjes MHD, Warlé MC, Hooijmans CR. Renal perfusion and function during pneumoperitoneum: a systematic review and meta-analysis of animal studies. PLoS One. 2016;11(9):e0163419.
35. Klop KWJ, Kok NFM, Dols LFC, Dor FJMF, Tran KTC, Terkivatan T, et al. Can right-sided hand-assisted retroperitoneoscopic donor nephrectomy be advocated above standard laparoscopic donor nephrectomy: a randomized pilot study. Transpl Int. 2014;27(2):162–9.
36. Wang K, Zhang P, Xu X, Fan M. Right versus left laparoscopic living-donor nephrectomy: a meta-analysis. Exp Clin Transplant Off J Middle East Soc Organ Transplant. 2015;13(3):214–26.
37. Tsoulfas G, Agorastou P, Ko D, Hertl M, Elias N, Cosimi AB, et al. Laparoscopic living donor nephrectomy: is there a difference between using a left or a right kidney? Transplant Proc. 2012;44(9):2706–8.

21

The risk factors of Urethrocutaneous fistula after hypospadias surgery in the youth population

Xujun Sheng[†], Ding Xu[†], Yu Wu, Yongjiang Yu, Jianhua Chen and Jun Qi[*]

Abstract

Background: The current research aims to evaluate the risk factors of urethrocutaneous fistula after hypospadias surgery among the youth in China.

Methods: One hundred twenty hypospadias patients were enrolled in our study. All of them were defined as Tanner 4 or 5. The information collected from the participants include age, urethral operation history, urinary comorbidities before operation, urine test before operation, body temperature before and after operation, type of surgical repair, chordee degree, urethral defect length and whether received vesicostomy after surgery or not. Independent t test, chi-square test and multivariate logistic regression were performed to evaluate the risk factor of urethrocutaneous fistula.

Results: Among the enrolled patients, 39 patients (32.5%) developed urethrocutaneous fistula after hypospadias repair. Our result showed significant association between the group with urethrocutaneous fistula and the group without urethrocutaneous fistula with respect to age, pyuria before operation, urethral defect length and the urethral operation history. The following logistic regression showed that urethral defect length and the urethral operation history were the risk factors of urethrocutaneous fistula.

Conclusions: Urethral defect length and urethral operation history should be taken into consideration before undergoing hypospadias surgery since our study discovered that the risk of developing urethrocutaneous fistula after hypospadias repair is associated with urethral defect length and urethral operation history. Age, surgical procedure, type of surgical repair, chordee degree and other factors were not obviously related to the development of urethrocutaneous fistula.

Keywords: Hypospadias, Urethrocutaneous fistula, Risk factor, Urethral defect length, Operation history

Background

Hypospadias, in which the urethral opening occurs on the ventral side of the penis, is the most common congenital condition of the penis. The incidence of hypospadias ranged from very low rate of 0.6/10,000 births (Malaysia) to extremely high rate of 464/10,000 births (Denmark). Low prevalence was also reported from China (0.7–4.5/ 10,000). However, the increasing trend in the prevalence has been shown [1]. Meanwhile, Hypospadias surgery has been in continuous evolution for many years with steadily improving reported results [2]. However, The results of hypospadias surgery are still frequently unfavourable with reported complication rate as high as 50% or above [3, 4]. The most common complications following hypospadias surgery accompany with urethrocutaneous fistula, meatal stenosis, urethral stricture, urethral diverticulum, glans dehiscence, breakdown, and cosmetic unfavorable outcome requiring redo-surgery [5]. Urethrocutaneous fistula, followed by hypospadias reconstruction, is one of the most common complications. Post-surgery fistula in children could occur as the result of one or more factors, such as meatal stenosis, urorethral stricture, hematoma, infection, poor surgical technique, etc. [6]. However, a lot of patients, especially those in the developing countries, go to

* Correspondence: qijun@xinhuamed.com.cn

[†]Xujun Sheng and Ding Xu contributed equally to this work.

Department of Urology, School of Medicine, Xinhua Hospital, Shanghai Jiao Tong University, 1665 Kongjiang Rd, XinHua Hospital, Shanghai 200092, China

outpatient department for treatment when they are grown up, possibly restrict to economic factors, unsuccessful surgery history or other reasons. There are a few other reports specifically concerning the hypospadias surgical outcomes among the youth population. Some studies reported higher complication rate occurs among adults than children using the same techniques [7], but another study argue against it [8]. Moreover, up to now, the risk factors of Urethrocutaneous fistula after hypospadias surgery in the youth are still unknown. The aim of this study is to evaluate these risk factors of Urethrocutaneous fistula after hypospadias surgery among youth population in China.

Methods

The retrospective study involved 120 patients who were treated in our department suffering from hypospadias from Jan 2002 to Dec 2013. Those who were defined as Tanner 4 or 5 and were followed up by their surgeons for evaluating the effect of operation from 6 months to 2 years (11.75 ± 3.89 months) were primarily focused in our study. This study was approved by the Ethics Committee of Xin Hua Hospital Affiliated to Shanghai Jiao Tong University School of Medicine [2014–007]. The information of the participants were collected on age, urethral operation history, urinary comorbidities before operation, infection before and after operation, type of surgical repair, chordee degree, urethral defect length and whether received vesicostomy or not after surgery. Urethral operation history was divided into 2 groups: one represented none; two represented the history of at least one urethral operations before the current surgery. Pyuria before surgery was defined as white blood cell> 5/HP in urine test. Infection after surgery was defined as body temperature > 38 °C. Chordee was quantified preoperatively by Horton test divided into mild (0–20°), moderate (30–40°) and severe (> 50°) [9]. Urethral defect length was measured after correction of chordee during the operation. The choice of the procedure was based on surgeon's experience and the characteristics of the urethral plate regardless of the meatal location. The hypospadias repairs can be classified into single-stage procedures and two-stage urethral plate substitution procedure (Bracka's repair). The single-stage procedures are (a) urethral plate tubularization (glanular approximation and Snodgrass repair) and (b) urethral plate augmentation (onlay lap and Snodgraft repair) [10]. All operations were conducted by four experienced urologists.

Statistical Package for Social Science(SPSS), version 13.0 was used for statistical analysis. The data was presented in the form of mean ± SD. Independent t-test was used to calculate the numerical parameters of two groups having significant difference when the parameter was consistent with normal distribution and Mann-Whitney U test was used when the parameter was consistent with nonparameter distribution. Chi-square test was analyzed in categorical parameters. Binary logistic regression was used in multivariate analysis to find the risk factors of urethrocutaneous fistula after hypospadias surgery in adults in China. For all statistical tests, a P-value < 0.05 was considered to be statistically significant.

Results

The median age of enrolled patients at surgery was 13.50 (11–42) years old. Thirty-nine patients developed urethrocutaneous fistula after surgical repair, which meant the complication rate was 32.5%. Five patients' hypospadias could not be completely repaired. Three patients met urethral stenosis. Seven patients met fistula associated with meatal stenosis while 1 patient met fistula associated with diverticulum. Among the enrolled patients, 62 patients (51.67%) received at least one hypospadias repair surgery before. The mean urethral defect length was 4.11 ± 2.70 cm. Sixteen patients (13.33%) received two-stage procedure and 18 patients (15%) received bladder stoma after the opreation. Table 1 shows that the age, the pyuria before operation, urethral defect length and urethral operation history had significant differences between the group with urethrocutaneous fistula and the group without urethrocutaneous fistula. The chordee showed no signicfant difference between two group from Table 2. With the following multivariate logistic regression, we found that two parameters, urethral defect length (OR1.215, 95%CI: 1.009–1.464) and urethral operation history (OR 2.469, 95% CI: 1.021–5.974) were the two independent risk factors of urethrocutaneous fistula. The correlation among all the parameters was summarized in Table 3.

Discussion

Hypospadias is the abnormal location of the urethra on the ventral surface of the penis with variable associations with the aborted development of the urethral spongiosum, ventral prepuce, and penile chordee [11]. Hypospadias surgery has been continuously evolving since its description by Celsius and Galen in the first and second centuries AD to improve suboptimal functional and cosmetic results. In spite of the advanced surgical techniques, the rates of complication after hypospadias repair remain high [12, 13]. One of the most common complications of hypospadias repair is urethrocutaneous fistula. Small-sized fistulas may disappear spontaneously, but most fistulas need surgical correction [14]. The incidence of urethrocutaneous fistula after hypospadias repair ranges from 6.20 to 38.8% [8, 9, 15–22], mostly during 10–20%. In the current study, the fistula rate was 32.5%, higher than the most studies. The possible reason was listed as below. Firstly, the most studies focused on the children while the enrolled patients in our study were defined as Tanner 4 or 5.

Table 1 The comparison of clinical parameters between the group with fistula and the group without fistula

	Without fistula (n = 81)	With fistula (n = 39)	P value
age	14.46 ± 3.80	16.82 ± 5.99	0.010*€
Pyuria before surgery	2.47% (2/81)	12.82% (5/39)	0.023*#
Urinary comorbidities before surgery	14.81% (12/81)	28.21% (11/39)	0.081#
Urethral defect length	3.75 ± 3.04 cm	4.86 ± 1.58 cm	0.034*€
Urethral operation history	43.21% (35/81)	69.23%(27/39)	0.008*#
urethral plate tubularization	59.26%(48/81)	46.15% (18/39)	0.177#
penis vascular pedicle flap	39.51% (32/81)	56.41% (22/39)	0.081#
free flap from oral cavity	6.17% (5/81)	0 (0/39)	0.113#
Two-stage surgical procedure	14.81% (12/81)	10.26% (4/39)	0.491#
bladder stoma	12.35% (10/81)	20.51% (8/39)	0.241#
Fever after surgery	9.88% (8/81)	23.08% (9/39)	0.052#

*$P < 0.05$ #chi-square test €independent t test

Secondly, in our study, the rate of at least one operation was 51.67%, obviously higher than that in other studies, indicating that urethral operation history plays an important role in development of the urethrocutaneous fistula.

The success of the hypospadias repair can be attributed to good tissue and vascular supply [19], which may be associated with patient age and the number of operations patients have undergone before. The rate of hypospadias repair complications ranges from 10.1 to 37.5% in adult patients undergoing a primary repair but more than doubles to between 27.5 and 63.6% [23, 24] in patients with at least one urethral operation. Urethral plate is a healthy tissue with an extensive vascular network and muscle support [25]. Therefore, urethral plate is the ideal material for hypospadias repair. The higher complication rate in patients undergoing at least one urethral operation may be due to lack of healthy urethral plate, which should be healed by scarring instead of epithelization [26]. In addition, previously repair lead to subsequent distortion of anatomy and vasculature. Urethrocutaneous fistula in these patients was probably associated with poor tissue quality and tissue ischemia [19].

Few studies have focused on the correlation between urethrocutaneous fistula and urethral defect length. Huang et al. [20] revealed that urethrocutaneous fistula occurred in 8.2% (5/61) patients with urethral defect length less than 2 cm, 12.8% (9/70) cases with urethral defect length of 2–3 cm and 22.6% (7/31) with urethral defect length of 3–4 cm. However, the 5 patients with urethral defect length > 4 cm did not developed urethrocutaneous fistula after surgical repair. The relatively small number of patients with urethral defect length > 4 cm may be responsible for it. Yildiz et al. [21] indicated that patients with mid-penile hypospadias had a 1.7-fold increase in surgical complications compared to those with distal hypospadias (18.4% vs 10.4%) and 1.3-fold increase in fistula complications (7.8 vs 5.9%). Khan et al. reached the similar result [9]. The current study suggested that urethral defect length may be another independent risk factors of urethrocutaneous fistula. It is suspected that the longer defect length need better tissue and richer vascular supply to repair and healing of two different kinds of tissues was relatively difficult [20].

From several studies, age is the risk factor for hypospadias repair. Huang et al. concluded that older children (> 6 years) with hypospadias repair were more subjected to urethrocutaneous fistula. Yildiz et al. [21] reported the rate of urethrocutaneous fistula was significantly higher in those aged over 10 years. Several potential explanations might account for it. First of all, erection was taken into consideration as evidenced by research on adult patient with hypospadias [27]. With the increasing age, erection occurred more frequently, resulted in postoperative bleeding and dehiscence, and affected the postoperative complications notably, especially for urethrocutaneous fistula [23]. Secondly, adolescent or adult hypospadias patients are much more likely to have undergone at least one urethral operation. In addition,

Table 2 The comparison of penile chordee between two groups

		Without fistula (n = 81)	With fistula (n = 39)	P value
Penile chordee	Mild (0–20°)	23	13	0.737
	Moderate (30–40°)	35	14	
	Severe (> 50°)	23	12	

$P < 0.05$

Table 3 The correlation among all the clinical parameters

		Age	Pyuria before surgery	Urinary comorbidities before surgery	Urethral defect length	Penile chordee	Urethral plate tubularization	Free flap from oral cavity	Penis vascular pedicle flap	Two-stage surgical procedure	bladder stoma	Fever after surgery	Urethral operation history
Age	r	1.000	0.125	0.179*	0.630**	−0.152	−0.217*	0.110	0.236**	0.300**	0.280**	0.135	0.475**
	P value	.	0.174	0.050	0.000	0.098	0.017	0.232	0.009	0.001	0.002	0.141	0.000
Pyuria before surgery	r	0.125	1.000	0.150	0.140	−0.090	−0.061	−0.052	0.061	−0.098	0.194*	0.205*	0.098
	P value	0.174	.	0.102	0.127	0.330	0.510	0.573	0.510	0.289	0.034	0.025	0.285
Urinary comorbidities before surgery	r	0.179*	0.150	1.000	0.105	−0.353**	−0.113	0.110	0.113	0.058	0.033	−0.016	0.471**
	P value	0.050	0.102	.	0.253	0.000	0.220	0.230	0.220	0.528	0.724	0.865	0.000
Urethral defect length	r	0.630**	0.140	0.105	1.000	0.042	−0.298**	0.227*	0.301**	0.389**	0.334**	0.160	0.461**
	P value	0.000	0.127	0.253	.	0.650	0.001	0.013	0.001	0.000	0.000	0.081	0.000
Penile chordee	r	−0.152	−0.090	−0.353**	0.042	1.000	0.077	−0.051	−0.143	0.195*	−0.117	0.004	−0.293**
	P value	0.098	0.330	0.000	0.650	.	0.404	0.578	0.120	0.033	0.203	0.962	0.001
Urethral plate tubularization	r	−0.217*	−0.061	−0.113	−0.298**	0.077	1.000	−0.231*	−0.899**	0.059	−0.136	−0.161	−0.204*
	P value	0.017	0.510	0.220	0.001	0.404	.	0.011	0.000	0.521	0.138	0.079	0.025
Free flap from oral cavity	r	0.110	−0.052	0.110	0.227*	−0.051	−0.231*	1.000	−0.021	0.164	0.029	0.035	0.202*
	P value	0.232	0.573	0.230	0.013	0.578	0.011	.	0.820	0.074	0.752	0.705	0.027
Penis vascular pedicle flap	r	0.236**	0.061	0.113	0.301**	−0.143	−0.899**	−0.021	1.000	−0.059	0.136	0.161	0.204*
	P value	0.009	0.510	0.220	0.001	0.120	0.000	0.820	.	0.521	0.138	0.079	0.025
Two-stage surgical procedure	r	0.300**	−0.0098	0.058	0.389**	0.195*	0.059	0.164	−0.059	1.000	0.041	−0.089	0.183*
	P value	0.001	0.289	0.528	0.000	0.033	0.521	0.074	0.521	.	0.655	0.333	0.045
bladder stoma	r	0.280**	0.194*	0.033	0.334**	−0.117	−0.136	0.029	0.136	0.041	1.000	0.097	0.219*
	P value	0.002	0.034	0.724	0.000	0.203	0.138	0.752	0.138	0.655	.	0.292	0.016
Fever after surgery	r	0.135	0.205*	−0.016	0.160	0.004	−0.161	0.035	0.161	−0.089	0.097	1.000	0.202*
	P value	0.141	0.025	0.865	0.081	0.962	0.079	0.705	0.079	0.333	0.292	.	0.027
Urethral operation history	r	0.475**	0.098	0.471**	0.461**	−0.293**	−0.204*	0.202*	0.204*	0.183*	0.219*	0.202*	1.000
	P value	0.000	0.285	0.000	0.000	0.001	0.025	0.027	0.025	0.045	0.016	0.027	.

*P < 0.05
**P < 0.01

adolescent or adult patients have different issues that may affect overall surgical success such as different skin and hair flora that may lead to perioperative infection [23]. Skin appendages, such as hair follicales, are potential microbial reservoirs [28]. Moreover, it is widely known that the healing ability of younger children is stronger than the older, which might be another reason for the lower incidence after successful surgical repair in younger patients [20]. In our study, patients with urethrocutaneous fistula were obviously older than patients without urethrocutaneous fistula. However, age was not the independent risk factor from the multivariate regression. Maybe prepuberty patients were excluded from our study and age was not so important among the patients defined as Tanner 4 or Tanner 5.

Despite the controversial status, a lot of the hypospadiologists favour the urinary diversion. From our study, urinary diversion after surgery had no significant difference between two groups.In addition, none of penile chordee, urinary comorbidities before operation, the pyuria before surgery, fever after surgery and surgical protocol had significant difference between two groups, which is different from the previous study [16]. It can be supposed our sample size is limited.

To sum up, our study also had some limitations. Because of the retrospective study, some parameters, such as surgical time, urethral plate width, glans size, urine culture result, GMS score and HOPE score evaluated before operation were not collected for analysis. GMS score could describe the severity of hypospadias with high inter-observer reliability [29] and have strong correlation with the risk of a surgical complication in the patients undergoing primary hypospadias repair [30]. Degree of chordee (S score) is independently prediction of fistula rate [30]. HOPE score was evaluated as an objective outcome measure of the cosmetic result after hypospadias surgery [31]. Furthermore, Confounding factors cannot completely excluded. In the further prospective study, the above limitation s will be taken into consideration.

Conclusions

Urethral defect length and urethral operation history should be taken into consideration when planning hypospadias surgery since our study discovered that the risk of developing urethrocutaneous fistula after hypospadias repair is associated with urethral defect length and urethral operation history. Age, surgical procedure, type of surgical repair, chordee degree and other factors were not obviously related to the development of urethrocutaneous fistula.

Abbreviations
AD: Anno Domini; OR: Odds ratio; SD: Standard deviation

Acknowledgements
The authors wish to thank the statistician named Xi Zhang for checking and revising statistical reporting.

Authors' contributions
Dr. XJS conceived of the study, and participated in its design and coordination. Dr. DX drafted the manuscript. Dr. YW carried out the acquisition of data, or analysis and interpretation of data. Dr. YJY revised the manuscript. Dr. JHC helped to the study coordination and draft the manuscript. Dr. JQ have given final approval of the version to be published. All authors read and approved the final manuscript.

Competing interests
The authors declare that they have no competing interest.

References
1. Springer A, van den Heijkant M, Baumann S. Worldwide prevalence of hypospadias. Journal of Pediatric Urology. 2016;12:152. e1–152.e7
2. Roberts J. Hypospadias surgery past, present and future. Curr Opin Urol. 2010;20:483–9.
3. Duckett JW. Hypospadias. In: Walsh PC, Petik AB, Vaughan ED, Wein AJ, editors. Campbell urology, vol. III. 7th ed. Philadelphia: W.B. Saunders Company; 1998. p. 2093–119.
4. Shukla AR, Patel RP, Canning DA. Hypospadias. Urol Clin North Am. 2004;31:445–60.
5. Springer A. Assessment of outcome in hypospadias surgery–a review. Frontiers in Pediatrics. 2014;2:1–7.
6. Agrawal K, Misra A. Unfavourable results in hypospadias. Indian J Plast Surg. 2013;46(2):419–27.
7. Hensle TW. Words of wisdom. Re: Treatment of adults with complications from previous hypospadias surgery. Eur Urol. 2013;63:180.
8. Snodgrass W, Villanueva C, Bush N. Primary and Reoperative hypospadias repair in adults: are results different than in children? J Urol. 2014;192(6):1730–3.
9. Khan M, Majeed A, Hayat W, et al. Hypospadias repair: a single Centre experience. Plastic Surgery Int. 2014;2014:453049.
10. Manzoni G, Bracka A, Palminteri E, Marrocco G. Hypospadias surgery: when, what and by whom ? BJU Int. 2004;94:1188–95.
11. Iqbal T, Nasir U, Khan M, et al. Frequency of complication in the snodgrass repair and its risk factors. Pakistan Journal of Surgery. 2011;27(3):188–93.
12. Nuininga JE, DE Gier RP, Verschuren R, Feitz WF. Long-term outcome of different types of 1-stage hypospadias repair. J Urol. 2005;174(4 Pt 2):1544–8.
13. Demirbilek S, Kanmaz T, Aydin G, Yucesan S. Outcomes of one-stage techniques for proximal hypospadias repair. Urology. 2001;58:267–70.
14. Waterman BJ, Renschler T, Cartwright PC, Snow BW, DeVries CR. Variables in successful repair of urethrocutaneous fistula af-ter hypospadias surgery. J Urol. 2002;168:726–30.
15. Sarhan OM, El-Hefnawy AS, Hafez AT, Elsherbiny MT, Dawaba ME, Ghali AM. Factors affecting outcome of tubularized incised plate (TIP) urethroplasty: sing le-center experience with 500 cases. J Pediatr Urol. 2009;5:378–82.
16. Kwon T, Song GH, Song K, Song C, Kim KS. Management of ure-thral fistulas and strictures af ter hypospadias repair. Korean J Urol. 2009;50:46–50.
17. Hwang JS, Jung GW, Cho WY. Outcome of tubularized incised plate urethroplasty for correction of hypospadias. Korean J Urol. 2003;44:1026–31.
18. Faasse MA, Johnson EK, Bowen DK, et al. Is glans penis width a risk factor for complications after hypospadias repair? J Pediatr Urol. 2016;12(4):202. e1–5
19. Ching CB, Wood HM, Ross JH, Gao T, Angermeier KW. The Cleveland Clinic experience with adult hypospadias patients undergoing repair: their presentation and a new classification system. BJU Int. 2011;107(7):1142–6.
20. Huang LQ, Ge Z, Tian J, et al. Retrospective analysis of individual risk factors for urethrocutaneous fistula after onlay hypospadias repair in pediatric patients.Ital. J Pediatr. 2015;41:35.
21. Yildiz T, Tahtali IN, Ates DC, Keles I, Ilce Z. Age of patient is a risk factor for urethrocutaneous fistula in hypospadias surgery. J Pediatr Urol. 2013; 9(6 Pt A):900–3.
22. Chung JW, Choi SH, Kim BS, Chung SK. Risk factors for the development of urethrocutaneous fistula after hypospadias repair: a retrospective study. Korean J Urol. 2012;53(10):711–5.
23. Hensle TW, Tennenbaum S, Reiley EA, Pollard J. Hypospadias repair in adults: adventures and misadventures. J Urol. 2001;165:77–9.
24. Senkul T, Karademir K, Iseri C, Erden D, Baykal K, Adayener C. Hypospadias in adults. Urology. 2002;60(6):1059–62.

25. Erol A, Kayikci A, Memik O, Cam K, Akman Y. Single vs. double dartos interposition flaps in preventing urethrocutaneous fistula after tubularized incised plate urethroplasty in primary distal hypospadias: a prospective randomized study. Urol Int. 2009;83(3):354–8.

26. Holland AJ, Smith GH. Effect of the depth and width of the urethral plate on tubularized incised plate urethroplasty. J Urol. 2000;164:489–91.

27. Wood HM, Kay R, Angermeier KW, Ross JH. Timing of the presentation of Urethrocutaneous fistulas after hypospadias repair in pediatric patients. J Urol. 2008;180:1753–6.

28. Lange-Asschenfeldt B, Marenbach D, Lang C, et al. Distribution of bacteria in the epidermal layers and hair follicles of the human skin. Skin Pharmacol Physiol. 2011;24:305–11.

29. Merriman LS, Arlen AM, Broecker BH, et al. The GMS hypospadias score: assessment of inter-observer reliability and correlation with post-operative complications. J Pediatr Urol. 2013;9(6 Pt A):707–12.

30. Arlen AM, Kirsch AJ, Leong T, et al. Further analysis of the Glans-Urethral Meatus-Shaft (GMS) hypospadias score: correlation with postoperative complications. J Pediatr Urol. 2015;11:71. e1–5

31. der Toorn v, de Jong TP, de Gier RP. Introducing the HOPE (Hypospadias Objective Penile Evaluation)-score: a validation study of an objective scoring system for evaluating cosmetic appearance in hypospadias patients. J Pediatr Urol. 2013;9(6 Pt B):1006–16.

miR-221-5p enhances cell proliferation and metastasis through post-transcriptional regulation of SOCS1 in human prostate cancer

Ning Shao[1†], Gui Ma[2†], Jinying Zhang[3*] and Wei Zhu[3*]

Abstract

Background: To investigate the effect of miR-221-5p on cell proliferaton and metastasis of human prostate cancer in vitro and vivo.

Methods: We established PC3 cell lines with stable overexpression or silencing of miRNA-221-5p via lentivirus infection. miRNA-221-5p and its target gene SOCS1 expression levels in the stable cells were analyzed by real-time polymerase chain reaction (RT-PCR) and western blotting. Using luciferase reporter assays to study the relationship between miR-221-5p and SOCS1. Cell proliferative activity was measured using the MTT assay and colony formation assay. Migration ability was assessed using wound-healing assay and transwell assay. To further study the function of miR-221-5p in human prostate cancer we established nude mice xenograft model in vivo.

Results: miR-221-5p regulates the proliferation, migration of prostate cancer cells in vitro and tumorigenesis in vivo by regulating socs1 expression through targeted its 3'UTR, and miR-221-5p regulates MAPK/ERK signaling pathway and EMT features in prostate cancer cells.

Conclusions: Up-regulation and silencing of miR-221-5p expression in prostate cancer cells are correlated with cell proliferation, migration and tumorigenesis, which suggest that miR-221-5p plays an important role in prostate cancer progression.

Keywords: Prostate cancer, miR-221-5p, SOCS1, Cell proliferation, Cell migration, Tumor xenograft

Background

Prostate cancer (PCa) is the most common malignant tumor in the human urinary system, and it is also the second major cause of death in the world. [1, 2]. Therapeutic approach includes radical prostatectomy, radiation therapy and androgen deprivation therapy (ADT) or combination therapy including ADT with radiation therapy. Many studies have confirmed that androgens play a crucial role in prostate cancer development and progression [3, 4]. ADT is an effective therapy to control prostate cancer progression by eliminating the level of androgens in the patients. However, most of patients eventually occur resistance after ADT and turn into castration-resistant prostate cancer (CRPC) [5]. Unfortunately, the majority of the patients enhance metastatic potential and the mortality of PCa patients has greatly increased [5–7]. Curable treatment method for CRPC is not established and it is not known that the mechanism of CRPC progression in detail. Additionally, many functional genes, such as tumor suppressors, oncogenes and transcription factors, have been demonstrated to play important roles in the progression of PCa [8–11]. Considering these circumstances, discovery of new therapy approach that inhibits the development of prostate cancer progression and prolongs survival time of the patients is very important in the field.

MicroRNAs (miRNAs), small non-coding single-stranded RNAs, are negative regulators for coding genes at the post-

---

* Correspondence: jinyingzhang2@163.com; zhuwei@njmu.edu.cn
†Equal contributors
3Department of Oncology, First Affiliated Hospital of Nanjing Medical University, Nanjing 210023, China
Full list of author information is available at the end of the article

transcriptional level to be master regulators of many important biological processes, such as cell growth, invasion, metastasis, and apoptosis, etc. all [12–14]. miRNAs can bind to complementary base-pairing sequences in the 3'untranslated regions (3'UTR) of their target gene mRNA, and results in mRNA translational inhibition or degradation [15]. Lots of studies indicate that miRNAs may play important roles in a wide range of important biological processes [16].

Accumulating evidence suggests that miRNAs can function as novel tumor oncogenes or suppressors, and the deregulation of specific miRNAs involved in many important biological processes, including proliferation, invasion, apoptosis, differentiation, angiogenesis and immune response, and lead to aberrant gene expression in various diseases [17, 18]. Gene microarray data have shown the abnormal expression and paradoxical roles of miR-221-5p in human prostate cancer tissues [19–21]. In earlier research, we find that the expression of miR-221-5p is significantly different between tumor tissues and adjacent tissues of prostate cancer patients. But the molecular mechanisms of miR-221-5p and the related target genes are largely unknown. In this study, we investigated the potential functions of miR-221-5p in prostate cancer and found that miR-221-5p can specific target SOCS1 (Suppressers of cytokine signaling (SOCS) family protein, which is tumor suppressor genes [22–25]. And we investigated that miR-221-5p accelerates cell growth, migration and tumor development of human prostate cancer cells in vitro and vivo, and miR-221-5p regulates MAPK/ERK signaling pathway and EMT features in prostate cancer cells.

Methods
Patient samples
For verification of miR-221-5p expression by polymerase chain reaction (PCR),20 tumor tissue and adjacent tissue samples were collected from patients with prostate cancer at Second People's Hospital of Wuxi Affiliated to Nanjing Medical University. At the time of sample collection, the histopathological types of the patient tumors were evaluated based on the pathological stages defined by the WHO. The collection of patient tumor tissues was approved by the hospital medical ethics committee, and informed consent was obtained from all patients.

Sample collection
The tumor tissues and adjacent tissues samples were collected from prostate cancer patients. The tissues are quickly stored in liquid nitrogen and record the patient's detailed information.

Cell culture
HEK293T cell and Human prostate cancer cell lines PC3,DU145 were purchased from the Institute of Cytobiology, Chinese Academy of Sciences. HEK293T cells were cultured in Dulbecco's Modified Eagle's Medium(DMEM) and PC3 cells were maintained in F12 K medium with 10% fetal bovine serum (Thermo Fisher Scientific) at 37°Cin a humidified air atmosphere containing 5% CO_2.

RNA extraction and quantitative real-time
Total RNA was purified using TRIZOL reagent (Invitrogen) and reverse transcribed to cDNA according to the PrimeScript RT reagent Kit (TaKaRa). The quantification of target gene transcripts was detected by RT-PCR using SYBR Premix Ex Taq (TaKaRa) and ABI Prism 7900 sequence detection system. GAPDH was used as a reference gene to analyze the target gene quantitatively. TaqMan miRNA Kit (Applied Biosystems) were used to detect the expression level of mature miR-221-5p with U6 small nuclear RNA as an internal control. The fold change was calculated by $2^{-\Delta\Delta Ct}$.

Construction of plasmids
The 3'UTR of SOCS1 was amplified from PC3 cells cDNA and inserted into the pMIR-REPORT Luciferase vector (Ambion). And the corresponding mutant plasmid was constructed through mutations in the seed regions of the miR-221-5p-binding sites. The miR-221-5p and miR-221-5p silencing sequence (TuD RNA, Tough Decoy (TuD) miRNA inhibitor) [26] were constructed into lentivirus plasmid pLKD-CMV-G&PR-U6-shRNA, establishing stable expression cell lines.

Lentivirus packaging and infection
miR-221-5p overexpression or silencing vector was co-transfected with the packaging plasmids pMD2.G and pSPAX2 into HEK293T cells using Lipofectamine 2000 (Invitrogen). For establishing cell lines with stable overexpression, PC3 and DU145 cells were cultured into 6-well plates, and then infected by lentivirus solution with polybrene (Sigma-Aldrich). After incubation for 72 h, the infection efficiency of lentivirus was evaluated by RT-PCR or fluorescence.

Cell proliferation assays
Cell viability was measured using a CellTiter Aqueous assay with MTT (Sigma–Aldrich) which convert MTT into a formazan-colored product and the absorbance was measured at a wavelength of 490 nm [27]. The cell cloning ability was measured using colony formation assay. Five hundred cells were seed into 6-well culture plates and cultured at 37 °C for 7–9 d. When colony formation was visible to the naked eye, the incubation

was terminated. Then the cells were stained with Crystal Violet and colonies were counted.

Cell migration assays

For wound healing assay, cells (2×10^5 cells/well) were seeded into a 6-well plates and incubated overnight. When the cells have grown to 90%, a wound was created by a micropipette tip. Then cells were cultured with serum-free medium after rinsing with PBS to remove floating cells. The wound mark were recorded at 0 h and 24 h later under a microscope (Olympus). For transwell migration assays, cells were seeded into the top transwell chambers with serum-free medium. Then the cells on the top chambers were fixed after 48 h, and cells that did not migrate were cleared by a cotton swab. The migration cells were stained by crystal violet and counted.

Luciferase reporter assays

Bioinformatic analysis of miR-221-5p target sites was performed using TargetScan website (http://www.targetscan.org/). For experiments, HEK293T cells plated on 96-well plates were co-transfected with miR-221-5p mimics or mimics NC, and with pMIR-REPORT-SOCS1–3'UTR(WT) or mutation plasmid pMIR-REPORT-SOCS 1–3'UTR(MUT) using Lipofectamine 2000 Transfection Reagent. The firefly luciferase and ranilla luciferase activities were quantified using Dual-Luciferase Reporter Assay system (Promega).

Antibodies and immunoblotting

The antibodies purchased were as follows: anti-GAPDH antibody, anti-phospho ERK1/2 from Cell Signaling Technology; anti-total ERK1/2 from Abcam Biotechnology. Protein lysates of cells were resolved by 10% SDS–polyacrylamide gel electrophoresis (SDS–PAGE) and transferred onto PVDF membranes. After the membranes were blocked by 5% nonfat milk, the membrane was incubated with specific antibodies as well as the secondary antibodies labeled with horseradish peroxidase and visualized by chemiluminescence [28].

Nude mice xenograft models

All animal procedures were performed in accordance to the protocols approved by the Institutional Animal Care and Use Committee at Second People's Hospital of Wuxi Affiliated to Nanjing Medical University. All animals were obtained from Shanghai SLAC Laboratory Animal Co.,Ltd. For xenograft models, the two PC3 cell lines were contributed, including miR-221-5p silencing cell and control cell lines. Two groups of cells in the logarithmic phase of growth were trypsinized and rinsed with PBS three times. Five nude mice per group (four-week-old male, total 10 mice) were injected with a clonal population of PC3 cell (5×10^6 cells) in 100ul PBS in the

upper right shoulders subcutaneous. Tumor volumes were measured every other days by digital callipers when the implantations were starting to grow bigger. The animals were then euthanized by intravenous injection of potassium chloride under general anesthesia. Tumor volumes were calculated using the formula: $V(mm^3) = length \times width^{2/2}$ [8, 28].

Statistical analysis

Statistical significance was assessed using Student's t test.

Results

miR-221-5p promotes cell proliferation of prostate cancer cells

A previous microarray data has shown that miRNAs are differentially expressed in prostate cancer tissues, borderline tissues and that some miRNAs, including miR-221-5p, are correlated with the progression of prostate cancer. And we have found that the expression of miR-221-5p is significantly different between tumor tissues and adjacent tissues of prostate cancer patients (Fig. 1a).Nevertheless the functions of these miRNAs in the progression of prostate cancer remained unexplored. We investigated whether miR-221-5p is effective on the growth of human prostate cancer cells. We established PC3 and DU145 cell lines stably expressing miR-221-5p via lentivirus infection. Successful overexpression of exogenous miR-221-5p was confirmed by RT-PCR (Fig. 1c).We next explored the changes in cell proliferation after stably expressing miR-221-5p by MTT and colony formation assays. As shown in Fig. 1e and f, the proliferation rate of PC3 and DU145 cells was significantly increased by stably expressing miR-221-5p cells in comparison with the control cells. Congruously, colony formation ability was also significantly increased. However,using the TuD RNA (Tough Decoy RNA) (Fig. 1b), we established PC3 cell lines that the activity of miR-221-5p is closed. We found that the proliferation rate of PC3 cells was significantly reduced as well as colony formation (Fig. 1g). Collectively, these data indicated that miR-221-5p has a positive effect on the growth of human prostate cancer cells.

miR-221-5p promotes the migration of prostate cancer cells

We next investigated whether miR-221-5p regulates cell migratory ability in prostate cancer cells. The transwell assay further confirmed that miR-221-5p regulates the migration of prostate cancer cells (Fig. 2a and b). Consistently, in wound healing assay, the migration rate was significantly increased with miR-221-5p overexpression (Fig. 2c). However, the migration rate was significantly reduced in the wound healing assay and the transwell assay when we silencing the activity of miR-221-5p by TuD RNA

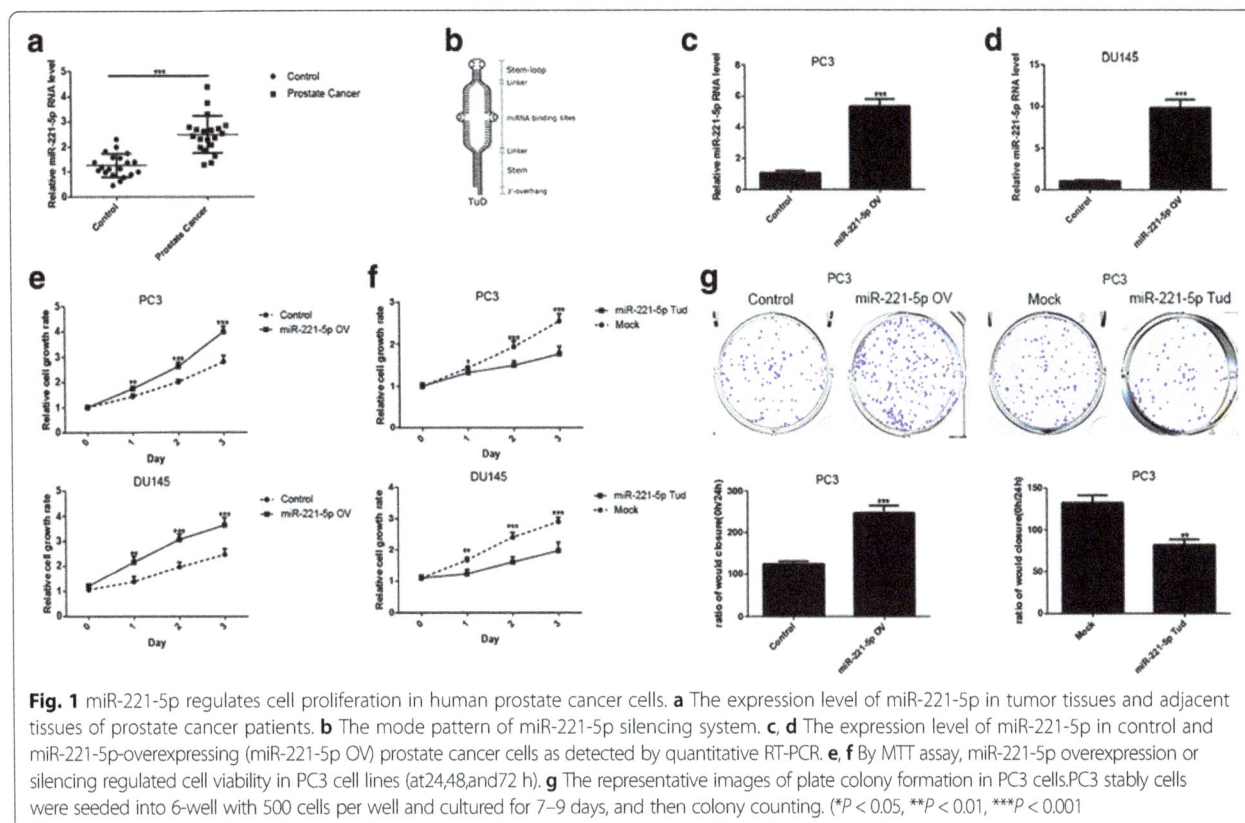

Fig. 1 miR-221-5p regulates cell proliferation in human prostate cancer cells. **a** The expression level of miR-221-5p in tumor tissues and adjacent tissues of prostate cancer patients. **b** The mode pattern of miR-221-5p silencing system. **c, d** The expression level of miR-221-5p in control and miR-221-5p-overexpressing (miR-221-5p OV) prostate cancer cells as detected by quantitative RT-PCR. **e, f** By MTT assay, miR-221-5p overexpression or silencing regulated cell viability in PC3 cell lines (at 24, 48, and 72 h). **g** The representative images of plate colony formation in PC3 cells. PC3 stably cells were seeded into 6-well with 500 cells per well and cultured for 7–9 days, and then colony counting. (*$P < 0.05$, **$P < 0.01$, ***$P < 0.001$

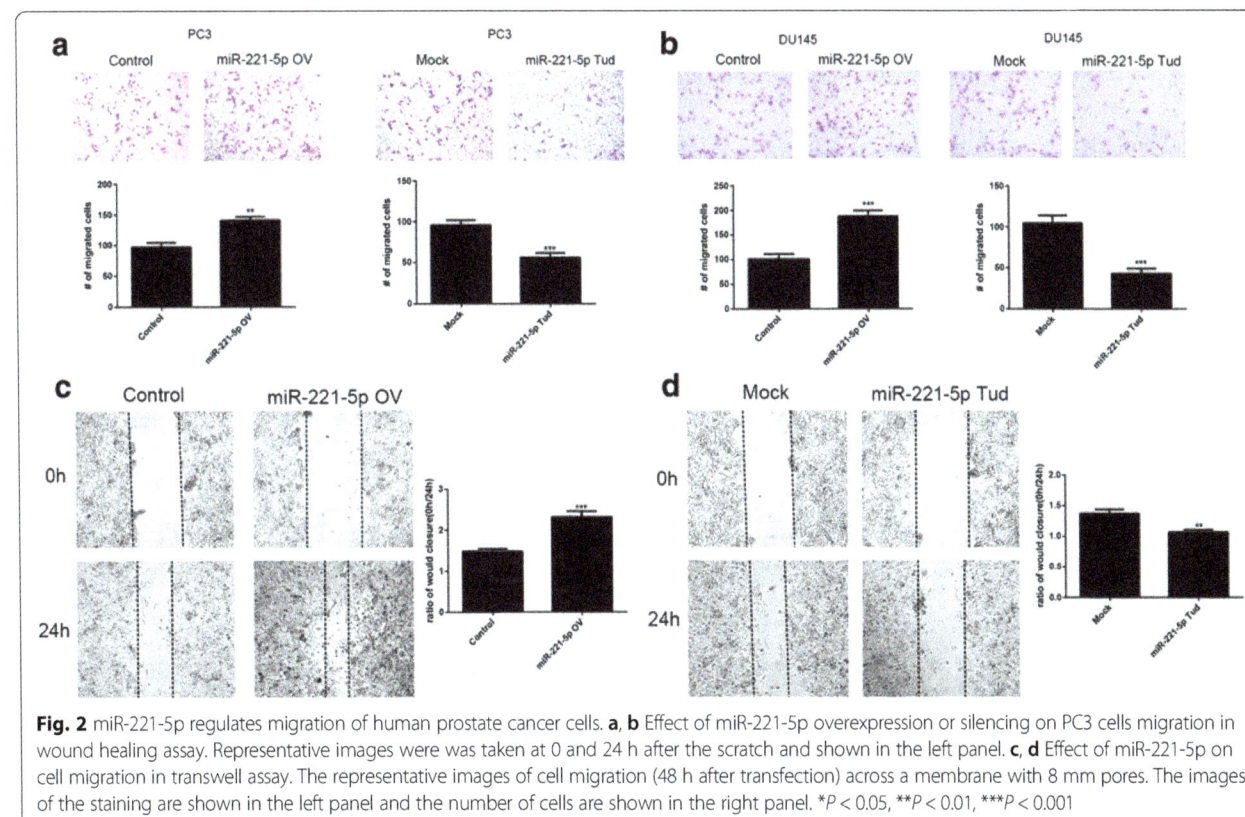

Fig. 2 miR-221-5p regulates migration of human prostate cancer cells. **a, b** Effect of miR-221-5p overexpression or silencing on PC3 cells migration in wound healing assay. Representative images were was taken at 0 and 24 h after the scratch and shown in the left panel. **c, d** Effect of miR-221-5p on cell migration in transwell assay. The representative images of cell migration (48 h after transfection) across a membrane with 8 mm pores. The images of the staining are shown in the left panel and the number of cells are shown in the right panel. *$P < 0.05$, **$P < 0.01$, ***$P < 0.001$

lentivirus (Fig. 2d).In conclusion, these data confirmed that miR-221-5p promotes the migration of prostate cancer cells.

miR-221-5p down-regulates SOCS1 expression by targeting its 3'UTR

SOCS1 as a tumor suppressor gene has been reported in previous researches, and found that SOCS1 has a lower expression level in patients with prostate cancer tissues than adjacent tissues (Fig. 3a). By TargetScan and miR-Base bioinformatics analyses, the 3'UTR of SOCS1 were identified as the potential binding site of miR-221-5p (Fig. 3b). To determine whether SOCS1 was regulated by miR-221-5p through direct binding to its 3'UTR, we inserted PCR products containing wild-type or mutant SOCS1 3'UTR binding sites into the pMIR-REPORT

Luciferase vector. The luciferase assays showed that miR-221-5p could significant reduce the luciferase activities of the 3'UTR of SOCS1, but the luciferase activity was not significant changed when SOCS1 3'UTR binding sites are mutated (Fig. 3c). This study indicates that miR-221-5p may suppress the expression of SOCS1 by targeting the binding 3'UTR sites of the SOCS1. Next, by RT-PCR and western blotting analysis, we found that overexpression of miR-221-5p significantly suppressed SOCS1 expression but silencing of miR-221-5p increased SOCS1 expression (Fig. 3d and e).

miR-221-5p regulates MAPK/ERK signaling pathway and EMT features in prostate cancer cells

The Ras/Raf/MEK/ERK signaling pathway plays an important role in cell proliferation. We next explored whether

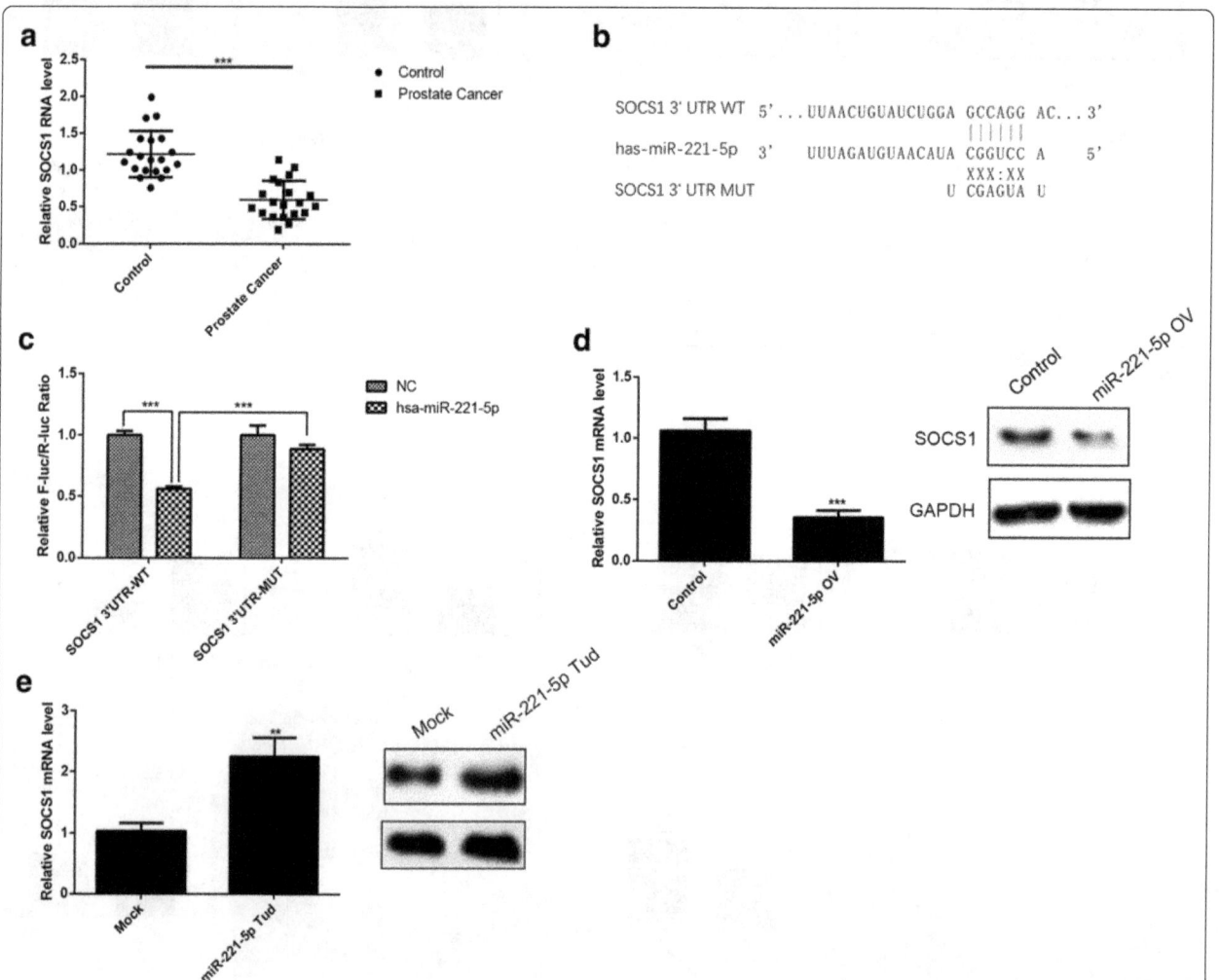

Fig. 3 SOCS1 is a direct downstream target for miR-221-5p. **a** The expression level of SOCS1 in tumor tissues and adjacent tissues of prostate cancer patients. **b** Model of the construction of wild-type or mutant SOCS1 3'UTR vectors. **c** Luciferase activity assays of luciferase vectors with wild-type or mutant SOCS1 3'UTR were performed after co-transfection with miR-221-5p mimic or negative control (NC). The luciferase activity was normalised to Renilla luciferase activity. **d, e** Western blot assays of SOCS1 protein in PC3 cells after infection with miR-221-5p overexpression or silening lentivirus. $*P < 0.05$, $**P < 0.01$, $***P < 0.001$

MAPK/ERK signaling pathway was also affected by miR-221-5p in prostate cancer cells. As expected, the serum was able to stimulate MAPK/ERK signaling pathways shown as increased phosphorylation of ERK in PC3 cells. We discovered that the phosphorylation of ERK was observably increased by overexpression of miR-221-5p in the prostate cancer cells (Fig. 4a). In contrast, silencing of miR-221-5p could inhibit serum-induced phosphorylation of ERK (Fig. 4b). These data indicated that Ras/Raf/MEK/ERK signaling pathway was regulated by miR-221-5p, likely explaining its effects on tumor-promoting activity in prostate cancer cells.

Epithelial-mesenchymal transition (EMT), a critical process for tumor migration and metastasis, was increased that shown as decrease of epithelial marker E-cadherin and increase of mesenchymal marker vimentin by overexpression of miR-221-5p (Fig. 4c). On the contrary, silencing of miR-221-5p promoted the expression of E-cadherin while suppress the expression of vimentin (Fig. 4d).

miR-221-5p promotes prostate cancer xenograft growth in vivo

In order to further demonstrate the tumor enhance activity of miR-221-5p in prostate cancers, we established a xenograft model to investigate the effects of miR-221-5p on tumor growth. PC3 cells, silencing of miR-221-5p or its control, were implanted into the nude mice (4 weeks). Then, the mice were sacrificed in 24 days when the tumor formation have significant difference (Fig. 5s and b). The growth of the PC3 cells in the nude mice as measured by tumor volume and tumor weight was significantly increased by silencing of miR-221-5p (Fig. 5c and d). Therefore, this clearly indicated that miR-221-5p has an effective activity to promote the xenograft of prostate cancer in vivo.

Discussion

miRNAs have been confirmed as important regulators of gene expression at the post transcriptional level, and these small non-coding RNAs molecules regulate a wide range of physiologicaland developmental processes [12–14]. Over the past several years, its mechanism become clear that regulates target gene expression of miRNAs contribute to the pathogenesis of most human cancers, where miRNAs has been proved to function as important regulators in tumorigenesis and development [13]. miRNA can regulate a variety of target genes, thus affecting the different physiological functions of cells.

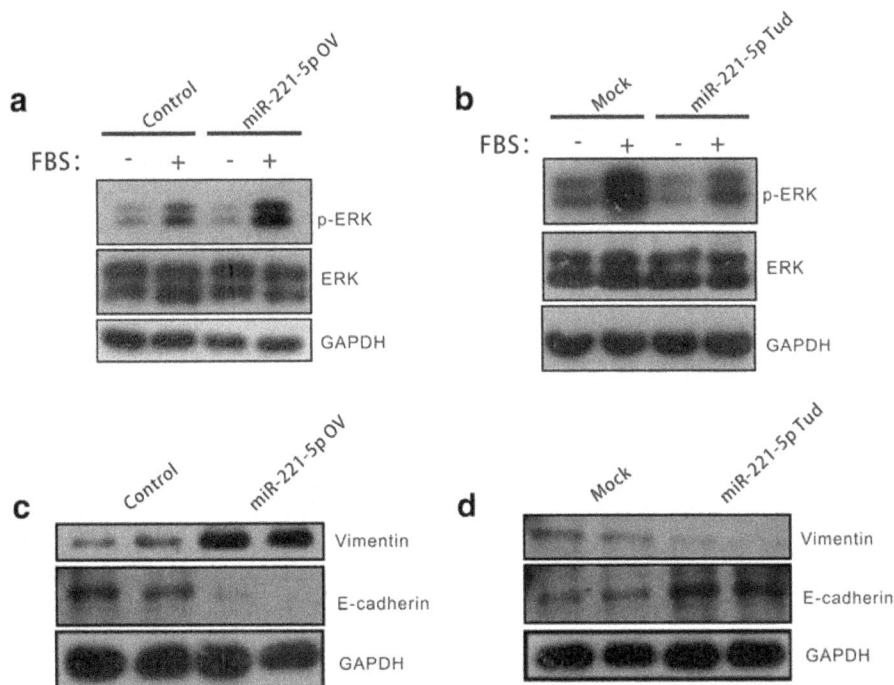

Fig. 4 miR-221-5p regulates MAPK/ERK signaling pathways and affects EMT features in human prostate cancer cells. **a** Overexpression of miR-221-5p enhances MAPK/ERK signaling pathways. After serum starvation for 16 h, PC3 cells with overexpression of miR-221-5p or control were stimulated with 10% FBS for 20 min and the cells were harvested for immunoblotting. **b** Silencing of miR-221-5p inhibits MAPK/ERK signaling pathways. PC3 stably cells of silencing miR-221-5p or control were serum-starved for 16 h, and cells were stimulated with 10% FBS for 20 min. Western blot analysis of MAPK/ERK signaling pathways proteins in the cell samples. **c, d** miR-221-5p promotes EMT features and regulates the expression of mesenchymal marker vimentin and epithelial marker E-cadherin

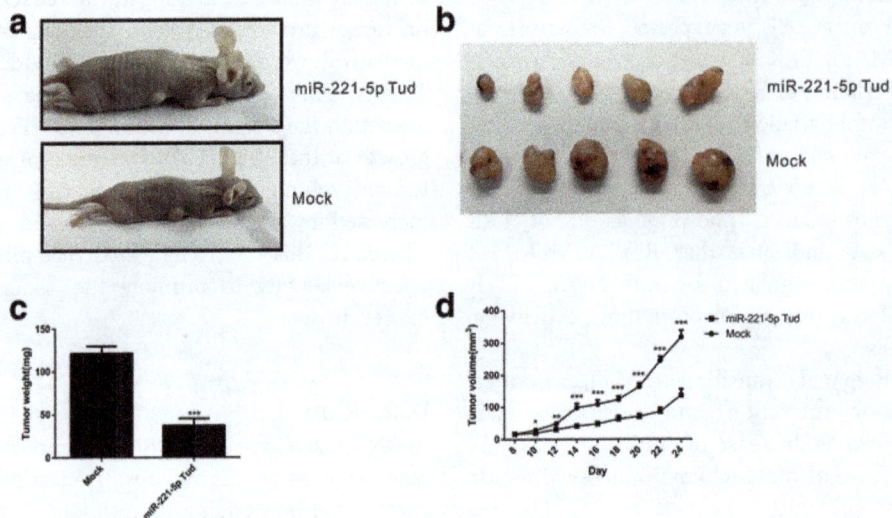

Fig. 5 Silencing of miR-221-5p enhances the growth of PC3 cell xenografts in nude mice model. **a** The subcutaneous tumors xenografts in nude mice derived from the silencing of miR-221-5p clones were smaller in size than control clones($n = 5$ each group). **b** Images of the tumors isolated from the nude mice($n = 5$ each group). **c** The weight of the tumors. **d** Tumor volume as calculated according to the formula: $V(mm^3) = length \times width^{2/2}$. *$P < 0.05$, **$P < 0.01$, ***$P < 0.001$

miRNA has obvious specificity in different cell, tissue and even different stages of tumor development, which makes miRNA play a complex and important role in the development of tumor [15–18].

Our studies have provided evidence that miR-221-5p can inhibit the expression of SOCS1 to control tumor proliferation, migration and tumorigenicity of prostate cancer cells both in vitro and in vivo. But Coarfa et al. [21] examined some publicly available, independent sets data and found that many of SIM-miRNAs were significantly downregulated in primary PC (compared with normal prostate),including miR-221-5p. Coarfa et al. found that miR-221-5p was associated with worse BCR-free survival in Taylor et al. [29] (GSE21036) according to their individual miRNA z-score (compared with normal prostate tissue).The results of our study with Coarfa et al. are inconsistent, and in order to find out why the results were inconsistent, We measured our collection of prostate cancer clinical sample, and found that in some tumor samples, the expression of miR-221-5p in the adjacent tissues was elevated and decreased in the cancer tissue, which is consistent with Coarfa et al's findings and indicated that the patient had obvious heterogeneity, but in the whole clinical data, miR-221-5p was positively correlated with prostate cancer. This suggests that miR-221-5p may have different effects at different stages of prostate cancer, but the number of prostate cancer samples currently collected is only 20, which is not enough to illustrate the problem. We will also collect more patient samples in subsequent trials to analyze the relationship between mir-221-5p and prostate cancer during different stages of development.

In this study, we found that miR-221-5p can specific target SOCS1, which is tumor suppressor genes,and suppress SOCS1 protein expression in PC3 and DU145 cells. But studies of Coarfa et al. show that miR-221-5p suppressed AR protein expression in LNCAP cells. This phenomenon further illustrates the complexity and specificity of miRNA functions in different tissues and cells.In subsequent studies, we will focus on the differences of miRNA in prostate cancer patients sample at different stages of tumor development or the different therapies, to discover more valuable information in the diagnosis and treatment of prostate cancer.

At the cellular level, by establishing the stably expression cell lines of overexpression or silencing miR-221-5p, we found that miR-221-5p regulates the cell proliferation, colony formation and migration of human prostate cancer cells. At the animal level, silencing of miR-221-5p inhibited significantly the tumorigenesis of prostate cancers in nude mice.

Given that the expression of SOCS1 is regulated at post-transcriptional level by miR-221-5p, detection the expression of miR-221-5p in cancer tissues would discover an effective approach to evaluate miR-221-5p as a potential prostate cancer biomarker. Extracellular signal regulated kinase (ERK) is a kinase regulating cell survival, growth and proliferation by promoting proline-induced protein phosphorylation, a critical process that controlling cell proliferation and metastasis [14]. SOCS1, a key inhibitory molecule of MAPK/ ERK signaling, can inhibit cell proliferation by suppressing cell cycle progression, promoting cell apoptosis, or promoting tumor cell metastasis and invasion when it is expressed aberrantly in cells [22–25]. In our studies, luciferase assays, qRT-PCR and western blotting demonstrated that miR-221-5p can target SOCS1 and regulates the expression in cells level. And miR-221-5p is able to regulate Ras/Raf/MEK/ERK signaling cascades in prostate cancer cells and such enhancement likely underlies its tumor-promoting activity in prostate cancer cells.

EMT as a critical step for tumor migration and metastasis has been demonstrated that miR-221-5p regulates EMT features in prostate cancer cells. As miR-221-5p is able to promote migration of prostate cancers, the association of miR-221-5p/SOCS1 with metastasis and EMT need to be addressed in the future. Theoretically, silencing the tumor promoting activity of miR-221-5p can stand out as an effective approach to inhibit cancer progression. Discovery of chemical molecules or other ways to regulate tumor promoting activity of miR-221-5p will have more effective to control tumor cells and inhibit tumor cell proliferation, tumor migration/metastasis. Future studies are needed to explore the association with miR-221-5p and SOCS1, and whether miR-221-5p/SOCS1 pair can be used as a new biomarker to diagnosis of prostate cancer, and whether it can be as a novel therapeutic target in prostate cancer treatment.

Conclusion

In conclusion, we find a new miR-221-5p/SOCS1 pair that may play an important role in progression of prostate cancer. And we also confirm that miR-221-5p enhances cell proliferation and metastasis through post-transcriptional regulation of SOCS1 by vitro and vivo experiments in human prostate cancer.

Abbreviations

3'UTR: 3'untranslated regions; ADT: Androgen deprivation therapy; CRPC: Castration-resistant prostate cancer; EMT: Epithelial-mesenchymal transition; ERK: Extracellular regulated protein kinases; GAPDH: Reduced glyceraldehyde-phosphate dehydrogenase; MAPK: Mitogen-activated protein kinase; MUT: Mutation; OV: Overexpression; PCa: Prostate cancer; RT-PCR: Quantitative real-time PCR; SOCS1: Suppressers of cytokine signaling (SOCS) family protein 1; TuD RNA: Tough Decoy (TuD) miRNA inhibitor; WT: Wild type

Acknowledgements
None.

Funding
No funding was obtained for this study.

Authors' contributions
Conceived and designed the study: JZ, WZ. Performed the experiments: NS, GM, JZ. Analyzed the data: JZ, WZ. Wrote the paper: NS, GM, JZ, WZ. All authors read and approved the final version of the manuscript.

Competing interests
The authors declare that they have no competing interests.

Author details
[1]Department of Urology, Fudan University Shanghai Cancer Center, Shanghai, China. [2]Department of Urology, Second People's Hospital of Wuxi, Nanjing Medical University, Wuxi, China. [3]Department of Oncology, First Affiliated Hospital of Nanjing Medical University, Nanjing 210023, China.

References
1. Siegel RL, Miller KD, Jemal A. Cancer statistics, 2016. CA Cancer J Clin. 2016;66(1):7–30.
2. Ferlay J, Soerjomataram I, Dikshit R, Eser S, Mathers C, Rebelo M, Parkin DM, Forman D, Bray F. Cancer incidence and mortality worldwide: sources, methods and major patterns in GLOBOCAN 2012. Int J Cancer. 2015;136(5):E359–86.
3. Shah RB, Mehra R, Chinnaiyan AM, Shen R, Ghosh D, Zhou M, Macvicar GR, Varambally S, Harwood J, Bismar TA, et al. Androgen-independent prostate cancer is a heterogeneous group of diseases: lessons from a rapid autopsy program. Cancer Res. 2004;64(24):9209–16.
4. Izumi K, Namiki M. Optimal treatment for castration-resistant prostate cancer. Asian J Androl. 2014;16(3):498.
5. Scher HI, Sawyers CL. Biology of progressive, castration-resistant prostate cancer: directed therapies targeting the androgen-receptor signaling axis. J Clin Oncol. 2005;23(32):8253–61.
6. Isaacs W, De Marzo A, Nelson WG. Focus on prostate cancer. Cancer Cell. 2002;2(2):113–6.
7. Collazo J, Zhu B, Larkin S, Martin SK, Pu H, Horbinski C, Koochekpour S, Kyprianou N. Cofilin drives cell-invasive and metastatic responses to TGF-beta in prostate cancer. Cancer Res. 2014;74(8):2362–73.
8. Huang W, Guo W, You X, Pan Y, Dong Z, Jia G, Yang C, Chen Y. PAQR3 suppresses the proliferation, migration and tumorigenicity of human prostate cancer cells. Oncotarget. 2016;8:53948–58.
9. Barbieri CE, Baca SC, Lawrence MS, Demichelis F, Blattner M, Theurillat JP, White TA, Stojanov P, Van Allen E, Stransky N, et al. Exome sequencing identifies recurrent SPOP, FOXA1 and MED12 mutations in prostate cancer. Nat Genet. 2012;44(6):685–9.
10. Lagos-Quintana M, Rauhut R, Lendeckel W, Tuschl T. Identification of novel genes coding for small expressed RNAs. Science. 2001;294(5543):853–8.
11. Le XF, Merchant O, Bast RC, Calin GA. The roles of MicroRNAs in the cancer invasion-metastasis Cascade. Cancer Microenviron. 2010;3(1):137–47.
12. Ferracin M, Veronese A, Negrini M. Micromarkers: miRNAs in cancer diagnosis and prognosis. Expert Rev Mol Diagn. 2010;10(3):297–308.
13. Bartel DP. MicroRNAs: genomics, biogenesis, mechanism, and function. Cell. 2004;116(2):281–29.
14. Luu HN, Lin HY, Sorensen KD, Ogunwobi OO, Kumar N, Chornokur G, Phelan C, Jones D, Kidd L, Batra J, et al. miRNAs associated with prostate cancer risk and progression. BMC Urol. 2017;17(1):18.
15. Esquela-Kerscher A, Slack FJ. Oncomirs - microRNAs with a role in cancer. Nat Rev Cancer. 2006;6(4):259–69.
16. Croce CM. Causes and consequences of microRNA dysregulation in cancer. Nat Rev Genet. 2009;10(10):704–14.
17. Yaman Agaoglu F, Kovancilar M, Dizdar Y, Darendeliler E, Holdenrieder S, Dalay N, Gezer U. Investigation of miR-21, miR-141, and miR-221 in blood circulation of patients with prostate cancer. Tumour Biol. 2011;32(3):583–8.
18. Hatakeyama S, Yoneyama T, Tobisawa Y, Ohyama C. Recent progress and perspectives on prostate cancer biomarkers. Int J Clin Oncol. 2017;22(2):214–21.
19. Zhang J, Li H, Yu JP, Wang SE, Ren XB. Role of SOCS1 in tumor progression and therapeutic application. Int J Cancer. 2012;130(9):1971–80.
20. Xu Y, Wang W, Gou A, Li H, Tian Y, Yao M, Yang R. Effects of suppressor of cytokine signaling 1 silencing on human melanoma cell proliferation and interferon-gamma sensitivity. Mol Med Rep. 2015;11(1):583–8.
21. Coarfa C, Fiskus W, Eedunuri VK, Rajapakshe K, Foley C, Chew SA, Shah SS, et al. Comprehensive proteomic profiling identifies the androgen receptor axis and other signaling pathways as targets of microRNAs suppressed in metastatic prostate cancer. Oncogene. 2016;35(18):2345–56.
22. Li Z, Metze D, Nashan D, Muller-Tidow C, Serve HL, Poremba C, Luger TA, Bohm M. Expression of SOCS-1, suppressor of cytokine signalling-1, in human melanoma. J Invest Dermatol. 2004;123(4):737–45.

23. Zhou H, Miki R, Eeva M, Fike FM, Seligson D, Yang L, Yoshimura A, Teitell MA, Jamieson CA, Cacalano NA. Reciprocal regulation of SOCS 1 and SOCS3 enhances resistance to ionizing radiation in glioblastoma multiforme. Clin Cancer Res. 2007;13(8):2344–53.

24. Haraguchi T, Ozaki Y, Iba H. Vectors expressing efficient RNA decoys achieve the long-term suppression of specific microRNA activity in mammalian cells. Nucleic Acids Res. 2009;37(6):e43.

25. Yoshioka T, Otero J, Chen Y, Kim YM, Koutcher JA, Satagopan J, Reuter V, Carver B, de Stanchina E, Enomoto K, et al. beta4 integrin signaling induces expansion of prostate tumor progenitors. J Clin Invest. 2013;123(2):682–99.

26. Taichman RS, Cooper C, Keller ET, Pienta KJ, Taichman NS, McCauley LK. Use of the stromal cell-derived factor-1/CXCR4 pathway in prostate cancer metastasis to bone. Cancer Res. 2002;62(6):1832–7.

27. Mosmann T. Rapid colorimetric assay for cellular growth and survival: application to proliferation and cytotoxicity assays. J Immunol Methods. 1983;65(1–2):55–63.

28. Feng L, Xie X, Ding Q, Luo X, He J, Fan F, Liu W, Wang Z, Chen Y. Spatial regulation of Raf kinase signaling by RKTG. Proc Natl Acad Sci U S A. 2007;104(36):14348–53.

29. Taylor BS, Schultz N, Hieronymus H, Gopalan A, Xiao Y, Carver BS, et al. Integrative genomic profiling of human prostate cancer. Cancer Cell. 2010;18:11–22.

23

Supportive interventions to improve physiological and psychological health outcomes among patients undergoing cystectomy

Helen Quirk[1]* (iD), Derek J. Rosario[2] and Liam Bourke[3]

Abstract

Background: Our understanding of effective perioperative supportive interventions for patients undergoing cystectomy procedures and how these may affect short and long-term health outcomes is limited.

Methods: Randomised controlled trials involving any non-surgical, perioperative interventions designed to support or improve the patient experience for patients undergoing cystectomy procedures were reviewed. Comparison groups included those exposed to usual clinical care or standard procedure. Studies were excluded if they involved surgical procedure only, involved bowel preparation only or involved an alternative therapy such as aromatherapy. Any short and long-term outcomes reflecting the patient experience or related urological health outcomes were considered.

Results: Nineteen articles (representing 15 individual studies) were included for review. Heterogeneity in interventions and outcomes across studies meant meta-analyses were not possible. Participants were all patients with bladder cancer and interventions were delivered over different stages of the perioperative period. The overall quality of evidence and reporting was low and outcomes were predominantly measured in the short-term. However, the findings show potential for exercise therapy, pharmaceuticals, ERAS protocols, psychological/educational programmes, chewing gum and nutrition to benefit a broad range of physiological and psychological health outcomes.

Conclusions: Supportive interventions to date have taken many different forms with a range of potentially meaningful physiological and psychological health outcomes for cystectomy patients. Questions remain as to what magnitude of short-term health improvements would lead to clinically relevant changes in the overall patient experience of surgery and long-term recovery.

Keywords: Bladder cancer, Cystectomy, Supportive intervention, Systematic review

Background

Perioperative complications from cystectomy and urinary diversion can be short- and long-term, physiological and psychological [1]. Postoperative morbidity and complication rates can lead to long hospital stays [2] and high readmission rates [3]. Surviving patients can experience emotional, physical and social challenges and changes in quality of life (QOL) [1]. The range of perioperative complications associated with cystectomy procedures requires a multidisciplinary approach to preoperative supportive care and postoperative rehabilitation [4].

Perioperative interventions should support patients' psychological health as much as physical health [5]. The optimal perioperative supportive interventions for cystectomy patients and associated health outcomes are currently uncertain. Evidence-based interventions have traditionally been non-standardised but have evolved into clinical pathways of care known as enhanced recovery after surgery (ERAS) protocols. ERAS protocols involve a series of perioperative care modifications and supportive interventions with the aim to achieve early recovery by

* Correspondence: h.quirk@shu.ac.uk
[1]Centre for Sport and Exercise Science, Sheffield Hallam University, S10 2BP, Sheffield, UK
Full list of author information is available at the end of the article

maintaining preoperative organ function and reducing physiological stress response following surgery [6]. ERAS protocols after cystectomy have had a low adoption [7], yet have been found to shorten hospital stay [3] without an increase postoperative morbidity [8]. Our understanding of the active ingredients of such protocols and how these may affect the overall patient experience in the long-term is limited and previous comprehensive reviews have involved non-randomised observational studies only [9] . Further exploration of the available evidence using rigorous systematic review methodology is required to develop our understanding of how to promote clinically relevant health outcomes for cystectomy patients.

The aim of this review is to summarise the available evidence base for any supportive interventions designed to improve short and/or long-term physiological and psychological health outcomes among patients undergoing cystectomy. Reviewing the literature of the wide range of perioperative supportive interventions and their related health outcomes will advance our understanding of what works for patients undergoing cystectomy.

Methods

A systematic review of the literature was performed in January 2018. Records were identified from MEDLINE, AMED, PsycInfo and EMBASE databases and the Cochrane collaboration. The search was limited to studies involving adult humans and published in the English language and not limited by date of publication. Literature search terms are available as supplementary material (see Additional file 1). Further searches were made for unpublished and grey literature. The http://www.clinicaltrials.gov website was searched for ongoing trials. The citation lists of included studies and previous systematic reviews were also checked to identify relevant studies.

Randomised controlled trials (RCTs) involving any non-surgical, perioperative interventions designed to support or improve the patient experience, including lifestyle, physical, medical and psychological treatments were considered for review. The intention was not to assess the effects of different forms of surgical diversion. Studies were eligible if they involved adults ≥18 years who were due to undergo or had undergone a cystectomy procedure and any method of urinary diversion. Supportive interventions could be implemented during diagnosis and treatment planning, the perioperative period, and during the length of hospital stay, follow-up and postoperative period. Interventions could be hospital-based or home-based. Comparison groups included those exposed to usual clinical care or standard procedure. Studies were excluded if they did not involve an intervention, or the intervention involved a surgical procedure only, bowel preparation only or an alternative therapy such as aromatherapy. Any outcomes reflecting the patient experience or related urological health

outcomes were considered and could be physiological, psychological, behavioural and social.

Data collection and analysis
Selection of studies
Following de-duplication, titles and abstracts of identified records were screened by one reviewer (HQ) and 10% were selected at random and checked independently by a second reviewer (LB). The full texts of potentially eligible records were retrieved and screened independently by the two reviewers (HQ, LB). Multiple records of the same study were linked together in the process. The study selection process is described in the PRISMA flow diagram (Fig. 1).

Data extraction and management
The full text of each article was read by two reviewers independently (HQ, LB) and after piloting of extraction tables, relevant data were extracted. Any discrepancies in data extraction between the two reviewers were resolved by discussion. The authors of included studies were contacted via email for clarification of unclear study methods or data wherever insufficient details were reported.

Assessment of risk of bias in included studies
The risk of bias of each included study was assessed by two reviewers (HQ, LB) working independently using the recommended tool in the Cochrane Handbook for Systematic Reviews of Intervention [10]. Any disagreements were resolved by discussion.

Dealing with missing data
Missing data and dropout rates for each of the included studies were assessed. When possible, all data extracted were relevant to an intention-to-treat analysis, in which participants were analysed in the groups to which they were assigned.

Assessment of heterogeneity and sensitivity analyses
Statistical methods for assessing heterogeneity and sensitivity analyses were planned, depending on the availability of data.

Data synthesis and statistical analysis
Meta-analyses were planned for wherever there was more than one RCT reporting the same outcome. Where meta-analyses were not feasible, a narrative synthesis approach was used [11].

Results
The search identified 63 articles meeting the inclusion criteria for full text screening (Fig. 1). In all, 44 articles were excluded and the reasons recorded. The remaining

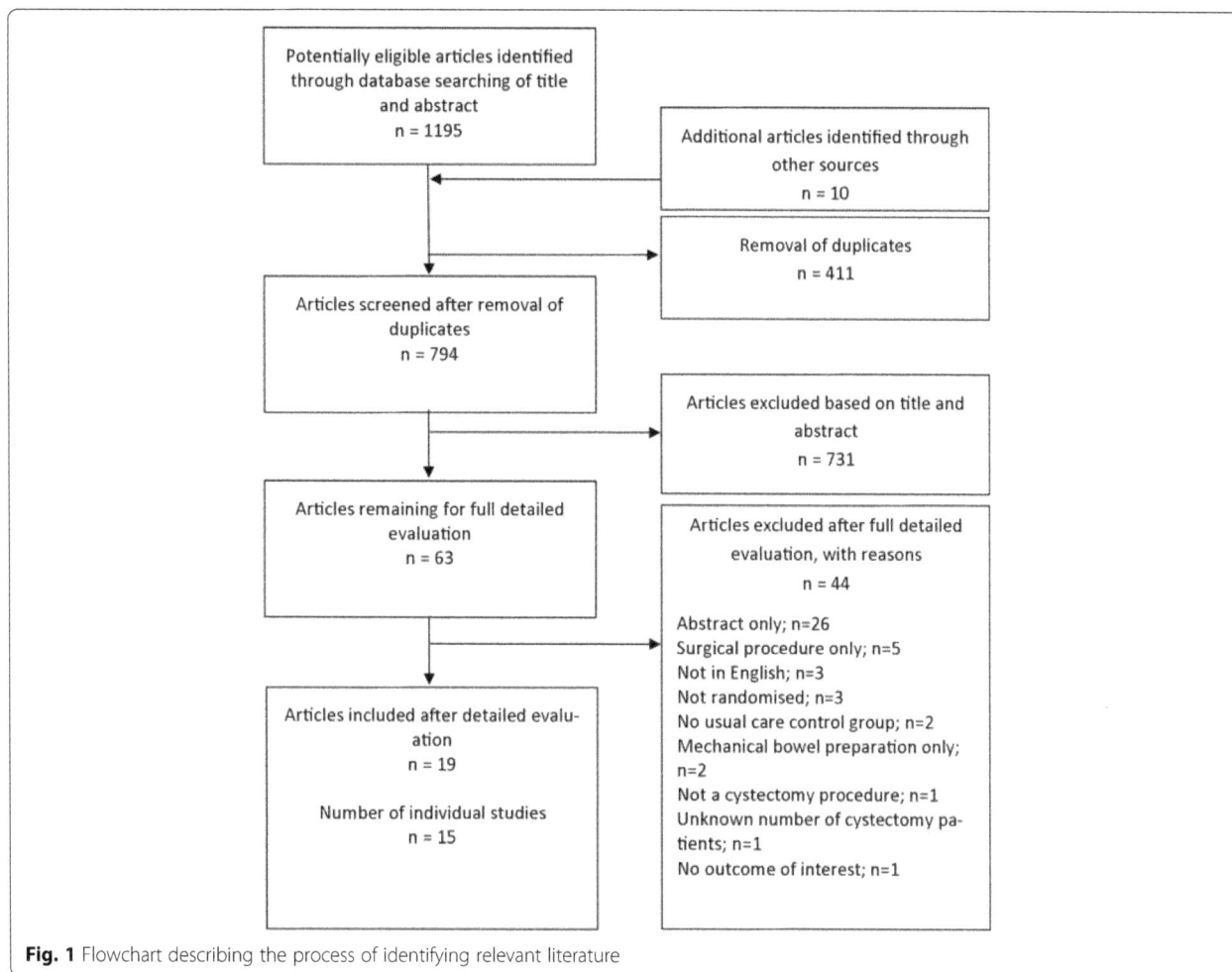

Fig. 1 Flowchart describing the process of identifying relevant literature

19 articles (representing 15 individual studies) were included in the review. Studies were published between 1989 [12] and 2017 [13–15] and were conducted in ten different countries; one was UK-based [14] (see Table 1).

Participants

Table 1 provides a summary of participant characteristics. All studies involved patients with bladder cancer undergoing radical cystectomy. Sample sizes ranged from 8 [15] to 280 [16], with a total of 1145 participants across all studies. The average age of participants ranged from 45.3 years (mean) [12] to 74.5 years (median) [15]. Most studies included both sexes, except two studies that included males only [15, 17]. Other patient characteristics, though not reported consistently included BMI, ethnicity, comorbidities, smoking history, and socio-economic data.

Interventions

See Table 2 for a summary of interventions included in this review.

Type

Intervention types included; exercise therapy [14, 18–21], pharmaceutical [16, 22, 23], ERAS protocol [17, 24, 25], psychological/educational [1, 12, 13, 15], chewing gum [26], and nutritional [27–29]. Interventions were delivered by exercise science staff [14], physiotherapists [18–21], Urological Enteral Stoma Therapy Nurses [13], trained nurse practitioners [15], hospital ward staff [27], and staff nurses [23], healthcare professionals [17] and study investigator [26]. Seven did not report who delivered the intervention [1, 12, 16, 22, 24, 25, 28]. Treatments to control group patients were determined by the standard procedure at the local hospital which may have involved some ERAS items [18–20, 25] and were not consistent across studies.

Recruitment and intervention setting

The majority of studies recruited participants via a single hospital urology department, two studies recruited across multiple centres [16, 28] and three did not report recruitment setting [1, 22, 24]. Intervention settings

Table 1 Summary of study details and participant characteristics

Reference and country	Sample size			Participant characteristics				Surgery procedure (as reported)	Urinary diversion type	Surgery type
	Total	INT	CONT	Age INT	Age CONT	Sex	Condition			
Ali et al., 1989 [12] Egypt	30	15	15	Mean 45.33 SD 5.9	Mean 45.86 SD 4.4	Male = 23 Female = 7	Bladder cancer	Urinary diversion	Not reported	Not reported
Banerjee et al., 2017 [14] UK	60	30	30	Mean 71.60 SD 6.80	Mean 72.5 SD 8.49	Male = 53 Female = 7	Bladder cancer	Radical cystectomy and urinary diversion	Not reported	Any surgical technique
Choi et al., 2011 [26] Korea	62	30	31	Mean 63.5 SD 4.5	Mean 64.5 SD 8.8	Not reported	Bladder cancer	Radical cystectomy and urinary diversion	Ileal conduit Orthotopic neobladder	Open and robot-assisted
Deibert et al., 2016 [28] USA	102	50	52	Not reported	Not reported	Male = 37 Female = 13	Bladder cancer	Radical cystectomy and urinary diversion	Ileal conduit Neobladder Pouch	Open and robot-assisted
Frees et al., 2017 [25] Canada	23	10	13	Mean 65.75 Range 49–86	Mean 70.40 Range 51–84	Male = 18 Female = 5	Bladder cancer	Radical cystectomy and urinary diversion	Ileal conduit Studer neobladder	Open and robot-assisted
Ghoneim & Hegazy, 2013 [22] Egypt	60	30	30	Mean 50.5 SD 11.2	Mean 49.4 SD 10.2	Male = 45 Female = 15	Bladder cancer	Radical cystectomy and urinary diversion	Not reported	Not reported
Jensen, Jensen et al., 2014, 2015, 2016, 2017 [13, 18–20] Denmark	107	65	64	Mean 68.5 SD 9.8	Mean 70.6 SD 9.2	Male = 79 Female = 28	Bladder cancer	Radical cystectomy	Ileal conduit Orthotopic neobladder Continent cutaneous reservoir	Open and robot-assisted
Karl et al., 2014 [24] Germany	101	62	39	Not reported	Not reported	Not reported	Bladder cancer	Radical cystectomy	Ileal conduit Orthotopic neobladder	Not reported
Lee et al., 2014 [16] USA	280	143	137	Mean 66 SD 10.9	Mean 64 SD 9.8	Male = 223 Female = 57	Bladder cancer	Radical cystectomy and urinary diversion	Orthotopic neobladder Continent cutaneous reservoir Noncontinent cutaneous reservoir	Open and robot-assisted
Månsson et al., 1997 [1] Sweden	57	24	26	Not reported	Not reported	Not reported	Bladder cancer	Radical cystectomy	Orthotopic neobladder	Not reported
Merandy et al., 2017 [15] USA	8	4	4	Median 74.5 IQR 73–81	Median 72 IQR 62–81.5	Male = 8 Female = 0	Bladder cancer	Radical cystectomy and urinary diversion	Orthotopic neobladder Incontinent conduit	Not reported
Mohamed et al., 2016 [23] Egypt	60	45 (15 per INT group)	15	Group 2 Mean 54.53 SD 8.56 Group 3 Mean 54.20 SD 10.65 Group 4 Mean 53.33 SD 10.0	Mean 47.80 SD 7.23	Male = 48 Female = 12	Bladder cancer	Radical cystectomy	Not reported	Not reported

Table 1 Summary of study details and participant characteristics *(Continued)*

Reference and country	Sample size			Participant characteristics			Condition	Surgery procedure (as reported)	Urinary diversion type	Surgery type
				Age		Sex				
	Total	INT	CONT	INT	CONT					
Olaru et al., 2015 [17] Romania	20	10	10	Median 62.5	Median 62.0	Male = 20 Female = 0	Bladder cancer	Radical cystectomy and ileal urinary diversion	Orthotopic neobladder Bricker diversion	Not reported
Porserud et al., 2014 [21] Sweden	18	9	9	Mean 72 SD 5	Mean 72 SD 4	Male = 14 Female = 4	Bladder cancer	Radical cystectomy and urinary diversion	Ileal conduit	Open
Roth et al., 2013 [27] Vidal et al., 2016 [29] Switzerland	157	74	83	Median 67 Range 34–80	Median 66 Range 30–86	Male = 106 Female = 51	Bladder cancer	Radical cystectomy, extended pelvic lymph node dissection, and ileal diversion	Ileal conduit Ileal orthotopic bladder substitute Catheterisable pouch	Not reported

CONT Control, *INT* Intervention, *SD* standard deviation

Table 2 Summary of intervention details and length of follow-up

Intervention type	Author and date	Recruitment and setting	Perioperative stage and delivery	Intervention content	Intervention time, duration, frequency	Length of follow-up
Exercise therapy	Banerjee et al., 2017 [14]	Patients recruited from a single hospital. Supervised intervention setting.	Preoperative intervention delivered by exercise science staff	Short-term preoperative vigorous intensity aerobic interval exercise on a cycle ergometer using the Borg Ratings of Perceived Exertion (RPE) Scale to control intensity. 5–10 warm up against light resistance (50 W), patients aimed to perform 6 × 5 min intervals to a target perceived exertion of 13–15 (somewhat hard to hard equating to 70–85% predicted max heart rate based on 220-age, with 2.5 min interpolated active rest intervals against light resistance (50 W). Instructed to maintain a steady pedalling cadence of 50–60 rev min-1 during intervals, and the exercise programme was progressed gradually adding more load to the flywheel to maintain the target perceived exertion. Followed by cool down against low resistance (50 W).	5–10 warm up.6 × 5 min intervals with 2.5 min interpolated active rest intervals. Twice weekly over preoperative period until surgery (3–6 weeks). Minimum of six sessions performed.	Until discharge
	Jensen, Jensen et al., 2014 [18] Jensen, Petersen et al., 2015 [20] Jensen, Laustsen et al., 2016 [19]	Patients recruited from a single hospital. Combined hospital and home-based intervention setting	Pre- and postoperative intervention delivered by physiotherapists	Preoperative standardised exercise training programme at home; step training on a step trainer and muscle strength and endurance exercises. Postoperative mobilisation and rehabilitation; instructions for getting out of bed, mobilisation and walking. Exercise-based rehabilitation in the hospital; respiratory and circulatory exercises, mobilisation, walking, supervised standardised progressive muscle strength and endurance training. Patients discharged with a home training exercise programme.	Preoperative 15 min step training and daily exercise programme consisting of six different exercises with individualised repetitions twice-daily. Postoperative mobilisation and exercise-based rehabilitation for 30 min twice-daily for the first seven postoperative days.	Day 35 and 4 months postoperatively
	Porserud et al., 2014 [21]	Patients recruited from a single hospital. Combined hospital and home-based intervention setting	Postoperative intervention delivered by physiotherapists	Postoperative group exercise training programme in the hospital; lower body strength and endurance training; walking and strengthening exercises, balance training, mobility training and stretching exercises. Music was used as inspiration. Participants were also instructed to take walks at a self-selected pace.	45 min twice a week for 12 weeks. Walks at a self-selected pace, 3–5 days a week for at least 15 min.	14 weeks and 1 year postoperatively

Table 2 Summary of intervention details and length of follow-up (Continued)

Intervention type	Author and date	Recruitment and setting	Perioperative stage and delivery	Intervention content	Intervention time, duration, frequency	Length of follow-up
Pharmaceutical	Ghoneim & Hegazy 2013 [22]	Recruitment setting not reported. Hospital based intervention	Preoperative intervention. Deliverer not reported	75 mg pregabalin orally.	2× day for 10 days prior to operation.	48 h postoperatively
	Lee et al., 2014 [16]	Patients recruited from multiple centres. Hospital based intervention	Pre- and postoperative intervention. Deliverer not reported	12 mg alvimopan before surgery and twice-daily doses postoperatively.	Single dose (12 mg) between 30 min and 5 h before surgery and twice-daily doses postoperatively until hospital discharge or a maximum of 7 days (15 in-hospital doses).	Until discharge and 30 days after discharge
	Mohamed et al., 2016 [23]	Patients recruited from single hospital. Hospital based intervention	Preoperative delivered by staff nurse	Group 2300 mg pregabalin orally 2 h preoperative Group 3300 mg pregabalin orally 2 h preoperative and 12 h thereafter Group 4600 mg pregabalin orally 2 h preoperative		24 h postoperatively
Fast-track/ERAS protocol	Frees et al., 2017 [25]	Patients recruited from single hospital. Hospital based intervention	Perioperative intervention. Deliverer not reported.	ERAS protocol (see original study for details).	Perioperative until discharge.	30 days postoperatively
	Karl et al., 2014 [24]	Recruitment setting not reported. Hospital based intervention	Perioperative intervention. Deliverer not reported	ERAS protocol (see original study for details).	Perioperative until discharge.	Day 3, day 7 postoperatively and until discharge
	Olaru et al., 2015 [17]	Patients recruited from a single hospital. Hospital based intervention	Perioperative intervention delivered by healthcare professionals	ERAS protocol (see original study for details).	Perioperative until discharge.	Until discharge
Psychological/ educational	Ali et al., 1989 [12]	Patients recruited from a single hospital. Hospital based intervention	Preoperative intervention. Deliverer not reported	Single, preoperative psychoeducational session provided to the patient and a significant other. Included explanation of the surgical procedure, site and appearance of stoma, device to be used postoperatively, reasons for wearing a collection device, and a visit from another "ostomate" who is functioning well. Patients encouraged to express fears and anxieties regarding social aspects of living with a stoma, including clothing, changes in body image, sexuality, exercise, activity, and odour.	1 × 30–60 min session.	Until discharge (approx. 12 days postoperatively)

Table 2 Summary of intervention details and length of follow-up *(Continued)*

Intervention type	Author and date	Recruitment and setting	Perioperative stage and delivery	Intervention content	Intervention time, duration, frequency	Length of follow-up
	Jensen, Kiesbye et al., 2017 [13]	Patients recruited from a single hospital. Combined hospital and home-based intervention setting	Pre- and postoperative intervention delivered by Urological Enteral Stoma Therapy Nurses	The education programme included basic skills to optimise the ability to perform independent stoma care. Patients encouraged to perform stoma care and change of appliance, both one-piece and two-piece system, at least twice at home providing them with training kits and appliances. The patient was educated about the urostomy and life with a urostomy related to the individual patient's life and life style. Every patient had a follow up prior to surgery where the Urological Enteral Stoma Therapy Nurse observed self-care skills regarding stoma care and change of appliance.	1 × education programme under supervision, 2 × practice at home, 1 × self-demonstration under observation prior to surgery.	Day 35 and 4 months and 12 months postoperatively
	Mansson et al, 1997 [1]	Recruitment setting not reported. Home based intervention	Postoperative intervention. Deliverer not reported	Psychosocial programme including weekly counselling, in the patient's home for 4 weeks, and thereafter by telephone. The discussion concerned consequences of the operation, practical and emotional problems, influences on mood and relations to partner and friends. The partner could be present at the interview.	Weekly counselling for 4 weeks then via telephone for 2 weeks.	3 months and 6 months postoperatively
	Merandy et al, 2017 [15]	Patients recruited from a single hospital. Hospital based intervention	Postoperative day 4, 5 or 6 delivered by trained nurse practitioners	Multimethod educational intervention was developed for each of the three different urinary diversions and included (a) a simplified medical illustration of participant-specific urinary diversion, (b) a step-by-step urinary diversion self-care instructional video, and (c) a pictorial Microsoft PowerPoint®. The content was driven by Bandura's (1977) four sources of self-efficacy and were based on first-hand observed difficulties experienced by patients with a urinary diversion. The video, PowerPoint, illustrations, and surveys were administered at the bedside by one of the investigators using a tablet computer. The intervention was enhanced by professional demonstration, followed by a chance for return demonstration.	1 × 1 h in duration, with an optional 30 min for participant questions	Immediately after intervention

Supportive interventions to improve physiological and psychological health outcomes among patients...

169

Table 2 Summary of intervention details and length of follow-up (*Continued*)

Intervention type	Author and date	Recruitment and setting	Perioperative stage and delivery	Intervention content	Intervention time, duration, frequency	Length of follow-up
Chewing gum	Choi et al., 2011 [26]	Patients recruited from a single hospital. Hospital based intervention	Postoperative intervention delivered by study investigators	Sugar-free chewing gum.	30 min chewing three times daily at 10 am, 3 pm and 8 pm until first flatus.	Discharge. Short term complications within 30 days
Nutritional	Deibert et al., 2016 [28]	Patients recruited from 2 hospital centres. Hospital based intervention.	Postoperative intervention. Deliverer not reported	Clear liquid diet on postoperative day 1 and access to a full regular diet from postoperative day 2 and beyond.	Postoperative until discharge	90 days postoperatively
	Roth et al., 2013 [27]	Patients recruited from a single hospital. Hospital based intervention	Postoperative intervention delivered by hospital ward staff	Total parenteral nutrition (TPN). Nutriflex special; a solution with a total energy of 1240 kcal/1000 ml and containing polyamino acids, glucose, and electrolytes. An additional 30 IU Actrapid HM and 1875 IU heparin per 24 h were added to the TPN solution.	Administered continuously for 5 days starting on postoperative day 1.	1, 3, 7, 12 days postoperatively and complications up to 30 days postoperatively
	Vidal et al., 2016 [29]					3, 6, 12, 18, 24, 30 and 36 months postoperatively

were hospital based [12, 15–17, 22–29], hospital and home based [13, 18–21], home-based [1] or supervised exercise setting [14].

Time, duration and frequency

Studies varied in time of intervention delivery; preoperative, postoperative or perioperative (see Table 2). Duration of intervention varied from 30 to 60 min for a single educational intervention [12, 15] to 12 weeks for the physical exercise intervention [21]. Six studies did not have standardised intervention duration; Banerjee et al.'s [14] exercise intervention took place preoperatively until surgery, Choi et al.'s [26] chewing gum intervention continued until first flatus, Deibert et al.'s [28] dietary intervention was postoperative until discharge, and those studies implementing ERAS protocols took place over the perioperative period until discharge [17, 24, 25]. Frequency of intervention administration differed depending on the intervention type (see Table 2).

Measurements

Methods of measuring outcomes varied across studies, making direct comparisons between studies difficult. Hospital records were used to measure length of stay (LOS) and readmission rate. Hospital measurements were used to assess functions such as bowel function and flatus, food tolerance and mobilisation. Complications were assessed using the standardised Clavien-Dindo classification system [14, 17, 20, 25–28] or via hospital reports. Symptoms (e.g., pain, fatigue, vomiting) tended to be self-reported using patient questionnaires. Three studies [18, 24, 25] used the validated European Organisation for Research and Treatment of Cancer (EORTC) [30] to assess quality of life (QOL) and in-patient satisfaction. Three studies used a visual analogue scale (VAS) to measure pain intensity [22, 23, 28], one study used Sickness Impact Profile (SIP) to measure sickness-related dysfunction and postoperative adjustment [1], two studies used the Short Form health survey (SF-36 and SF-12) to evaluate health-related QOL [21, 29], one used the Functional Assessment of Cancer Therapy- Bladder Cancer (FACT-BL) questionnaire to measure QOL [25] and one used the State-Trait Anxiety Inventory (STAI) to measure state anxiety [12]. Self-care was measured using the Urostomy Education Scale (UES) [13]. Self-efficacy was measured using the six-item Self-Efficacy to Manage Chronic Disease (SES6G) scale [15].

Outcome measurement (length of follow-up) tended to be short term (up to 30 days postoperatively) in the majority of articles reviewed ($n = 11$), and ranged between 24 h postoperatively [23] to a median of 50 months after surgery (IQR 21–62 months) [29] (See Table 2).

Effect of interventions

The outcomes used to measure the effect of interventions are summarised in Table 3. Differences in definitions and measurements of outcomes across studies meant that meta-analyses were not possible.

Length of stay and readmission

Length of stay (LOS) was reported in 11 articles [1, 14, 16, 17, 20, 21, 24–28]. The most common definition of LOS was total hospital stay duration in days. Two studies defined it as postoperative days (from surgery until discharge) [1, 16]. Median LOS ranged from 7 [14] to 21 days [1]. Frees et al. [25] and Lee et al. [16] found a significant difference in LOS between intervention and control groups. Frees et al. found LOS was significantly shorter in the patients receiving ERAS protocol compared to standard procedure (mean 6.1 days vs. 7.39 days; $p = 0.020$). Lee et al. found mean LOS was significantly shorter in patients given alvimopan compared to placebo controls (alvimopan, 7.44 days; control 10.07 days; $p < 0.01$).

Frequency of readmission to hospital after discharge was measured as an outcome in five studies [16, 20, 21, 25, 28]. No study reported significant results for readmission rates after supportive intervention compared to controls.

Physiological adjustment after surgery

Bowel function and flatus Nine studies measured bowel function [18, 20, 27, 28], also defined as time to first defecation or bowel movement [17, 25, 26], constipation [24] and lower gastrointestinal function [16]. Statistically significant reductions in average time until first bowel movement were found in four studies after the intervention; ERAS protocol [25], chewing gum [26], physical exercise [18] and alvimopan [16]. Time to first flatus was measured in five studies [17, 18, 25–27] and three found statistically significant reductions in time after ERAS protocol [25], chewing gum [26] and physical exercise [18]. Frees et al. [25] found significant reduction in time to first flatulence in the ERAS group compared to the standard procedure controls (2.5 days compared to 3.62 days) ($p = 0.011$).

Food tolerance Six studies measured food tolerance, defined at nutritional intake [20], appetite loss [24], gastrointestinal recovery/tolerance of solid food [16], early feeding [17] and resumption of full diet [27]. Deibert et al. [28] found time to full diet tolerance was the same in both early diet and control arms, respectively (5.84 days vs 6.71 days, $p = 0.27$). Lee et al. [16] found mean time to gastrointestinal recovery was 1.3 days shorter for the alvimopan group (5.5 days) compared with

Table 3 Summary of outcomes measured and statistically significant findings

			LOS & readmission		Physiological outcomes													Psychological outcomes							
	Intervention	Date	LOS	Readmission	Bowel function/Defecation	Appetite / food tolerance	Pain	Flatus	Nausea and vomiting	Physical function	Mobilisation	Strength/power	Dyspnea	Insomnia	Fatigue	Sexual function	Balance	HRQOL	Social functioning	Emotional functioning	Self-care	Self-efficacy	Vitality	Mental Health	Anxiety
Exercise therapy	Banerjee et al.	2017	•									**													
	Jensen et al.	2014			**		•	**	•	•			**	**	•	•		•	•	•					
	Jensen et al.	2015	•	•	•	•					**												**		
	Jensen et al.	2016										**													
	Porserud et al.	2014	•	•			•			•	**	•					•	•	•	•					
Pharmaceutical	Ghoneim & Hegazy	2013					**		•																
	Lee et al.	2014	**	•	**	**																			
	Mohamed et al.	2016					**																		
Fast-track/ERAS protocol	Frees et al.	2017	**	•	**		**	**	•									•	•	•					
	Karl et al.	2014	•		•	**	•		•	**	**		•	•	**			•	•	**					
	Olaru et al.	2015	•		•	•		•																	
Psychological / educational	Ali et al.	1989																							**
	Jensen et al.	2017																			**	•			
	Mansson et al.	1997	•																		•	•			
	Merandy et al.	2017																			•			•	
Chewing gum	Choi et al.	2010	•		**			**																	
Nutritional	Deibert et al.	2016	•	•	•	**																			
	Roth et al.	2013	•		•	•		•																	
	Vidal et al.	2016														•		•							
Total studies measuring that outcome			11	5	9	6	6	5	4	3	3	3	2	2	2	2	1	5	4	4	3	2	1	1	1

	Not measured		•	Measured and not statistically significant	**	Measured and statistically significant

the placebo control group (6.8 days; 95% CI, 1.4 to 2.3; $p < 0.0001$). Karl et al. [24] found that the amount of food consumed in relation to the amount of food offered on postoperative day 3 was significantly higher in the ERAS group compared to standard procedure controls ($p = 0.02$).

Nausea and vomiting Four studies measured vomiting [22], nausea [25] or both [18, 24] and none reported any significant differences between intervention and control groups after the intervention.

Pain Six studies measured pain [18, 21–25]. Three studies reported statistically significant pain outcomes. Ghoneim and Hegazy [22] found VAS score to be significantly lower postoperatively until 32 h in the intervention group receiving preoperative pregabalin compared to the control group ($p < 0.05$), but found no significant difference 32–48 h postoperatively. Mohamed et al. [23] found a significant reduction in VAS score in intervention groups who received preoperative pregabalin in comparison with the control group immediately after surgery, and 2 h postoperatively ($p < 0.05$). Frees et al. [25] found ERAS patients reported a reduction in VAS score every day after surgery until day 7 compared to patients undergoing

standard procedure. This difference reached statistical significance on the day of surgery ($p = 0.017$) and from postoperative days 2 ($p = 0.014$) to 4 ($p = 0.039$), where pain intensity was nearly doubled for patients who received standard procedure.

Fatigue Two studies measured fatigue using the EORTC symptom scale [18, 24]. Jensen et al. [18] found the control group (no physical exercise intervention) demonstrated a clinically relevant reduction in fatigue symptoms at 4 months follow-up that was not statistically significant. Karl et al. [24] reported significant differences in fatigue scores between the ERAS and control group at day 7 ($p = 0.014$) and discharge ($p = 0.003$), but did not report the group data.

Mobilisation, strength/power and balance Three studies measured mobilisation [20, 21, 24], defined as the distance walked during the first seven postoperative days [20], mobilisation and walking distance [24] and distance walked in the 6 min walk test [21]. Jensen et al. [20] reported significantly longer average walking distance in the intervention group after the physical exercise intervention (4806 m walked; 95% CI, 4075 to 5536 m), compared to the control group (2906 m walked; 95% CI, 2408 to 3404 m; $p < 0.001$). Karl et al. [24] reported that patients in the ERAS group covered significantly greater walking distances by postoperative day 3 compared to controls ($p = 0.039$). Porserud et al. [20, 21] found that after the 12 week exercise training period, both the intervention and the control group patients had increased the distance walked ($p = 0.043$ and $p = 0.012$, respectively), but the increase was higher among the intervention group ($p = 0.013$) who had exercised postoperatively. One year later, the exercise group continued to have increased walking distance compared to controls ($p = 0.010$).

The three studies using exercise therapy measured strength or power. Jensen et al. [19] measured strength as muscle leg power (W/kg) using a leg extensor power test and found that the prehabilitation physical exercise programme led to a significant improvement in muscle power in the intervention group of 0.35 W/kg (95% CI, 0.12 to 0.54) at time for surgery compared to baseline ($p < 0.002$) with a significant difference between intervention and control group. Banerjee et al. [14] implemented a short-term preoperative vigorous intensity aerobic interval exercise programme on a cycle ergometer and showed that after 3–6 weeks of training, statistically significant differences in peak power output (W) were found between the exercise group (148 ± 41; 95% CI, 132 to 165) compared to non-exercising controls (129 ± 44; 95% CI, 111 to 147; $p < 0.001$) [14]. Porserud et al. [21] measured lower body strength using a 30-s chair stand test and found no significant differences between the intervention and control group. Porserud et al. also measured balance by asking patients to walk two laps in a figure of eight drawn on the floor, with a walking aid if necessary and found no significant differences between intervention and control group post-intervention or 1 year later [20].

Physical function Three studies measured physical function, two using the EORTC-QLQ-30 [18, 24] and one using the SF-36 [21]. No statistical differences were found, except for Karl et al.'s [24] study, which found statistically higher physical functioning scores on postoperative day 3 for patients in the ERAS group.

Dyspnoea Dyspnoea was measured in two studies using the EORTC-QLQ-30 [18, 24]. Jensen et al. [18] found a 10% significant decrease in symptoms of dyspnoea in the intervention group (physical exercise rehabilitation) compared with the control group at 4 month follow-up. Karl et al. [24] reported no significant differences between intervention and control group after the ERAS protocol.

Insomnia Insomnia was measured in two studies using the EORTC-QLQ-30 [18, 24] and no significant differences between intervention and control groups were found after the intervention.

Sexual function Two studies measured sexual function [18, 29]. Jensen et al. [18] found an improvement of 7% in sexual interest and activity in the control group 4 months after the intervention, which they described as clinically relevant though it was not statistically significant. Vidal et al. [29] measured sexual function as a long-term follow-up to the TPN nutritional intervention described by Roth et al. [27] and found no statistically significant differences between intervention and control group at 0, 3, 12 and 24 month follow-ups.

Psychological adjustment after surgery

Social and emotional functioning Four studies measured social and emotional functioning using EORTC-QLQ-30 [18, 24], the SF-36 [21] and the SIP questionnaire [1]. No study found statistically significant differences between intervention and control groups after the intervention except Karl et al. [24] who found a stable emotional functioning score during hospitalisation in the control group and continuous improvement in emotional functioning until discharge in patients exposed to the ERAS protocol (no data reported) [24].

Health related quality of life Five studies measured QOL, one using the FACT-BL [25], two using global health-related QOL from the EORTC-QLQ-30 and functional subscales [18, 24] and two using the SF-12 or 36 [21, 29]. Porserud et al. [21] found no statistically significant differences between intervention and control group in the QOL domains. Jensen et al. [18] found the physical rehabilitation intervention group demonstrated a clinically relevant decrease compared to the control group on role function and cognitive function at the 4 month follow-up, although differences were not statistically significant. Frees et al. [25] and Vidal et al. [29] found no statistically significant differences between intervention and control groups in QOL scores.

Self-care and self-efficacy Three studies measured self-care [13, 15, 20] and two measured self-efficacy [13, 15] as outcomes of the intervention. Jensen et al. [20] found the ability to independently perform personal activities of daily living was significantly reduced by 1 day in the intervention group after pre-and postoperative physical exercise intervention compared to controls (3 days vs 4 days; $p \leq 0.05$). Jensen et al. [13] found no statistical significant difference ($p = 0.35$) in mean self-efficacy score between treatment groups on admission to surgery. However, a significant increase in the total stoma self-care score of 2.7 points (95% CI, 0.9 to 4.5) was found in the intervention group compared to the standard procedure group at postoperative day 35, and differences continued at day 120 (4.3 95% CI, 2.1 to 6.5) and 365 (5.1 95% CI, 2.3 to 7.8). Merandy et al. [15] found that the single preoperative educational intervention was not associated with self-care independence scores ($p = 0.4286$) and brought about no significant change in self-care or self-efficacy scores.

Other outcomes Other outcome measures explored in isolation included vitality and mental health [21] and anxiety [12]. Porserud et al. [21] found no significant differences between intervention and control group in vitality and mental health scores as measured by the SF-36. Ali and Khalil [12] found patients who received psychoeducational preparation prior to surgery showed less state anxiety on the third day postoperatively than the control group ($p < 0.00$ [sic]) and before discharge ($p < 0.00$ [sic]) compared to controls. Through a qualitative analysis, Ali and Khalil [12] also found that patients fears and worries before surgery concerned i) cancer, ii) mutilation and body image distortion, and iii) impact on social/marital relationships.

Complications

Eleven studies reported complications associated with the surgical procedures, seven using the standardised Clavien-Dindo classification system [14, 17, 20, 25–28] (See Additional file 2). Generally, interventions were not found to substantially increase the normal complication rate, with the exception of one study that was terminated prematurely due to high gastrointestinal complications in patients exposed to total parenteral nutrition (TPN) for 5 days postoperatively [27].

Adherence and fidelity

Adherence to the intervention was reported in eight articles. Table 4 gives a summary of the adherence reported in each of the articles under review. Eleven articles did not report adherence to the intervention. Fidelity of the intervention delivery was not reported in any article.

Risk of bias

Figure 2 shows the risk of bias summary table for the studies included. The standard of reporting was generally low, with many articles omitting Consolidated Standards of Reporting Trials (CONSORT) details [31]. Low reporting quality meant the majority of studies were judged to have unclear risk of bias on at least one domain. All studies were described as having randomised designs, but only ten articles reported the randomisation procedure (e.g., web-based block randomisation [18]). In

eight articles, it was unclear how participants were randomised. One study was described as randomised but did not describe a true randomisation procedure, therefore considered high risk of bias [15]. Seven studies were rated low risk for 'selection bias', because they referred to allocation concealment in their reporting of the randomisation procedure [13, 18–21, 23]. Studies tended to be rated as unclear or high risk for 'performance bias' and 'detection bias' because it was unclear whether patients, study personnel or outcome assessors were blind to the treatment group. Double-blind RCTs are difficult, if not impossible for many non-pharmaceutical intervention studies, exposing most of the studies to performance bias. Two studies included in the review were described as double-blind [16, 23]. All studies were judged to be at high risk of some 'other bias'. This included, use of a single centre [12], different surgical and treatment procedures across different sites [16], LOS being influenced by hospital discharge rules (rather than health outcomes) [26], small sample sizes [1, 12, 17, 21, 22, 26], change over time in surgical procedure [18–20], intervention and control group patients being treated on the same hospital ward [18–20], use of male patients only [17], not recruiting the target sample size [21, 28] and premature termination of the study [27, 29].

Heterogeneity and sensitivity analyses

Differences in the included studies, particularly in types of interventions, definitions of outcomes and tools used to measure outcomes meant sensitivity analyses could not be conducted and heterogeneity could not be assessed statistically.

Discussion

Supportive interventions for cystectomy patients have included exercise therapy, pharmaceuticals, ERAS protocols, psychological/educational programmes, chewing gum and nutrition delivered at various stages over the perioperative period. It is difficult to make clear recommendations for clinical practice, especially for potential long-term benefits to patient health, but this review can offer suggestions for potential short-term benefits of interventions.

Review findings suggest that integrating exercise therapy into the pre- or postoperative care of cystectomy patients could have clinically important benefits for bowel function, physical function, strength/power, mobilisation and QOL but is not always feasible for patients. The findings align with other reviews demonstrating the positive effects of exercise for bladder cancer patients [32]. Exercise can be challenging for cancer patients and requires careful consideration with respect to patient age and comorbidities [18, 33]. Research exploring the optimal type of exercise therapy would be informative, as intensive exercise

Table 4 Adherence to the intervention

Paper	Adherence
Ali et al., 1989 [12]	Not reported
Banerjee et al., 2017 [14]	The median number of supervised exercise sessions attended by patients in the exercise arm was 8 (range 1–10) over a preoperative period of 3–6 weeks. The average number of aerobic intervals achieved in the first week of exercise was 5.5 (range 3.5–6.0), whereas all patients were achieving six intervals per session in the fourth week.
Choi et al., 2011 [26]	Not reported
Deibert et al. 2016 [28]	Not reported
Frees et al., 2017 [25]	Not reported
Ghoneim & Hegazy, 2013 [22]	100% adherence to pregabalin
Jensen et al., 2014 [18]	A total of 66% (95% confidence interval (CI) 51; 78) adhered more than 75% of the recommended progressive standardised exercise program.
Jensen et al., 2016 [19]	A total of 66% (95% confidence interval (CI) 51; 78) adhered more than 75% of the recommended progressive standardised exercise program.
Jensen et al., 2015 [20]	A total of 66% (95% confidence interval (CI) 51; 78) adhered more than 75% of the recommended progressive standardised exercise program.
Jensen et al., 2017 [13]	Not reported
Karl et al., 2014 [24]	Not reported
Lee et al., 2014 [16]	119 out of 143 (83%) patients completed the alvimopan
Mansson et al., 1997 [1]	Not reported
Merandy et al., 2017 [15]	Not reported
Mohamed et al., 2016 [23]	Not reported
Olaru et al., 2015 [17]	Counselling and education was implemented in 90% of patients
Porserud et al., 2014 [21]	Participants attended a median of 76% (range 67–95%) of the group exercise training sessions and patients self-reported daily walks on 87% (56–100%) of the days during the 12-week period, averaging 3.5 h (2–11.5%) per week
Roth et al., 2013 [27]	Not reported
Vidal et al., 2016 [29]	Not reported

may not always be appropriate [21] or accessible [14] for patients undergoing cystectomy.

Cystectomy patients may benefit from pharmaceutical intervention for pain relief and physical function in the immediate postoperative period, which is likely to have a positive impact on length of hospital stay, QOL, the patient experience and healthcare costs. However, the effect on pain management might be short-lived and side-effects such as the sedative effect of pregabalin should be considered [22, 23].

Only three of the included studies used ERAS protocols [17, 24, 25], supporting the observation that the adoption of ERAS protocols in urological procedures to date has been low [6]. The findings suggest that ERAS protocols have the potential to offer widest range of benefits for cystectomy patients. However, it is hard to identify what actually works within each context and the quality and quantity of the evidence needs improvement. Tyson and Chang [9] systematically reviewed 13 studies comparing ERAS after cystectomy versus standard care with a meta-analysis of effectiveness. ERAS

protocols were investigated within observational studies only and were found to reduce the LOS, time-to-bowel function, and rate of complications after cystectomy, but the pooled estimates were biased in favour of ERAS and each perioperative pathway was different within each study [9]. If ERAS protocols are to be adopted, then high-quality multicentre studies are needed to accumulate evidence supporting the short and long-term impact of their use.

The findings demonstrate that psychologically-supportive and educational interventions are less common than physical or medical interventions, but could reduce postoperative anxiety and promote postoperative adjustment, self-care and coping in cystectomy patients. Such outcomes are likely to benefit QOL and positive adjustments with clinical relevance [13], but are likely to require a longer and more individualised approach than those implemented in the studies included in this review. The findings are consistent with a previous systematic review of exercise and psychosocial rehabilitation interventions to improve health-related

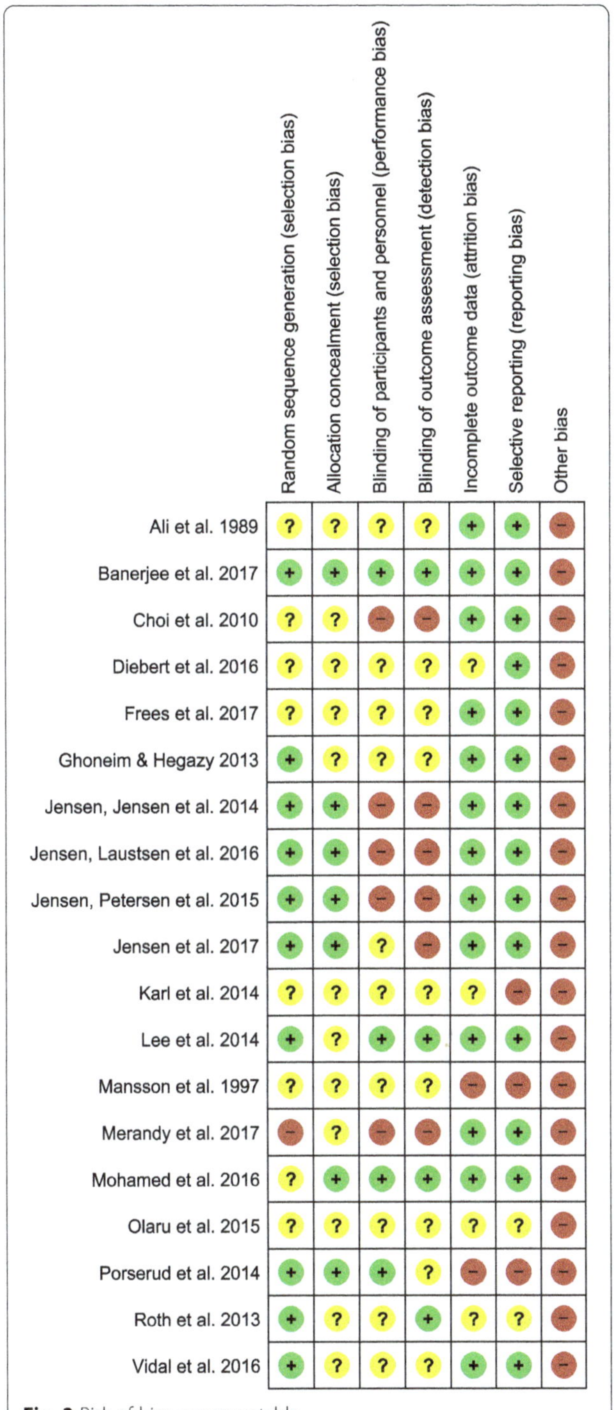

	Random sequence generation (selection bias)	Allocation concealment (selection bias)	Blinding of participants and personnel (performance bias)	Blinding of outcome assessment (detection bias)	Incomplete outcome data (attrition bias)	Selective reporting (reporting bias)	Other bias
Ali et al. 1989	?	?	?	?	+	+	-
Banerjee et al. 2017	+	+	+	+	+	+	-
Choi et al. 2010	?	?	-	-	+	+	-
Diebert et al. 2016	?	?	?	?	?	+	-
Frees et al. 2017	?	?	?	?	+	+	-
Ghoneim & Hegazy 2013	+	?	?	?	+	+	-
Jensen, Jensen et al. 2014	+	+	-	-	+	+	-
Jensen, Laustsen et al. 2016	+	+	-	-	+	+	-
Jensen, Petersen et al. 2015	+	+	-	-	+	+	-
Jensen et al. 2017	+	+	?	-	+	+	-
Karl et al. 2014	?	?	?	?	?	-	-
Lee et al. 2014	+	?	+	+	+	+	-
Mansson et al. 1997	?	?	?	?	-	-	-
Merandy et al. 2017	-	?	-	-	+	+	-
Mohamed et al. 2016	?	+	+	+	+	+	-
Olaru et al. 2015	?	?	?	?	?	?	-
Porserud et al. 2014	+	+	+	?	-	-	-
Roth et al. 2013	+	?	?	+	?	?	-
Vidal et al. 2016	+	?	?	?	+	+	-

Fig. 2 Risk of bias summary table

outcomes in patients with bladder cancer undergoing radical cystectomy, which found limited evidence for beneficial effects of psychosocial interventions [32]. Given that poor preoperative mental health has been associated with complications after cystectomy [34] and postoperative problems can have a significant impact on QOL [5], assessing perioperative psychological health status could help identify those patients who may be in need of extra support. Further research is required to explore the best approach to provision of psychological support for patients to ensure that patients are not only surviving, but surviving well.

Asking cystectomy patients to chew gum postoperatively may have benefits for bowel function and is unlikely to have any adverse effects. The early introduction of diet was feasible and safe, but TPN was associated with an increased rate of infectious complications, impaired bowel function, as well as higher costs [27].

Some level of bias was present in all studies included in this review, with most of the uncertainty in judging bias coming from lack of clarity of randomisation and blinding procedures. Methodological details were underreported and future publications should adequately report high quality research. No study reported fidelity of intervention delivery meaning it was unclear whether the treatment was delivered as intended. Additionally, the surgical procedure, including form of urinary diversion to control group patients varied across studies (see Table 1), introducing potentially confounding factors. This makes it difficult to show whether any health benefits were related to the supportive intervention or to determine the optimal 'dosage' or exposure to the intervention required to bring about health benefits. Many of the studies lacked statistical power due to small sample sizes meaning statistical significance should be interpreted with caution.

Recommendations for future research

Implications for clinical practice have been difficult to make, suggesting that future research should explore the clinical relevance of the outcomes found in research studies. Maintenance data through longer follow-ups are essential to explore i) long-term complications and readmissions and ii) whether short-term health outcomes are sustained over time. Adequately powered clinical trials are required to explore the long-term effects of physical prehabilitation and rehabilitation for cystectomy survivors. More research exploring psychologically-supportive interventions would be informative because the current findings highlight that psychological and behavioural outcomes (e.g., self-care behaviour and behaviour change) are scarcely studied and poorly understood. Standards of reporting must be improved, including details of fidelity and adherence.

Conclusions

This review provides a broad overview of the non-surgical supportive interventions available to help optimise the health outcomes of patients undergoing cystectomy procedures. It has shown that supportive interventions have taken many different forms with a range of potentially meaningful physiological and psychological health outcomes for patients in the short and long term after surgery. Questions remain as to what magnitude of improvements in the physiological and psychological health outcomes reported would lead to actual changes in the patient experience of surgery and recovery. Whilst this review can offer suggestions for potential benefits of interventions, clarification is required to understand what forms of support are most effective in improving the long-term quality of life of cystectomy patients.

Abbreviations
CONSORT: Consolidated Standards of Reporting Trials; EORTC-QLQ-30: European Organisation for Research and Treatment of Cancer - Quality of life of cancer patients; ERAS: Enhanced recovery after survey; FACT-BL: Functional Assessment of Cancer Therapy- Bladder Cancer; LOS: Length of stay; QOL: Quality of life; RCT: Randomised controlled trial; SES6G: Self-Efficacy to Manage Chronic Disease scale; SF-36 and SF-12: Short Form health survey; SIP: Sickness Impact Profile; STAI: State-Trait Anxiety Inventory; UES: Urostomy Education Scale; VAS: Visual analogue scale

Funding
The review was funded by the Urostomy Association. The Urostomy Association commissioned researchers to conduct the review and had no role in the design, collection, analysis, or interpretation of data or writing of this manuscript.

Authors' contributions
LB obtained funding and made substantial contributions to the conception of the review. HQ and LB contributed to the literature search, screening, data extraction and analysis of the data. DR and LB made substantial contributions to the interpretation of data and critical revision of the manuscript for important intellectual content. HQ drafted the manuscript and all authors have read, contributed to and approved the final version.

Competing interests
The authors declare that they have no competing interests.

Author details
[1]Centre for Sport and Exercise Science, Sheffield Hallam University, S10 2BP, Sheffield, UK. [2]Department of Oncology, University of Sheffield, Sheffield, UK. [3]Faculty of Health and Wellbeing, Sheffield Hallam University, Sheffield, UK.

References
1. Månsson Å, Colleen S, Hermeren G, Johnson G. Which patients will benefit from psychosocial intervention after cystectomy for bladder cancer? Br J Urol. 1997;80(1):50–7.
2. Baumgartner RG, Wells N, Chang SS, Cookson MS, Smith JA Jr. Causes of increased length of stay following radical cystectomy. Urol Nurs. 2002;22(5):319.
3. Altobelli E, Buscarini M, Gill HS, Skinner EC. Readmission Rate and Causes at 90-Day after Radical Cystectomy in Patients on Early Recovery after Surgery Protocol. Bladder Cancer. 2017;3(1):51–6.
4. Kehlet H. Multimodal approach to control postoperative pathophysiology and rehabilitation. Br J Anaesth. 1997;78(5):606–17.
5. Palapattu GS, Haisfield-Wolfe ME, Walker JM, Brintzenhofeszoc K, Trock B, Zabora J, Schoenberg M. Assessment of perioperative psychological distress in patients undergoing radical cystectomy for bladder cancer. J Urol. 2004; 172(5):1814 7.
6. Azhar RA, Bochner B, Catto J, Goh AC, Kelly J, Patel HD, Pruthi RS, Thalmann GN, Desai M. Enhanced recovery after urological surgery: a contemporary systematic review of outcomes, key elements, and research needs. Eur Urol. 2016;70(1):176–87.
7. Cerantola Y, Valerio M, Persson B, Jichlinski P, Ljungqvist O, Hubner M, Kassouf W, Muller S, Baldini G, Carli F. Guidelines for perioperative care after radical cystectomy for bladder cancer: Enhanced Recovery After Surgery (ERAS®) society recommendations. Clin Nutr. 2013;32(6):879–87.
8. Daneshmand S, Ahmadi H, Schuckman AK, Mitra AP, Cai J, Miranda G, Djaladat H. Enhanced recovery protocol after radical cystectomy for bladder cancer. J Urol. 2014;192(1):50–6.
9. Tyson MD, Chang SS. Enhanced Recovery Pathways Versus Standard Care After Cystectomy: A Meta-analysis of the Effect on Perioperative Outcomes. Eur Urol. 2016;70(6):995–1003.
10. Higgins J, Green S. Cochrane handbook for systematic reviews of interventions In., vol. Version 5.1.0 [updated March 2011]: The Cochrane Collaboration; 2011: Available from http://handbook.cochrane.org.
11. Popay J, Roberts H, Sowden A, Petticrew M, Arai L, Rodgers M, Britten N: Guidance on the conduct of narrative synthesis in systematic reviews: A product from the ESRC Methods Programme. In., vol. Version 1. Lancaster University, Lancaster; 2006: b92.
12. Ali NS, Khalil HZ. Effect of psychoeducational intervention on anxiety among Egyptian bladder cancer patients. Cancer Nurs. 1989;12(4):236–42.
13. Jensen B, Sondergaard I, Kiesbye B, Jensen J, Kristensen S. Efficacy of preoperative uro-stoma-education on self-efficacy after radical cystectomy; Secondary outcome from a prospective randomized controlled trial. Eur J Oncol Nurs. 2017;28:41–6.
14. Banerjee S, Manley K, Shaw B, Lewis L, Cucato G, Mills R, Rochester M, Clark A, Saxton JM. Vigorous intensity aerobic interval exercise in bladder cancer patients prior to radical cystectomy: a feasibility randomised controlled trial. Support Care Cancer. 2017;26(5):1515–23.
15. Merandy K, Morgan MA, Lee R, Scherr DS. Improving self-efficacy and self-care in adult patients with a urinary diversion: A pilot study. Oncol Nurs Forum. 2017;44(3):e90–e100.
16. Lee CT, Chang SS, Kamat AM, Amiel G, Beard TL, Fergany A, Karnes RJ, Kurz A, Menon V, Sexton WJ, et al. Alvimopan accelerates gastrointestinal recovery after radical cystectomy: a multicenter randomized placebo-controlled trial. Eur Urol. 2014;66(2):265–72.
17. Olaru V, Gingu C, Baston C, Manea I, Domnisor L, Preda A, Voinea S, Stefan B, Dudu C, Sinescu I. Applying fast-track protocols in bladder cancer patients undergoing radical cystectomy with ileal urinary diversions-early results of a prospective randomized controlled single center study. Rom J Urol. 2015;14(4):58.
18. Jensen BT, Jensen JB, Laustsen S, Petersen AK, Søndergaard I, Borre M. Multidisciplinary rehabilitation can impact on health-related quality of life outcome in radical cystectomy: secondary reported outcome of a randomized controlled trial. J Multidiscip Healthc. 2014;7:301.
19. Jensen B, Laustsen S, Jensen J, Borre M, Petersen A. Exercise-based prehabilitation is feasible and effective in radical cystectomy pathways-secondary results from a randomized controlled trial. J Urol. 2016;195:e652.
20. Jensen B, Petersen A, Jensen J, Laustsen S, Borre M. Efficacy of a multiprofessional rehabilitation programme in radical cystectomy pathways: a prospective randomized controlled trial. Scand J Urol. 2015;49:133–41.
21. Porserud A, Sherif A, Tollbäck A. The effects of a physical exercise programme after radical cystectomy for urinary bladder cancer. A pilot randomized controlled trial. Clin Rehabil. 2014;28(5):451–9.
22. Ghoneim AA, Hegazy MM. The analgesic effect of preoperative pregabalin in radical cystectomy for cancer bladder patients. Chinese-German J Clin Oncol. 2013;12(3):113–7.
23. Mohamed MA, Othman AH, Abd El-Rahman AM. Analgesic efficacy and safety of peri-operative pregabalin following radical cystectomy: A dose grading study. Egypt J Anaesth. 2016;32(4):513–7.
24. Karl A, Buchner A, Becker A, Staehler M, Seitz M, Khoder W, Schneevoigt B, Weninger E, Rittler P, Grimm T. A new concept for early recovery after surgery for patients undergoing radical cystectomy for bladder cancer: results of a prospective randomized study. J Urol. 2014;191(2):335–40.
25. Frees S, Aning J, Black P, Struss W, Bell R, Gleave M, So A. A prospective randomized single-centre trial evaluating an ERAS protocol versus a standard protocol for patients treated with radical cystectomy and urinary diversion for bladder cancer. Eur Urol Suppl. 2017;16(3):e1024.

26. Choi H, Kang SH, Yoon DK, Kang SG, Ko HY, Moon DG, Park JY, Joo KJ, Cheon J. Chewing gum has a stimulatory effect on bowel motility in patients after open or robotic radical cystectomy for bladder cancer: a prospective randomized comparative study. Urology. 2011;77(4):884–90.

27. Roth B, Birkhäuser FD, Zehnder P, Thalmann GN, Huwyler M, Burkhard FC, Studer UE. Parenteral nutrition does not improve postoperative recovery from radical cystectomy: results of a prospective randomised trial. Eur Urol. 2013;63(3):475–82.

28. Deibert CM, Silva MV, RoyChoudhury A, McKiernan JM, Scherr DS, Seres D, Benson MC. A Prospective Randomized Trial of the Effects of Early Enteral Feeding After Radical Cystectomy. Urology. 2016;96:69–73.

29. Vidal Faune A, Arnold N, Vartolomei M, Kiss B, Burkhard FC, Thalmann GN, Roth B. Does postoperative parenteral nutrition after radical cystectomy impact oncological and functional outcomes in bladder cancer patients? European Urology. Supplements. 2016;15(3):e515.

30. Sprangers M, Cull A, Groenvold M, Bjordal K, Blazeby J, Aaronson NK. The European Organization for Research and Treatment of Cancer approach to developing questionnaire modules: an update and overview. Qual Life Res. 1998;7(4):291–300.

31. Begg C, Cho M, Eastwood S, Horton R, Moher D, Olkin I, Pitkin R, Rennie D, Schulz KF, Simel D. Improving the quality of reporting of randomized controlled trials: the CONSORT statement. Jama. 1996;276(8):637–9.

32. Rammant E, Decaestecker K, Bultijnck R, Sundahl N, Ost P, Pauwels NS, Deforche B, Pieters R, Fonteyne V. A systematic review of exercise and psychosocial rehabilitation interventions to improve health-related outcomes in patients with bladder cancer undergoing radical cystectomy. Clin rehabil. 2017;32(5):594–606.

33. Bourke L, Smith D, Steed L, Hooper R, Carter A, Catto J, Albertsen PC, Tombal B, Payne HA, Rosario DJ. Exercise for men with prostate cancer: a systematic review and meta-analysis. Eur Urol. 2016;69(4):693–703.

34. Sharma P, Henriksen CH, Zargar-Shoshtari K, Xin R, Poch MA, Pow-Sang JM, Sexton WJ, Spiess PE, Gilbert SM. Preoperative patient reported mental health is associated with high grade complications after radical cystectomy. J Urol. 2016;195(1):47–52.

24

Perioperative outcomes of zero ischemia radiofrequency ablation-assisted tumor enucleation for renal cell carcinoma: results of 182 patients

Chengwei Zhang[1†], Xiaozhi Zhao[1†], Suhan Guo[2], Changwei Ji[1], Wei Wang[1] and Hongqian Guo[1*]

Abstract

Background: To evaluate the perioperative outcomes of zero ischemia radiofrequency ablation-assisted tumor enucleation.

Methods: Patients undergoing zero ischemia radiofrequency ablation-assisted tumor enucleation were retrospectively identified from July 2008 to March 2013. The tumor was enucleated after RFA treatment. R.E.N.A.L., PADUA and centrality index (C-index) score systems were used to assess each tumor case. We analyzed the correlation of perioperative outcomes with these scores. Postoperative complications were graded with Clavien-Dindo system. Multivariate logistic regression analyses were used to assess risk of complications.

Results: Among 182 patients assessed, median tumor size, estimated blood loss, hospital stay and operative time were 3.2 cm (IQR 2.8–3.4), 80 ml (IQR 50–120), 7 days (IQR 6–8) and 100 min (IQR 90–120), respectively. All three scoring systems were strongly correlated with estimated blood loss, hospital stay and operative time. We found 3 (1.6%) intraoperative and 23 (12.6%, 13 [7.1%] Grade 1 and 10 [5.5%] Grade 2 & 3a) postoperative complications. The median follow-up was 55.5 months (IQR 45–70). Additionally, the complexities of R.E.N.A.L., PADUA and C-index scores were significantly correlated with complication grades ($P < 0.001$; $P < 0.001$; $P < 0.001$; respectively). As the representative, R.E.N.A.L. score was an independent predictive factor for postoperative complications and patients with a high complexity had an over 24-fold higher risk compared to those with a low complexity (OR 24.360, 95% CI 4.412–134.493, $P < 0.001$).

Conclusions: Zero ischemia radiofrequency ablation-assisted tumor enucleation is considered an effective nephron-sparing treatment. Scoring systems could be useful for predicting perioperative outcomes of radiofrequency ablation-assisted tumor enucleation.

Keywords: Zero ischemia, Radiofrequency ablation, Tumor enucleation, Renal cell carcinoma, Nephrometry scoring systems

Background

Increasing numbers of small and incidental renal tumors have been detected with the enhancement of imaging technology. The estimated incidence of renal cancers is 5% among all tumors for males and 3% for females [1]. Nephron-sparing surgery (NSS) has been the recommended method to treat cT1a and T1b renal tumors to preserve renal function [2, 3]. However, traditional NSS is considered to have some concerns, including hemostasis, tumor margin status, the collecting system invasion, renal vasculature clamping and hypothermia deployment.

Excision of the tumor with a substantial margin of normal parenchyma is the standard technique in partial nephrectomy and may reduce the risk of local recurrence [4]. To preserve more kidney parenchyma and avoid major bleeding, simple tumor enucleation (TE) was introduced in 2006. TE is a safe and acceptable

---

* Correspondence: dr.ghq@nju.edu.cn
†Equal contributors
[1]Department of Urology, Nanjing Drum Tower Hospital, Medical School of Nanjing University, 321 Zhongshan Rd., Nanjing 210008, People's Republic of China
Full list of author information is available at the end of the article

treatment for NSS [5]. Moreover, the oncologic result with TE is similar to that with radical nephrectomy for treatment of both T1a and T1b renal cell carcinoma (RCC) [6].

As a result of hilar clamping, renal function will be influenced to a certain extent after ischemia with traditional NSS or simple TE, which is more important to the patients who suffer from solitary kidney. Radiofrequency ablation (RFA) has been used in medical field for more than 75 years [7]. The combination of RFA and NSS began in 2003, with no need for clamping the renal pedicle [8]. We reported our technique of RFA-assisted TE for renal tumors in 2012. Hemorrhage can be controlled to some extent and ischemia can be avoided to better protect renal function [9]. Therefore, we can achieve zero ischemia within our TE process.

Nephrometry scoring systems were recently created to predict surgical outcomes after partial nephrectomy. The R.E.N.A.L. and PADUA nephrometry scoring systems contain analogous elements, including tumor size, tumor depth, proximity or aggressiveness to the collecting system, tumor position (anterior or posterior plane) and tumor location in terms of polarity or relation to renal hilum [10, 11]. Differently, The centrality index (C-Index) indicates tumor size and proximity relative to the renal hilum, which provides a measurement of tumor centrality [12]. Both R.E.N.A.L and C-index were found associated with decreased estimated glomerular filtration rate (eGFR) after partial nephrectomy [13, 14]. Satasivam et al.'s report figured out R.E.N.A.L score would predict histological features of tumor aggressiveness [15]. As a vital variable of standard NSS surgery, ischemia time was proved to have strong relationship with all three nephrometry score systems [16, 17]. In spite TE has been widely approved for treatment of RCC, few studies focus on nephrometry scores to evaluate clinical outcomes after TE.

Therefore, we attempt to evaluate the perioperative outcomes of RFA-assisted TE for RCC in our single institute and associate the use of nephrometry scoring systems for predicting the perioperative complications.

Methods
Patients
We retrospectively identified consecutive patients who underwent RFA-assisted TE via an open or laparoscopic approach for a single renal tumor in our institution between July 2008 and March 2013. Patients with pathologically confirmed RCC were included. In addition to RFA assisted TE, simple TE and simple RFA are both our choices in the treatment for RCC. In this study all the selected patients were undergoing RFA assisted TE. All patients were informed of the option and all provided signed informed consent to

be in the study, which was approved by the local ethics committee.

Measurements
Preoperatively, all tumors seen on enhanced computerized tomography (CT) or magnetic resonance imaging (MRI) were scored by three senior urologists with different degrees of expertise in terms of the scoring systems. Final scores had interobserver concordance. Tumor stage was determined by the 2010 tumor-node-metastasis classification [4]. Ultrasonography and CT or MRI of the abdomen were performed preoperatively, as was chest X-ray, testing for serum creatinine level and other examinations. The eGFR was calculated by the modified Modification of Diet in Renal Disease equation (MDRD) before and after surgery [18]. Estimated blood loss, operative time and hospital stay were recorded.

Complexity levels of each nephrometry scoring system were defined as follows: R.E.N.A.L Scores ranged from 4 to 12 points. A score of 4, 5 or 6 indicated a lesion of low complexity, and 10, 11 or 12 indicated the highest complexity [10]. PADUA scores ranged from 6 to 14. Tumor with a score of 6 or 7 was considered as low complexity while a score above 9 was high complexity [11]. For the C-index system, tumors were separated into 2 categories of greater than 2.5 (low complexity) or less than 2.5 (high complexity) [13].

Zero ischemia RFA-assisted TE
Our zero ischemia RFA-assisted TE technique was previously described [9]. All patients were under general anesthesia. The laparoscopic or open approach was via a retroperitoneal or transperitoneal route. The kidney was completely separated from perirenal fat and the renal pedicle was isolated. We localized the tumor by direct vision or intraoperative open or laparoscopic ultrasonography. Before RFA the tumor was biopsied percutaneously (17-gauge TruCore).

The electrode was inserted into the tumor via a percutaneous or laparoscopic approach, under the guidance of intraoperative ultrasonography. RFA was performed by the Cool-tip system, which was controlled by a feedback algorithm. One to three cycles were used, depending on tumor size and depth.

TE was performed with an open or laparoscopic approach with the renal hilum not clamped. Toward the pseudocapsule (PS), we incised the kidney capsule next to the lesion. The surgical plane was determined by the surgeon's choice. Blunt dissection was used to enucleate the tumors. The rim of the normal renal parenchyma was not visible. Bleeding control involved bipolar coagulation with a 1-cm electrode for several minutes. The parenchymal defect remained open but covered with fibrin glue; the opening of the calyces was ligated by running or single suture with 3-zero monofilament. A single surgeon (HG) performed all surgeries.

Follow-up

The follow-up protocol at our institution comprised a clinical visit and physical examination, as well as contrast enhanced CT at 7 days, 3, 6 months and then every 6 months thereafter sequentially. Patients with renal insufficiency or contrast agent allergy were followed by enhanced MRI.

Statistical analysis

Data are presented as mean (SD), median (interquartile range [IQR]) or number (%). All demographic data, including continuous and variables, was analyzed by independent chi-square test. Multivariate logistic regression analysis was used to determine variables predicting perioperative incidences of complications. Odds ratios (ORs) and 95% confidence intervals (95% CIs) were calculated. Spearman's nonparametric method was used for correlation analysis because of nonnormal distribution of scores. All statistical analyses involved use of SPSS 18.0 (SPSS Inc., Chicago, IL). $P < 0.05$ was considered statistically significant.

Results

Patients' demographics are demonstrated in Table 1. We identified 182 patients with perioperative imaging data (125 men [68.7%]; mean [SD] age 57.6 [SD 11.0]; mean body mass index 23.3 kg/m^2 [SD 4.2]); the approach was laparoscopic for 170 patients (93.4%) and open for 12 (6.6%); 115 (63.2%) patients suffered from American Society of Anesthesiologists (ASA) scores of I or II and 67 (36.8%) was scores of III. The median (IQR) tumor size was 3.2 cm (2.8–3.9) and most (73.1%, $n = 133$) were more than 50% exophytic. The median (IQR) operative time was 100 min (90–120 min), median estimated blood loss 80 ml (50–120 ml) and median hospital stay 7 days (6–8 days). No residual tumor was found on enhanced CT or MRI after surgery. Additionally, for most patients (n = 133, 73.1%), tumors were clear-cell RCC on histopathology. No viable tumor cells were identified on the parenchymal side and the PS was undamaged in all cases. The median follow-up was 55.5 months (IQR 45–70). Totally there were 11 deaths occurring during the follow-up period, in which 2 were related to renal cancer. Distant metastasis developed in five patients at 18 and 35 months after surgery and they died at 38 and 55 months after surgery, respectively. Three patients suffered from lung metastasis and the other two were bone metastasis.

After calculating tumor scores on preoperative imaging, we associated the R.E.N.A.L., PADUA and C-Index scores with some clinical variables (Table 2). For all three scoring

Table 1 Characteristics of patients undergoing radiofrequency ablation (RFA)-assisted tumor enucleation (TE) for renal cell carcinoma ($n = 182$)

Age, years, mean (SD)	57.6 (11.0)
Male gender	125 (68.7)
Body mass index, kg/m^2, mean (SD)	23.3 (4.2)
Operative time, min, median (IQR)	100 (90–120)
Estimated blood loss, ml, median (IQR)	80 (50–120)
Hospital stay, days, median (IQR)	7 (6–8)
Tumor size, cm, median (IQR)	3.2 (2.8–3.9)
Right tumor laterality	102 (55.7)
Follow-up, months, median (IQR)	55.5 (45–70)
ASA score	
< II	115 (63.2)
> III	67 (36.8)
eGFR, ml/min/1.73m^2, mean (SD)	
Pre-operation	64.3 (18.1)
12 months post-operation	60.8 (17.3)
Tumor location	
> 50% exophytic	133 (73.1)
< 50% exophytic	41 (22.5)
Entirely endophytic	8 (4.4)
Tumor position	
Anterior	85 (46.7)
Posterior	97 (53.3)
Surgical approach	
Laparoscopic	170 (93.4)
Open	12 (6.6)
Histology, no. patients	
Clear cell renal cell carcinoma	133
Papillary	13
Oncocytoma	10
Angiomyolipoma	15
Chromophobe renal cell cancer	8
Unclassified renal cell cancer	3

Data are no. (%) unless indicated. *IQR* Interquartile range, *ASA* American Society of Anesthesiologists, *eGFR* Estimated glomerular filtration rate

systems, in which R.E.N.A.L. score complexity played the most significant role ($P < 0.001$), estimated blood loss, operative time and hospital stay but not eGFR change differed by score complexity. All scores and their complexities were strongly correlated with estimated blood loss, operative time and hospital stay (Table 3). However, correlation coefficients with eGFR change in absolute value or percentage were less than 0.2, suggesting a weak correlation.

We evaluated perioperative complications, found 3 intraoperative complications and 23 postoperative ones.

Table 2 Association between nephrometry scores and clinical outcome variables

Nephrometry scores	No. (%)	Estimated blood loss, ml, median (IQR)	Operative time, min, median (IQR)	Hospital stay, days, median (IQR)	Change in eGFR, median (IQR)
R.E.N.A.L. score					
Low (4–6)	132	70 (50,100)	100 (90,110)	6 (5.25,8)	−4.05 (−6.88,-1.3)
Moderate (7–9)	43	120 (75,160)	120 (100,130)	8 (6,9)	−3.7 (−5.3,−0.9)
High (10–12)	7	210 (170,250)	150 (120,160)	10 (8,10)	-0.9 (− 3.3,1.3)
P value		**< 0.001**	**< 0.001**	**< 0.001**	0.136
PADUA score					
Low (6–7)	108	70 (50,90)	100 (90,110)	6 (5.25,8)	− 4.2 (− 6.72,-1.3)
Moderate (8–9)	64	100 (61.25,148.75)	102.5 (90,127.5)	8 (6,9)	− 3.4 (− 6.05,-1.12)
High (10–13)	10	190 (127.5220)	130 (103.75,156.25)	8.5 (6.5,10)	−1.25 (− 3.35,1.95)
P value		**< 0.001**	**0.002**	**0.005**	0.112
C-index score					
Low (> 2.5)	116	70 (50,100)	100 (90,113.75)	6 (5,8)	− 3.8 (− 6.72,-0.95)
High (< 2.5)	66	102.5 (75,162.5)	102.5 (95,130)	7.5 (6,9)	− 3.75 (− 5.98,-0.9)
P value		**< 0.001**	**0.005**	**0.006**	0.921

Boldface means the data is significant ($P < 0.05$)

All the postoperative complications were classified by the Clavien-Dindo grading system, which included 17 (74%) Grade 1–2 complications (Grade 1: 18, Grade 2: 1) and 6 (26%) Grade 3a complications (Table 4). The major complications (Grade 3a) contained urinary leakage and perinephric urinoma. At the same time, we identified strong correlation of complexities between postoperative complications and all the three systems ($P < 0.001$, Table 5), which meant high systems score was significantly associated with high incidence of complications. R.E.N.A.L. score had a most significant correlation coefficient ($\rho = 0.376$). To evaluate potential preoperative risk factors associated with postoperative complications, multivariate logistic regression analysis was performed. As the representative of score systems, R.E.N.A.L. score was the only independent predictive factor of the occurrence of postoperative complications (Table 6). Patients with a high complexity (R.E.N.A.L. score 10–12) had an over 24-fold higher risk compared with those with a low complexity (R.E.N.A.L. score 4–6).

Discussion

We succeeded to perform zero ischemia RFA-assisted TE in 182 patients. We evaluated the follow-up of our

RFA-assisted TE and the association of these scoring systems with perioperative outcomes. All three scoring systems were strongly correlated with estimated blood loss, hospital stay and operative time. The complexity of the scoring systems was significantly associated with postoperative complication grades. Additionally, R.E.N.A.L. scores were an independent predictive factor for postoperative complications and patients with a high complexity had an over 24-fold higher risk compared to those with a low complexity (OR 24.360, 95% CI 4.412–134.493, $P < 0.001$). Zero ischemia RFA-assisted TE is considered a safe and effective nephron-sparing treatment. Scoring systems could be useful for predicting perioperative outcomes of RFA-assisted TE.

Simple TE has been found a safe and acceptable NSS treatment. Carini et al. evaluated the safety and efficacy of simple TE as a conservative treatment in the early twentieth century: among 232 patients undergoing TE for sporadic, unilateral, pathologically confirmed pT1a RCC, no major complications were found [5]. Likewise, TE was associated with the same progression-free survival and cancer-specific survival as with racial nephrectomy (RN) for both T1a and T1b RCC [6]. In terms of adverse events, the rate was 16%,

Table 3 Correlation between nephrometry scores and clinical outcomes

Tumor characteristics and scores	Estimated blood loss	Operative time	Hospital stay	Absolute change in eGFR	Percentage change in eGFR
R.E.N.A.L. score	0.438**	0.252**	0.210*	0.072	0.077
PADUA score	0.373**	0.264**	0.241**	0.087	0.105
C-Index Score	0.407**	0.311**	0.203*	0.007	0.035

Data are Spearman correlation coefficients, ρ
*$P < 0.05$
**$P < 0.001$

Table 4 Perioperative complications characteristics

Complications	No. patients
Intraoperative complications	3
Blood loss requiring transfusion	2
Conversion	1
Postoperative complications	23
Clavien-Dindo Grade 1	13
Pain	10
Hematuria	2
Renal infarction	1
Clavien-Dindo Grade 2	4
Limited hematoma	1
Postoperative Fever	3
Clavien-Dindo Grade 3a	6
Urinary leakage (stent)	5
Perinephric urinoma (drainage)	1

Table 6 Multivariate logistic regression predicting incidences of postoperative complications in patients undergoing RFA-assisted TE

Variable	OR	95% CI	P value
Age	0.997	0.954–1.042	0.897
Gender	1.875	0.512–6.868	0.343
BMI	1.955	0.672–6.118	0.169
ASA score	1.817	0.735–5.160	0.278
Laterality	2.499	0.657–9.501	0.179
Surgical approach (laparoscopic vs open)	1.744	0.832–2.011	0.461
R.E.N.A.L Score			
Low (4–6)	Reference		
Moderate (7–9)	7.062	2.566–19.436	**< 0.001**
High (10–12)	24.360	4.412–134.493	**< 0.001**

OR Odds ratio, *95% CI* 95% confidence interval, *BMI* Body mass index, *ASA* American Society of Anesthesiologists
Boldface means the data is significant (*P* < 0.05)

with only 3% needing re-intervention [19]. TE and RN showed oncologic equivalence in a large cohort (about 1000 patients undergoing RN and 500 TE) in 16 centers [20].

The width of surgical margin seems the most striking difference between TE and traditional NSS. Continuous PS determines the oncologic safety of TE. In general, TE is performed by blunt dissection by using the natural cleavage plane between the tumor and the normal parenchyma. Among 90 consecutive patients undergoing TE, 67% tumors were intact and uninvaded. Although the remaining patients showed signs of penetration within layers, only 6 showed penetration on the perirenal fat tissue side. The surgical margin was negative after TE in all cases [21].

Table 5 Correlation between nephrometry score complexity and postoperative complication grade

Nephrometry scores	Complication Grade			ρ^a	P value
	Absent	Grade 1	Grade 2 and 3a		
R.E.N.A.L. score					
Low (4–6)	125	4	3	0.376	**< 0.001**
Moderate (7–9)	31	7	5		
High (10–12)	3	2	2		
PADUA score					
Low (6–7)	103	3	2	0.372	**< 0.001**
Moderate (8–9)	53	7	4		
High (10–13)	3	3	4		
C-Index score					
Low (> 2.5)	110	2	4	0.290	**< 0.001**
High (< 2.5)	49	11	6		

[a]pearman correlation coefficients
Boldface means the data is significant (*P* < 0.05)

RFA is considered a minimally invasive technique to treat renal tumor. In the past 10 years, percutaneous RFA was an effective treatment for patients, who survived with a small renal mass but had poor surgical condition [3]. Our institute started to treat renal tumors with RFA in 2005 [22]. We have identified that R.E.N.A. L. score is independently associated with occurrence of complications after RFA [23].

RFA-assisted TE has many advantages as compared with simple RFA or NSS. We have achieved zero ischemia during resection of renal tumors with RFA-assisted TE, which maximizes the prevention or delay of decreased renal function. Huang J reported a randomized clinical trial in 2016 and compared the renal functional outcome between RFA assisted TE and conventional laparoscopic partial nephrectomy. Results showed zero ischemia RFA assisted TE presented better renal function preservation. Our results in this article proved that the functional outcomes were also associated with the nephrometry scores [24]. With RFA as a single procedure, our technique allows surgeons to remove the entire tumor, which can provide an accurate pathological result to identify positive or negative surgical margins. According to our previous report, we have proved the oncological safety for the technique of RFA assisted TE. No patient showed positive surgical margins. Microscopy revealed that the pseudocapsule was intact in all cases and no viable tumor cells were identified on the parenchymal side of the tumor [9].

Since our technique is performed without hilar clamping, we did not achieve good intraoperative bleeding control. However, we found little incidence of blood transfusion after surgery because of the superiority of RFA for hemostasis. In contrast, the incidence of urinary leakage seemed high as compared with conventional NSS or TE. We found 5 patients with prolonged urinary leakage, which might occur when the tumor was close to the calyces. We found that the nephrometry scoring systems could predict the incidence of complications. As the result, communication and counseling to patients with high nephrometry scores is important. Rosevear et al. similarly showed an association of the R.E.N.A.L. score and complications for patients undergoing partial nephrectomy [25]. Bruner et al. reported an association between R.E.N.A.L. score and urinary leakage after partial nephrectomy [26], which also could be concluded from our research. On the basis of Minervini's report about TE, PADUA score was associated with complications, especially Clavien-Dindo grade 3 surgical complications [27].

Our study has some limitations. Because of the short follow-up, we cannot evaluate the 5-years OS or CSS of RFA-assisted TE. Secondly, our study was retrospective. Randomized controlled studies about RFA-assisted TE should be performed to study this technique further.

Conclusions
Zero ischemia RFA-assisted TE is considered an oncologically safe technique to treat renal cancer, for both protect of renal function and low rate of perioperative complications. Nephrometry scoring systems represent a multifactorial approach to evaluate the renal masses and categorize patients undergoing RFA-assisted TE. From the strong relationship we found, scoring systems may give pertinent information about perioperative outcomes. Zero ischemia RFA-assisted TE is an effective option to treat renal carcinoma.

Abbreviations
95% CI: 95% confidence interval; C-Index: Centrality index; CT: Computerized tomography; eGFR: Estimated glomerular filtration rate; HR: Hazard ratio; MRI: Magnetic resonance imaging; NSS: Nephron-sparing surgery; OR: Odds ratio; PS: Pseudocapsule; RCC: Renal cell carcinoma; RFA: Radiofrequency ablation; RN: Racial nephrectomy; TE: Tumor enucleation

Authors' contributions
CZ: Protocol development, Acquisition of data, Statistical analysis, Manuscript writing. XZ: Protocol development, Acquisition of data, Statistical analysis, Manuscript editing. SG: Manuscript editing. CJ: Acquisition of data. WW: Acquisition of data. HG: Protocol development, Manuscript editing. All authors read and approved the final manuscript.

Competing interests
The authors declare that they have no competing interests.

Author details
[1]Department of Urology, Nanjing Drum Tower Hospital, Medical School of Nanjing University, 321 Zhongshan Rd., Nanjing 210008, People's Republic of China. [2]School of Public Health, Nanjing Medical University, Nanijng 210029, People's Republic of China.

References
1. Siegel R, Ma J, Zou Z, Jemal A. Cancer statistics, 2014. CA Cancer J Clin. 2014;64(1):9–29.
2. Uzzo RG, Novick AC. Nephron sparing surgery for renal tumors: indications, techniques and outcomes. J Urol. 2001;166(1):6–18.
3. Zagoria RJ, Pettus JA, Rogers M, Werle DM, Childs D, Leyendecker JR. Long-term outcomes after percutaneous radiofrequency ablation for renal cell carcinoma. Urology. 2011;77(6):1393–7.
4. Ljungberg B, Cowan NC, Hanbury DC, Hora M, Kuczyk MA, Merseburger AS, Patard JJ, Mulders PF, Sinescu IC, European Association of Urology Guideline G. EAU guidelines on renal cell carcinoma: the 2010 update. Eur Urol. 2010; 58(3):398–406.
5. Carini M, Minervini A, Masieri L, Lapini A, Serni S. Simple enucleation for the treatment of PT1a renal cell carcinoma: our 20-year experience. Eur Urol. 2006;50(6):1263–8. discussion 1269-1271
6. Minervini A, Serni S, Tuccio A, Siena G, Vittori G, Masieri L, Giancane S, Lanciotti M, Khorrami S, Lapini A, et al. Simple enucleation versus radical nephrectomy in the treatment of pT1a and pT1b renal cell carcinoma. Ann Surg Oncol. 2012;19(2):694–700.
7. Triadafilopoulos G. The great beyond: radiofrequency ablation for hemostasis. Endoscopy. 2014;46(11):925–6.
8. Jacomides L, Ogan K, Watumull L, Cadeddu JA. Laparoscopic application of radio frequency energy enables in situ renal tumor ablation and partial nephrectomy. J Urol. 2003;169(1):49–53. discussion 53
9. Zhao X, Zhang S, Liu G, Ji C, Wang W, Chang X, Chen J, Li X, Gan W, Zhang G, et al. Zero ischemia laparoscopic radio frequency ablation assisted enucleation of renal cell carcinoma: experience with 42 patients. J Urol. 2012;188(4):1095–101.
10. Kutikov A, Uzzo RG. The R.E.N.A.L. nephrometry score: a comprehensive standardized system for quantitating renal tumor size, location and depth. J Urol. 2009;182(3):844–53.
11. Ficarra V, Novara G, Secco S, Macchi V, Porzionato A, De Caro R, Artibani W. Preoperative aspects and dimensions used for an anatomical (PADUA) classification of renal tumours in patients who are candidates for nephron-sparing surgery. Eur Urol. 2009;56(5):786–93.
12. Simmons MN, Ching CB, Samplaski MK, Park CH, Gill IS. Kidney tumor location measurement using the C index method. J Urol. 2010;183(5):1708–13.
13. Samplaski MK, Hernandez A, Gill IS, Simmons MN. C-index is associated with functional outcomes after laparoscopic partial nephrectomy. J Urol. 2010; 184(6):2259–63.
14. Kwon T, Jeong IG, Ryu J, Lee C, Lee C, You D, Kim CS. Renal function is associated with Nephrometry score after partial nephrectomy: a study using diethylene Triamine Penta-acetic acid (DTPA) renal scanning. Ann Surg Oncol. 2015;22(Suppl 3):1594–600.
15. Satasivam P, Sengupta S, Rajarubendra N, Chia PH, Munshey A, Bolton D. Renal lesions with low R.E.N.A.L nephrometry score are associated with more indolent renal cell carcinomas (RCCs) or benign histology: findings in an Australian cohort. BJU Int. 2012;109(Suppl 3):44–7.
16. Spaliviero M, Poon BY, Aras O, Di Paolo PL, Guglielmetti GB, Coleman CZ, Karlo CA, Bernstein ML, Sjoberg DD, Russo P, et al. Interobserver variability of R.E.N.A.L., PADUA, and centrality index nephrometry score systems. World J Urol. 2015;33(6):853–8.
17. Bylund JR, Gayheart D, Fleming T, Venkatesh R, Preston DM, Strup SE, Crispen PL. Association of tumor size, location, R.E.N.A.L., PADUA and centrality index score with perioperative outcomes and postoperative renal function. J Urol. 2012;188(5):1684–9.
18. Levey AS, Bosch JP, Lewis JB, Greene T, Rogers N, Roth D. A more accurate method to estimate glomerular filtration rate from serum creatinine: a new prediction equation. Modification of diet in renal disease study group. Ann Intern Med. 1999;130(6):461–70.
19. Minervini A, Vittori G, Lapini A, Tuccio A, Siena G, Serni S, Carini M. Morbidity of tumour enucleation for renal cell carcinoma (RCC): results of a single-Centre prospective study. BJU Int. 2012;109(3):372–7. discussion 378
20. Minervini A, Ficarra V, Rocco F, Antonelli A, Bertini R, Carmignani G, Cosciani Cunico S, Fontana D, Longo N, Martorana G, et al. Simple enucleation is equivalent to traditional partial nephrectomy for renal cell carcinoma: results of a nonrandomized, retrospective, comparative study. J Urol. 2011;185(5):1604 10.
21. Minervini A, di Cristofano C, Lapini A, Marchi M, Lanzi F, Giubilei G, Tosi N, Tuccio A, Mancini M, della Rocca C, et al. Histopathologic analysis of peritumoral pseudocapsule and surgical margin status after tumor enucleation for renal cell carcinoma. Eur Urol. 2009;55(6):1410–8.

22. Ji C, Li X, Zhang S, Gan W, Zhang G, Zeng L, Yan X, Liu T, Lian H, Guo H. Laparoscopic radiofrequency ablation of renal tumors: 32-month mean follow-up results of 106 patients. Urology. 2011;77(4):798–802.

23. Chang X, Ji C, Zhao X, Zhang F, Lian H, Zhang S, Liu G, Zhang G, Gan W, Li X, et al. The application of R.E.N.A.L. nephrometry scoring system in predicting the complications after laparoscopic renal radiofrequency ablation. J Endourol. 2014;28(4):424–9.

24. Huang J, Zhang J, Wang Y, Kong W, Xue W, Liu D, Chen Y, Huang Y. Comparing zero ischemia laparoscopic radio frequency ablation assisted tumor enucleation and laparoscopic partial nephrectomy for clinical T1a renal tumor: a randomized clinical trial. J Urol. 2016;195(6):1677–83.

25. Rosevear HM, Gellhaus PT, Lightfoot AJ, Kresowik TP, Joudi FN, Tracy CR. Utility of the RENAL nephrometry scoring system in the real world: predicting surgeon operative preference and complication risk. BJU Int. 2012;109(5):700–5.

26. Bruner B, Breau RH, Lohse CM, Leibovich BC, Blute ML. Renal nephrometry score is associated with urine leak after partial nephrectomy. BJU Int. 2011; 108(1):67–72.

27. Minervini A, Vittori G, Salvi M, Sebastianelli A, Tuccio A, Siena G, Masieri L, Gacci M, Lapini A, Serni S, et al. Analysis of surgical complications of renal tumor enucleation with standardized instruments and external validation of PADUA classification. Ann Surg Oncol. 2013;20(5):1729–36.

Long-term outcomes of total ureterectomy with ileal-ureteral substitution treatment for ureteral cancer: a single-center experience

Yin-Chien Ou[†], Che-Yuan Hu[†], Hong-Lin Cheng and Wen-Horng Yang[*]

Abstract

Background: To explore the feasibility and long-term outcomes of renal preservation in a retrospective cohort of patients with ureteral urothelial carcinoma undergoing total ureterectomy with ileal-ureteral substitution.

Methods: A retrospective review of the data from patients treated with total ureterectomy with ileal-ureteral substitution from 1988 to 2016 was performed. The pre-operative oncological status, long-term oncological outcome, long-term renal functional outcome, early and late complications were analyzed.

Results: A total of eight patients with a median age of 70 years were included. The median follow-up time was 109 months. Six patients had multi-focal tumor involvement over the target ureter, and six patients had bilateral upper tract involvement. Only one patient encountered the upper-tract recurrence. The 2 and 5-year cancer-specific survival rates were 87.5 and 75.0%, respectively. The renal function was well-preserved in most patients, with only one patient needed life-long postoperative hemodialysis. Five patients experienced early complications and four patients experienced late complications. No perioperative mortality happened.

Conclusions: A total ureterectomy with an ileal-ureteral substitution is feasible for treating ureteral urothelial carcinoma when a renal-sparing procedure is indicated. It provides good long-term oncological outcomes over the upper tract, and it also preserves the renal function.

Keywords: Upper urinary tract urothelial carcinoma, Total ureterectomy, Ileum, Reconstructive surgical procedures

Background

Upper-tract urothelial carcinoma (UTUC) is a high-incidence disease in southern Taiwan. It has been associated with arsenic exposure and consumption of Chinese herbal products that contain aristolochic acid [1, 2]. Radical nephroureterectomy with bladder cuff excision provides durable oncological control, and remains the gold standard for treating UTUC [3]. However, kidney sparing surgery may take an important role in the arsenic or aristolochic acid endemic area, because the incidence of bilateral upper tract involvement was reported around 8–10% in the geographical region of aristolochic acid nephropathy [4, 5]. Also, the recurrence of UCs in the contralateral upper tract was reported to occur in 2–6% [6, 7]. Since the incidence of ureteral urothelial carcinoma (UC) is twice higher than the renal pelvic UC over the endemic area of arsenic exposure [2], kidney sparing surgeries are now considered reasonable alternatives in selected patients with chronic renal insufficiency, a solitary functional kidney, synchronous bilateral UTUCs or high risk of contralateral upper urinary tract recurrence.

Some researchers [8–10] have reported technical feasibility and good oncologic outcome in patients with ureteral UCs, using kidney sparing procedures such as endoscopic ablation and segmental ureterectomy (SU). However, endoscopic management may carry risks of under-staging, under-grading, or increased risk of recurrence, where SU may not be feasible in multifocal disease or in the case of long segment of tumor involvement [8]. Both procedures also encounter certain risk of recurrence on the remaining ureter [11, 12].

* Correspondence: solarex333@gmail.com
[†]Yin-Chien Ou and Che-Yuan Hu contributed equally to this work.
Department of Urology, National Cheng Kung University Hospital, No.138, Sheng Li Road, Tainan 704, Taiwan, Republic of China

Total ureterectomy provides a maximal resection of the diseased ureter from uretero-pelvic junction to bladder cuff, which is also a reasonable alternative for patients with multifocal ureteral disease. Some case series [13–15] have reported that the combination of a total ureterectomy and renal auto-transplantation with a pyelocystostomy eliminates a potential multifocal ureteral UCs over the entire ureter. However, graft function and vascular complications are the major concerns of this procedure [13, 16–18]. Ileal-ureteral substitution was designed to bridge a huge ureteral defect, and the safety was showed in some studies [19–21]. However, only small case series and case reports discussed about the combination of total ureterectomy with ileal-ureteral substitution in treating ureteral UC [12, 22, 23]. Besides, these studies did not focus on the long-term functional and oncological outcome specifically for this procedure. We present a single-center's experience of the total ureterectomy with ileal-ureteral substitution for ureteral UC patients in southern Taiwan over the last two decades after a long-term follow up.

Methods
Study design
We retrospectively reviewed the medical records of all patients who had a total ureterectomy with an ileal-ureteral substitution for ureteral UC at our center from January 1988 through December 2016. Approval from our hospital's Institutional Review Board had been obtained before the commencement of the study (IRB number: A-ER-105-059). The patients' underlying diseases, baseline renal function, surgical planning, pathology reports, early complications, late complications, long-term renal function, and the oncological outcomes were collected. The baseline renal function was evaluated using serum creatinine levels 1 day before surgery. The estimated glomerular filtration rate (eGFR) was calculated using the Modification of Diet in Renal Disease equation, and the patients were classified into different stages of chronic kidney disease (CKD). The pathology reports for these patients were reviewed by a single pathologist, and were translated into clinical grading and staging based on the *AJCC Cancer Staging Manual, 7th edition*. Complications were taken into consideration only if they were related to the surgery. Early complications were defined as those that occurred within 30 days after surgery, and late complications were defined as those at least 30 days after surgery. Early complications were rated major or minor based on the Clavien-Dindo classification of surgical complications [24]. Upper tract recurrence was defined as any documented radiographic or pathological evidence of cancer recurrence inside the ileal ureter, the ipsilateral renal pelvis, or over the surgical field. Bladder recurrence and distant metastasis data

were also collected for oncological outcomes. Overall recurrence was defined as the combination of local recurrence, bladder recurrence, and any detectable distant metastasis.

Surgical procedures
All patients underwent surgeries with similar technique by two surgeons. The main surgical steps were described as follows. A midline incision was made to approach into the abdominal cavity. Enter the retroperitoneal cavity and wide dissection to expose the renal pelvis and ureter. En bloc resection from ureteropelvic junction till bladder cuff was performed to remove the pathologic ureter. An ileal segment about 20 to 25 cm was harvested at least 15 cm away from the ileocecal valve. The ileal graft was lying in the isoperistaltic direction, with end-to-end pyelo-ileal anastomosis, and end-to-side reimplantation into the posterior wall of the urinary bladder. A double-J ureteral stent was placed before completion of the anastomosis. Retroperitonization of the reconstructed ileal segment was done to avoid urine leakage or tumor seeding into peritoneal cavity. No anti-reflux system was performed due to the concern of any obstructive condition in the solitary kidney patients. A suction drain is positioned in retroperitoneum close to anastomotic sites. A Foley catheter was inserted in the bladder and left for at least 1 week postoperatively.

Follow-up for outcomes
All patients were regularly followed-up in our hospital after the total ureterectomy with ileal-ureteral substitution. Chest X-ray, renal ultrasonography, intravenous urography, and abdominal computed tomography imaging were done at regular intervals to evaluate any evidence of anastomotic obstruction, local recurrence, or distant metastasis. All patients underwent cystoscopy and semi-rigid ureteroscopy evaluation every 3 months during the first 2 years, every 6 months for the following 2 years, and then annually. Renal function was closely monitored based on serum creatinine levels. Metabolic derangements were monitored via biochemical blood tests including serum bicarbonate and chloride levels.

Statistical analysis
SPSS 17.0 (SPSS Inc., Chicago, IL, USA) was used for all statistical analyses. The data are presented as median values due to small numbers and wide ranges.

Results
Population
Eight patients, including two men and six women, underwent total ureterectomy with ileal-ureteral substitution for ureteral UC. The median age for these patients were 70 years (range: 37–78) when they received the surgery. Substantial follow-up data were available for all patients,

with a median follow-up period of 109 months (range: 23–167). All the resected ureters, six from right side and two from left side, were confirmed to have ureteral UCs. Four of them had pTa tumors, one had a pT1 tumor, and another three had pT2 tumors. All the surgical margins were free from tumor involvement.

Two patients (patient #1 and #8) presented with bilateral synchronous UTUCs. For them, a nephroureterectomy with bladder cuff excision for one side and a total ureterectomy with ileal-ureteral substitution for the other side were done as a single surgery. Patient #8 also had a pT2 bladder UC near left ureteral orifice, which was grossly removed by transurethral resection prior to this surgery. She insisted to preserve her bladder, and refused the suggestion of radical cystectomy. Therefore, a concomitant partial cystectomy was done along with the left nephroureterectomy, and the final pathology report revealed a pT3 disease with free surgical margin for her bladder specimen.

Four patients (patient #4, #5, #6, and #7) presented with bilateral asynchronous UTUCs. They all had received nephroureterectomy with bladder cuff excision for the contralateral kidney, and had lived with a solitary functional kidney before receiving the total ureterectomy with ileal-ureteral substitution. Beside the ureteral tumor, Patient #6 also presented with an upper calyceal tumor. He insisted to keep him away from hemodialysis as long as possible, and therefore a concomitant partial nephrectomy was performed for his upper calyceal lesion.

Two patients (patient #2 and #3) presented with unilateral UTUC. Patient #2 had lived with a solitary functional kidney due to a prior radical nephrectomy for contralateral renal cell carcinoma. Patient #3 had multifocal ureteral UC, but he favored kidney-sparing surgery after fully understanding the pros and cons of the procedure.

Four patients had previous history of bladder UC. All of them had received appropriate management and follow-up before this surgery. No patient had evidence of lymph node involvement according to pre-operative abdominal computed tomography scan. The clinical characteristics and oncological status of these eight patients are showed in Table 1.

Early and late complications

Four major (Clavien grade III–IV) and two minor (Clavien grade I–II) early complications developed in four patients. Two of the four major complications required a secondary surgical exploration for the leakage of pyelo-ileal anastomosis (patients #2 and #6), and the other two required temporary hemodialysis because of blood clot obstructions in the renal pelvis (patients #4 and #6). The two minor complications, including one self-limited urine leakage (patient #3) and one urinary tract infection (patient #2), were conservatively treated. There was no perioperative mortality.

Four patients had late complications throughout the follow-up period. Patient #6 had recurrent episodes of gross hematuria, and deteriorating renal function that finally required long-term hemodialysis. The patient's remaining kidney and ileal-ureter were resected 1 year after the total ureterectomy. Both the resected kidney and the ileal-ureter were free of tumor recurrence. Patients #5 and #7 had recurrent urinary tract infections, and were managed with oral antibiotics on an outpatient basis. Long-term prophylaxis antibiotics were not necessary in both patients. Hyperchloremic metabolic acidosis was diagnosed in patient #1 and #5, with serum bicarbonate levels less than 20 mmol/l and serum chloride levels exceeding 107 mmol/l. They both had adequate respiratory compensation, and no medication was given throughout the follow-up period. The complications of each patient are listed in Table 2. The Clavien classifications and managements for the complications are showed in Table 3.

Long-term outcome of renal function

The baseline renal function of our patients included one with CKD stage II, three with CKD stage III, three with

Table 1 The clinical characteristics and oncological status of the patients

Patient No.	Age (years)	Sex	OP side	UC involvement of the target ureter (Sections involved)	Pathology of the ureter (stage/grade)	Extension of UTUC	Previous history of bladder UC
1	75–80	F	Rt	Multifocal (upper and lower)	pTa/High	Bilateral synchronous	
2	70–75	F	Rt	Multifocal (upper to lower)	pT2/High	Unilateral	
3	35–40	M	Lt	Multifocal (upper to lower)	pTa/Low	Unilateral	
4	70–75	F	Rt	Unifocal (middle)	pTa/High	Bilateral asynchronous	V
5	70–75	F	Rt	Multifocal (upper)	pT1/Low	Bilateral asynchronous	V
6	55–60	M	Lt	Multifocal (upper to lower)	pTa/High	Bilateral asynchronous	V
7	55–60	F	Rt	Unifocal (lower)	pT2/High	Bilateral asynchronous	
8	70–75	F	Rt	Multifocal (middle to lower)	pT2/High	Bilateral synchronous	V

OP operation, *UC* urothelial carcinoma, *UTUC* upper tract urothelial carcinoma

Table 2 The oncological outcome, renal function, and complications of the patients

Patient No.	F/u period (mo)	Time to recurrence (mo)	Site of recurrence	Pre-operative CKD stage (eGFR, mL/min)	Long-term CKD stage (eGFR, mL/min)	Early complications	Late complications
1	137	Nil		IV (22.94)	IV (21.27)		Metabolic acidosis
2	41	12	Bladder	III (39.51)	II (65.23)	Urine leakage	
3[a]	157	Nil		II (80.06)	I (106.14)	Urine leakage	
4[a]	167	Nil		III (58.26)	III (36.95)	Acute kidney injury	
5[a]	81	Nil		IV (27.21)	V (10.88)		Recurrent UTI Metabolic acidosis
6	141	23	Bladder	V (12.21)	H/D	Urine leakage Acute kidney injury	Recurrent hematuria
7[b]	56	42	Upper tract[c]	IV (15.81)	III (32.26)		Recurrent UTI
8[b]	23	12	Bladder	III (51.47)	III (57.14)	UTI	

F/u follow-up, *CKD* chronic kidney disease, *H/D* Hemodialysis, *UTI* urinary tract infection, *eGFR* estimated glomerular filtration rate
[a]Patients who are still alive
[b]Patients who had distant metastasis during follow-up
[c]Urothelial carcinoma recurrence was found over pelvic-ileal anastomosis

CKD stage IV, and one with CKD stage V. At the end of the follow-up, renal function improved in three patients, remained stable in three patients, and deteriorated in two patients. Only patient #6 required long-term hemodialysis. The baseline and long-term renal functions for each patient are listed in Table 2.

Oncological outcome

Seven patients showed no evidence of upper tract recurrence on follow-up images. Patient #7 developed pyelo-ileal anastomotic stenosis 42 months after her ureterectomy. She subsequently underwent a pyeloplasty, and UC recurrence over the stenotic site was confirmed. She was the only patient with upper tract recurrence after the total ureterectomy with the ileal-ureteral substitution. Regular cystoscopy examinations showed that three patients had bladder UC recurrence; two of them had a previous history of bladder UC.

Two patients had distant metastasis. Patient #7 had an upper tract recurrence, and eventually died of UC with liver metastasis 56 months after the surgery. Patient #8 had a bladder recurrence during the follow-up, and she died of UC with bone metastasis 23 months after the surgery. The 5-year upper tract RFS rate were 87.5%. The 2 and 5-year recurrence-free survival (RFS) rates were 62.5 and 50%, respectively, and the 2 and 5-year cancer-specific survival (CSS) rates were 87.5 and 75.0%, respectively. Time to recurrence and location of recurrence for each patient are listed in Table 2.

Discussion

Multifocal occurrence and frequent recurrence are well-known features of UTUC. Treating UTUC with radical nephroureterectomy and bladder cuff excision provides optimal tumor control and is now accepted as the gold standard [3]. However, resecting a kidney will cause excessive loss of renal function, which increases the risks of death and cardiovascular events [25]. Moreover, health-related quality of life progressively declines with more advanced stages of CKD [26]. Kidney-sparing procedures were designed to provide adequate local tumor control while preserving the kidney, and they are especially important in patients who will require dialysis if they receive nephroureterectomy. Five of our patients already lived with a solitary functional kidney preoperatively, and another two had synchronous bilateral diseases. For them, hemodialysis would have been inevitable without kidney-sparing procedures.

Several kidney-sparing procedures have been developed and evaluated for their pros and cons for treating UTUCs. Endoscopic management provides survival outcomes equivalent to that of a nephroureterectomy only in well selected patients with low-grade tumors [9]. Five-year CSS rates for SU were reported comparable to those of nephroureterectomy only in patients without proximal, long segment, or multifocal tumors [10]. Six patients in our series presented with multifocal diseases within the target ureter. Besides, the pathology report revealed that six patients had high grade tumors and five patients have a stage higher than Ta. Endoscopic management or SU are certainly not a good choice for these patients.

Total ureterectomy with renal autotransplantation has the advantage of complete resection for the pathological ureter. Cheng et al. [13] also reported the benefit of transurethral resection directly through the pyelocystostomy for renal pelvis recurrence after autotransplantation. However, this procedure also carries certain surgical risks. Delayed graft function and vascular complications including pseudoaneurysm, thrombosis, arterial stenosis, and hemorrhage

Table 3 The early and late complications, the Clavien-Dindo classification, and subsequent managements

Complications	Patients (n)	Management	Clavien-Dindo Classification
Early complications			
Self-limited urinary leakage	1	Conservative treatment	I
Urinary tract infection	1	Medical treatment	II
Leakage of anastomosis	2	Explore laparotomy	III
Acute kidney injury	2	Emergency hemodialysis	IV
Late complications			
Recurrent hematuria	1	Resection of the kidney and ileal ureter (after hemodialysis)	
Recurrent urinary tract infection	2	Medical treatment	
Mild hyperchloremic metabolic acidosis	2	No need of treatment	

have been reported [13, 16, 17]. Eisenberg et al. [18] concluded that renal autotransplantation has a higher rate of vascular complications than does allotransplantation. Seven of our patients had a baseline CKD stage III or above, and five of them were aged 70 or over. The complications that mentioned above might be catastrophic for them. Besides, the pyelocystostomy might create a route for ascending tumor seeding from the bladder to the renal pelvis, which, in turn, might compromise the oncological outcome and renal function preservation. Four patients in our series had a previous history of bladder UC, we thought it was not appropriate to link the renal pelvis directly to the bladder for these patients.

Using ileal-ureteral substitution for ureteral reconstruction was first described by Shoemaker in 1906, and was most commonly used for ureteral stricture after genitourinary surgery [22]. Other common indications include iatrogenic ureteral injury during a urological procedure, retroperitoneal fibrosis, and recurrent ureteropelvic junction obstruction [19–21]. The long-term safety for this procedure was well-discussed in previous studies [19–21]. A total ureterectomy with ileal-ureteral substitution not only provides maximal ureteral excision as wide as in renal autotransplantation, but avoids the devastating vascular complications. According to our review, only a few studies [12, 22, 23] used the total ureterectomy and ileal ureteral-substitution to treat ureteral UC. The present study, which focuses on the outcome of total ureterectomy with ileal-ureteral substitution in treating ureteral UCs, has the largest sample and the longest follow-up.

Most of the patients in our series had multifocal, invasive, and high grade UCs over their target ureters. Besides, six patients had bilateral upper tract diseases, and four of them also had bladder involvement. Our study presents a good oncological outcome for these patients with a median follow-up period of 109 months. Only one patients had an upper-tract recurrence over the pelvic-ileal anastomotic site 42 months postoperatively. Three patients, two

with a history of bladder UC before, had bladder recurrence. The 2-year RFS and CSS rates were 62.5 and 87.5%, respectively, and the 5-year rates were 50.0 and 75.0%, respectively. Distant metastasis occurred in two patients, however one of whom (patient #8) had a pT3 bladder UC at the time of her total ureterectomy. Gadzinski et al. [9] reported excellent survival outcomes for endoscopic management in well-selected patients. The 5-year CSS rate for low-grade tumor was 100%, and for high-grade tumor was 85.7% in their group. However, Raymundo et al. [8] reported a 32% of under-staging and a 43% of upper tract recurrence in endoscopically managed patients. For properly selected patients treated with SU, the 2 and 5-year CSS rates were 92.2 and 86.8%, respectively [10], and the 5-year RFS rate (combining upper tract and bladder recurrence) was 37% [27]. Hung et al. [28] reported that the bladder recurrence, upper tract recurrence, and distant metastasis rates after SU were 34.2, 14.3, and 8.6%, respectively. Our literature review showed only some small series without long-term survival outcomes for UTUC treated with total ureterectomy and renal autotransplantation. In addition to the overall recurrence and survival outcomes, we focused on upper tract recurrence because subsequent treatment is much more complicated than it is for bladder recurrence. Total ureterectomy provided excellent local oncological control, that seven of our eight patients were upper tract recurrence-free for 5 years. However, the urothelium remaining over the ipsilateral renal pelvis still has some risk of cancer recurrence, and this is the limitation for the procedure. Detailed and scheduled image follow-ups to detect any abnormal filling defect or anastomotic stenosis is extremely important for these patients.

Besides oncological control, maintaining residual renal function is the core concept of using kidney-sparing procedures to treat ureteral UCs in patients with a solitary kidney, bilateral tumors, or poor renal function. Most studies that focus on endoscopic management or SU provide no information about the maintenance of renal function. A recent review article reported that 74.7% of patients treated with ileal-ureteral substitution had reduced or stable postoperative serum creatinine levels [22]. In our patients, the ileal ureter was used to repair the huge defect between the renal pelvis and the urinary bladder after a total ureterectomy. All of our patients had stage II or higher baseline CKD. Six patients had stable or improved renal function during the long-term follow-up. We thought the improvement might be related to the relatively broad lumen after substitution of ileum to the pathologic ureter. Only one patient required postoperative life-long dialysis. He had a solitary kidney with CKD stage V at baseline, and he underwent a concomitant partial nephrectomy for upper calyceal UC. He underwent temporary hemodialysis because of a perioperative blood clot obstruction in his renal pelvis, and thereafter his renal function gradually deteriorated.

Using the ileum to replace the ureter carries certain risks: anastomotic complications, bowel complications, and wound infection [19–22]. Our patients had four major and two minor early complications but no surgically related mortality. In the literature, anastomotic urine leakage was the most common perioperative complication, and recurrent urinary tract infection was the most frequently mentioned long-term complication [19–22]. We present a similar result that two recurrent urinary tract infections during the long-term follow up. Several studies had mentioned about the hyperchloremic metabolic acidosis after the ileal ureteral substitution [19, 20, 22, 29]. The metabolic disorders seem more prevalent in patients with poor renal function, using excessive size of the ileal graft, or increasing the exposure of the bowel mucosa to urine. All our patients had relatively broad lumen after substitution of ileum, and they underwent regular image follow up to ensure the patency and fast flow of the urine from the renal pelvis down into the bladder. We propose that the urine is exposed to the bowel mucosa in a very limited time span. Therefore, only two patients in our series were found to have metabolic acidosis. Both of them tolerated the condition well under adequate respiratory compensation. This results implied that ileal interposition in individuals with poor preoperative renal function may still be feasible when the substitution is made only to the ureter, and the bladder is remained as a reservoir of urine.

This study has certain limitations. First, this study is retrospectively designed without a control group. The unique preoperative characteristics of these patients such as multifocal ureteral UCs, simultaneous or non-simultaneous bilateral upper tract involvement, high grade disease which is not suitable for conventional nephroureterectomy or other renal preservation surgeries, make it difficult to provide a matched case-control study. Second, statistical analysis is not feasible in a relatively small sample size. Nevertheless, we introduce a safe renal conservation surgery with good control of oncological outcome in such a special cohort of patients. Further research in a multicenter prospective randomized controlled design may help to draw a more explicit conclusion.

Conclusions

Total ureterectomy with ileal ureteral substitution is a feasible choice of renal conservation surgery in treating ureteral UC. It is especially indicated in CKD patients having multi-focal ureteral UCs or long segment ureteral UC, when traditional renal conservation surgeries cannot have adequate tumor control. In our experience, this method not only provided maximal local excision of the involved ureter with a good long-term oncological outcome, but also preserved the residual renal function without remarkable complications.

Abbreviations
CKD: Chronic kidney disease; CSS: Cancer-specific survival; eGFR: estimated glomerular filtration rate; RFS: Recurrence-free survival; SU: Segmental ureterectomy; UC: Urothelial carcinoma; UTUC: Upper-tract urothelial carcinoma

Acknowledgments
The work was supported by grants from National Cheng Kung University Hospital (NCKUH-10704013).

Authors' contributions
WHY made substantial contributions to conception and design, analysis and interpretation of data, he gave final approval of the version to be published. HLC made substantial contributions to conception and design, and acquisition of data. CYH made substantial contributions to conception and design, was involved in drafting the manuscript and revising it critically for important intellectual content. YCO made substantial contributions to acquisition of data, analysis and interpretation of data, and was a major contributor in writing the manuscript. All authors above have read and approve of this final version.

Competing interests
The authors declare that they have no competing interests.

References
1. Chen CH, Dickman KG, Moriya M, Zavadil J, Sidorenko VS, Edwards KL, et al. Aristolochic acid-associated urothelial cancer in Taiwan. Proc Natl Acad Sci U S A. 2012;109(21):8241–6. PubMed PMID: 22493262. Pubmed Central PMCID: 3361449
2. Yang MH, Chen KK, Yen CC, Wang WS, Chang YH, Huang WJ, et al. Unusually high incidence of upper urinary tract urothelial carcinoma in Taiwan. Urology. 2002;59(5):681–7. PubMed PMID: 11992840. Epub 2002/05/07. eng
3. Margulis V, Shariat SF, Matin SF, Kamat AM, Zigeuner R, Kikuchi E, et al. Outcomes of radical nephroureterectomy: a series from the upper tract urothelial carcinoma collaboration. Cancer. 2009;115(6):1224–33. PubMed PMID: 19156917

Long-term outcomes of total ureterectomy with ileal-ureteral substitution treatment for ureteral cancer...

191

4. Dragicevic D, Djokic M, Pekmezovic T, Micic S, Hadzi-Djokic J, Vuksanovic A, et al. Survival of patients with transitional cell carcinoma of the ureter and renal pelvis in Balkan endemic nephropathy and non-endemic areas of Serbia. BJU Int. 2007;99(6):1357–62. PubMed PMID: 17346272. Epub 2007/03/10. eng

5. Colin P, Koenig P, Ouzzane A, Berthon N, Villers A, Biserte J, et al. Environmental factors involved in carcinogenesis of urothelial cell carcinomas of the upper urinary tract. BJU Int. 2009;104(10):1436–40. PubMed PMID: 19689473

6. Novara G, De Marco V, Dalpiaz O, Galfano A, Bouygues V, Gardiman M, et al. Independent predictors of contralateral metachronous upper urinary tract transitional cell carcinoma after nephroureterectomy: multi-institutional dataset from three European centers. Int J Urol. 2009;16(2):187–91. PubMed PMID: 19054165

7. Li WM, Shen JT, Li CC, Ke HL, Wei YC, Wu WJ, et al. Oncologic outcomes following three different approaches to the distal ureter and bladder cuff in nephroureterectomy for primary upper urinary tract urothelial carcinoma. Eur Urol. 2010;57(6):963–9. PubMed PMID: 20079965

8. Roupret M, Hupertan V, Traxer O, Loison G, Chartier-Kastler E, Conort P, et al. Comparison of open nephroureterectomy and ureteroscopic and percutaneous management of upper urinary tract transitional cell carcinoma. Urology. 2006;67(6):1181–7. PubMed PMID: 16765178

9. Gadzinski AJ, Roberts WW, Faerber GJ, Wolf JS Jr. Long-term outcomes of nephroureterectomy versus endoscopic management for upper tract urothelial carcinoma. J Urol. 2010;183(6):2148–53. PubMed PMID: 20399468

10. Jeldres C, Lughezzani G, Sun M, Isbarn H, Shariat SF, Budaus L, et al. Segmental ureterectomy can safely be performed in patients with transitional cell carcinoma of the ureter. J Urol. 2010;183(4):1324–9. PubMed PMID: 20171666. Epub 2010/02/23. eng

11. Suriano F, Brancato T. Nephron-sparing Management of Upper Tract Urothelial Carcinoma. Rev Urol. 2014;16(1):21–8. PubMed PMID: 24791152. Pubmed Central PMCID: PMC4004281

12. Pedrosa JA, Masterson TA, Rice KR, Kaimakliotis HZ, Monn MF, Bihrle R, et al. Oncologic outcomes and prognostic impact of urothelial recurrences in patients undergoing segmental and total ureterectomy for upper tract urothelial carcinoma. Can Urol Assoc J. 2015;9(3–4):E187–92. PubMed PMID: 26085878. Pubmed Central PMCID: PMC4455638

13. Cheng YT, Flechner SM, Chiang PH. The role of laparoscopy-assisted renal autotransplantation in the treatment of primary ureteral tumor. Ann Surg Oncol. 2014;21(11):3691–7. PubMed PMID: 25015030

14. Pettersson S, Brynger H, Henriksson C, Johansson SL, Nilson AE, Ranch T. Treatment of urothelial tumors of the upper urinary tract by nephroureterectomy, renal autotransplantation, and pyelocystostomy. Cancer. 1984;54(3):379–86. PubMed PMID: 6375852

15. Holmang S, Johansson SL. Tumours of the ureter and renal pelvis treated with resection and renal autotransplantation: a study with up to 20 years of follow-up. BJU Int. 2005;95(9):1201–5. PubMed PMID: 15892801

16. Orlic P, Vukas D, Drescik I, Ivancic A, Blecic G, Budiselic B, et al. Vascular complications after 725 kidney transplantations during 3 decades. Transplant Proc. 2003;35(4):1381–4. PubMed PMID: 12826165

17. Webster JC, Lemoine J, Seigne J, Lockhart J, Bowers V. Renal autotransplantation for managing a short upper ureter or after ex vivo complex renovascular reconstruction. BJU Int. 2005;96(6):871–4. PubMed PMID: 16153220. Epub 2005/09/13. eng

18. Eisenberg ML, Lee KL, Zumrutbas AE, Meng MV, Freise CE, Stoller ML. Long-term outcomes and late complications of laparoscopic nephrectomy with renal autotransplantation. J Urol. 2008;179(1):240–3. PubMed PMID: 18001789. Epub 2007/11/16. eng

19. Wolff B, Chartier-Kastler E, Mozer P, Haertig A, Bitker MO, Roupret M. Long-term functional outcomes after ileal ureter substitution: a single-center experience. Urology. 2011;78(3):692–5. PubMed PMID: 21741686. Epub 2011/07/12. eng

20. Verduyckt FJ, Heesakkers JP, Debruyne FM. Long-term results of ileum interposition for ureteral obstruction. Eur Urol. 2002;42(2):181–7. PubMed PMID: 12160591. Epub 2002/08/06. eng

21. Chung BI, Hamawy KJ, Zinman LN, Libertino JA. The use of bowel for ureteral replacement for complex ureteral reconstruction: long-term results. J Urol. 2006;175(1):179–83. Discussion 83-4. PubMed PMID: 16406903. Epub 2006/01/13. eng

22. Armatys SA, Mellon MJ, Beck SD, Koch MO, Foster RS, Bihrle R. Use of ileum as ureteral replacement in urological reconstruction. J Urol. 2009; 181(1):177–81. PubMed PMID: 19013597. Pubmed Central PMCID: PMC2667902. Epub 2008/11/18. eng

23. Banerji JS, George AJ. Total ureterectomy and ileal ureteric replacement for TCC ureter in a solitary kidney. Can Urol Assoc J. 2014;8(11–12):E938–40. PubMed PMID: 25553174. Pubmed Central PMCID: PMC4277541

24. Dindo D, Demartines N, Clavien PA. Classification of surgical complications: a new proposal with evaluation in a cohort of 6336 patients and results of a survey. Ann Surg. 2004;240(2):205–13. PubMed PMID: 15273542. Pubmed Central PMCID: PMC1360123. Epub 2004/07/27. eng

25. Go AS, Chertow GM, Fan D, McCulloch CE, Hsu CY. Chronic kidney disease and the risks of death, cardiovascular events, and hospitalization. N Engl J Med. 2004;351(13):1296–305. PubMed PMID: 15385656

26. Mujais SK, Story K, Brouillette J, Takano T, Soroka S, Franek C, et al. Health-related quality of life in CKD patients: correlates and evolution over time. Clin J Am Soc Nephrol. 2009;4(8):1293–301. PubMed PMID: 19643926. Pubmed Central PMCID: PMC2723973. Epub 2009/08/01. eng

27. Zincke H, Neves RJ. Feasibility of conservative surgery for transitional cell cancer of the upper urinary tract. Urol Clin North Am. 1984;11(4):717–24. PubMed PMID: 6506376. Epub 1984/11/01. eng

28. Hung SY, Yang WC, Luo HL, Hsu CC, Chen YT, Chuang YC. Segmental ureterectomy does not compromise the oncologic outcome compared with nephroureterectomy for pure ureter cancer. Int Urol Nephrol. 2014; 46(5):921–6. PubMed PMID: 24202956. Pubmed Central PMCID: PMC4012151. eng

29. Shokeir AA. Interposition of ileum in the ureter: a clinical study with long-term follow-up. Br J Urol. 1997;79(3):324–7. PubMed PMID: 9117208. Epub 1997/03/01. eng

26

Triptorelin relieves lower urinary tract symptoms in Chinese advanced prostate cancer patients: a multicenter, non-interventional, prospective study

Le-Ye He[1†], Ming Zhang[2†], Zhi-Wen Chen[3], Jian-Lin Yuan[4], Ding-Wei Ye[5], Lu-Lin Ma[6], Hui Wei[7], Jiang-Gen Yang[8], Shan Chen[9], Ben Wan[10], Shu-Jie Xia[11], Zhi-Liang Weng[12], Xiang-Bo Kong[13], Qiang Wei[14], Feng-Shuo Jin[15], Xiang-Hua Zhang[16], Wei-Qing Qian[17], Shu-Sheng Wang[18], Ying-He Chen[19], Hong-Shun Ma[20], Ying-Hao Sun[21*] and Xu Gao[21*]

Abstract

Background: Although triptorelin is increasingly used in China for biochemical castration, its effects on primary prostate cancer symptoms remain unclear. This study aimed to assess the prevalence of lower urinary tract symptoms (LUTS) in Chinese prostate cancer patients and the effectiveness of triptorelin on LUTS.

Methods: In this 48-week multicenter, non-interventional, prospective study, we enrolled patients with locally advanced or metastatic prostate cancer. Patients received triptorelin (15 mg) intramuscularly at baseline and at weeks 12, 24, and 36 with symptom assessment using the International Prostate Symptoms Score (IPSS). The primary endpoints were the prevalence of LUTS at baseline per IPSS categories and the percentage of patients with moderate to severe LUTS (IPSS > 7) at baseline, having at least a 3-point reduction of IPSS score at week 48.

Results: A total of 398 patients were included; 211 (53.0%) and 160 (40.2%) among them had severe and moderate LUTS, respectively. Of the patients with IPSS scores available at baseline and at week 48 ($n = 213$), 81.2% achieved a reduction in IPSS of at least 3 points. Of the patients with moderate to severe LUTS at baseline and IPSS scores available at baseline and at week 48 ($n = 194$), 86.6% achieved a total IPSS reduction of at least 3 points.

Conclusions: The vast majority of Chinese patients with locally advanced or metastatic prostate cancer scheduled to receive triptorelin as part of their standard treatment have severe or moderate LUTS. Triptorelin therapy resulted in sustained improvement of LUTS in these patients.

Keywords: Prostate cancer, Lower urinary tract symptoms (LUTS), Prevalence, International prostate symptoms score (IPSS), Triptorelin

Background

The incidence of prostate cancer is increasing in China due to an aging population and changes in diet over the previous decades [1, 2]. Despite considerable improvements in the control of localized disease, one third of patients diagnosed with prostate cancer will progress to an advanced or metastatic stage requiring systemic therapy [3]. Androgen suppression by surgical or medical castration is the treatment of choice for these patients [4, 5], leading to a dramatic involution of the primary cancer and metastases in more than 95% of all cases [4, 5]. With the development of injectable depot formulations of gonadotropin-releasing hormone (GnRH) agonists, chemical castration has become a viable alternative to surgical castration [6].

Triptorelin is an agonist of natural GnRH with increased duration of action and higher affinity for the pituitary

* Correspondence: sunyhsmmu@126.com; gaoxu.changhai@foxmail.com
†Equal contributors
[21]Department of Urology, Changhai Hospital, Second Military Medical University, 168 Changhai Road, Shanghai 200433, China
Full list of author information is available at the end of the article

receptor compared with the parent compound [7]. It downregulates GnRH receptors and causes a post-receptor desensitization of gonadotrophic cells, resulting in reversible biochemical castration [8]. After initial stimulation, gonadotropin secretion is inhibited by prolonged administration of triptorelin, thereby suppressing testicular function [9].

Triptorelin pamoate (Diphereline®) 3-month depot formulation has been marketed in China since 2010. However, the effect of biochemical castration by triptorelin on the primary symptoms of prostate cancer has not yet been studied in this specific population. Early prostate cancer often does not cause symptoms; although some patients do present with symptoms, the actual incidence of this malignancy is unknown. We carried out this multicenter, non-interventional, prospective study to evaluate the prevalence of lower urinary tract symptoms (LUTS) in Chinese prostate cancer patients scheduled to receive triptorelin and to examine the effectiveness of triptorelin on LUTS.

Methods

Patients

This study enrolled patients at 21 centers across China (Appendix 1) between June 2010 and December 2012. Men with locally advanced or metastatic prostate cancer (at least T3 stage), scheduled to receive triptorelin pamoate and mentally and physically fit to answer the questionnaire, were included in this study. The included subjects could have had a history of surgery. Patients were excluded if they had hypersensitivity to triptorelin or one of its excipients, if they were at risk of a serious complication in case of a tumour flare, had received another experimental drug over the last 3 months before the study, had received a luteinizing hormone-releasing hormone (LHRH) analogue in the preceding 6 months, or had a life expectancy < 12 months.

The study protocol was approved by the institutional review boards of each participating center, and the study was performed in compliance with Good Pharmacoepidemiology Practice. All participating centers followed Good Clinical Practice. Written informed consent was obtained from all participants.

Therapeutic regimen

The decision to prescribe triptorelin was taken by attending physicians before enrolment, and not influenced by participation in the study. Each eligible patient received an intramuscular injection of triptorelin (15 mg) at baseline and at weeks 12, 24, and 36. Patients received concomitant anti-androgen treatment to prevent flares at treatment initiation according to locally accepted guidelines and standard practice.

Patient evaluation

Urinary symptoms were assessed at baseline, and at 24 and 48 weeks after the start of triptorelin treatment using the International Prostate Symptoms Score (IPSS). The seven symptom questions have a severity scale of 0 to 5, and the total IPSS ranges between 0 and 35. Higher scores reflect greater severity. Total IPSS values of 0, 1-7, 8-19, and 20-35 indicate none, mild, moderate and severe urinary symptoms, respectively. The obstructive (voiding) subscore ranges between 0 and 20, and the irritative (storage) subscore between 0 and 15. PSA (ng/mL) was recorded at baseline and at weeks 24 and 48, only as part of standard care. The subjects' quality of life (QoL) due to urinary symptoms was assessed by the QoL question of the IPSS.

Statistical analysis

A sample size of 500 patients was chosen based on feasibility, which would allow estimating the prevalence of LUTS in locally advanced or metastatic prostate cancer patients [(based on a two-sided 95% confidence interval (CI)], with a maximum precision of 0.044 for an estimated prevalence of 0.50. Summary statistics [n, mean, standard deviation (SD)], range, and frequency counts) were provided for demographic and baseline characteristics, including age, height, weight, time since first prostate cancer diagnosis, Gleason score, and indication to start triptorelin treatment. Statistical analyses were pre-specified with the inclusion of all patients with total IPSS baseline data. The full analysis set, i.e. effectiveness population, included all patients who received at least one triptorelin injection with at least one post baseline IPSS assessment. The per-protocol set included all patients from the full set who were not excluded for protocol violation. Unless otherwise specified, all effectiveness results reported herein were based on the full analysis set; for patients who withdrew or were lost to follow-up, the last observation performed was used.

The primary endpoints were the prevalence of LUTS at baseline per IPSS categories and the percentage of patients with moderate to severe LUTS (IPSS > 7) at baseline and having at least 3-point reduction of IPSS score at week 48. Major secondary outcomes were changes from baseline of IPSS total score and obstructive and irritative subscores, changes from baseline of total IPSS categories, changes of PSA and PSA categories from baseline and QoL.

All statistical tests were exploratory and two-sided, at the 5% significance level. Approximate binomial CIs were produced using the Agresti-Coull method. All statistical analyses were performed with the Statistical Analysis System® (SAS®) software version 9.1.3 and 9.2 (SAS Institute, Cary, NC, USA). For the overall analysis based on IPSS categories, the Bhapkars test was used to assess differences between baseline and post-baseline visit distributions. Paired t-test was used to assess if changes from baseline at week 24 and 48 differed from 0 for PSA levels as well as total and each of the IPSS subscores. Pearson's correlation analysis was performed to assess the association between total IPSS and PSA. Shift tables were also used to describe distribution changes in IPSS categories at week 24 and 48 versus baseline.

Results

Patient demographic and baseline characteristics

The study flowchart is shown in Fig. 1. The study intended to enroll 500 locally advanced or metastatic prostate cancer patients scheduled to receive triptorelin, but enrollment was terminated prematurely because of poor recruitment. In total, 399 patients were finally enrolled. One participant was excluded because baseline International Prostate Symptoms Score (IPSS) was not available, and 398 patients were included in the study population. The demographic and baseline characteristics of the study population are shown in Table 1. They were 72.2 ± 8.5 years old, and weighted 65.9 ± 8.9 kg. Slightly more than half (53.1%) of the patients had Gleason scores ≥ 8; 34.0% and 12.9% had Gleason scores of 7 and ≤ 6, respectively.

The majority of the patients were diagnosed with T3 (259 patients) or T4 (77 patients) advanced and/or metastatic prostate cancer. The mean time from first prostate cancer diagnosis to baseline was 0.1 ± 0.7 years. Triptorelin was first-line therapy for most patients (90.9%). Two hundred and thirty-nine patients (60.1%) took all four injections of triptorelin and 75 (18.8%) patients took only one injection.

The majority of patients (75.6%) took medications before they entered the study. Bicalutamide was the

Table 1 Demographic and baseline characteristics of the study population

Variables	Study Population ($N = 398$)
Age (years)	
Mean ± SD (Range)	72.2 ± 8.5(47, 93)
Height (cm)	
Mean ± SD (Range)	169.2 ± 5.5(145, 186)
Weight (kg)	
Mean ± SD (Range)	65.9 ± 8.9(44, 102)
Gleason score	
N (%)	341 (85.7)
≤ 6	44 (12.9)
7	116 (34.0)
≥ 8	181 (53.1)
TNM stage, n (%)	
T3N0M0	97 (24.4)
T4N0M0	10 (2.5)
T(any)N(any)M+	168 (42.2)
Regional lymph nodes status (N+)	22 (5.5)
Other[a]	101 (25.4)
Time since first prostate cancer diagnosis (years)[b]	
Mean ± SD (Range)	0.1 ± 0.7(0, 8)
Indications to Start Triptorelin Treatment, n (%)	
First line therapy	
Locally advanced prostate cancer	228 (57.3)
Metastatic prostate cancer	134 (33.7)
Others[a]	36(9.1)
Any anti-androgen therapy, n (%)	
Yes	389 (97.7)
Any surgical history, n (%)	
Yes	66 (16.6)
Prior radiotherapy, n (%)	
Yes	16 (4.0)
Prior endocrine therapy for prostate cancer, n (%)	
Yes	14 (3.5)
Any prior medication, n (%)	
Yes	301 (75.6)
Prior endocrine therapy, n (%)	
Yes	299 (75.1)
Bicalutamide	259 (65.1)
Flutamide	40 (10.1)
Goserelin	1 (0.3)
Any concomitant medication, n (%)	
Yes	101 (25.4)
Concomitant endocrine therapy, n (%)	
Yes	95 (23.9)
Bicalutamide	79 (19.8)
Flutamide	17 (4.3)

[a]TNM stage not re-evaluated for disease recurrence after radical treatment
[b]Time since first prostate cancer diagnosis (years) defined as (baseline visit date – date of first prostate cancer diagnosis)/365.25 and rounded to the largest number that was less than or equal to the calculated value

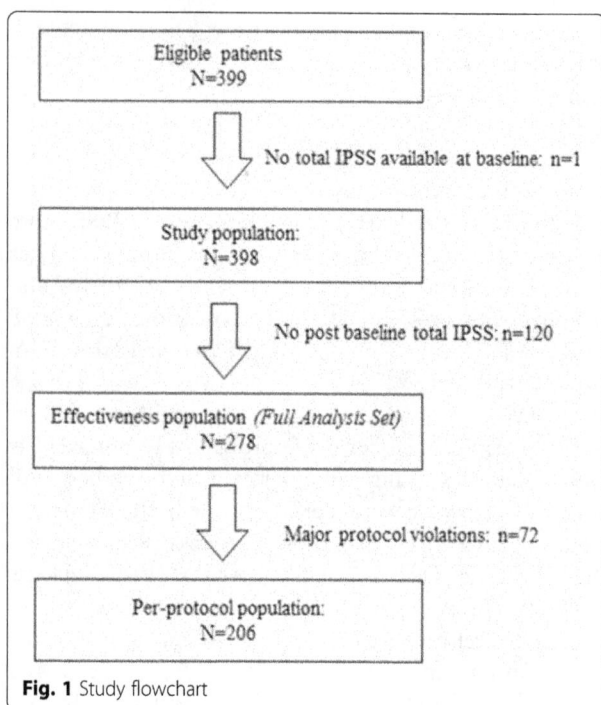

Fig. 1 Study flowchart

Eligible patients
N=399

No total IPSS available at baseline: n=1

Study population:
N=398

No post baseline total IPSS: n=120

Effectiveness population (Full Analysis Set)
N=278

Major protocol violations: n=72

Per-protocol population:
N=206

most commonly used drug. During the study, 101 (25.4%) patients took concomitant medications. Endocrine therapy (n = 95; 23.9%), bicalutamide (n = 79; 19.8%), Flutamide (n = 17; 4.3%), urologicals (n = 7; 1.8%), Alfuzosin (n = 3; 0.8%), flavoxate hydrochloride (n = 1; 0.3%), Tamsulosin (n = 1; 0.3%), terazosin (n = 1; 0.3%), and tolterodine L-tartrate (n = 1; 0.3%) were also administered. Among the 398 patients assessed, 66 (16.6%) had a history of surgery, mostly radical or transurethral prostatectomies.

IPSSs during the treatment were missing for 120 participants (30.1%), and 278 patients were included in the full analysis set. There were 72 cases of major protocol violations, and 206 patients were included in the per-protocol set.

Primary outcome measures
Prevalence of LUTS
In the study population, 211 (53.0%), 160 (40.2%), and only 26 (6.5%) patients had severe, moderate and mild LUTS at baseline, respectively.

Effectiveness of triptorelin therapy in reducing total IPSS.

Effectiveness of triptorelin therapy in reducing total IPSS is shown in Table 2. In the full analysis population, 277 patients had LUTS at baseline, including 213 with total IPSS available at week 48. The vast majority (81.2%; 95%CI 75.4, 85.9) achieved an IPSS reduction of at least 3 points with triptorelin therapy at week 48. Moreover, 255 (91.7%) patients had moderate to severe LUTS at baseline, including 194 with total IPSS available at week 48, of which 168 (86.6; 95%CI 81.0, 90.7) patients had a total IPSS reduction of at least 3 points after 48 weeks of triptorelin therapy. Furthermore, 212 (83.1%) patients with moderate to severe LUTS at baseline had non-operated prostate cancer. At week 24, 57.1% (145/254) of the non-operated prostate cancer patients achieved a total IPSS reduction of at least 3 points, which further increased to 70.1% (136/194; 95%CI 63.3, 76.1) at week 48.

Secondary outcome measures
IPSS total score, obstructive and irritative subscores
The mean total IPSS was 21.2 ± 6.7 at baseline for 255 patients who had moderate to severe LUTS at baseline, which decreased to 13.7 ± 6.9 at week 24, with a mean change of − 7.5 ± 7.2 from baseline (95%CI, − 8.4 to − 6.6) (Fig. 2a). The mean total IPSS further decreased to 12.1 ± 6.4 at week 48, with a mean change of − 9.0 ± 7.3 from baseline (95%CI, − 10 to − 8.0). The mean baseline IPSS obstructive subscore for patients with moderate to severe LUTS at baseline was 11.9 ± 4.3, which was reduced to 7.4 ± 4.3, with a mean change of − 4.5 ± 4.7 from baseline at week 24 (95%CI, − 5.0 to − 3.9) (Fig. 2b). The mean IPSS obstructive subscore was further reduced to 6.5 ± 4.0, with a mean change of − 5.3 ± 4.7 from baseline at week 48 (95%CI, − 6.0 to − 4.6). The mean baseline IPSS irritative subscore for patients with moderate to severe LUTS at baseline was 9.3 ± 3.0, which declined to 6.3 ± 3.0, with a mean change of − 3.0 ± 3.2 from baseline at week 24 (95%CI, − 3.4 to − 2.6) (Fig. 2c). The mean IPSS irritative subscore was further reduced to 5.6 ± 2.8, with a mean change of − 3.7 ± 3.3 from baseline at week 48 (95%CI, − 4.2 to − 3.2).

Changes in total IPSS categories
In the full analysis population, 146 (57.3%) patients had severe symptoms at baseline, which decreased to 18.9% at week 24, and 11.9% at week 48 (Fig. 3). More than 20% of patients with moderate to severe LUTS at baseline had improvements to mild LUTS after triptorelin therapy (21.7% and 24.2% at weeks 24 and 48, respectively). At week 48, 12/65 (18.5%) patients with moderate symptoms at baseline improved to mild symptoms, 68/97 (70.1%) patients with severe symptoms at baseline improved to moderate symptoms, and 8/97 (8.3%) patients improved to mild symptoms. A similar trend was observed at week 24.

Changes in PSA levels
At baseline, 89.3% of patients had PSA levels ≥10 ng/mL, 5.1% with PSA 0 to < 4 ng/mL, and 5.5% with PSA ≥4 to 10 ng/mL. At week 48, most (83.9%) patients had PSA levels from 0 to < 4 ng/mL while only 11.7% of patients had PSA levels ≥10 ng/mL (Fig. 4). Mean PSA change from baseline to week 24 and 48 was − 286.6 ± 1095.7 ng/mL (95%CI, − 429.2 to − 143.9) and − 259.9 ± 986.2 ng/mL (95%CI, − 405.3 to − 114.4), respectively. All patients who had a PSA level of ≥4 to < 10 ng/mL at baseline had their PSA revert back to < 4 ng/mL from week 24

Table 2 Effectiveness of triptorelin therapy in reducing total IPSS (full analysis population)

		LUTS at baseline (N = 277) and IPSS data at week 48 (N = 213)	Moderate to severe LUTS at baseline (N = 255) and IPSS data at week 48 (N = 194)	Moderate to severe LUTS at baseline with non-operated prostate cancer (N = 212) and IPSS data at week 48 (N = 194)
LUTS at baseline and ≥ 3 point reduction in IPSS	N (%)	173 (81.2)	168 (86.6)	136 (70.1)
	95% CI	(75.4, 85.9)	(81.0, 90.7)	(63.3, 76.1)

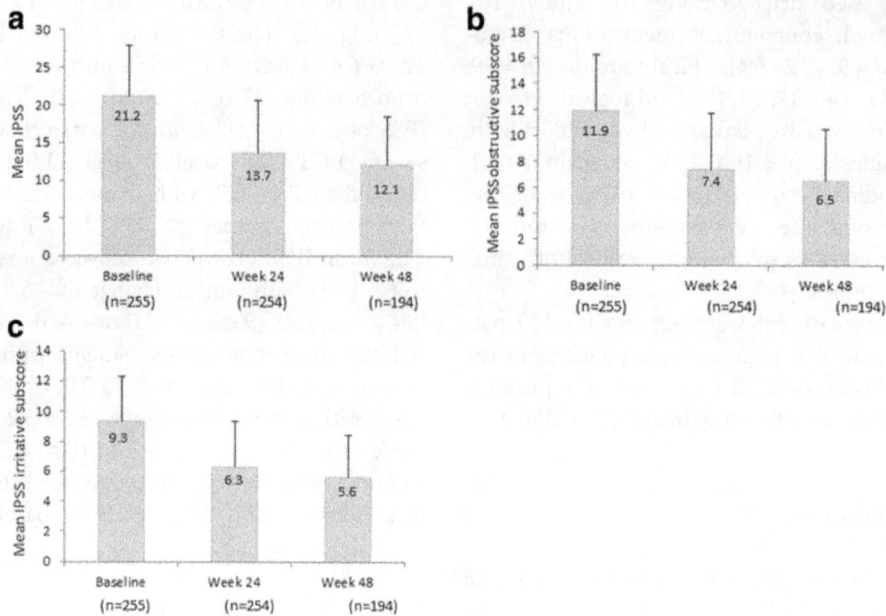

Fig. 2 Mean change from baseline at weeks 24 and 48 in patients with moderate to severe LUTS and prostate cancer receiving triptorelin therapy. **a** Total IPSS, (**b**) IPSS obstructive (voiding) subscore, (**c**) IPSS irritative (storage) subscore. Error bars represent standard deviations. IPSS, International Prostate Symptoms Score; LUTS, lower urinary tract symptoms

except one patient who had an increased PSA level at week 24. Pearson's correlation analysis revealed no correlation between PSA changes and total IPSS changes from baseline at weeks 24 (rho = −0.046; P = 0.532) and 48 (rho = 0.087; P = 0.289).

QoL

At baseline, the majority of prostate cancer patients with urinary symptoms were unhappy (30.6%), mostly dissatisfied (31.8%), or terribly dissatisfied (14.9%) with their QoL; only 1.2% of the assessed patients were pleased

and 5.1% mostly satisfied with their QoL (Table 3). After 48 weeks of treatment with triptorelin, 10.8% of patients were delighted, with 12.9% pleased, 30.4% mostly satisfied, and 26.8% equally satisfied and dissatisfied with their QoL. Only 5.7% of the tested patients were unhappy, with 12.9% mostly dissatisfied; only 1 patient (0.5%) was terribly dissatisfied with their QoL.

Discussion

This 48-week multicenter, non-interventional, prospective study assessed the baseline LUTS rates of patients

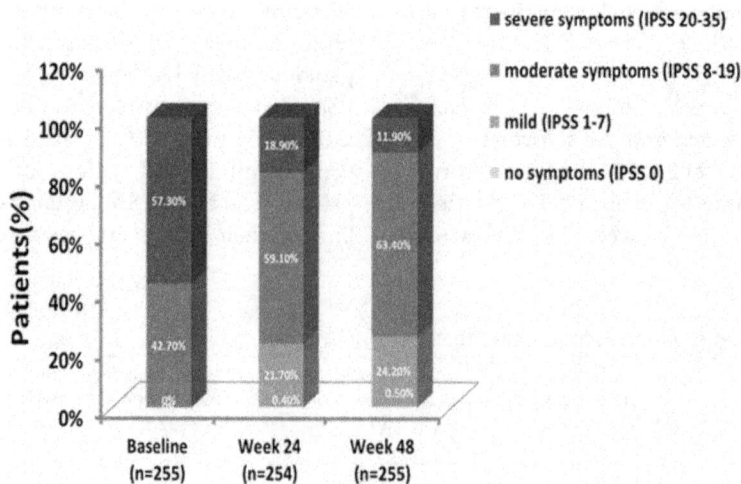

Fig. 3 Proportions of triptorelin-treated patients with no, mild, moderate or severe LUTS at baseline, and at weeks 24 and 48. LUTS, lower urinary tract symptoms

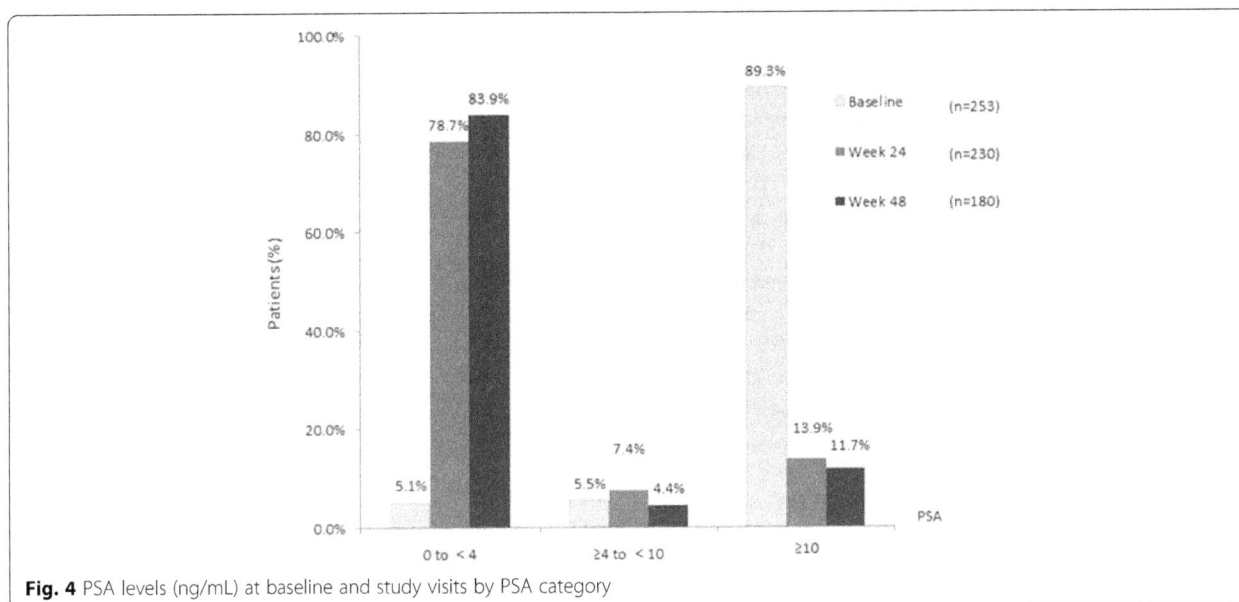

Fig. 4 PSA levels (ng/mL) at baseline and study visits by PSA category

with locally advanced or metastatic prostate cancer. Of these patients, 93.2% had severe to moderate LUTS, a noticeably higher proportion than in a Belgian population study (61.5%) [10] and a recent observational grouped analysis (52.1%) [11]. Total mean IPSS and mean irritative /obstructive scores were also higher in our study than those reported in the Belgian study (total mean IPSS: 21.1 vs. 14.0; mean irritative score: 9.3 vs. 6.5; mean obstructive score: 11.9 vs. 7.5) [10]. These findings suggest that more attention should be focused on the high prevalence of LUTS in Chinese patients with prostate cancer, and highlight the differences in severity of LUTS between Chinese and European populations.

Androgens act via the androgen receptor to regulate the proliferation of cells in the prostate as well as prostate cancer cells, and the effectiveness of androgen deprivation in treating prostate cancer is clear evidence

for their importance in driving disease progression [12]. Triptorelin is a GnRH agonist that results in reversible biochemical castration, and its role in treating patients with prostate cancer is well established [13, 14]; however, its efficacy on the primary symptoms of prostate cancer, such as LUTS, has not yet been extensively studied [9, 11, 15, 16]. Our study revealed that Chinese patients with locally advanced or metastatic prostate cancer scheduled to receive triptorelin as part of standard treatment achieved clinically meaningful improvements in LUTS (IPSS reduction > 3) from baseline, maintained throughout the study. Most patients with moderate to severe LUTS at baseline had a total IPSS reduction of at least 3 points after 48 weeks of triptorelin therapy (86.6%). Triptorelin was also effective in patients with non-operated prostate cancer; most of them achieved a total IPSS reduction of at least 3 points at week 48

Table 3 Quality of life of patients with prostate cancer and moderate to severe LUTS by visit

	Baseline	Week 24	Week 48	Last Available Visit
No.	255	254	194	255
Quality of life due to urinary symptom, n (%)				
0 – delighted	0	13 (5.1)	21 (10.8)	21 (8.2)
1 – pleased	3 (1.2)	35 (13.8)	25 (12.9)	32 (12.5)
2 – mostly satisfied	13 (5.1)	54 (21.3)	59 (30.4)	72 (28.2)
3 – mixed – about equally satisfied and dissatisfied	42 (16.5)	73 (28.7)	52 (26.8)	72 (28.2)
4 – mostly dissatisfied	81 (31.8)	61 (24.0)	25 (12.9)	43 (16.9)
5 – unhappy	78 (30.6)	12 (4.7)	11 (5.7)	12 (4.7)
6 – terrible	38 (14.9)	6 (2.4)	1 (0.5)	3 (1.2)

IPSS international prostate symptom score, *LUTS* lower urinary tract symptoms

(70.1%), which was seen as early as week 24 in more than half (57.1%) of the patients.

At weeks 24 and 48, improvements from baseline in mean total IPSS were achieved for patients with moderate to severe LUTS at baseline (21.2, 13.7 and 12.1, respectively). Although there is no direct comparison with other GnRH agonists for efficacy on LUTS for prostate cancer patients, the reductions in total IPSS appear to be similar to those reported among patients receiving goserelin in previous studies [17]. Additionally, there were improvements in mean IPSS irritative and obstructive subscores at week 48 in these patients. Improvements in LUTS were associated with QoL benefits for patients with locally advanced or metastatic prostate cancer. At baseline, the majority of patients with moderate to severe LUTS were unhappy or mostly dissatisfied with their QoL due to urinary symptoms. After 48 weeks of treatment with triptorelin, more than half of patients were delighted, pleased, or satisfied with their QoL.

Consistent with previous studies [13, 14], decreases in PSA levels from baseline to weeks 24 and 48 were observed with triptorelin therapy in this study. In patients with moderate to severe LUTS at baseline who had PSA levels ≥10 ng/mL at baseline (89.3%), PSA decreased to < 4 ng/mL by the end of the study (83.9%). However, we found no correlation between PSA change from baseline and total IPSS change from baseline.

The present analysis reported a high prevalence of LUTS for prostate cancer patients in China and confirmed the efficacy of triptorelin on LUTS for Chinese patients. However, the present study had limitations. First, it failed to recruit the intended number of participants, and enrolment was terminated prematurely. In addition, nearly one third of patients (30.1%, $n = 120$) had no post baseline total IPSS and thus were excluded from the full analysis. Meanwhile, some medications administered concomitantly with triptorelin might affect LUTS, biasing our analysis. The prevalence of LUTS reported in this study may be higher than in routine clinical practice. Nevertheless, the severity of LUTS and the high rate of advanced prostate cancer reported in this study should serve to increase our awareness of this disease, and highlight the importance of its timely diagnosis and management.

Conclusions

In conclusion, nine out of ten Chinese patients with locally advanced or metastatic cancer had severe or moderate LUTS at baseline, which negatively impacts their QoL. Triptorelin therapy improved LUTS in these prostate cancer patients; these effects were maintained during the study, leading to clinically meaningful improvements in QoL.

Appendix

Table 4 List of participating institutions

NO.	Hospital	Investigator	Location
1	Changhai Hospital, Second Military Medical University	Ying-Hao Sun	Shanghai
2	Third Xiangya Hospital, Central South University	Le-Ye He	Changsha
3	The Second Hospital of Jilin University	Ming Zhang	Changchun
4	Southwest Hospital, Third Military Medical University	Zhi-Wen Chen	Chongqing
5	Xjiing Hospital, The Fourth Military Medical University	Jian-Lin Yuan	Xi'an
6	Fudan University Shanghai Cancer Center	Ding-Wei Ye	Shanghai
7	Peking University Third Hospital	Lu-Lin Ma	Beijing
8	Shenzhen Zhongshan Urological Hospital	Hui Wei	Shenzhen
9	Shenzhen People's Hospital, The Second Clinical Medical College of Ji'nan University	Jiang-GenYang	Shenzhen
10	Beijing Tongren Hospital Capital Medical University	Shan Chen	Beijing
11	Beijing Hospital of the Ministry of Health	Ben Wan	Beijing
12	Shanghai First People's Hospital Affiliated to Shanghai Jiaotong University	Shu-Jie Xia	Shanghai
13	The First Affiliated Hospital of Wenzhou Medical College	Zhi-Liang Weng	Wenzhou
14	China-Japan Union Hospital, Jilin University	Xiang-Bo Kong	Changchun
15	West China Hospital, Sichuan University	Qiang Wei	Chengdu
16	Daping Hospital, Third Military Medical University	Feng-Shuo Jin	Chongqing
17	Shougang Hospital of Peking University	Xiang-Hua Zhang	Beijing
18	Huadong Hospital, Fudan University	Wei-Qing Qian	Shanghai
19	Guangdong Provincial Hospital of Chinese Medicine, Guangzhou University of Chinese Medicine	Shu-Sheng Wang	Guangzhou
20	Second Affiliated Hospital of Wenzhou Medical College	Ying-He Chen	Wenzhou
21	Tianjin First Central Hospital	Hong-Shun Ma	Tianjin

Abbreviations

CI: Confidence interval; GnRH: Gonadotropin-releasing hormone; IPSS: International Prostate Symptoms Score; LHRH: Luteinizing hormone-releasing hormone; LUTS: Lower urinary tract symptoms; QoL: Quality of life; SAS: Statistical Analysis System; SD: Standard deviation

Acknowledgements

All 21 participating centers are acknowledged for their contribution in this study: Changhai Hospital in Shanghai (Dr. Ying-Hao Sun, Xu Gao), Third Xiangya

Hospital in Changsha (Dr. Le-Ye He), The Second Hospital of Jilin University in Changchun (Dr. Ming Zhang), Southwest Hospital in Chongqing (Dr. Zhi-Wen Chen), Xijing Hospital in Xi'an (Dr. Jian-Lin Yuan), Fudan University Shanghai Cancer Center in Shanghai (Dr. Ding-Wei Ye), Peking University Third Hospital in Beijing (Dr. Lu-Lin Ma), Shenzhen Zhongshan Urological Hospital in Shenzhen (Dr. Hui Wei), Shenzhen People's Hospital in Shenzhen (Dr. Jiang-Gen Yang), Beijing Tongren Hospital in Beijing (Dr. Shan Chen), Beijing Hospital of the Ministry of Health in Beijing (Dr. Ben Wan), Shanghai First People's Hospital in Shanghai (Dr. Shu-Jie Xia), The First Affiliated Hospital of Wenzhou Medical College in Wenzhou (Dr. Zhi-Liang Weng), China-Japan Union Hospital in Changchun (Dr. Xiang-Bo Kong), West China Hospital in Chengdu (Dr. Qiang Wei), Daping Hospital in Chongqing (Dr. Feng-Shuo Jin), Shougang Hospital in Beijing (Dr. Xiang-Hua Zhang), Huadong Hospital in Shanghai (Dr. Wei-Qing Qian), Guangdong Provincial Hospital of Chinese Medicine in Guangzhou (Dr. Shu-Sheng Wang), Second Affiliated Hospital of Wenzhou Medical College in Wenzhou (Dr. Ying-He Chen) and Tianjin First Central Hospital in Tianjin (Dr. Hong-Shun Ma). The authors wish to thank Bo Cui, MD, PhD (Aiwei Med-pharmaceutical Technology, Ltd, China) for assistance in drafting the manuscript.

Funding
These studies and this analysis were funded by Ipsen. Writing assistance in the preparation of this manuscript was supported by Ipsen.

Authors' contributions
LH and MZ analyzed and interpreted the patient data. YS and XG carried out the statistical analysis and were the major contributors in writing the manuscript. All authors contributed to designing the protocol, provided input on the manuscript, and read and approved the final manuscript.

Competing interests
All the authors have no financial interest or financial conflict with the subject matter or materials discussed in the paper. Ipsen assumed all costs associated with the medical writing and publication of the paper.

Author details
[1]Department of Urology, Third Xiangya Hospital, Central South University, Changsha, Hunan, China. [2]Department of Urology, the Second Hospital of Jilin University, Changchun, China. [3]Department of Urology, Southwest Hospital, Third Military Medical University, Chongqing, China. [4]Department of Urology, Xijing Hospital, the Fourth Military Medical University, Xi'an, China. [5]Department of Urology, Fudan University Shanghai Cancer Center, Shanghai, China. [6]Department of Urology, Peking University Third Hospital, Beijing, China. [7]Department of Urology, Shenzhen Zhongshan Urological Hospital, Shenzhen, China. [8]Department of Urology, Shenzhen People's Hospital, The Second Clinical Medical College of Ji'nan University, Shenzhen, China. [9]Department of Urology, Beijing Tongren Hospital Capital Medical University, Beijing, China. [10]Department of Urology, Beijing Hospital of the Ministry of Health, Beijing, China. [11]Department of Urology, Shanghai First People's Hospital Affiliated to Shanghai Jiaotong University, Shanghai, China. [12]Department of Urinary Surgery, the First Affiliated Hospital of Wenzhou Medical College, Wenzhou, China. [13]Department of Urology, China-Japan Union Hospital, Jilin University, Changchun, China. [14]Departmentof Urology, West China Hospital, Sichuan University, Chengdu, Sichuan, China. [15]Department of Urinary Surgery, Institute of Surgery Research, Daping Hospital, Third Military Medical University, Chongqing, China. [16]Department of Urology, Shougang Hospital of Peking University, Beijing, China. [17]Department of Urology, Huadong Hospital, Fudan University, Shanghai, China. [18]Department of Urology, Guangdong Provincial Hospital of Chinese Medicine, Guangzhou University of Chinese Medicine, Guangzhou, China. [19]Department of Urology, Second Affiliated Hospital of Wenzhou Medical College, Wenzhou, China. [20]Department of Urology, Tianjin First Central Hospital, Tianjin, China. [21]Department of Urology, Changhai Hospital, Second Military Medical University, 168 Changhai Road, Shanghai 200433, China.

References
1. Ye D, Li C. Epidemiological trends of prostate cancer: retrospect and prospect. China Oncology. 2007;17:177–80.
2. Tao ZQ, Shi AM, Wang KX, Zhang WD. Epidemiology of prostate cancer: current status. Eur Rev Med Pharmacol sci. 2015;19:805–12.
3. Shore ND, Karsh L, Gomella LG, Keane TE, Concepcion RS, Crawford ED. Avoiding obsolescence in advanced prostate cancer management: a guide for urologists. BJU Int. 2015;115:188–97.
4. Yang CS, Feng Q. Chemo/dietary prevention of cancer: perspectives in China. J Biomed Res. 2014;28:447–55.
5. Siddiqui E, Mumtaz FH, Gelister J. Understanding prostate cancer. J R Soc Promot Heal. 2004;124:219–21.
6. Lundstrom EA, Rencken RK, van Wyk JH, Coetzee LJ, Bahlmann JC, Reif S, Strasheim EA, Bigalke MC, Pontin AR, Goedhals L, et al. Triptorelin 6-month formulation in the management of patients with locally advanced and metastatic prostate cancer: an open-label, non-comparative, multicentre, phase III study. Clin Drug Investig. 2009;29:757–65.
7. Kirby RS, Fitzpatrick JM, Clarke N. Abarelix and other gonadotrophin-releasing hormone antagonists in prostate cancer. BJU Int. 2009;104:1580–4.
8. Han J, Zhang S, Liu W, Leng G, Sun K, Li Y, Di X. An analytical strategy to characterize the pharmacokinetics and pharmacodynamics of triptorelin in rats based on simultaneous LC-MS/MS analysis of triptorelin and endogenous testosterone in rat plasma. Anal Bioanal Chem. 2014;406:2457–65.
9. Peltier A, Aoun F, De RV, Cabri P, Van VR. Triptorelin in the relief of lower urinary tract symptoms in advanced prostate Cancer patients: the RESULT study. Prostate Cancer. 2015;2015:117–24.
10. Folkerd EJ, Dowsett M. Influence of sex hormones on cancer progression. J Clin Oncol. 2010;28:4038–44.
11. Gil T, Aoun F, Cabri P, Maisonobe P, van Velthoven R. A prospective, observational grouped analysis to evaluate the effect of triptorelin on lower urinary tract symptoms in patients with advanced prostate cancer. Ther Adv Urol. 2015;7:116–24.
12. Heyns CF, Simonin MP, Grosgurin P, Schall R, Porchet HC. South African Triptorelin study G. Comparative efficacy of triptorelin pamoate and leuprolide acetate in men with advanced prostate cancer. BJU Int. 2003;92:226–31.
13. Teillac P, Heyns CF, Kaisary AV, Bouchot O, Blumberg J. Pharmacodynamic equivalence of a decapeptyl 3-month SR formulation with the 28-day SR formulation in patients with advanced prostate cancer. Horm Res. 2004;62: 252–8.
14. Zhong K, Li W, Gui M, Long Z, He L. Improvement of lower urinary tract symptoms in patients with prostate cancer treated with maximal androgen blockade. Zhong nan da xue xue bao Yi xue ban = Journal of Central South University Medical sciences. 2011;36:849–53.
15. Gil T, Aoun F, Cabri P, Perrot V, van Velthoven R. Triptorelin for the relief of lower urinary tract symptoms in men with advanced prostate cancer: results of a prospective, observational, grouped-analysis study. Ther Adv Urol. 2017; 9:179–90.
16. Woo HH, Murphy DG, Testa GM, Grummet JP, Chong M, Stork AP. Effect of triptorelin on lower urinary tract symptoms in Australian prostate cancer patients. Res Rep Urol. 2017;9:27–35.
17. Axcrona K, Aaltomaa S, da Silva CM, Ozen H, Damber JE, Tanko LB, Colli E, Klarskov P. Androgen deprivation therapy for volume reduction, lower urinary tract symptom relief and quality of life improvement in patients with prostate cancer: degarelix vs goserelin plus bicalutamide. BJU Int. 2012;110:1721–8.

27

Characterizing the transcutaneous electrical recruitment of lower leg afferents in healthy adults: implications for non-invasive treatment of overactive bladder

Eshani Sharan[1], Kelly Hunter[1], Magdy Hassouna[3] and Paul B. Yoo[1,2*]

Abstract

Background: As a potential new treatment for overactive bladder (OAB), we investigated the feasibility of non-invasively activating multiple nerve targets in the lower leg.

Methods: In healthy participants, surface electrical stimulation (frequency = 20 Hz, pulse width = 200 μs) was used to target the tibial nerve, saphenous nerve, medial plantar nerve, and lateral plantar nerve. At each location, the stimulation amplitude was increased to define the thresholds for evoking (1) cutaneous sensation, (2) target nerve recruitment and (3) maximum tolerance.

Results: All participants were able to tolerate stimulation amplitudes that were 2.1 ± 0.2 (range = 2.0 to 2.4) times the threshold for activating the target nerve.

Conclusions: Non-invasive electrical stimulation can activate neural targets at levels that are consistent with evoking bladder-inhibitory reflex mechanisms. Further work is needed to test the clinical effects of stimulating one or more neural targets in OAB patients.

Keywords: Transcutaneous electrical nerve stimulation, Bladder neuromodulation, Overactive bladder, Tibial nerve, Saphenous nerve, Plantar nerve

Background

Overactive bladder (OAB) is characterized by symptoms of frequency and urgency that may or may not result in urinary incontinence [1]. Unlike cases of neurogenic bladder with known etiology (e.g., spinal cord injury or multiple sclerosis), OAB is commonly diagnosed in otherwise healthy individuals. OAB can affect up to 16% of adults and can adversely affect an individual's ability to perform everyday tasks, social interactions, and sleeping habits, all of which can be quantified by significant decreases in quality of life measures [2, 3]. Widely accepted clinical therapies include behavioural modification [4], drugs, intravesical Botox [5], and sacral

neuromodulation [6]. However, long-term therapeutic efficacy can be limited. Up to 80% of patients discontinue drugs within the first 6 months [7], Botox injection can cause urinary retention, and sacral neuromodulation is an expensive and relatively invasive treatment option.

As an alternative, patients may be provided with percutaneous tibial nerve stimulation (PTNS) therapy, which is a procedure performed in a clinical setting. It involves the insertion of a 34G stainless needle above the medial malleolus, through which electrical pulses are used to stimulate the tibial nerve. Nerve activation is confirmed by movement of the toes or a sensation radiating along the sole of the foot. Weekly clinical visits are repeated for 3 months, and if the patient responds to treatment, maintenance PTNS is provided every 3 weeks thereafter [8, 9].

Studies suggest that transcutaneous electrical nerve stimulation (TENS) of the tibial nerve (TN) could also

* Correspondence: paul.yoo@utoronto.ca
[1]Institute of Biomaterials and Biomedical Engineering, University of Toronto, 164 College Street, Room 407, Toronto, ON M5S 3G9, Canada
[2]Department of Electrical and Computer Engineering, University of Toronto, Toronto, ON, Canada
Full list of author information is available at the end of the article

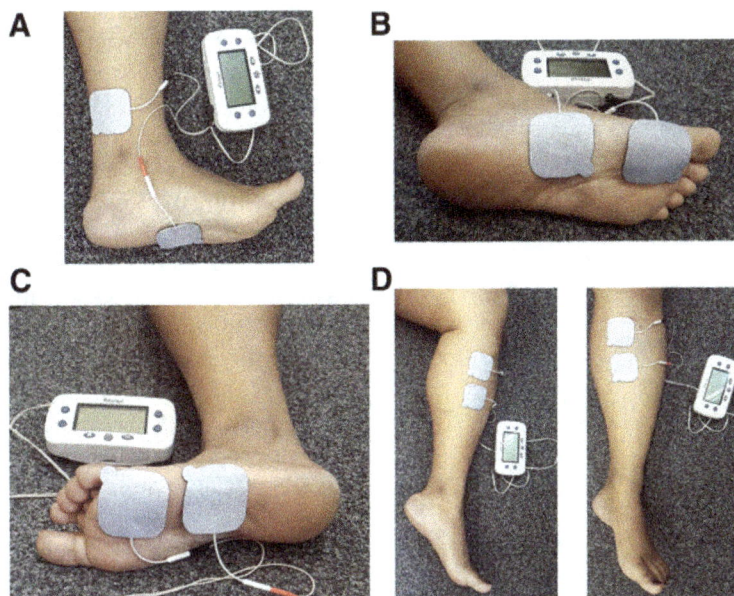

Fig. 1 Captured images of surface electrodes used to target the 4 neural targets. **a** The tibial nerve (TN) configuration involved the cathode being placed 3 finger widths above and 1 finger width posterior to the medial malleolus, and the anode placed at the midsole of the foot. **b** The medial plantar nerve (MPN) was targeted by placing both electrodes along the medial side of the plantar foot surface: the cathode is placed at the base of the hallux and the anode is placed 2 finger widths from the cathode. **c** The lateral plantar nerve (LPN) was targeted by placing both electrodes along the lateral side of the foot. **d** The saphenous nerve (SAFN) configuration involved positioning the cathode 2 finger widths below the medial condyle of the tibia, and the anode 2 fingers widths inferior to the cathode

provide an effective means of treating OAB. It is non-invasive, relatively inexpensive, and could allow patients to self-administer treatment at home. Since the first clinical report on the therapeutic effects of TN stimulation [10], multiple studies have demonstrated the feasibility of using TENS in OAB patients. For example, Ammi et al. showed that daily TENS applied near the ankle can significantly improve the quality of life in patients [11], and Manriquez et al. demonstrated that TENS applied twice a week can achieve clinical efficacy that is comparable to bladder medication [12]. Despite these findings, optimal therapeutic use of TENS remains unclear [13].

As a potential solution for improving the clinical efficacy, we have begun to investigate the feasibility of using TENS to electrically activate multiple nerve targets. Bladder-inhibitory responses evoked by TN stimulation is a well-documented phenomenon that has been demonstrated in anesthetized animals [14–16], and also in human participants subjected to surface stimulation of the plantar surface of the foot [17, 18]. It has also been shown in anesthetized rats that electrical stimulation of the medial and lateral plantar nerves can evoke reflexes that (1) inhibit the bladder during electrical stimulation (i.e. acute effect) or (2) cause bladder inhibition that is sustained even after the stimulus has been turned off (i.e., prolonged effect), respectively [19]. In addition, there is evidence that electrical stimulation of the saphenous nerve (SAFN) can also modulate bladder function.

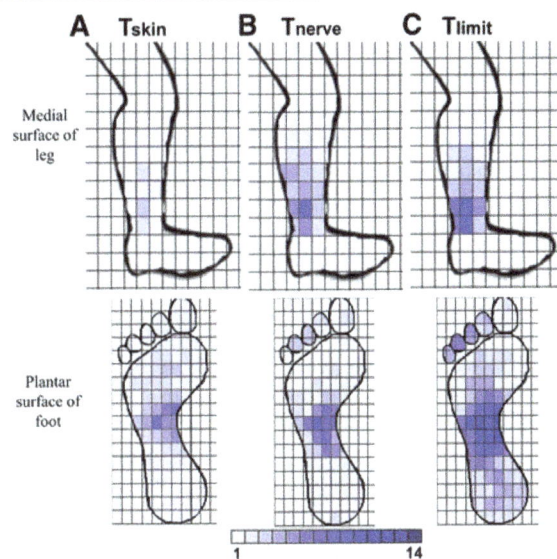

Fig. 2 Shaded anatomical plot of the sensation perceived during TN stimulation. The color of each square within the grid represents the cumulative number of participants that felt stimulation at that location. Progressive spread of the perceived sensation occurred as the stimulation amplitude was increased: (**a**) T_{skin}, (**b**) T_{nerve}, and (**c**) T_{limit}. There were increases in the 'activated' areas both on the plantar foot surface and the medial aspect of the lower leg. It is noted that the color scale (1 to 14) indicates that not all 15 participants shaded in the same pixels in response to stimulation. (same as in Fig. 3)

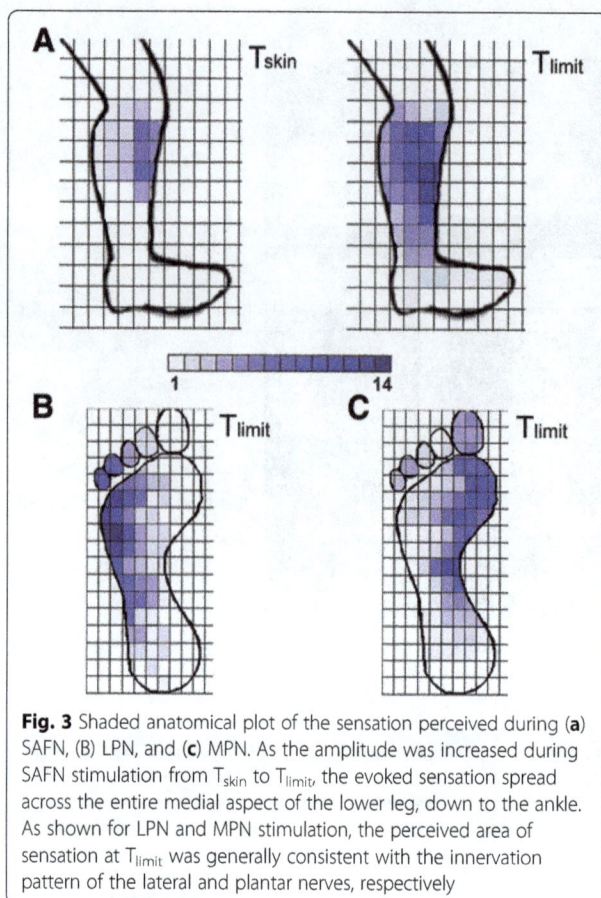

Fig. 3 Shaded anatomical plot of the sensation perceived during (**a**) SAFN, (**B**) LPN, and (**c**) MPN. As the amplitude was increased during SAFN stimulation from T_{skin} to T_{limit}, the evoked sensation spread across the entire medial aspect of the lower leg, down to the ankle. As shown for LPN and MPN stimulation, the perceived area of sensation at T_{limit} was generally consistent with the innervation pattern of the lateral and plantar nerves, respectively

By implanting a nerve cuff electrode around the SAFN (immediately below the knee) in anesthetized rats [20], we showed that prolonged bladder-inhibitory responses can be evoked in a frequency-dependent manner (10 Hz to 20 Hz). And in a small cohort of OAB patients [21], we have observed significant improvements in both OAB symptoms and quality of life measures following 12 weeks of percutaneous SAFN stimulation.

In this study, we investigated the feasibility of using TENS to selectively activate multiple nerve targets located in the lower leg (tibial nerve, saphenous nerve, medial plantar nerve, and lateral plantar nerve). A commercially available TENS device was used to electrically stimulate each target in healthy participants. The primary goal was to systematically characterise the electrical recruitment of each target nerve by defining: (1) the threshold amplitude for eliciting cutaneous sensation, (2) the threshold amplitude for activating the target nerve, and (3) the maximum stimulation amplitude tolerated by participants.

Methods

In accordance with the protocol approved by the research ethics board (REB, Approval #32461) of the University of Toronto, the study was conducted in 15

healthy participants (10 female, age = 23.9 ± 2.5 years, range = 19–28 years) who provided written consent prior to beginning each experiment. Participants were recruited using posters placed around the university campus, and e-mails sent to the students and faculty at the University of Toronto.

The experiment involved a one-hour session, during which a total of 11 stimulation trials were conducted. Following skin sterilization with alcohol wipes, a pair of 5 cm × 5 cm self-adhesive surface electrodes (STIM-CARE, DJO Global, Vista, California) were placed on the lower leg to activate different neural targets (Fig. 1): tibial nerve (TN), medial plantar nerve (MPN), the lateral plantar nerve (LPN), and the saphenous nerve (SAFN). Both electrodes were connected to a hand-held TENS unit (Empi Continuum™, DJO Global, Vista, California), where the stimulation frequency (20 Hz) and pulse width (200 µs) were set at constant values.

The electrical activation of each neural target involved a series of 3 stimulation trials, where the amplitude was increased from 0 mA up to a pre-defined endpoint. The first trial was terminated at the cutaneous sensory threshold, where the participant felt the stimulation at the surface electrode (T_{skin}). The second trial was terminated at the threshold for activating the target nerve (T_{nerve}), where the participant for example began to feel paresthesia radiate distally along the medial surface of the leg. Finally, the third trial was terminated when the participant could no longer tolerate TENS stimulation (T_{limit}). The 4 neural targets were tested in randomized order by conducting a set of stimulation trials on one leg (e.g., TN + right leg) and then switching to the contralateral leg to test another nerve (e.g., MPN + left leg). Any potential carry-over effects of stimulation were minimized by alternating neural targets between each leg. The nerve activation threshold (T_{nerve}) was confirmed by either a foot motor response (TN, LPN, and MPN) or a cutaneous sensation that radiated down the medial aspect of the lower leg (SAFN). Immediately following each trial, the participant was provided a questionnaire that asked the individual to quantify the perceived intensity of surface stimulation using a visual analogue scale (VAS range = 1 to 5), where 1 indicated the least comfortable sensation (Additional file 1). The questionnaire also instructed each participant to indicate the perceived area of stimulation by shading in an anatomical grid of the lower leg. All raw data involving nerve activation thresholds and VAS scores are provided in this manuscript (Additional file 2).

Data analysis

The stimulation amplitudes that achieved threshold activation of the skin (T_{skin}), target nerve (T_{nerve}), and maximum tolerance (T_{limit}) were summarized across all

Table 1 Summary of TENS activation thresholds: mean ± SD (range)

Target Nerve	T_{skin} (mA)	T_{nerve} (mA)	T_{limit} (mA)
TN	10.2 ± 2.8 (6–17)	19.7 ± 4.4 (9–30)	42.2 ± 2.5 (22–64)
SAFN	8.7 ± 2.3 (6–15)	25.7 ± 7.4 (17–41)	47.7 ± 9.3 (28–62)
LPN	13.6 ± 3.7 (6–22)	25.5 ± 6.1 (19–41)	50.2 ± 15.5 (28–85)
MPN	11.6 ± 4.2 (3.5–19)	21.7 ± 5.9 (15–39)	50.1 ± 23.0 (25–100)

participants and represented as the mean ± standard deviation. Since each participant exhibited different cutaneous thresholds, the T_{nerve} and T_{limit} values for each nerve target were normalized to the participant's T_{skin}. Data obtained from the questionnaire was used to summarize the perceived intensity of stimulation (VAS scores), and to also generate anatomical plots that show the spatial distribution of stimulation-evoked 'sensation'. An anatomical plot for each neural target was created by summing the total number of participants that shaded in a particular pixel within the grid (maximum = 15), and then assigning a color intensity that was proportional to the number of participants who perceived stimulation in that particular pixel (Fig. 2). Statistical analysis was conducted by performing a one-way ANOVA followed by a pair-wise Tukey-Kramer multi-comparisons (JMP, SAS Institute Inc.©, Cary, NC). A p-value less than 0.05 was considered statistically significant.

Results

Transcutaneous electrical activation of the 4 neural targets (TN, SAFN, MPN, and LPN) was achieved in all 15 healthy participants. Each participant was able to indicate graphically the anatomical representation of electrical stimulation that was perceived at T_{skin} and T_{limit}. As shown in Fig. 2, the perceived sensation of electrical pulses applied at T_{skin} was spatially limited to the location of the surface electrodes. At T_{limit}, the anatomical plots show notable spread of sensation radiating away from the

surface electrodes. Participants receiving TN stimulation indicated the evoked sensation spread up the medial aspect of the lower leg and also across a larger area of the ventral foot surface. Participants receiving SAFN stimulation indicated that the evoked sensation consistently radiated down to the medial malleolus (Fig. 3a). In contrast, electrical stimulation of the MPN and LPN at T_{limit} resulted in perceived 'sensations' that were consistent with selective nerve activation (i.e., minimal spillover into adjacent innervation area, Fig. 3b-c).

As shown in Table 1, the average stimulation amplitude needed to evoke a cutaneous sensation using any of the 4 configurations ranged from 8.7 mA to 13.6 mA. The SAFN configuration exhibited the lowest T_{skin}, which was significantly lower than T_{skin} for MPN and LPN stimulation ($p < 0.05$). The stimulation amplitude required to activate the underlying target nerve (T_{nerve}) increased substantially from T_{skin}, where the amplitude needed to activate the TN was found to be significantly lower than that for SAFN and LPN activation ($p < 0.05$). The average stimulation amplitude at which maximum tolerance was achieved (T_{limit}) ranged between 42.2 mA to 50.2 mA, with no statistical difference among the four targets.

When comparing T_{nerve} and T_{limit} (both normalized with respect to T_{skin}), we found that the SAFN configuration required larger amplitudes to recruit the underlying nerve bundle (Fig. 4a), and to also reach maximum tolerance (Fig. 4b). As indicated in Table 1, these findings were primarily due to the significantly lower T_{skin}

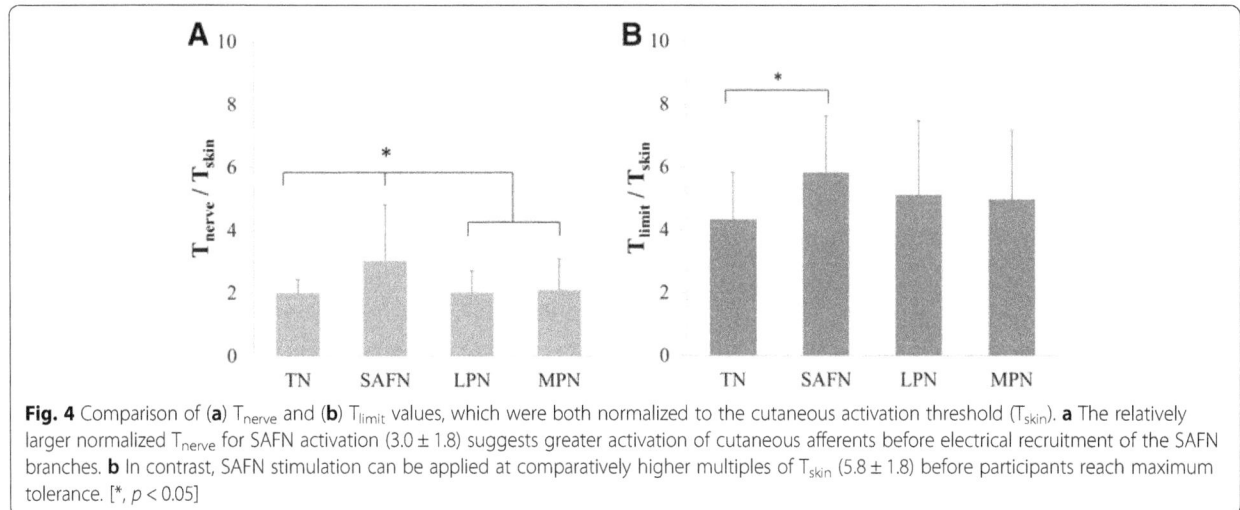

Fig. 4 Comparison of (**a**) T_{nerve} and (**b**) T_{limit} values, which were both normalized to the cutaneous activation threshold (T_{skin}). **a** The relatively larger normalized T_{nerve} for SAFN activation (3.0 ± 1.8) suggests greater activation of cutaneous afferents before electrical recruitment of the SAFN branches. **b** In contrast, SAFN stimulation can be applied at comparatively higher multiples of T_{skin} (5.8 ± 1.8) before participants reach maximum tolerance. [*, $p < 0.05$]

achieved by TENS activation of the SAFN. However, regardless of the stimulation configuration, TENS was able to provide electrical stimulation up to 2.1 ± 0.2 (range = 2.0 to 2.4) times the nerve activation threshold (Fig. 5). The summarized VAS scores quantitatively confirmed the significantly larger sensations (e.g. lower VAS scores) perceived by participants when TENS was applied at T_{limit} relative to T_{skin} (Fig. 6). The perceived level of intensity was similar across the different stimulation sites.

Discussion

In this study, we characterized the electrical activation of 4 different nerve targets which may be considered for providing non-invasive treatment of OAB. In healthy adult subjects, we found that selective activation of the MPN, LPN and SAFN was possible up to approximately 2.1 times the target nerve activation threshold (T_{nerve}). Similar to our previous computational study of PTNS [22], co-activation of SAFN fibers was observed in every participant when TENS was used to target the TN trunk. The level of target nerve activation that was achieved in this study are consistent with the stimulation amplitudes required to evoke bladder-inhibitory responses in anesthetized animals [16, 23], and also for achieving therapeutic effects with PTNS [8, 9, 24]. It was recently shown clinically that both plantar nerves can be simultaneously stimulated to elicit bladder-inhibitory responses [17, 18, 25].

Multiple studies show that transcutaneous TN stimulation can elicit therapeutic effects in OAB patients. One of the most common electrode configurations used to stimulate the TN involves one electrode being placed

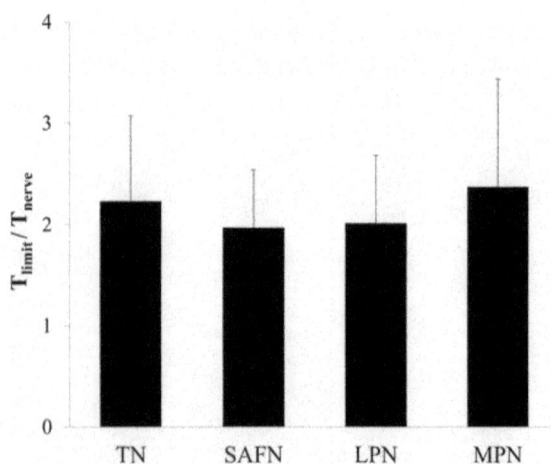

Fig. 6 The sensations evoked by transcutaneous stimulation were quantified with visual analogue score (VAS) measurements taken at T_{skin} and T_{limit}. Regardless of the stimulation configuration, the average VAS scores were consistent with cutaneous activation and maximum tolerance: TN (4.8 ± 0.4, 1.7 ± 0.8), MPN (4.9 ± 0.5, 1.7 ± 0.8), LPN (5.0 ± 0.1, 1.5 ± 0.5), SAFN (4.7 ± 0.6, 1.5 ± 0.6), respectively. [*, $p < 0.05$]

immediately posterior to the medial malleolus and the return electrode placed 5 cm to 10 cm cephalad to the first [11, 26, 27]. In these studies, the authors reported treatment success rates ranging between 53% and 87% of patients. Patidar et al. used a different TN configuration (one electrode just above the medial malleolus and the second electrode placed 5 cm cephalad to the first) to achieve a comparable 71% response rate in a group of pediatric OAB patients [28]. Whereas, other researchers achieved TN stimulation by placing surface electrodes in similar fashion to PTNS (one above the medial malleolus and the other below) [12, 29].

The anatomical sensory maps generated by TN stimulation in this study (Fig. 2) indicate that co-activation of subsets of SAFN fibers occurs at and above the TN activation threshold (T_{nerve}). These results are consistent with computational simulations of PTNS [22, 30] and further support the notion that electrical activation of SAFN fibers can potentially contribute to the clinical effects of PTNS therapy. Given the disparate spinal projections of the SAFN (L2-L4) and TN (L5-S4) in humans, it is likely that both neural inputs involve different neural mechanisms. However, it is currently unclear whether co-activation of TN and SAFN afferents will have any significant effect on treating OAB symptoms, when compared to TN stimulation alone.

Non-invasive TENS has the advantage of being a low risk (minimal side-effects), low cost, and convenient technology that can help patients chronically manage OAB symptoms. Although limited in number, published clinical trials involving TENS of the TN demonstrate

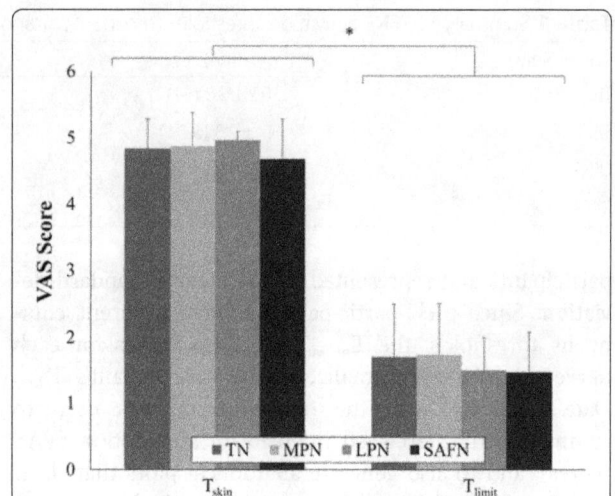

Fig. 5 Transcutaneous recruitment of the target nerve was expressed in relation to the maximum tolerable stimulation amplitude reported by each participant. The range of normalized T_{nerve} values was consistent across all 4 stimulation configurations: 2.1 ± 0.2 (range = 2.0 to 2.4). Statistically, there was no significant difference among the different neural targets ($p = 0.48$)

therapeutic response rates that are relatively consistent with those achieved by PTNS [31]. However, optimization of long-term TENS therapies will require further work in determining the proper electrode size that will enable maximum tolerable stimulation amplitudes [32], allowing patients to find their most effective or comfortable set of stimulation parameters (e.g, frequency), and also assessing different types of clinical support (e.g., urology clinic, physiotherapy clinic) that will maximize patient compliance.

Conclusion

This study shows the feasibility of non-invasively stimulating neural targets in the lower leg that are aimed at treating OAB. In healthy adult subjects, we confirmed that each targeted nerve (TN, SAFN, MPN, LPN) achieved activation levels that are relevant to evoking bladder-inhibitory reflexes. Further clinical studies are necessary to determine whether individual or co-activation of these neural targets with TENS can be used to treat OAB patients.

Abbreviations

LPN: Lateral plantar nerve; MPN: Medial plantar nerve; OAB: Overactive bladder; PTNS: Percutaneous tibial nerve stimulation; SAFN : Saphenous nerve; TENS: Transcutaneous tibial nerve stimulation; TN: Tibial nerve; VAS: Visual analog scale

Acknowledgements

The authors also acknowledge Dr. M Sasha John and Ms. Donna Shukaris for reviewing this manuscript.

Funding

The authors acknowledge financial support from the Canadian Institutes of Health Research (CIHR) Proof of Principle grant (345331) for acquiring materials used in this study (stimulator and electrodes), and from the AGE-WELL Strategic Investment Program (A16015) for HQP (highly qualified personnel) training (ES).

Authors' contributions

ES and KH participated in data collection, analysis, and preparing manuscript. PBY, MH supervised the research and edited the manuscript. All authors provided final approval of the manuscript.

Competing interests

The author PBY has filed intellectual property regarding treatment of overactive bladder using peripheral nerve stimulation.

Author details

[1]Institute of Biomaterials and Biomedical Engineering, University of Toronto, 164 College Street, Room 407, Toronto, ON M5S 3G9, Canada. [2]Department of Electrical and Computer Engineering, University of Toronto, Toronto, ON, Canada. [3]Division of Urology, Toronto Western Hospital, Toronto, ON, Canada.

References

1. Abrams P, et al. The standardisation of terminology in lower urinary tract function: report from the standardisation sub-committee of the international continence society. Urology. 2003;61(1):37–49.
2. Stewart WF, et al. Prevalence and burden of overactive bladder in the United States. World J Urol. 2003;20(6):327–36.
3. Rogers RG, Abrams P, Kelleher CJ, Kerr LA. Overactive bladder significantly affects quality of life. Am J Manag Care. 2000;6(11 Suppl):S580–90.
4. Burgio KL, et al. Behavioral training with and without biofeedback in the treatment of urge incontinence in older women: a randomized controlled trial. JAMA. 2002;288(18):2293–9.
5. Schmid DM, et al. Experience with 100 cases treated with Botulinum-a toxin injections in the Detrusor muscle for idiopathic overactive bladder syndrome refractory to Anticholinergics. J Urol. 2006;176(1):177–85.
6. Hassouna MM, et al. Sacral neuromodulation in the treatment of urgency-frequency symptoms: a multicenter study on efficacy and safety. J Urol. 2000; 163(6):1849–54.
7. Yu YF, Nichol MB, Yu AP, Ahn J. Persistence and adherence of medications for chronic overactive bladder/urinary incontinence in the california medicaid program. Value Health. 2005;8(4):495–505.
8. Peters KM, Carrico DJ, Wooldridge LS, Miller CJ, MacDiarmid SA. Percutaneous tibial nerve stimulation for the long-term treatment of overactive bladder: 3-year results of the STEP study. J Urol. 2013;189(6):2194–201.
9. MacDiarmid SA, et al. Long-term durability of percutaneous tibial nerve stimulation for the treatment of overactive bladder. J Urol. 2010;183(1):234–40.
10. McGuire EJ, et al. Treatment of motor and sensory detrusor instability by electrical stimulation. J Urol. 1983;129(1):78–9.
11. Ammi M, Chautard D, Brassart E, Culty T, Azzouzi AR, Bigot P. Transcutaneous posterior tibial nerve stimulation: evaluation of a therapeutic option in the management of anticholinergic refractory overactive bladder. Int Urogynecol J Pelvic Floor Dysfunct. 2014;25(8): 1065–9.
12. Manríquez V, et al. Transcutaneous posterior tibial nerve stimulation versus extended release oxybutynin in overactive bladder patients. A prospective randomized trial. Eur J Obstet Gynecol Reprod Biol. 2016;196:6–10.
13. Booth J, Connelly L, Dickson S, Duncan F, Lawrence M. The effectiveness of transcutaneous tibial nerve stimulation (TTNS) for adults with overactive bladder syndrome: a systematic review. Neurourol Urodyn. 2017;
14. Matsuta Y, Roppolo JR, de Groat WC, Tai C. Poststimulation inhibition of the micturition reflex induced by tibial nerve stimulation in rats. Physiol Rep. 2014;2(1):e00205.
15. Su X, Nickles A, Nelson DE. Comparison of neural targets for neuromodulation of bladder micturition reflex in the rat. Am J Physiol Ren Physiol. 2012;303(8):F1196–206.
16. Tai C, Shen B, Chen M, Wang J, Roppolo JRR, de Groat WCC. Prolonged poststimulation inhibition of bladder activity induced by tibial nerve stimulation in cats. Am J Physiol Ren Physiol. 2011;300(2):F385–92.
17. Chen ML, Chermansky CJ, Shen B, Roppolo JR, de Groat WC, Tai C. Electrical stimulation of somatic afferent nerves in the foot increases bladder capacity in healthy human subjects. J Urol. 2014;191(4):1009–13.
18. Chen G, Liao L, Miao D. Electrical stimulation of somatic afferent nerves in the foot increases bladder capacity in neurogenic bladder patients after sigmoid cystoplasty. BMC Urol. 2015;15:26–8.
19. Kovacevic M, Yoo PB. Reflex neuromodulation of bladder function elicited by posterior tibial nerve stimulation in anesthetized rats. Am J Physiol. 2015; 308(4):F320–9.
20. Moazzam Z, Yoo PB. Frequency-Dependent Inhibition of Periodic Bladder Contractions by Saphenous Nerve Stimulation in Anesthetized Rats. Neurourol Urodyn. 2017.
21. MacDiarmid SA, John MS, Yoo PB. A pilot feasibility study of treating overactive bladder patients with percutaneous saphenous nerve stimulation. Neurourol Urodyn. In press.
22. Elder CW, Yoo PB. Co-activation of saphenous nerve fibers: A potential therapeutic mechanism of percutaneous tibial nerve stimulation? In: 2016 38th Annual International Conference of the IEEE Engineering in Medicine and Biology Society (EMBC). Orlando: 2016. p. 3129–32. https://doi.org/10.1109/EMBC.2016.7591392.
23. Moazzam Z, Yoo PB. Frequency-dependent inhibition of bladder function by saphenous nerve stimulation in anesthetized rats. Neurourol Urodyn. 2017. In press.
24. Govier FE, et al. Percutaneous afferent neuromodulation for the refractory overactive bladder: results of a multicenter study. J Urol. 2001;165(4):1193–8.

25. Ferroni MC, et al. Transcutaneous electrical nerve stimulation of the foot: results of a novel at-home, noninvasive treatment for nocturnal enuresis in children. Urology. 2017;101:80–4.
26. Schreiner L, dos Santos TG, Knorst MR, da Silva Filho IG. Randomized trial of transcutaneous tibial nerve stimulation to treat urge urinary incontinence in older women. Int Urogynecol J Pelvic Floor Dysfunct. 2010;21(9):1065–70.
27. Booth J, et al. A feasibility study of Transcutaneous posterior Tibial nerve stimulation for bladder and bowel dysfunction in elderly adults in residential care. J Am Med Dir Assoc. 2013;14(4):270–4.
28. Patidar N, Mittal V, Kumar M, Sureka SK, Arora S, Ansari MS. Transcutaneous posterior tibial nerve stimulation in pediatric overactive bladder: a preliminary report. J Pediatr Urol. 2015;11(6):351.e1–6.
29. De Sèze M, et al. Transcutaneous posterior tibial nerve stimulation for treatment of the overactive bladder syndrome in multiple sclerosis: results of a multicenter prospective study. Neurourol Urodyn. 2011;30(3):306–11.
30. Elder CW and Yoo PB. A Finite Element Modeling Study of Peripheral Nerve Recruitment by Percutaneous Tibial Nerve Stimulation in the Human Lower Leg. Med Eng Phys. (In press).
31. Burton C, Sajja A, Latthe PMPM, Sajja A, Latthe PM. Effectiveness of percutaneous posterior tibial nerve stimulation for overactive bladder: a systematic review and meta-analysis. Neurourol Urodyn. 2012;31(8):1206–16.
32. Lyons GM, Leane GE, Clarke-Moloney M, O'Brien JV, Grace PA. An investigation of the effect of electrode size and electrode location on comfort during stimulation of the gastrocnemius muscle. Med Eng Phys. 2004;26(10):873–8.

28

Impact of endoscopic enucleation of the prostate with thulium fiber laser on the erectile function

Dmitry Enikeev[1]* (iD), Petr Glybochko[1], Leonid Rapoport[1], Zhamshid Okhunov[2], Mitchel O'Leary[2], Natalya Potoldykova[1], Roman Sukhanov[1], Mikhail Enikeev[1], Ekaterina Laukhtina[1] and Mark Taratkin[1]

Abstract

Background: The impact of number of endoscopic enucleation of the prostate techniques (holmium laser enucleation - HoLEP for example) on erectile function have already been investigated. However, the thulium-fiber laser, in this setting remains unstudied. In this study, we compared sexual function outcomes in patients with benign prostatic hyperplasia (BPH) treated with transurethral resection of the prostate (TURP) or thulium-fiber laser enucleation (ThuFLEP).

Methods: We performed a retrospective analysis of patients who underwent transurethral resection and endoscopic enucleation of the prostate for BPH; inclusion criteria was the presence of infravesical obstruction (IPSS > 20, Qmax < 10 mL/s). Erectile function (EF) was assessed using the International Index of Erectile Function (IIEF-5) both prior to endoscopic examination, and six months after.

Results: A total of 469 patients with BPH were included in the study; of these, 211 underwent to ThuFLEP, and 258 TURP. Preoperative IIEF-5 in TURP and ThuFLEP groups were 11.7 ($\pm$4.5) and 11.1 ($\pm$5.0), respectively ($p = 0.17$). At six month the IIEF-5 score was unchanged ($p = 0.26$ and $p = 0.08$) and comparable in both groups ($p = 0.49$). However, mean IIEF-5 score shown significant increase of 0.72 in ThuFLEP group, comparing to decrease of 0.24 in TURP patients ($p < 0.001$).

Conclusions: Both TURP and ThuFLEP are effective modalities in the management of infravesical obstruction due to BPH. At six months follow-up after surgery, both techniques lead to comparable IIEF-5 score. However, our results demonstrated that the ThuFLEP is more likely to preserve the erectile function leading to increase of IIEF-5 at six months in contrast to TURP which lead to slight drop in IIEF-5 score.

Keywords: Thulium fiber laser, Endoscopic enucleation of the prostate, BPH, Erectile function, ThuFLEP

Background

Benign prostatic hyperplasia (BPH) is expected to afflict 50% of men over the age of 50 [1]. It has been demonstrated [2–4] that there is an association between BPH and erectile dysfunction (ED). BPH has also been shown to deteriorate the existing erectile disturbances or to become one of the causes of its development [2]. Conversely, timely surgical treatment of BPH (i.e. transurethral resection of the prostate (TURP)) has been shown to perturb the development of erectile dysfunction [4]. As the BPH in most cases is not a life-threatening condition, the main

outcomes of it is treatment not only the improvement in an international prostate symptom score (IPSS) (as the outcome that shows the micturition quality), but the men's quality of life after surgery. With significant sexual activity of aging males the question of the effect of transurethral surgery on erectile function is prominent [5].

The impact of number of endoscopic enucleation of the prostate techniques on erectile function has already been investigated [6, 7]. A study assessing the influence of a thulium fiber laser (Tm-fiber) enucleation of the prostate (ThuFLEP), however, is currently lacking. Different from widely used Tm:YAG laser (in ThuLEP and ThuVEP techniques), Tm-fiber laser allows to minimize penetration depth (2-times in comparison to Tm:YAG), which reduces tissue damage and allows to perform precise incisions [8].

* Correspondence: dvenikeev@gmail.com
[1]Institute for Urology and Reproductive Health, Sechenov University, Moscow, Russia
Full list of author information is available at the end of the article

This is possible due to Tm-fiber laser wavelength of 1940 nm (vs 2010 nm of Tm:YAG), which leads to increase of laser energy absorption in tissue, allowing to decrease the penetration depth and leading to instantaneous vaporization [9, 10]. Also, it is believed that the use of Tm-fiber laser may to decrease the carbonization rate, comparing to Tm:YAG lasers [9]. Unlike the Tm:YAG laser which consists of several flash-lamp pumped Tm:YAG crystals the Tm-fiber laser use in it is construction the laser fiber pumped by diode laser, which leads to difference in wavelength and smaller size of the laser device.

The objective of this study was to assess the efficacy and safety of the Tm-fiber laser and evaluate its impact on erectile dysfunction (ED) in patients who underwent ThuFLEP comparing to patients, who underwent the standard monopolar TURP.

Methods

Patient identification and data collection

We performed a retrospective analysis of patients who underwent ThuFLEP or TURP for infravesical obstruction due to BPH between December 2012 and February 2018. Inclusion criteria was the presence of infravesical obstruction (defined as IPSS > 20, Qmax < 10 mL/s). Patients were excluded from analysis if they had prostate cancer, urethral strictures, or bladder calculi.

Surgical technique

We used the Urolase (NTO IRE-Polus, Russia) (120 W) Tm-fiber laser with wavelength of 1940 nm and a 600-μm laser fiber, and a 26 Ch resectoscope (Karl Storz, Germany) with continuous irrigation (0.9% saline). All ThuFLEP procedures were performed as previously described [11]. In ThuFLEP technique (Tm fiber laser) we usually perform 70% of the surgery dissecting the tissue with laser energy and only 30% of the surgery are usually done in blunt enucleation, in contrast to ThuLEP technique (Tm:YAG laser) with exact opposite ratio of blunt and laser dissection.

Instantaneous vaporization of the tissue and small penetration depth of Tm-fiber laser allows to perform fast and precise incisions with minimal need for coagulation of bleeding vessels. All procedure steps, except the incision at veromontanum was performed in 60 W (1.5 J) power setting, however at veromontanum we decreased the energy to 30 W. We suggest that it may preserve the sphincter zone and decrease the incontinence rate. Adenomatous tissue was retrieved using a 5-mm cystoscope and a morcellator (Piranha, Richard Wolf, Germany). Monopolar TURP (5% glucose) with Ch 24 resectoscope (Karl Storz, Germany) was performed on 258 patients whose ages varied between 54 and 83 years (average 68.0 ± 6.7 years). Prostatic vessels were coagulated with a roller electrode (if necessary).

Study outcomes

Primary outcome of the study was to assess the difference in erectile function (EF), which was measured using the five-item version of the International Index of Erectile Function (IIEF-5) both prior to surgery and six months after. Secondary outcome of the study was decrease of infravesical obstruction severity, which was assessed using International Prostate Symptom Score (IPSS) and the maximum flow rate (Qmax).

Statistical analysis

Baseline characteristics, perioperative data, and descriptive statistics from the procedures were collected. Continuous variables were compared by one-way ANOVA test. Categorical variables were compared by via Chi square tests. Nonparametric variables were compared with Kolmogorov–Smirnov and Kruskall-Wallis tests. Post Hoc analysis was performed with Mann-Whitney U Test. Propensity score matching for comparison of patients with different prostate volume and surgery time was done (with SPSS Propensity score matching). All statistical analyses were carried out using SPSS Statistics 23.0 (SPSS Inc., Chicago, IL, USA). A p-value < 0.05 was considered to indicate statistical significance.

Results

A total of 469 patients were included in the study. The mean age of the patients subjected to ThuFLEP (211) was 67 ± 7.4 years. The average prostate volume in this group was 90 ± 42.9 cc (30–250 cc), with an average PSA of 4.7 ± 2.7 ng/mL. The mean age in TURP group (258) was 68 ± 6.7 average prostate volume in TURP group was 63.0 ± 17.1 cc (30–89 cc), with a total PSA level of 4.2 ± 2.3 ng/mL (Table 1). The larger prostate volume in ThuFLEP group was not suggested as the limitation, because both groups were comparable in preoperative IPSS, Qmax and IIEF-5 scores ($p = 0.22$; $p = 0.06$; $p = 0.17$) (Table 2) (additional analyses with propensity score matching was done).

The average operative time was 72 min in the ThuFLEP group, and 54 min in the TURP group. A urethral catheter was left in place for 1–2 days in the ThuFLEP group, and 3–4 days in the TURP group. Average hospital stay was 3 and 5 days for the ThuFLEP and TURP groups, respectively. The ThuFLEP duration was longer than TURP ($p < 0,001$) (due to larger prostate volume

Table 1 Patients demographics and clinical characteristics

	ThuFLEP (n = 211)	TURP (n = 258)	p
Age (years, mean, range)	67 ± 7.4	68 ± 6.7	0.22
Prostate volume (cc, mean, range)	90 ± 42.9	63 ± 17.1	< 0.001*
PSA (ng/ml, mean, range)	4.7 ± 2.7	4.2 ± 2.3	0.03*

*statistically significant difference. Data given as mean ± SD

Table 2 Pre- and postoperative functional results at six months

	ThuFLEP (n = 211)	TURP (n = 258)	p
IPSS – preop. (score)	21.8 (± 1.6)	21.6 (±1.7)	0.22
IPSS – postop. (score)	10.9 (± 3.0)	10.6 (±3.2)	0.35
p	< 0.001*	< 0.001*	
QoL – preop. (score)	4.0 (± 0.8)	3.9 (±0.8)	0.23
QoL – postop. (score)	1.8 (± 0.6)	1.7 (±0.6)	0.38
p	< 0.001*	< 0.001*	
Qmax – preop. (ml/s)	7.5 (± 1.7)	7.8 (±1.9)	0.06
Qmax – postop. (ml/s)	16.2 (± 3.3)	16.6 (±1.5)	0.08
p	< 0.001*	< 0.001*	
PVR – preop. (ml)	70.1 (± 28.7)	68.7 (±21.5)	0.08
PVR – postop. (ml)	17.3 (± 11.7)	15.3 (±13.6)	0.08
p	< 0.001*	< 0.001*	
IIEF-5 – preop. (score)	11.1 ± 5.0	11.7 ± 4.5	0.17
IIEF-5 – postop.(score)	11.7 ± 4.7	11.5 ± 4.7	0.49
p	0.08	0.26	
IIEF-5 change	▲0.72 ± 1.6	▼0.24 ± 2.2	p < 0.001*

*statistically significant difference; ▲ – increase of score; ▼ – decrease of score. Data given as mean ± SD

and technical aspects of techniques). The catheterization length and hospital stay were in favor of ThuFLEP ($p < 0,001$). At six months follow up, each group had a significant improvement in the IPSS, QoL and Qmax (Table 2).

IIEF-5 score in TURP group remained stable (average preoperative value: $11.7 ± 4.5$; average postoperative value: $11.5 ± 4.7$). EF following TURP was unchanged in 43% of patients; improved EF - 21% of patients and impaired EF in 34% of patients. De novo erectile dysfunction (mild) was found in 5 (2%) patients.

Similarly, no significant change in EF was seen in patients subjected to ThuFLEP. The average IIEF-5 value before surgery was $11.1 ± 5.0$, and that 6 months after surgery was $11.7 ± 4.7$. The EF following ThuFLEP remained stable in 56%, improve in 26% of patients and decreased in 18% of patients. There was no de novo ED in patients within the ThuFLEP group. Therefore, both techniques, were comparable in postoperative IIEF-5. However, mean increase of IIEF-5 score in ThuFLEP group was about $0.72 ± 1.6$ while the IIEF-5 score in TURP group show decrease of $0.24 ± 2.2$ (Table 2). This difference between the two techniques was statistically significant ($p < 0.001$) (Fig. 1). Due to difference in the preoperative prostate volume and operative time we did propensity score matching, which has confirmed our results with mean decrease of IIEF-5 in TURP patients of 0.24 and increase in ThuFLEP group of 0.7 ($p < 0.001$), no difference were found in pre- and postoperative IIEF-5 scores between two groups ($p = 0.09$ and $p = 0.77$, respectively).

Our next step was to compare the erectile function change in groups of patients with different stages of ED (assessed with IIEF-5 score) (Fig. 2). In patients with severe ED (1–7) no difference between TURP and ThuFLEP ($p = 0.76$) was observed, moreover both techniques allowed slight, yet significant increase of EF ($p < 0.001$). In moderate ED group (8–11) ThuFLEP showed no influence on EF, whereas TURP led to slight decrease ($p = 0.05$), with significant difference between the techniques ($p = 0.002$). In patients with mild-moderate ED (12–16) ThuFLEP led to increase ($p = 0.04$) and TURP to decrease of EF ($p = 0.031$) with significant difference between the techniques ($p = 0.001$). In patients with mild ED (12–16) or without ED (22–25) ThuFLEP showed no influence on IIEF-5 score ($p = 0.617$ and $p = 0.192$, respectively), whereas TURP decreased IIEF-5 score in patients with mild ED (p = 0.04) and had no influence on the patients without ED ($p = 0.08$).

To estimate the possible influence of other EF-affecting diseases and disorders we compared the IIEF-5 differences in patients with obesity (ThuFLEP – 55 and TURP – 68), cardiovascular diseases (ThuFLEP 40 and TURP 65) and diabetes mellitus (ThuFLEP 15 and TURP 17). We did not observe increase or decrease of EF for such patients in both in ThuFLEP and TURP groups ($p = 0.1$, $p = 0.1$ and $p = 0.257$, respectively).

Among short-term complications most frequent was clot retention, which was found in 17 (6.6%) and 9 (4.3%) patients after TURP and ThuFLEP, respectively (0.373). In three patients (1.4%) after ThuFLEP we encounter superficial bladder wall damage with the morcellator. One patient after TURP necessitated blood transfusion (0.4%), and one had TURP-syndrome (0.4%). Six months after surgery 10 (3.9%) patients in TURP group and 2 (0.9%) in ThuFLEP group had urinary incontinence ($p = 0.9$); urethral stricture was found in 3 (1.2%) after TURP and 1 (0.5%) after ThuFLEP (0.806), the bladder neck sclerosis was found in 5 (1.9) and 1 (0.5) patient ($p = 0.088$) after TURP and ThuFLEP, respectively.

Discussion

At six months, both surgical modalities were equally efficacious in eliminating infravesical obstruction due to BPH. A longer thulium enucleation time demonstrated in our study (72 min versus 54 min) is mostly attributed to a larger BPH volume within the ThuFLEP group (90 cc on average) compared to the TURP group (BPH is 63 cc on average). However, propensity score matching allowed to rule out it is influence on the results.

The results of recent meta-analyses and systematic reviews show endoscopic enucleation to be highly efficacious in the treatment of BPH, and to have comparable postoperative outcomes to TURP [12–14]. Both techniques are very effective regarding IPSS and Qmax outcomes, however, the

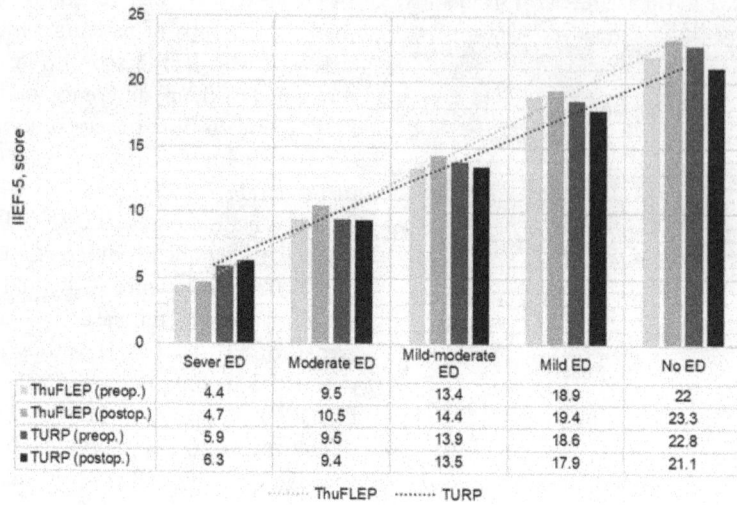

Fig. 1 IIEF-5 prior and six months after the surgery

	Sever ED	Moderate ED	Mild-moderate ED	Mild ED	No ED
ThuFLEP (preop.)	4.4	9.5	13.4	18.9	22
ThuFLEP (postop.)	4.7	10.5	14.4	19.4	23.3
TURP (preop.)	5.9	9.5	13.9	18.6	22.8
TURP (postop.)	6.3	9.4	13.5	17.9	21.1

effect of surgical treatment of benign prostatic enlargement (BPE) on EF after surgery remain the subject of discussion amongst Urologists. Certain authors [15] suggest that ED is function of age; others relate it to preexisting ED [16]. Hanbury et al. [17] suggest that erectile dysfunction may be caused by intraoperative injury of the prostatic capsule and the adjacent neurovascular bundles during TURP. According to the data of different investigations [15, 18, 19], ED as a consequence of TURP occurs in up to 35% of patients. Nevertheless, it should be mentioned that certain decrease of EF in these patients is frequently diagnosed before surgical intervention [15].

In our work, the erectile function following TURP remained intact in 43% of cases. EF was restored in 21% of patients, and impaired in 36% of patients. No statistically significant differences between the pre- and postoperative means were noted according to IIEF-5 score assessment. These facts may indicate that the EF did not change significantly after TURP. Similar data was obtained by Muenter et al. [20]. They note that TURP did not lead to changes in EF within 52% of patients, and that EF improved, albeit insignificantly, in 29%. Moreover, EF was shown to decrease in only 19% of their patients. The authors believed, however, that the reason

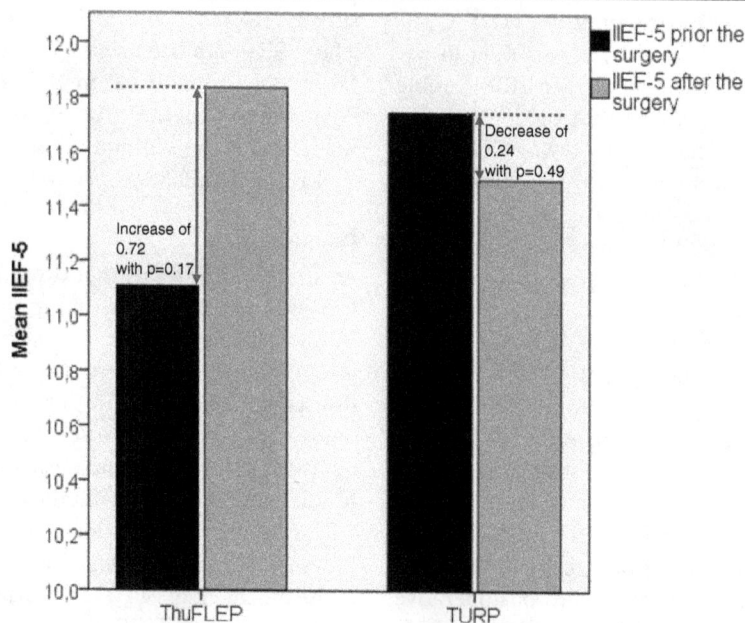

Fig. 2 IIEF-5 score in patients with different stages of ED

for such decrease is the neurovascular bundles damage, because of the generated monopolar current passed in close proximity to the prostatic capsule [20]. This theory was in part confirmed by Li et al. [21], as they indicated in their meta-analysis a predominantly small EF decrease during a short-term follow-up. However, at a follow-up of 12 months after TURP, the average EF values returned to normal and did not differ from those recorded preoperatively, especially in patients presenting with an initially high EF value [21].

In turn, the holmium and thulium lasers are distinguished by a smaller tissue penetration depth when compared to the electrocoagulation used in TURP [10]. According to EAU guidelines on laser technologies [10], the application of thulium laser enhances hemostasis, minimizes the degree of damage to the underlying tissues, and allows the capsule and the neurovascular bundles intimately adjacent to the posterolateral surface of the prostate to remain intact. Tiburtius et al. [22] demonstrated the action of a thulium:YAG laser on the erectile function, and found a small but significant increase (from 19 to 20) in the IIEF-5 score at a follow-up of 12 months. This finding was attributed to the shallow penetration depth of Tm:YAG energy.

According to our data, the average outcomes as assessed by IIEF-5 before and after surgery did not change substantially. However, it was shown that in contrast to TURP, ThuFLEP allows to significantly increase IIEF-5 score. Fried et al. suggested that the shallow laser penetration depth of a Tm-fiber laser is due to its wavelength being close to that of the water absorption peak [9]. Prostate tissues contain a considerable amount of water, and the energy is transmitted to tissues more effectively at such a wavelength [9, 10]. Thus, safer incisions can be made at a lower risk of perforating the surgical capsule and damaging the neurovascular bundles intimately adjacent to the posterolateral surface of the prostate. Another possible explanation may be that enucleation procedure itself allows significant increase of urinary function and faster rehabilitation, which together with increase of quality of life may facilitate EF recovery.

This suggestion for thulium laser is supported by Iacono et al. [23]: at 12 months after surgery, the erectile function was completely restored in all the patients enrolled in the study, a finding linked to the low probability of perforation of the surgical capsule found with employing a thulium laser. This reduces the risk of erectile dysfunction by means of an injury to the neurovascular bundles. Similar data was obtained by Chung et al. [24] who described EF to decline three months after ThuLEP performance. ED was revealed in both patients with already existing erectile disturbances, and in those without erectile complaints. Close correlation was observed between the IIEF-5 score assessment and the age of the patients. It was noted that the older the patient, the more marked the decline in EF was.

At 12 months of follow-up, however, the functional outcomes as assessed by the IIEF-5 returned to the preoperative level in both groups. This led them to conclude that ThuLEP does not have a long-term negative impact on erectile function [24]. However Iacono et al. and Chung et al. studies were conducted with Tm:YAG laser, which is different from Tm-fiber laser technology and ThuFLEP procedure [23, 24].

In our study, the erectile function after ThuFLEP remained unchanged in 56% of patients. The functional outcomes as assessed by the IIEF-5 score after surgery improved in 26% of patients and decreased in 18% of observations. In most patients, no changes in the erectile function were noted. As for the patients with obesity, cardiovascular diseases and diabetes mellitus, no change in EF was noted, which may signify that in such patients EF was affected not with urination disorders/BPH, but with other pathology. In groups of the patients with different stages of preoperative ED (from "sever ED" to "No ED") we found that ThuFLEP allowed to preserve EF in all groups and even increase it in patients with severe and mild-moderate ED. TURP led to increase of EF in patients with severe ED, showed no influence on the patients without ED and decreased EF in all other groups. Generally, the IIEF-5 decrease in TURP by 0.24 and increased by 0.72 in ThuFLEP group. Such a slight difference between two techniques, may not be of high clinical significance, still it shows that ThuFLEP is more likely to increase or preserve EF in contrast to TURP. Which in turn mean, that laser enucleation with Tm-fiber laser may be considered as one of the possible techniques of choice for patients who concerned of theirs EF. Still, this statement is theoretical, and further investigation is necessary.

Among main limitations of the study were its retrospective nature and absence of long-term data (up to 12 months). Another limitation was use of the simplified IIEF version – IIEF-5 questionnaire, which did not allow us to precisely estimate changes in the different components of erectile function.

Conclusions

Both TURP and ThuFLEP have shown to be effective in the management of infravesical obstruction due to BPH. Despite the absence of statistically significant differences in the IIEF-5 assessments before and after surgery, the application of a Tm-fiber laser in 26% of patients with significant ED resulted in the improvement in EF. In contrast to TURP it allowed to perform slight, but significant increase of IIEF-5. ThuFLEP can be considered to retain, and in certain cases, increase the erectile function.

Abbreviations
BPH: Benign prostatic hyperplasia; ED : Erectile dysfunction; EF: Erectile function; HoLEP: Holmium laser enucleation; IIEF-5: International Index of Erectile Function; IPSS: International prostate symptom score; QoL: Quality of

life; ThuFLEP : Tm-fiber laser enucleation; ThuLEP : Thulium laser enucleation; Tm-fiber: Thulium fiber laser; TURP: Transurethral resection of the prostate

Authors' contributions
DV - Manuscript writing/editing, Protocol/project development; PG - Protocol/project development; LR - Protocol/project development, acquisition of funding; ZO - Manuscript writing/editing, protocol/project development; MO - Manuscript writing/editing, collection of data, data analysis; NP - Data analysis, data obtaining; RS – Data obtaining, data analysis; ME – Manuscript editing; Protocol development; EL - Manuscript writing, data analysis; MT- Manuscript writing/editing; Protocol/project development; Data analysis. All authors read and approved the final manuscript.

Competing interests
The authors declare that they have no competing interests.

Author details
[1]Institute for Urology and Reproductive Health, Sechenov University, Moscow, Russia. [2]Department of Urology, University of California, Irvine; Orange, CA, USA.

References
1. Vuichoud C, Loughlin KR. Benign prostatic hyperplasia: epidemiology, economics and evaluation. Can J Urol. 2015;22(Suppl 1):1–6.
2. Rosen R, Altwein J, Boyle P, Kirby RS, Lukacs B, Meuleman E, O'Leary MP, Puppo P, Robertson C, Giuliano F. Lower urinary tract symptoms and male sexual dysfunction: the multinational survey of the aging male (MSAM-7). Eur Urol. 2003;44(6):637–49.
3. Gacci M, Bartoletti R, Figlioli S, Sarti E, Eisner B, Boddi V, Rizzo M. Urinary symptoms, quality of life and sexual function in patients with benign prostatic hypertrophy before and after prostatectomy: a prospective study. BJU Int. 2003;91(3):196–200.
4. Park HJ, Won JE, Sorsaburu S, Rivera PD, Lee SW. Urinary tract symptoms (LUTS) secondary to benign prostatic hyperplasia (BPH) and LUTS/BPH with erectile dysfunction in Asian men: a systematic review focusing on Tadalafil. World J Mens Health. 2013;31(3):193–207.
5. Becher EF, McVary KT. Surgical procedures for BPH/LUTS: impact on male sexual health. Sex Med Rev. 2014;2(1):47–55.
6. Elshal AM, El-Assmy A, Mekkawy R, Taha DE, El-Nahas AR, Laymon M, El-Kappany H, Ibrahiem EH. Prospective controlled assessment of men's sexual function changes following holmium laser enucleation of the prostate for treatment of benign prostate hyperplasia. Int Urol Nephrol. 2017;49(10):1741–9.
7. Saredi G, Pacchetti A, Pirola GM, Martorana E, Berti L, Scroppo FI, Marconi AM. Impact of thulium laser enucleation of the prostate on erectile, ejaculatory and urinary functions. Urol Int. 2016;97(4):397–401.
8. Enikeev DV, Glybochko PV, Okhunov Z, Alyaev YG, Rapoport LM, Tsarichenko D, Enikeev ME, Sorokin NI, Dymov AM, Taratkin MS. Retrospective analysis of short-term outcomes after monopolar versus laser endoscopic enucleation of the prostate: a single center experience. J Endourol. 2018;32(5):417–23.
9. Fried NM, Murray KE. High-power thulium fiber laser ablation of urinary tissues at 1.94 microm. J Endourol. 2005;19(1):25–31.
10. Herrmann TR, Liatsikos EN, Nagele U, Traxer O, Merseburger AS. EAU guidelines panel on lasers T: EAU guidelines on laser technologies. Eur Urol. 2012;61(4):783–95.
11. Enikeev D, Glybochko P, Rapoport L, Gahan J, Gazimiev M, Spivak L, Enikeev M, Taratkin M. A randomized trial comparing the learning curve of three endoscopic enucleation techniques (HoLEP, ThuFLEP and MEP) for BPH using mentoring approach - initial results. Urology. 2018. https://doi.org/10.1016/j.urology.2018.06.045.
12. Becker B, Netsch C, Glybochko P, Rapoport L, Taratkin M, Enikeev D. A feasibility study utilizing the thulium and holmium laser in patients for the treatment of recurrent benign prostatic hyperplasia after previous prostatic surgery. Urol Int. 2018;101(2):212–8.
13. Netsch C, Engbert A, Bach T, Gross AJ. Long-term outcome following thulium VapoEnucleation of the prostate. World J Urol. 2014;32(6):1551–8.
14. Cornu JN, Ahyai S, Bachmann A, de la Rosette J, Gilling P, Gratzke C, McVary K, Novara G, Woo H, Madersbacher S. A systematic review and meta-analysis of functional outcomes and complications following transurethral procedures for lower urinary tract symptoms resulting from benign prostatic obstruction: an update. Eur Urol. 2015;67(6):1066–96.
15. Soderdahl DW, Knight RW, Hansberry KL. Erectile dysfunction following transurethral resection of the prostate. J Urol. 1996;156(4):1354–6.
16. Tscholl R, Largo M, Poppinghaus E, Recker F, Subotic B. Incidence of erectile impotence secondary to transurethral resection of benign prostatic hyperplasia, assessed by preoperative and postoperative snap gauge tests. J Urol. 1995;153(5):1491–3.
17. Hanbury DC, Sethia KK. Erectile function following transurethral prostatectomy. Br J Urol. 1995;75(1):12–3.
18. Taher A. Erectile dysfunction after transurethral resection of the prostate: incidence and risk factors. World J Urol. 2004;22(6):457–60.
19. Miner M, Rosenberg MT, Perelman MA. Treatment of lower urinary tract symptoms in benign prostatic hyperplasia and its impact on sexual function. Clin Ther. 2006;28(1):13–25.
20. Muntener M, Aellig S, Kuettel R, Gehrlach C, Sulser T, Strebel RT. Sexual function after transurethral resection of the prostate (TURP): results of an independent prospective multicentre assessment of outcome. Eur Urol. 2007;52(2):510–5.
21. Li Z, Chen P, Wang J, Mao Q, Xiang H, Wang X, Wang X, Zhang X. The impact of surgical treatments for lower urinary tract symptoms/benign prostatic hyperplasia on male erectile function: a systematic review and network meta-analysis. Medicine (Baltimore). 2016;95(24):e3862.
22. Tiburtius C, Knipper S, Gross AJ, Netsch C. Impact of thulium VapoEnucleation of the prostate on erectile function: a prospective analysis of 72 patients at 12-month follow-up. Urology. 2014;83(1):175–80.
23. Iacono F, Prezioso D, Di Lauro G, Romeo G, Ruffo A, Illiano E, Amato B. Efficacy and safety profile of a novel technique, ThuLEP (thulium laser enucleation of the prostate) for the treatment of benign prostate hypertrophy. Our experience on 148 patients. BMC Surg. 2012;12(Suppl 1):S21.
24. Chung JS, Park SH, Oh CK, Kim SC, Kim TS, Kang PM, Seo WI, Kim WS, Yoon JH, Kang DI, et al. Longitudinal changes in erectile function after thulium: YAG prostatectomy for the treatment of benign prostatic obstruction: a 1-year follow-up study. Lasers Med Sci. 2017;32(7):1517–23.

29

Pre- and intra-operative predictors of postoperative hospital length of stay in patients undergoing radical prostatectomy for prostate cancer in China: a retrospective observational study

Qingmei Huang, Ping Jiang, Lina Feng, Liping Xie, Shuo Wang, Dan Xia, Baihua Shen, Baiye Jin, Li Zheng and Wei Wang[*]

Abstract

Background: Hospital length of stay (LOS) has recently been receiving increasing attention as a marker of medical resource consumption. Identifying predictors of longer LOS can better equip doctors to counsel patients and facilitate more efficient patient flow and utilization of medical resources. The objective of this study was to identify pre- and intra-operative risk factors for postoperative hospital LOS in patients who had undergone radical prostatectomy in China.

Methods: We retrospectively analyzed data of 793 eligible patients with prostate cancer who had undergone radical prostatectomy in our institution between January 2011 and March 2016. Relevant preoperative variables, including patient characteristics, medical comorbidities, prostate cancer disease-specific variables, urinary tract symptoms, preoperative laboratory values, and intraoperative variables including operation type, operation duration, and blood loss, were analyzed. The outcome was postoperative length of stay which was calculated as the time from the date of operation to the date of discharge. Multiple linear regression analysis was used to identify predictors of this outcome.

Results: The mean postoperative LOS was 11.7 days (±4.6 days) and the median 10 days (range, 5–46 days). According to univariate and multivariate analysis, operation type (open or laparoscopic), blood loss, Gleason score (≥8) and preoperative laboratory values of white blood count (WBC) were found to be the main explanatory predictors of postoperative LOS of patients with prostate cancer in our institution. Additionally, open surgery was the strongest significant predictor of longer LOS according to the standardized coefficients in this model.

Conclusions: Our findings indicate that significant predictors of longer postoperative LOS in patients who have undergone radical prostatectomy in China include both preoperative variables of Gleason score, WBC and intraoperative variables of operation type (open or laparoscopic), blood loss. To shorten hospital LOS in patients with prostate cancer and optimize utilization of Chinese medical resources, efforts should be made to improve the intraoperative process and reduce the prevalence of preoperative risk factors.

Keywords: Prostate cancer, Radical prostatectomy, Predictor, Length of stay, China

* Correspondence: wangw2005@zju.edu.cn
Department of Urology, The First Affiliated Hospital, College of Medicine, Zhejiang University, 79 Qingchun Road, Hangzhou 310003, Zhejiang, China

Background

Prostate cancer is the commonest cancer in men [1] and radical prostatectomy is one of the main treatments for clinically localized prostate cancer [2]. With increasing aging of China's population, the number of patients with newly diagnosed prostate cancer has been increasing continuously in recent years [3, 4], challenging Chinese medical institutions to provide adequate care despite limited medical resources. In recent years, hospital length of stay (LOS) has been increasingly used as a marker for medical resource consumption [5–7]. Prolonged LOS is not only associated with higher medical costs and resource consumption [5, 8], but may also place patients at greater risk of complications, including hospital-acquired infections and deep vein thrombosis [9, 10]. In China, there is another important consideration regarding LOS, especially for patients who are to undergo elective surgery, including radical prostatectomy. The limited number of hospital beds means that such patients must wait for a bed to become available, which frequently depends on other patients being discharged. Thus, it is important to identify risk factors for prolonged LOS and provide strategies for shortening LOS and reducing unnecessary resource utilization.

Numerous risk factors are associated with prolonged LOS, including preoperative and intraoperative factors and postoperative complications [11]. Studies focusing on preoperative risk factors have pointed out that some of them are important predictors of LOS [12]. One recent study evaluating factors that predict longer hospital stay in patients who have undergone robot-assisted radical prostatectomy (RARP) identified patient comorbidity as the only independent preoperative predictor of prolonged hospital LOS [13]. Previous studies exploring both pre- and intra-operative risk factors for prolonged LOS after commonly-performed urologic surgery, including prostatectomy, have identified some with significant impact, including older age, low hematocrit, high creatinine, operation duration, and intraoperative transfusion [11, 14]. However, because these researchers did not analyze disease-specific variables, these factors remain unexplored for patients with prostate cancer.

Elucidating risk factors that are significantly associated with LOS may help physicians to identify patients at greater risk for prolonged LOS and thus provide more appropriate counseling [12], as well as ultimately facilitating more efficient patient flow and operations management. However, the findings of studies conducted in Western countries may not be applicable to Chinese men with prostate cancer [15]. As far as we know, no studies have explored risk factors related to prolonged hospital LOS in Chinese inpatients who have undergone radical prostatectomy for prostate cancer. We therefore comprehensively collected possible risk factors, including patient characteristics, comorbidities, disease-specific variables, urinary tract symptoms, preoperative laboratory values, and intra-operative variables, with the aim of examining pre- and intra-operative predictors of prolonged LOS for prostate cancer patients in China.

Methods

Study sample

Between January 2011 and March 2016, 836 consecutive patients with localized prostate cancer underwent radical prostatectomy and were discharged from our institution. Only patients with the pathological diagnosis of prostatic adenocarcinoma were included in this study, those with sarcoma of the prostate being excluded. Patients who had undergone transurethral resection of the prostate or another operation for concomitant diseases during the period of hospitalization were also excluded. Additionally, patients for whom equal to or more than three study variables were unavailable were also excluded from the final analysis. All patients' data were extracted by a trained clinical reviewer from electronic medical records maintained in a secure clinical database at our institution. After applying inclusion and exclusion criteria, 793 inpatients were included in the final analysis. The flowchart of screening for eligibility for the study is shown in Fig. 1.

Dependent variable: Postoperative LOS

The primary outcome variable was postoperative LOS in days, which was calculated from the date of operation to the date of discharge. Because the data of LOS in days were not normally distributed, these data were subjected to reciprocal transformation to meet the model assumption of a normal distribution. The reciprocally transformed LOS was then used as the dependent variable in the subsequent multiple linear regression analysis.

Independent variables measured

In this study, 32 variables were assessed. Preoperative variables included patient characteristics, comorbidities, prostate cancer disease-specific variables, urinary tract symptoms, and preoperative laboratory values. Patient characteristics assessed included age, body mass index (BMI), marital status, smoking and drinking status, and family history of prostate cancer. Comorbidities, including hypertension requiring medication; diabetes requiring either oral medication or insulin injections or both; and history of cardiovascular and cerebrovascular disease were combined into one variable because of the small positive sample size. History of cardiovascular and cerebrovascular disease was treated as a dichotomous variable and defined as positive in the presence of a history of myocardial infarction, coronary artery disease before or after coronary stent implantation, arrhythmia, transient ischemic attack, or cerebrovascular accident such as cerebral embolism, cerebral thrombosis, or

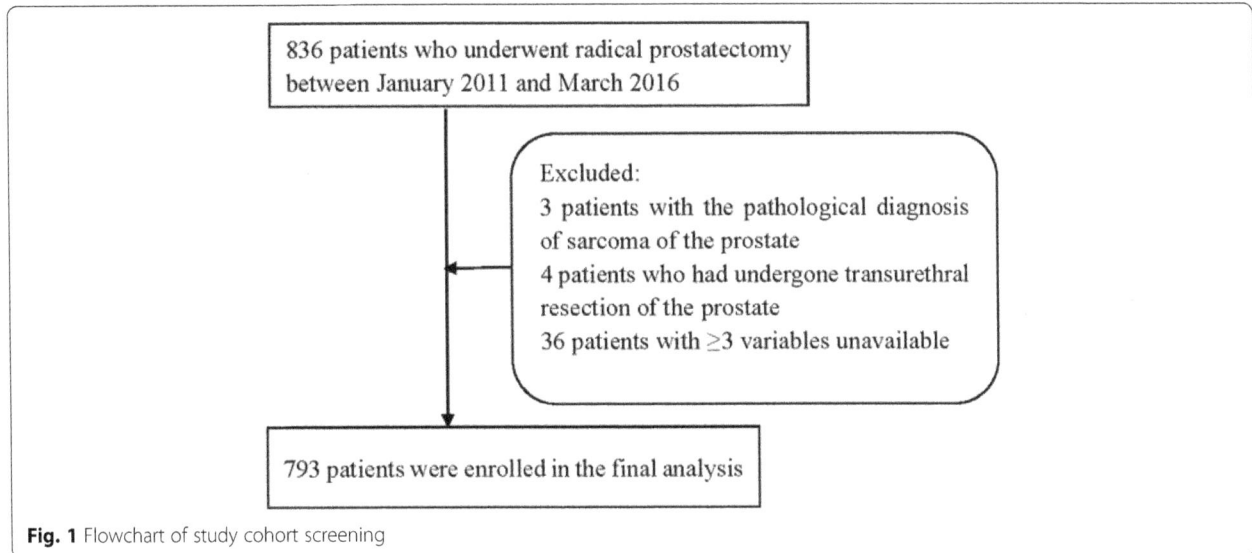

Fig. 1 Flowchart of study cohort screening

cerebral hemorrhage. The above information was abstracted from preoperative medical records. Inclusion of the disease-specific variable of prostate specific antigen (PSA) was considered essential; the most recent PSA value prior to surgery was used in the analysis. Biopsy Gleason scores were acquired from prostate biopsy reports. Prostate volume was calculated by using the following formula: transverse diameter × vertical diameter × longitudinal diameter × $\pi/6$; the diameters were measured by color ultrasound. Urinary tract symptoms, including dysuria, pain or burning on urination, frequent urination, urgent urination, and hematuria, were assessed as dichotomous variables and abstracted from medical records of symptoms reported by patients. Preoperative laboratory values closest to the day of surgery were also recorded, including white blood count ($\times 10^9$/L) (WBC), neutrophil count (%), hemoglobin, hematocrit, platelet count ($\times 10^9$/L), albumin, glutamic-pyruvic transaminase (GPT), serum total bilirubin, creatinine, serum potassium, serum calcium, and blood glucose. Intraoperative variables, including operation duration (h), blood loss (L), and operation type were collected from operation notes and operation logs. The type of surgery performed (open radical prostatectomy [ORP], laparoscopic radical prostatectomy [LRP], or robot-assisted radical prostatectomy [RARP]) was selected by each patient after discussion with the surgeon.

Statistical analysis

Continuous data are presented as mean ± standard deviation or median (interquartile range) and categorical data as frequency and percentage. Correlations between each variable and LOS were tested by univariate analysis, including the Mann–Whitney U test for variables with two subgroups, Kruskal–Wallis test for variables with

multiple subgroups and Spearman correlation analysis for continuous variables. Variables that were found to be significantly associated with LOS ($p \leq 0.1$; two-sided probability) in the univariate analysis were included in the subsequent multiple linear regression analysis by using stepwise selection methods. $P < 0.05$ was set as the criterion for inclusion of a variable in the final model. There were missing data in the variables of BMI, Prostate volume and Operation duration, while the extent of cases with one or two missing variables in the 793 patients was less than 3% and there were no statistically difference in LOS between cases with versus without missing data. Missing data were imputed by mean substitution and were included in the data analysis. All statistical analyses were performed using SPSS software (version 17.0, SPSS).

Results

The mean postoperative LOS for the entire sample was 11.7 days (± 4.6 days), and the median 10 days (range: 5–46 days; Fig. 2). The mean age of the 793 study patients was 67.0 ± 6.8 years and the mean BMI 23.7 ± 2.8 kg/m². The mean preoperative PSA value was 17.0 ± 22.3 ng/mL (range: 0.009–363.3 ng/mL), with 191 patients' (24.1%) value being in the high-risk range (PSA > 20 ng/mL). As to type of surgery, 325 patients (41.0%) had undergone ORP, 257 (32.4%) LRP, and 211 (26.6%) RARP. The mean operation time (hours) was 3.0 ± 0.9 h. Details of patient characteristics and pre- and intra-operative variables are listed in Table 1.

Table 1 shows variables significantly associated with LOS in days according to univariate analysis (P value ≤0.1). Both some pre- and intra-operative variables were associated with longer postoperative LOS; namely, the prostate cancer disease-specific variables of preoperative PSA value and

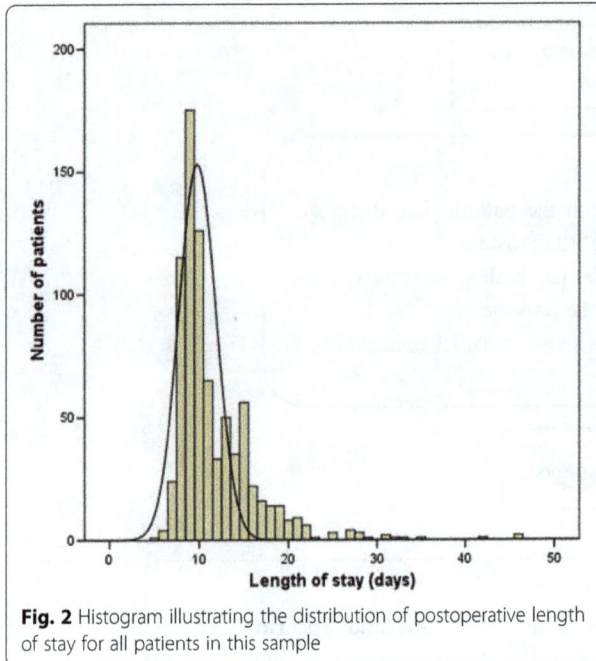

Fig. 2 Histogram illustrating the distribution of postoperative length of stay for all patients in this sample

biopsy Gleason score, urinary tract symptoms of dysuria, preoperative laboratory values for WBC, platelet count, serum calcium and blood glucose, and intraoperative variables of operation type, and blood loss. However, patient age was not a risk factor for longer LOS. Additionally, the intraoperative variable of operation duration was not found to be significantly associated with longer postoperative LOS. The same results were obtained when reciprocal-transformed LOS was subjected to univariate analysis.

Table 2 summarizes the results of multiple linear regression analysis. The intraoperative variables of operation type (open or laparoscopic) and blood loss, the disease-specific variable of Gleason score, and preoperative laboratory values of WBC were found to be the main explanatory factors for postoperative LOS of prostate cancer patients in our institution. Of the above variables, the operation type of open was the strongest significant predictor for longer LOS ($\beta = -0.325$), followed by blood loss ($\beta = -0.205$) according to the standardized coefficients (negative coefficients corresponding to longer LOS because of the reciprocal transformation). In addition, the disease-specific variable of Gleason score was an important predictor of longer postoperative LOS. The variable of WBC was inversely associated with LOS, which means that a lower preoperative white blood count is associated with a longer postoperative LOS. The R-squared value (indicator of fit) for the entire model is 20.5%, indicating that all of the significant variables in the model account for 20.5% variance in the postoperative LOS of men undergoing surgery for prostate cancer in China. In order to easily interpret the effect of the unstandardized coefficients of

the significant factors on LOS in days, we take the 50th percentile of LOS (10 days) for example. Specifically, if the open operation was conducted, the length of hospital stay would be prolonged to be 12.05 days, increased about 2 days compared with operation of RARP. While the operation of laparoscopic would increase LOS by 0.87 day or in other words more than a half day but less than 1 day. Additionally, 1 unit (L) greater blood loss would prolong the 50th percentile of LOS to be 12.99 days, increased by about 3 days and Gleason score ≥ 8 would increase LOS by about 1 day compared to the reference category of Gleason score ≤ 6. However, for the effect of WBC, one unit decrease in WBC would slightly increase the 50th percentile of LOS by 0.2 day.

Discussion

The expected increasing numbers of patients with prostate cancer will inevitably increase the demand for access to hospitalization; it is therefore important to optimize medical resource utilization in an attempt to meet this demand. Hospital LOS, an important indicator of resource utilization, has been increasingly investigated in the face of limited medical resources and increasing pressure for cost containment [5, 7, 15]. Identifying risk factors that influence LOS of patients with prostate cancer in China will enable more accurate prediction of bed flow and access and thus facilitate more efficient resource allocation. In our study, we found that the preoperative variables of biopsy Gleason score (≥ 8) and WBC and intraoperative variables of operation type (open or laparoscopic), and blood loss are significant predictors of longer LOS for post-radical prostatectomy patients with prostate cancer in China.

In our study, the median postoperative LOS of our patient cohort was 10 days, which is much longer than that reported from Western countries, where the median postoperative LOS after radical prostatectomy is reportedly only one day [13, 14]. This discrepancy is likely attributable to the huge differences in healthcare systems, medical insurance status, admission/discharge policies, and sociocultural factors between China and these countries [16]. First, in China, the lack of post-hospitalization care such as that provided by rehabilitation centers and clinician's follow-up checks, which are commonly available in Western countries [15, 17], lengthens the LOS. In China, most post-radical prostatectomy patients stay in hospital until they have achieved stable physical fitness. For example, the discharge criteria in our institution include normal vital signs, return of bowel function, ambulation without assistance, and removal of pelvic drainage tubes, unlike the criteria in Western hospitals [13]. What's more, the structure of healthcare financing may also contribute to the longer LOS in China than in Western countries. For example, the USA Medicare prospective payment system and

Table 1 Characteristics of the 793 patients and variables associated with LOS by univariate analysis

Variables	Mean ± SD or n (%)	LOS		P value
		Mean ± SD	Median (25th–75th percentile)	
Patient demographics				
Age (y)	67.0 ± 6.8	11.7 ± 4.6	10.0 (9.0–14.0)	0.693[a]
Body mass index (kg/m^2)	23.7 ± 2.8	11.7 ± 4.6	10.0 (9.0–14.0)	0.407[a]
Marital status				0.877[c]
Married	771 (97.2%)	11.7 ± 4.6	10.0 (9.0–14.0)	
Widowed	16 (2.0%)	11.8 ± 6.1	10.0 (9.0–11.8)	
Single	6 (0.8%)	11.8 ± 3.7	10.0 (9.0–16.3)	
Smoking				0.612[b]
No	511 (64.4%)	11.8 ± 4.5	10.0 (9.0–14.0)	
Yes	282 (35.6%)	11.6 ± 4.8	10.0 (9.0–13.3)	
Drinking				0.678[b]
No	621 (78.3%)	11.7 ± 4.5	10.0 (9.0–13.5)	
Yes	172 (21.7%)	11.7 ± 5.2	10.0 (9.0–14.0)	
Family history of Prostate cancer				0.752[b]
No	580 (73.1%)	11.7 ± 4.8	10.0 (9.0–14.0)	
Yes	213 (26.9%)	11.7 ± 4.3	10.0 (9.0–13.0)	
Medical comorbidities				
Hypertension				0.798[b]
No	434 (54.7%)	11.8 ± 5.1	10.0 (9.0–13.3)	
Yes	359 (45.3%)	11.6 ± 4.1	10.0 (9.0–14.0)	
Diabetes				0.487[b]
No	718 (90.5%)	11.8 ± 4.8	10.0 (9.0–13.0)	
Yes	75 (9.5%)	11.3 ± 3.5	10.0 (8.0–14.0)	
Cardiovascular & cerebrovascular diseases				0.705[b]
No	734 (92.6%)	11.7 ± 4.6	10.0 (9.0–13.0)	
Yes	59 (7.4%)	12.0 ± 5.0	10.0 (9.0–15.0)	
Prostate cancer disease-specific variables				
Biopsy Gleason score				**< 0.001**[c]
≤ 6	254 (32.0%)	11.1 ± 4.2	10.0 (9.0–12.0)	
7	344 (43.4%)	11.7 ± 5.0	10.0 (9.0–13.0)	
≥ 8	195 (24.6%)	12.6 ± 4.5	11.0 (9.0–15.0)	
Preoperative PSA	17.0 ± 22.3	11.7 ± 4.6	10.0 (9.0–14.0)	**0.036**[a]
Prostate Volume (ml)	34.0 ± 19.6	11.7 ± 4.6	10.0 (9.0–14.0)	0.214[a]
Urinary tract problems				
Dysuresia				**0.032**[b]
No	667 (84.1%)	11.6 ± 4.7	10.0 (9.0–13.0)	
Yes	126 (15.9%)	12.3 ± 4.3	11.0 (9.0–15.0)	
Pain or burning on urination				0.416[b]
No	761 (96.0%)	11.7 ± 4.7	10.0 (9.0–13.0)	
Yes	32 (4.0%)	11.9 ± 3.6	10.5 (9.0–15.0)	
Frequent urination				0.169[b]
No	633 (79.8%)	11.7 ± 4.9	10.0 (9.0–13.0)	
Yes	160 (20.2%)	11.8 ± 3.7	10.0 (9.0–14.0)	

Table 1 Characteristics of the 793 patients and variables associated with LOS by univariate analysis *(Continued)*

Variables	Mean ± SD or n (%)	LOS Mean ± SD	Median (25th–75th percentile)	P value
Urgent urination				0.912[b]
No	690 (87.0%)	11.8 ± 4.8	10.0 (9.0–14.0)	
Yes	103 (13.0%)	11.4 ± 3.6	10.0 (9.0–14.0)	
Hematuria				0.545[b]
No	776 (97.9%)	11.7 ± 4.7	10.0 (9.0–14.0)	
Yes	17 (2.1%)	11.1 ± 3.8	10.0 (8.0–12.5)	
Preoperative laboratory values				
White blood count (×10⁹/L)	5.8 ± 1.5	11.7 ± 4.6	10.0 (9.0–14.0)	**< 0.001**[a]
Neutrophil (%)	57.0 ± 8.9	11.7 ± 4.6	10.0 (9.0–14.0)	0.467[a]
Hemoglobin (g/L)	143.3 ± 13.4	11.7 ± 4.6	10.0 (9.0–14.0)	0.713[a]
Hematocrit (%)	42.1 ± 3.6	11.7 ± 4.6	10.0 (9.0–14.0)	0.387[a]
Platelet count (× 10⁹/L)	186.9 ± 49.3	11.7 ± 4.6	10.0 (9.0–14.0)	**0.005**[a]
Albumin (g/L)	43.2 ± 4.2	11.7 ± 4.6	10.0 (9.0–14.0)	0.475[a]
GPT (U/L)	23.6 ± 21.2	11.7 ± 4.6	10.0 (9.0–14.0)	0.170[a]
Serum total bilirubin (ummol/L)	12.3 ± 5.0	11.7 ± 4.6	10.0 (9.0–14.0)	0.402[a]
Creatinine (ummol/L)	78.4 ± 13.2	11.7 ± 4.6	10.0 (9.0–14.0)	0.106[a]
Serum potassium (mmol/L)	4.2 ± 0.4	11.7 ± 4.6	10.0 (9.0–14.0)	0.309[a]
Serum calcium (mmol/L)	2.3 ± 0.1	11.7 ± 4.6	10.0 (9.0–14.0)	**0.008**[a]
Blood glucose (mmol/L)	5.0 ± 0.9	11.7 ± 4.6	10.0 (9.0–14.0)	**0.053**[a]
Intraoperative variables				
Operation type[&]				**< 0.001**[c]
Open	325 (41.0%)	13.3 ± 5.1	12.0 (10.0–15.0)	
Laparoscopic	257 (32.4%)	11.0 ± 3.8	10.0 (9.0–12.0)	
Robot assisted	211 (26.6%)	10.1 ± 4.1	9.0 (8.0–10.0)	
Blood loss (L)	0.2 ± 0.2	11.7 ± 4.6	10.0 (9.0–14.0)	**< 0.001**[a]
Operation duration (h)	3.0 ± 0.9	11.7 ± 4.6	10.0 (9.0–14.0)	0.177[a]

SD, standard deviation; LOS, length of stay; PSA, prostate specific antigen; GPT, Glutamic-pyruvic transaminase
Bold values indicate significant *p* values (*p* ≤ 0.1)
[&]A LSD post hoc test revealed that all three subgroups were significantly different from each other
[a]Spearman correlation analysis
[b]Mann-Whitney *U* test
[c]Kruskal-Wallis H(K) test

diagnosis-related group-based payment system for hospitalization provide a financial incentive for earlier hospital discharge [18], whereas China's healthcare system generally provides treatments and care independent of LOS or costs [16, 19]. Indeed, the cost per night (bed expense: about $4.43) is much lower in our hospitals than in Western countries [20]. Traditionally, many patients are willing to stay longer in hospital, where medical treatment and nursing care are easily accessible, to ensure they are in good physical condition before discharge rather than agreeing to earlier discharge with the attendant risks of developing complications outside hospital. Another noteworthy point is that Chinese doctors tend to be more conservative and cautious in ensuring that patients achieve a stable state before discharging them from hospital, their motivation being to avoid potential challenges, legal action, or even threats from patients or their families, as have occurred in association with tense doctor–patient relationships in China, especially in recent years [21, 22]. All the above reasons likely contribute to the much longer LOS for both patients with prostate cancer and those with other diseases [15, 17, 23] in China than in Western studies.

Being one of the main treatments for clinically localized prostate cancer, three types of radical prostatectomy are available in our institution, namely open, laparoscopic, and robotic prostatectomy. Many previous studies comparing operative outcomes of the three types of surgery, have reported that minimally invasive (laparoscopic or robotic) surgery is associated with a significantly shorter LOS than open surgery [24–28]. Our findings were consistent with

Table 2 The results of multiple linear regression analysis

Variables	Unstandardized coefficient[a]	Standardized coefficient (β)[a]	t value	P value
Operation type				
Robot assisted	REF	–	–	–
Open	−0.017	−0.325	−7.259	**< 0.001**
Laparoscopic	−0.008	−0.146	−3.730	**< 0.001**
Blood loss (L)	−0.023	−0.205	−5.438	**< 0.001**
Gleason score				
≤ 6	REF	–	–	–
7	−0.003	−0.061	− 1.668	0.096
≥ 8	−0.009	−0.152	−4.115	**< 0.001**
White blood count ($\times 10^9$/L)	0.002	0.089	2.775	**0.006**
Preoperative PSA	8.222E-6	0.007	0.208	0.835
Dysuresia	−0.002	−0.027	−0.826	0.409
Platelet count ($\times 10^9$/L)	2.816E-5	0.053	1.550	0.122
Serum calcium (mmol/L)	−0.012	− 0.058	−1.797	0.073
Blood glucose (mmol/L)	0.001	0.043	1.352	0.177

REF, referent; —, not applicable

Bold items indicate factors significantly associated with LOS (*p* values < 0.05)

[a]negative coefficients corresponding to longer LOS because of the reciprocal transformation

this in that patients undergoing open radical prostatectomy had longer LOS than both patients undergoing LRP and RARP. In fact, undergoing open radical prostatectomy was the strongest predictor of LOS according to multivariate analysis in our study. It is noteworthy that operation type of laparoscopic was also a significant predictor of LOS by multivariate analysis and a post hoc comparison between the three operation types revealed a significantly longer LOS for patients undergoing LRP than RARP on univariate analysis. Previous studies have highlighted the advantages of RARP over ORP [24–28] and LRP [29, 30]; specifically, less blood loss, lower transfusion rate, lower complication rates, and better functional outcomes [24–30]. Shorter hospital stay of RARP over ORP have also been widely reported [24–28] while our study identified that not only for ORP but also for LRP, RARP has shorter LOS, which differs from reports from Western countries [29]. Relevant point to this discrepancy is that a large proportion of patents in our study had undergone ORP (41.0%) or LRP (32.4%), only 26.6% patients having undergone RARP, unlike in Western countries, where much greater proportion of patients reportedly undergo RARP [13, 14, 31]. This may be another explanation for postoperative LOS being so much longer for patients with prostate cancer in China than for those in Western countries. Although RARP has many advantages over LRP and ORP [24–30], it is much more costly than the other two options [20, 27]. Therefore, RARP may be the optimal choice for affluent patients.

We also found the intraoperative variable of blood loss to be an important predictor of longer LOS after radical prostatectomy. This result is consistent with previous studies [11, 14] that analyzed data from the National Surgery Quality Improvement Program database to explore the risk factors for prolonged LOS after commonly performed urologic surgical procedures, including nephrectomy and prostatectomy, and concluded that intraoperative transfusion is significantly associated with longer postoperative LOS. In addition, the above studies [11, 14] and other related studies [31–33] were consistent in finding that the intraoperative variable of operation duration is also significantly associated with longer LOS. However, our findings were inconsistent with these in that operation duration was not a significant predictor of longer LOS. In this context, it is noteworthy that one recent study exploring risk factors for hospital LOS in patients undergoing RARP drew a contradictory conclusion [13], reporting a shorter operative time with prolonged hospital LOS on univariate analysis but lack of support for this finding by multivariate analysis, indicating that the variable of operation duration as predictor of LOS after radical prostatectomy may need further investigation.

In one previous study [13], the disease-specific variable of Gleason score was also evaluated but not found to be significant, which conflicts with our findings. In our study, we abstracted and analyzed the prostate cancer disease-specific variables of preoperative PSA, biopsy Gleason score, and prostate volume and found that preoperative PSA and biopsy Gleason score were both associated with LOS by univariate analysis. However, only Gleason score ≥ 8 was an important predictor of longer LOS by multivariate analysis. Patients with higher biopsy

Gleason scores (≥ 8) may thus be at risk of longer postoperative LOS after radical prostatectomy. To the best of our knowledge, this is the first report of a significant association between this variable and hospital LOS in post-prostatectomy patients. However, there are few studies on the impact of prostate cancer disease-specific risk factors on hospital LOS. Further prospective research is needed to validate the significance of Gleason score as a predictor of prolonged LOS.

Studies investigating predictors of LOS in other surgical disciplines have also highlighted that preoperative laboratory values such as low hematocrit, high creatinine, or low albumin are significant indicators of prolonged LOS [12, 14, 34]. We also abstracted these preoperative laboratory values, but found that hematocrit, creatinine or albumin were not significantly associated with LOS in our patient cohort, whereas white blood count, platelet count, serum calcium and blood glucose were. However, of these variables, only white blood count persisted into the final model after multiple linear regression analysis. It makes intuitive sense that higher white blood counts would indicate tissue infection and inflammation that would likely lengthen hospital stay. However, in our study the results were contradictory in that WBC was inversely associated with LOS, meaning that lower preoperative WBC were associated with longer postoperative LOS. To better understand this puzzling result, we made a further analysis by categorizing the variable of WBC as abnormal low, normal, abnormal high on the basis of clinical cutoff points. And results showed that the percent of patients with abnormal low WBC was six-fold greater than the percent of patients with abnormal high WBC and a post hoc comparison revealed that patients with abnormal low WBC had significant longer LOS than patients with normal WBC while no statistically significant difference exist between patients with abnormal high WBC and patients with normal WBC. This confusing result may indicate that prostate cancer patients may be more easily in an underling condition. Because the lower WBC may be an indication of that patients were with severe infections, or radiotherapy/chemotherapy or other unfitness physical state [35, 36], which may result in longer postoperative LOS. However, given the limitations of few studies exploring the relationship between this variable and LOS in prostate cancer patients, more studies are needed to further verify or refute this result of our study.

We here identified several important predictors of longer LOS for post-prostatectomy patients with prostate cancer in China. In particular, we added the disease-specific variable of Gleason score as a risk factor for longer LOS. However, several limitations of our study should be noted. First, it was a retrospective analysis and data were collected from a single institution in Zhejiang, China, thus limiting the generalizability of these finding to other countries or even other institutions in China. Second, we only analyzed preoperative and intraoperative variables and the R^2 value in the final regression model was 0.205; such a small R^2 value suggests that postoperative variables such as complications may play major roles in postoperative LOS. Previous studies have reported strong associations between postoperative adverse events and prolonged LOS [11]. Hence, future analyses should include postoperative variables to enable more comprehensive exploration of risk factors that impact LOS after radical prostatectomy in China. Third, the radical prostatectomies of the 793 patients analyzed were performed by different surgeons in our institution. Because we could not quantify the levels of skill of the surgeons involved, we were unable to draw conclusions about their influence on LOS. Last but not least, because countries differ greatly in their healthcare policies, our results should be considered in the context of country-specific healthcare systems and medical–cultural environments when comparing them with results from other countries. Additionally, the influence of doctors' and patients' attitudes to LOS should not be ignored because the doctor–patient relationship tends to be more strained in China than in Western countries.

Conclusions

Elucidating the risk factors for longer LOS will enable better patient counseling and more efficient management of medical resources. In our study, we found that both some preoperative and intraoperative variables are significant predictors of longer postoperative LOS after radical prostatectomy in China. Measures should be taken to improve intraoperative procedures and reduce the prevalence of preoperative risk factors without sacrificing the quality of medical care with the aim of shortening hospital LOS and improving the efficiency of utilization of Chinese medical resources.

Abbreviations
BMI: Body mass index; GPT: Glutamic-pyruvic transaminase; LOS: Length of stay; LRP: Laparoscopic radical prostatectomy; ORP: Open radical prostatectomy; PSA: Prostate specific antigen; RARP: Robot-assisted radical prostatectomy; REF: Referent; SD: Standard deviation; SE: Standard error; WBC: White blood count

Acknowledgements
We thank Qiqi Mao and Zhenghui Hu very much for their work on language editing and manuscript revision. And we thank Dr. Trish Reynolds, MBBS, FRACP, from Liwen Bianji, Edanz Group China, for editing the English text of a draft of this manuscript.

Authors' contributions
QH participated in the study design, data collection and analysis, and wrote the manuscript. PJ participated in the data collection and helped perform

the statistical analysis of the data. LF participated in the data collection and management. LX, SW, DX, BS and BJ provided the clinical data and revised the manuscript. LZ participated in the collection of data. WW participated in the study design, data interpretation and revised the manuscript. All authors have read and approved the final version of the manuscript.

Competing interests

The authors declare that they have no competing interests.

References

1. Resnick MJ, Lacchetti C, Bergman J, Hauke RJ, Hoffman KE, Kungel TM, et al. Prostate cancer survivorship care guideline: American Society of Clinical Oncology clinical practice guideline endorsement. J Clin Oncol. 2015;33:1078–85.
2. Heidenreich A, Bastian PJ, Bellmunt J, Bolla M, Joniau S, van der Kwast T, et al. EAU guidelines on prostate cancer. Part 1: screening, diagnosis, and local treatment with curative intent-update 2013. Eur Urol. 2014;65:124–37.
3. Ye D, Zhu Y. Epidemiology of prostate cancer in China: an overview and clinical implication. Zhonghua Wai Ke Za Zhi. 2015;53:249–52.
4. Qi D, Wu C, Liu F, Gu K, Shi Z, Lin X, et al. Trends of prostate cancer incidence and mortality in shanghai, China from 1973 to 2009. Prostate. 2015;75:1662–8.
5. McMullan R, Silke B, Bennett K, Callachand S. Resource utilisation, length of hospital stay, and pattern of investigation during acute medical hospital admission. Postgrad Med J. 2004;80:23–6.
6. Polverejan E, Gardiner JC, Bradley CJ, Holmes-Rovner M, Rovner D. Estimating mean hospital cost as a function of length of stay and patient characteristics. Health Econ. 2003;12:935–47.
7. Rotter T, Kinsman L, James E, Machotta A, Gothe H, Willis J, et al. Clinical pathways: effects on professional practice, patient outcomes, length of stay and hospital costs. Cochrane Database Syst Rev. 2010; https://doi.org/10.1002/14651858.CD006632.pub2.
8. Bolenz C, Gupta A, Roehrborn CG, Lotan Y. Predictors of costs for robotic-assisted laparoscopic radical prostatectomy. Urol Oncol. 2011;29:325–9.
9. Saleh SS, Callan M, Therriault M, Landor N. The cost impact of hospital-acquired conditions among critical care patients. Med Care. 2010;48:518–26.
10. Glance LG, Stone PW, Mukamel DB, Dick AW. Increases in mortality, length of stay, and cost associated with hospital-acquired infections in trauma patients. Arch Surg. 2011;146:794–801.
11. Collins TC, Daley J, Henderson WH, Khuri SF. Risk factors for prolonged length of stay after major elective surgery. Ann Surg. 1999;230:251–9.
12. Lorentz CA, Leung AK, AB DR, Perez SD, Johnson TV, Sweeney JF, et al. Predicting length of stay following radical nephrectomy using the National Surgical Quality Improvement Program Database. J Urol. 2015;194:923–8.
13. Potretzke AM, Kim EH, Knight BA, Anderson BG, Park AM, Sherburne Figenshau R, et al. Patient comorbidity predicts hospital length of stay after robot-assisted prostatectomy. J Robot Surg. 2016;10:151–6.
14. Wallner LP, Dunn RL, Sarma AV, Campbell DA, Wei JT. Risk factors for prolonged length of stay after urologic surgery: the National Surgical Quality Improvement Program. J Am Coll Surg. 2008;207:904–13.
15. Li Q, Lin Z, Masoudi FA, Li J, Li X, Hernández-Díaz S, et al. National trends in hospital length of stay for acute myocardial infarction in China. BMC Cardiovasc Disord. 2015;15:9.
16. Ma Y, Liu Y, Fu HM, Wang XM, Wu BH, Wang SX, et al. Evaluation of admission characteristics, hospital length of stay and costs for cerebral infarction in a medium-sized city in China. Eur J Neurol. 2010;17:1270–6.
17. Wu Q, Ning GZ, Li YL, Feng HY, Feng SQ. Factors affecting the length of stay of patients with traumatic spinal cord injury in Tianjin, China. J Spinal Cord Med. 2013;36:237–42.
18. Felder S. The variance of length of stay and the optimal DRG outlier payments. Int J Health Care Finance Econ. 2009;9:279–89.
19. Zhang L, Cheng X, Liu X, Zhu K, Tang S, Bogg L, et al. Balancing the funds in the new cooperative medical scheme in rural China: determinants and influencing factors in two provinces. Int J Health Plann Manag. 2010;25:96–118.
20. Bolenz C, Gupta A, Hotze T, Ho R, Cadeddu JA, Roehrborn CG, et al. Cost comparison of robotic, laparoscopic, and open radical prostatectomy for prostate cancer. Eur Urol. 2010;57:453–8.
21. Ending violence against doctors in China. Lancet. 2012;379:1764.
22. Jingang A. Which future for doctors in China? Lancet. 2013;382:936–7.
23. Chen D, Liu S, Tan X, Zhao Q. Assessment of hospital length of stay and direct costs of type 2 diabetes in Hubei Province. China BMC Health Serv Res. 2017;17:199.
24. Basto M, Sathianathen N, Te Marvelde L, Ryan S, Goad J, Lawrentschuk N, et al. Patterns-of-care and health economic analysis of robot-assisted radical prostatectomy in the Australian public health system. BJU Int. 2016;117:930–9.
25. Trinh Q, Sammon J, Sun M, Ravi P, Ghani KR, Bianchi M, et al. Perioperative outcomes of robot-assisted radical prostatectomy compared with open radical prostatectomy: results from the nationwide inpatient sample. Eur Urol. 2012;61:679–85.
26. Liu J, Maxwell BG, Panousis P, Chung BI. Perioperative outcomes for laparoscopic and robotic compared with open prostatectomy using the National Surgical Quality Improvement Program (NSQIP) database. Urology. 2013;82:579–83.
27. Leow JJ, Chang SL, Meyer CP, Wang Y, Hanske J, Sammon JD, et al. Robot-assisted versus open radical prostatectomy: a contemporary analysis of an all-payer discharge database. Eur Urol. 2016;70(5):837–45.
28. Alemozaffar M, Sanda M, Yecies D, Mucci LA, Stampfer MJ, Kenfield SA. Benchmarks for operative outcomes of robotic and open radical prostatectomy: results from the health professionals follow-up study. Eur Urol. 2015;67:432–8.
29. Huang X, Wang L, Zheng X, Wang X. Comparison of perioperative, functional, and oncologic outcomes between standard laparoscopic and robotic-assisted radical prostatectomy: a systemic review and meta-analysis. Surg Endosc. 2017;31:1045–60.
30. Tewari A, Sooriakumaran P, Bloch DA, Seshadri-Kreaden U, Hebert AE, Wiklund P. Positive surgical margin and perioperative complication rates of primary surgical treatments for prostate cancer: a systematic review and meta-analysis comparing retropubic, laparoscopic, and robotic prostatectomy. Eur Urol. 2012;62:1–15.
31. Monn MF, Jain R, Kaimakliotis HZ, Flack CK, Koch MO, Boris RS. Examining the relationship between operative time and hospitalization time in minimally invasive and open urologic procedures. J Endourol. 2014;28:1132–7.
32. Procter LD, Davenport DL, Bernard AC, Zwischenberger JB. General surgical operative duration is associated with increased risk-adjusted infectious complication rates and length of hospital stay. J Am Coll Surg. 2010;210:60–5. e61–62
33. Huang KH, Kaplan AL, Carter SC, Lipsitz SR, Hu JC. The impact of radical prostatectomy operative time on outcomes and costs. Urology. 2014;83:1265–71.
34. Ad N, Holmes SD, Shuman DJ, Pritchard G, Massimiano PS, Rongione AJ, et al. Potential impact of modifiable clinical variables on length of stay after first-time cardiac surgery. Ann Thorac Surg. 2015;100:2102–7.
35. Bonilla MA, Menell JS. Chapter 13–Disorders of White Blood Cells. In: Lanzkowsky's Manual of Pediatric Hematology and Oncology. Sixth ed. London: Academic Press; 2016. p. 209–38.
36. Feher J. White Blood Cells and Inflammation. In: Quantitative Human Physiology-An Introduction. London: Academic Press; 2012. p. 437–45.

30

Mannitol reduces nephron loss after warm renal ischemia in a porcine model

José A. Damasceno-Ferreira[1,2], Leonardo A. S. Abreu[1,3], Gustavo R. Bechara[1], Waldemar S. Costa[1], Marco A. Pereira-Sampaio[1,4], Francisco J. B. Sampaio[1] and Diogo B. De Souza[1*]

Abstract

Background: Mannitol has been employed to ameliorate renal warm ischemia damage during partial nephrectomy, however, there is limited scientific evidence to support the use of mannitol during partial nephrectomy. The objective of the present study was to investigate the glomerular number after renal warm ischemia, with and without the use of mannitol in a Pig Model.

Methods: Twenty-four male pigs were assigned into three groups. Eight animals were allocated to the sham group that was subjected to laparoscopic dissection of the left renal hilum, without renal ischemia. Eight animals were allocated to the ischemia group that had the left renal hilum clamped for 30 min through laparoscopic access. Eight animals received mannitol (250 mg/kg) before the occlusion of renal hilum for 30 min. The kidneys were collected after the euthanasia of the pigs 21 days post surgery. The right kidney was utilized as a self-control for each animal. Serum creatinine, urea levels, the weight and volume of the kidneys were measured. Glomerular volumetric density, volume-weighted glomerular volume, and cortical volume were quantified through stereological methods and employed to determine the number of nephrons per kidney. Student's t test and ANOVA were used for statistical analysis.

Results: In the ischemia group, the left kidney recorded a reduction of 24.6% (290, 000 glomeruli) in the number of glomeruli in comparison to the right kidney. Kidneys subjected to ischemia also displayed decreased weight and volume in comparison to the sham and mannitol groups. No difference was observed between the left and right kidneys from the sham and mannitol groups. Further, no distinction in serum creatinine and urea among the groups was observed.

Conclusion: The use of mannitol significantly reduces nephron loss during warm ischemia in pigs.

Keywords: Kidney, Mannitol, Partial nephrectomy, Warm ischemia, Swine

Background

Despite the development of new techniques for minimally invasive partial nephrectomy, renal warm ischemia is often necessary to obtain an adequate operative field [1]. However, renal ischemia during partial nephrectomy is associated with post-operative functional decline [2].

A maximum duration of 25 min for warm ischemia has been proposed for preventing renal damage [3]. Furthermore, recent studies have shown that the quality and quantity of remnant renal parenchyma is of great importance to predict renal function [4]. Thus, various methods have been employed to prevent damage to the remnant kidney parenchyma after prolonged warm renal ischemia [5–8].

Mannitol has been employed to ameliorate the renal damage caused by warm ischemia during partial nephrectomies. Although there is limited scientific evidence to validate the application of mannitol to preserve kidney function during partial nephrectomy, almost 80% of groups that perform partial nephrectomy routinely apply mannitol as an ameliorating agent [9]. According to some investigations, renal function exhibits no difference in relation to mannitol administration during renal ischemia in

* Correspondence: diogobenchimol@gmail.com
[1]Urogenital Research Unit, Rio de Janeiro State University, Rio de Janeiro, RJ, Brazil
Full list of author information is available at the end of the article

partial nephrectomy [10, 11]. However, there is a lack of quantitative morphological studies exploring the effects of mannitol to ameliorate damage caused during renal warm ischemia. For this experiment, swine was employed as an animal model, since it is considered the most adequate model for comparison with human kidney's anatomy and physiology [12, 13] Thus, the aim of this study was to investigate the number of glomeruli, applying an unbiased stereological method, post renal warm ischemia with and without the administration of mannitol, in a porcine model.

Methods

Twenty-four male domestic pigs weighing 25 kg were included in this study. All experiments were performed in adherence to the Brazilian law for scientific use of animals, and this project was formally approved by the local Ethics Committee for animal experimentation (CEUA-048-2011). Animals were accommodated in groups of six in appropriate facilities, with air conditioning, food, and water ad libitum.

The animals were randomly assigned into three experimental groups of eight animals each. Group sham (S) was subjected to kidney and hilar dissection but not renal ischemia. Group ischemia (I) was subjected to 30 min of renal warm ischemia. Group mannitol (M) was also subjected to 30 min of renal warm ischemia, but mannitol (250 mg/kg, IV) [14] was administrated 15 min before the pedicle clamping.

The left kidney was accessed laparoscopicaly with a transperitoneal approach under general anesthesia and aseptic technique, [12]. Renal vessels were clamped *en bloc* in groups I and M with a laparoscopic Satinsky clamp. After 30 min of ischemia, the vascular clamp was removed, and the normal color of the kidney was verified through observation. In the sham group, all steps (except the hilar clamping) were performed; subsequent to the dissection of the renal pedicle, the animals were maintained under anesthesia for 30 min without renal ischemia. The right kidneys were not manipulated during the experiment and were served as controls. The animals were administered a single dose of penicillin benzathine (Benzetacil, Eurofarma, São Paulo, Brazil) at 400, 000 UI/Kg subsequent to anesthetic induction and tramadol hydrochloride (Tramal, Pfizer, Guarulhos, Brazil) at 4 mg/Kg twice a day for 48 h post surgery. Food and water were offered ad libitum six hours after the procedure. The recovery to normal ambulation required up to four hours after the surgery. Serum creatinine and urea levels were determined before surgery and on postoperative days 10 and 21 to assess renal function. For this purpose, animals were restrained and blood was collected through venipuncture. Serum was separated

through the technique of centrifugation and stored at $-20°$ C until analysis.

The animals were evaluated on a daily basis for 21 days after surgery, and subsequent to this period, were euthanized through anesthetic overdose (sodium thiopental 200 mg/kg IV). The kidneys were harvested, weighed, and their volumes were measured with the Scherle's method [15]; subsequently, the organs were fixed by immersion in 4% buffered formaldehyde for stereological analyses. All histological analyses were performed by a blinded observer. Samples were randomly collected from the cortical region of these 48 kidneys and were processed through routine histological methods. The specimens were paraffin-embedded, sectioned at 5-µm thickness, and stained with hematoxylin and eosin. The cortical-medullar ratio was estimated employing the point-counting-method according to the Cavalieri principle [16]. The absolute cortical volume (CV) was achieved through the product of the cortical-medullar ratio and renal volume.

From each kidney, 25 histological fields obtained from different sections of the renal cortex were photographed with a digital camera (DP70, Olympus, Tokyo, Japan) coupled to a microscope (BX51, Olympus). Glomerular volumetric density (Vv [glom]) was estimated by the point-counting technique with a M42 test-system [17, 18].

The volume-weighted mean glomerular volume (VWGV) was estimated using the point-sampled intercept method [16, 17, 19], analyzing 50 glomeruli per kidney.

The estimation of the total number of glomeruli per kidney was achieved through the product of CV and Vv [glom] and the division of the quotient by the VWGV [16, 19].

For each stereological parameter, left kidneys were compared with the right organs of each group with the Student's t test. Mean creatinine and urea serum levels were compared between groups by employing one-way ANOVA and between different experimental instances (0, 10, and 21 days respectively) through repeated measures ANOVA. For all comparisons, $p < 0.05$ was considered significant. Data were expressed as mean ± standard deviation. Analyses were performed using GraphPad Prism 5.0 (GraphPad Software, San Diego, USA).

Results

All animals recovered effectively from the surgeries and were included for the evaluation of allanalyzed parameters. No adverse events were observed. No variations in serum creatinine and urea levels were observed among the studied groups (Table 1).

The weight and volume of the left kidney for group I reduced by 6.2% and 6.3% respectively, in comparison to the right kidney. For group S as well as group M, no

Table 1 Serum creatinine levels of pigs subjected to sham surgery or to renal ischemia with or without mannitol administration

Creatinine		Preoperative	10 days Post-operative	21 days Post-operative	p value
	Sham	1.52 ± 0.4	1.10 ± 0.1	1.39 ± 0.7	0.62
	Ischemia	1.13 ± 0.3	1.13 ± 0.2	1.20 ± 0.3	0.85
	Mannitol	1.3 ± 0.5	0.92 ± 0.2	0.91 ± 0.1	0.10
	p value	0.31	0.16	0.16	
		Preoperative	10 days Post-operative	21 days Post-operative	p value
Urea	Sham	37.0 ± 1.4	38.2 ± 8.2	41.0 ± 6.8	0.63
	Ischemia	41.9 ± 8.2	41.2 ± 7.2	42 ± 7.2	0.98
	Mannitol	33.4 ± 4.9	35.7 ± 9.0	35.9 ± 7.0	0.82
	p value	0.09	0.45	0.21	

Data expressed as mean ± S.D.

difference was observed between the weight and volume of the kidneys.

The cortical-medullar ratio and absolute CV were the only factors that recorded a difference among left and right kidneys of group I, with the left kidney displaying a 2.3% and 8.3% decrease in these parameters respectively. For the other groups, no difference was noted regarding these parameters. Regarding Vv [glom] and VWGV, no difference was found across all groups.

Finally, the total number of glomeruli in left kidneys of group I, a 24.6% decrease in comparison to the right kidneys was observed. This represented a loss of approximately 290, 000 glomeruli caused by warm ischemia for 30 min (Fig. 1). However, in the group subjected to the same duration of ischemia exposure, but received mannitol pre-treatment, no difference was observed, along with group S. All stereological data are listed in Table 2.

Discussion

Warm ischemia was identified as the "ultimate enemy" for partial nephrectomy [20], and several methods to ameliorate its negative aspects have been proposed [5–8]. Although mannitol is largely employed for this purpose [9], its effects for ischemia protection during partial nephrectomy were only recently investigated [10, 11]. This is the first study that shows the beneficial effects of mannitol for preserving the renal functional units post warm ischemia.

Both previous studies on this issue indicated that the use of mannitol during partial nephrectomies does not affect clinically significant improvements in renal function preservation [10, 11]. They were retrospective studies that presented the results of estimated glomerular filtration rate of patients subjected to partial nephrectomy with or without mannitol administration. Therefore, their negative results may be due to the heterogeneity of the patients and laboratory analysis. Although the animal model presents certain limitations, the present study was randomly conducted with several appropriate control factors that

may affect the results, such as age, weight, and nutritional status, warm ischemia time, mannitol dosage, and performed analysis.

Furthermore, in the present study, we used unbiased stereological methods to determine the number of glomeruli on each kidney that could be considered equal to the number of nephrons [16, 19]. As a "nephron-sparing surgery," the main objective of partial nephrectomy is the treatment of the renal tumor while sparing as most nephrons as possible. In accordance with this objective, one of the most adequate measurements to study the impact of warm ischemia for partial nephrectomy would be the determination of the number of nephrons [17].

The preservation of renal nephrons following warm ischemia by mannitol usage may rely on different mechanisms. Mannitol is most recognized as an osmotic diuretic, and diuretics (not only mannitol but also furosemide) are known to inhibit tubular reabsorption and decrease parenchymal oxygen demand [21]. Thus,

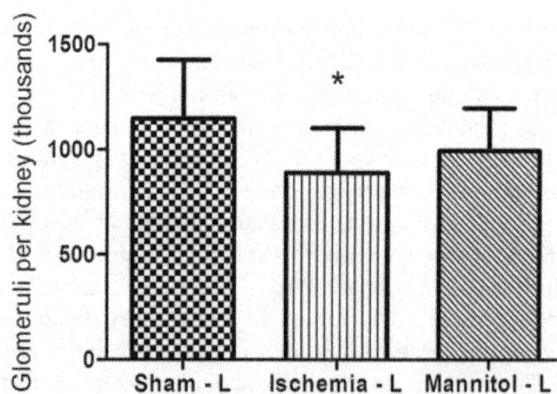

Fig. 1 Number of glomeruli in the left kidneys of pigs subjected to sham surgery or warm ischemia for 30 min with and without mannitol pre-treatment. *$p < 0.05$ in comparison to contra lateral control. Data are expressed as mean (boxes) ± standard deviation (error bars)

Table 2 Stereological data of right and left kidneys of pigs subjected to sham surgery or to left renal ischemia with or without mannitol administration

	Sham			Ischemia			Mannitol		
	Right	Left	p-value	Right	Left	p-value	Right	Left	p-value
Kidney weight (g)	56.8 ± 4.9	58.2 ± 8.5	0.52	59.2 ± 10.9	55.5 ± 11.0	0.008	58.5 ± 10.4	55.4 ± 8.5	0.06
Kidney volume (ml)	54.4 ± 4.1	55.2 ± 7.7	0.70	56.6 ± 9.8	53.0 ± 10.5	0.007	55.4 ± 9.8	52.5 ± 8.1	0.09
Cortical-medullar ratio (%)	71.6 ± 2.3	70.4 ± 4.1	0.32	71.8 ± 2.4	70.1 ± 2.2	0.04	71.4 ± 4.0	71.9 ± 3.3	0.72
Cortical volume (ml)	38.9 ± 3.3	38.9 ± 6.5	0.98	40.6 ± 7.4	37.2 ± 7.9	0.002	39.3 ± 5.9	37.8 ± 6.2	0.17
Vv [glom] (%)	3.79 ± 0.5	3.72 ± 0.5	0.68	3.59 ± 0.4	3.08 ± 0.9	0.16	4.06 ± 0.9	3.72 ± 0.8	0.37
VWGV (10^5 μm^3)	13.4 ± 1.6	12.7 ± 1.1	0.25	12.5 ± 2.4	12.4 ± 1.2	0.94	14.1 ± 3.9	14.3 ± 3.9	0.86
Glomeruli (millions)	1.10 ± 0.1	1.14 ± 0.2	0.68	1.18 ± 0.2	0.89 ± 0.2	0.04	1.18 ± 0.4	0.99 ± 0.2	0.18

Data expressed as mean ± S.D.

different diuretics have been employed before renal warm ischemia [9]. Moreover, mannitol is an intravascular volume expander, associated with the increased renal blood flow [22]. As more blood flows into the kidney, more oxygen is delivered to renal cells, and this is considered beneficial for an organ supposed to be subjected to ischemia. Finally, mannitol is also considered an antioxidant, capable of scavenging the hydroxyl radical, thus reducing oxidant-derived injury in several organs [23, 24]. As reactive oxygen species are largely produced during renal warm ischemia, the group that received mannitol in the present study may experience nonsignificant reduction in the number of nephrons due to the antioxidant properties of mannitol.

Despite the potential advantages of the use of mannitol during warm ischemia for partial nephrectomy displayed in the present study, some issues should be addressed. As stated by Omae et al., [10] omitting the use of mannitol offers some advantages, including reduction of operative time and procedural costs. Further, some complications with mannitol administration during partial nephrectomy have been reported [25]. Thus, we should note that mannitol usage is not free of charge. However, we should emphasize that mannitol infusion can be planned during surgery to reduce operative time, and also, the cost of mannitol is minimal, especially when compared to the overall costs of laparoscopic partial nephrectomy.

The results of our study support the application of mannitol as a renal warm ischemia protective agent to be employed during partial nephrectomy. Regardless, further evidence confirming or refuting these results is required. The effects of mannitol should be studied in other experimental situations such as single kidney models, renal insufficiency, and selective clamping techniques. Further, this is an animal study, and its results should not be directly transposed to humans. Although the swine constitutes the most adequate model for comparison with human kidney's anatomy and physiology [12, 13], is the fact remains that this is study was conducted in an experimental setting and different from clinical practice.

Conclusion

In conclusion, we discovered that warm ischemia of 30 min in a Pig Model determined a loss of nearly one quarter of renal nephrons. However, the application of mannitol prevented significant nephron loss during warm ischemia.

Abbreviations
CV: Absolute cortical volume; I: Group ischemia; M: Group mannitol; S: Group sham; Vv [glom]: Glomerular volumetric density; VWGV: Volume-weighted mean glomerular volume

Funding
This study was supported by grants from the National Council for Scientific and Technological Development (CNPq), the Coordination for the Improvement of Post-Graduate Students (CAPES), and the Foundation for Research Support of Rio de Janeiro (FAPERJ), Brazil. These foundations did not interfere in the design of the study and collection, analysis, and interpretation of data and in writing the manuscript.

Authors' contributions
JAD contributed to the study design, participated in all experiments and stereological analysis, and data interpretation. LASA participated in all experiments and contributed in data interpretation. GRB participated in all experiments and contributed in the process of data interpretation. WSC contributed to the study design, stereological analysis, and data interpretation. MAP contributed to the study design, participated in all experiments, data interpretation, and manuscript drafting. FJBS contributed to the study design and data interpretation. DBS contributed to the study design, participated in all experiments and stereological analysis, data interpretation, and manuscript drafting. All authors read and approved the final manuscript.

Competing interests
The authors declare that they have no competing interests.

Author details

[1]Urogenital Research Unit, Rio de Janeiro State University, Rio de Janeiro, RJ, Brazil. [2]Department of Veterinary Clinical Pathology, Fluminense Federal University, Niterói, RJ, Brazil. [3]Faculty of Medicine, Estacio de Sá University, Rio de Janeiro, RJ, Brazil. [4]Department of Morphology, Fluminense Federal University, Niteroi, RJ, Brazil.

References

1. Haber GP, Gill IS. Laparoscopic partial nephrectomy: contemporary technique and outcomes. Eur Urol. 2006;49:660–5.
2. Mir MC, Ercole C, Takagi T, Zhang Z, Velet L, Remer EM, Demirjian S, Campbell SC. Decline in renal function after partial nephrectomy: etiology and prevention. J Urol. 2015;193:1889–98.
3. Rod X, Peyronnet B, Seisen T, Pradere B, Gomez FD, Verhoest G, Vaessen C, De La Taille A, Bensalah K, Roupret M. Impact of ischaemia time on renal function after partial nephrectomy: a systematic review. BJU Int. 2016;
4. Thompson RH, Lane BR, Lohse CM, Leibovich BC, Fergany A, Frank I, Gill IS, Blute ML, Campbell SC. Renal function after partial nephrectomy: effect of warm ischemia relative to quantity and quality of preserved kidney. Urol. 2012;79:356–60.
5. Cohen J, Dorai T, Ding C, Batinic-Haberle I, Grasso M. The administration of renoprotective agents extends warm ischemia in a rat model. J Endourol. 2013;27:343–8.
6. Gill IS, Patil MB, Abreu AL, Ng C, Cai J, Berger A, Eisenberg MS, Nakamoto M, Ukimura O, Goh AC, et al. Zero ischemia anatomical partial nephrectomy: a novel approach. J Urol. 2012;187:807–14.
7. Keel CE, Wang Z, Colli J, Grossman L, Majid D, Lee BR. Protective effects of reducing renal ischemia-reperfusion injury during renal hilar clamping: use of allopurinol as a nephroprotective agent. Urol 2013, 81. 210:e215–0.
8. Wang Z, Colli JL, Keel C, Bailey K, Grossman L, Majid D, Lee BR. Isoprostane: quantitation of renal ischemia and reperfusion injury after renal artery clamping in an animal model. J Endourol. 2012;26:21–5.
9. Cosentino M, Breda A, Sanguedolce F, Landman J, Stolzenburg JU, Verze P, Rassweiler J, Van Poppel H, Klingler HC, Janetschek G, et al. The use of mannitol in partial and live donor nephrectomy: an international survey. W J urol. 2013;31:977–82.
10. Omae K, Kondo T, Takagi T, Iizuka J, Kobayashi H, Hashimoto Y, Tanabe K. Mannitol has no impact on renal function after open partial nephrectomy in solitary kidneys. Int J Urol. 2014;21:200–3.
11. Power NE, Maschino AC, Savage C, Silberstein JL, Thorner D, Tarin T, Wong A, Touijer KA, Russo P, Coleman JA. Intraoperative mannitol use does not improve long-term renal function outcomes after minimally invasive partial nephrectomy. Urol. 2012;79:821–5.
12. de Souza DB, Abilio EJ, Costa WS, Sampaio MA, Sampaio FJ. Kidney healing after laparoscopic partial nephrectomy without collecting system closure in pigs. Urol. 2011;508(**77**):e505–9.
13. Pereira-Sampaio MA, Favorito LA, Sampaio FJ. Pig kidney: anatomical relationships between the intrarenal arteries and the kidney collecting system. Applied study for urological research and surgical training. J Urol. 2004;172:2077–81.
14. Khoury W, Namnesnikov M, Fedorov D, Abu-Gazala S, Weinbroum AA. Mannitol attenuates kidney damage induced by xanthine oxidase-associated pancreas ischemia-reperfusion. J Surg Res. 2010;160:163–8.
15. Ribeiro CT, Milhomem R, De Souza DB, Costa WS, Sampaio FJ, Pereira-Sampaio MA. Effect of antioxidants on outcome of testicular torsion in rats of different ages. J Urol. 2014;191:1578–84.
16. Souza DB, Costa WS, Cardoso LE, Benchimol M, Pereira-Sampaio MA, Sampaio FJ. Does prolonged pneumoperitoneum affect the kidney? Oxidative stress, stereological and electron microscopy study in a rat model. Int Braz J Urol. 2013;39:30–6.
17. de Souza DB, de Oliveira LL, da Cruz MC, Abilio EJ, Costa WS, Pereira-Sampaio MA, Sampaio FJ. Laparoscopic partial nephrectomy under warm ischemia reduces the glomerular density in a pig model. J Endourol. 2012; 26:706–10.
18. de Souza DB, Silva D, Cortez CM, Costa WS, Sampaio FJ. Effects of chronic stress on penile corpus cavernosum of rats. J Androl. 2012;33:735–9.
19. Benchimol de Souza D, Silva D, Marinho Costa Silva C, Barcellos Sampaio FJ, Silva Costa W, Martins Cortez C. Effects of immobilization stress on kidneys of Wistar male rats: a morphometrical and stereological analysis. Kidney & blood pressure research. 2011;34:424–9.
20. Pignot G, Bouliere F, Patard JJ. Warm ischaemia: the ultimate enemy for partial nephrectomy. Eur Urol. 2010;58:337–9.
21. Gelman S. Does mannitol save the kidney. Anesth Analg. 1996;82:899–901.
22. Zager RA, Mahan J, Merola AJ. Effects of mannitol on the postischemic kidney. Biochemical, functional, and morphologic assessments. Laboratory investigation; a journal of technical methods and pathology. 1985;53:433–42.
23. England MD, Cavarocchi NC, O'Brien JF, Solis E, Pluth JR, Orszulak TA, Kaye MP, Schaff HV. Influence of antioxidants (mannitol and allopurinol) on oxygen free radical generation during and after cardiopulmonary bypass. Circulation. 1986;74:III134–7.
24. Haraldsson G, Sorensen V, Nilsson U, Pettersson S, Rashid M, Schersten T, Akerlund S, Jonsson O. Effect of pre-treatment with desferrioxamine and mannitol on radical production and kidney function after ischaemia-reperfusion. A study on rabbit kidneys. Acta Physiol Scand. 1995;154:461–8.
25. Erickson BA, Yap RL, Pazona JF, Hartigan BJ, Smith ND. Mannitol extravasation during partial nephrectomy leading to forearm compartment syndrome. Int Braz J Urol. 2007;33:68–71. discussion 71.

31

The location of the bladder neck in postoperative cystography predicts continence convalescence after radical prostatectomy

Susumu Kageyama*⬛, Tetsuya Yoshida, Masayuki Nagasawa, Shigehisa Kubota, Keiji Tomita, Kenichi Kobayashi, Ryosuke Murai, Teruhiko Tsuru, Eiki Hanada, Kazuyoshi Johnin, Mitsuhiro Narita and Akihiro Kawauchi

Abstract

Background: This study was conducted to determine whether the location of the bladder neck in postoperative cystography predicts recovery of continence after radical prostatectomy.

Methods: Between 2008 and 2015, 203 patients who underwent laparoscopic radical prostatectomy (LRP, $n = 99$) and robot assisted radical prostatectomy (RARP, $n = 104$) were analyzed. The location of the bladder neck was visualized by postoperative routine cystography, and quantitative evaluation of the bladder neck position was performed according to the bladder neck to pubic symphysis (BNPS) ratio proposed by Olgin et al. (J Endourol, 2014). Recovery of continence was defined as no pad use or one security pad per day. To determine the predictive factors for recovery of continence at 1, 3, 6 and 12 months, several parameters were analyzed using logistic regression analysis, including age (≤ 68 vs. > 68, BMI (≤ 23.4 vs. > 23.4 kg/m^2), surgical procedure (LRP vs. RARP), prostate volume (≤ 38 vs. > 38 mL), nerve-sparing technique, vesico-urethral anastomosis leakage, and BNPS ratio (≤ 0.59 vs. > 0.59).

Results: The mean postoperative follow-up was 1131 days (79–2880). At 1, 3, 6 and 12 months after surgery, continence recovery rates were 25, 53, 68 and 81%, respectively. Although older age (> 68) and RARP were significant risk factors for incontinence within 3 months, neither was significant after 6 months. A high BNPS ratio (> 0.59) was the only significant risk factor for the persistence of incontinence at all observation points, up to 12 months.

Conclusions: A lower bladder neck position after prostatectomy predicts prolonged incontinence.

Keywords: Bladder neck location, Radical prostatectomy, Continence recovery

Background

Rates of detection of localized prostate cancer have increased with early detection using serum PSA screening and this in turn has led to increased numbers of radical prostatectomies. Postoperative urinary incontinence may occur in a proportion of patients who undergo radical prostatectomy and is one of the most serious complications impacting the quality of life of patients. Several clinical characteristics have been reported to be critical factors predicting postoperative continence recovery, including the patient's age [1–3], BMI [2, 4], prostate size [2], nerve-sparing technique [5], vesico-urethral anastomosis leakage [6], and so on. Various procedures have been reported to prevent postoperative incontinence, however, surgeons have not been able to overcome this complication completely [7].

In some institutions, postoperative cystography is performed routinely before removing the Foley catheter to confirm no vesico-urethral anastomosis leakage. Several physicians have reported that the postoperative cystogram findings predict continence after radical

* Correspondence: kageyama@belle.shiga-med.ac.jp
Department of Urology, Shiga University of Medical Science, Seta Tsukinowa-cho, Otsu, Shiga 520-2192, Japan

prostatectomy [8–12]. In their prostatectomy series, Jeong et al. reported that the vesico-urethral anastomosis location (VUAL) visualized by routine postoperative cystography correlated with early recovery of postoperative continence [9]. They showed a higher location of the bladder neck was correlated with better recovery of continence. Olgin et al. also reported a similar finding, using their original quantitative evaluation of the bladder neck position in a routine cystography after RARP [10].

In this study we investigated whether the location of the bladder neck in postoperative cystography in our LRP and RARP series predicted recovery of continence within 12 months of surgery.

Methods

Two hundred and three patients who underwent LRP (*n* = 99) and RARP (*n* = 104) for clinically localized prostate cancer in the Shiga University of Medical Science Hospital from 2008 to 2015 were evaluated. All clinical, pathological and radiographical data were collected from medical records. The patients' demographics are presented in Table 1. This retrospective observational study was approved by the internal ethical committee of Shiga University of Medical Science.

The surgical procedure briefly is as follows: The Retzius space was approached extraperitoneally (LRP) or transperitoneally (RARP) and an antegrade radical prostatectomy was performed with bilateral pelvic lymph node dissection. A nerve-sparing technique was indicated individually according to various conditions, including PSA value, Gleason score, number and location of positive cores and the patient's desire to preserve sexual function. Bilateral and unilateral nerve-sparing techniques were performed in 10 (12%) and 24 (30%) cases, respectively. The vesico-uretharal anastomosis was performed with a Van Velthoven running suture. All patients underwent posterior and anterior reconstructions.

Cystography was carried out routinely six days after surgery. Images were obtained in the supine position without abdominal straining and the bladder was filled with ~ 100 mL of diluted contrast medium. A Foley catheter was advanced a few centimeters into the bladder in order to visualize the bladder neck clearly. When vesico-urethral anastomosis leakage was observed, catheter removal was delayed and a repeat cystography was performed every week until the leakage resolved. To evaluate the position of the bladder neck quantitatively, we calculated the bladder neck to pubic symphysis (BNPS) ratio, as proposed by Olgin et al. [10]. The BNPS ratio was calculated by measuring the distance from the superior edge of the pubic symphysis to the bladder neck and dividing this by the total pubic symphysis length in the cystogram. A representative cystogram is shown in Fig. 1. A single physician (SKa), who was blinded to the clinical data of the patients,

Table 1 Patients' characteristics and operative data

Mean age (range)	67.7 (48–76)
Mean BMI (kg/m2), (range)	23.7 (16.6–33.2)
Mean preoperative PSA (ng/mL), (range)	9.21 (2.24–43.20)
Clinical T stage, (%)	
T1b	3 (1.5)
T1c	122 (60.1)
T2a	45 (22.1)
T2b	15 (7.4)
T2c	18 (8.9)
D'Amico Risk Criteria, (%)	
Low risk	40 (19.7)
Intermediate risk	108 (53.2)
High risk	55 (27.1)
Operation procedure, (%)	
Laparoscopic	99 (48.8)
Robot-assisted	104 (51.2)
Nerve-sparing, (%)	
Bilateral	24 (11.8)
Unilateral	61 (30.0)
Non-sparing	118 (58.1)
Mean operative time (min), (range)	257 (137–612)
Mean estimated blood loss (g), (range)	378 (10–2431)
Mean prostate volume (mL), (range)	41 (18–92)
Positive surgical margin, (%)	56 (27.5)
Vesicourethral anastomosis leakage, (%)	16 (7.9)
Mean Postoperative followup (days)	1131 (79–2880)

evaluated cystograms and determined the BNPS ratio. Recovery of continence was defined as wearing no pad or using one safety pad per day.

Univariate analyses were performed using student t-test or the chi-square test. Uni- and multivariate logistic regression analyses were also performed. When *p*-values were less than 0.25 in univariate logistic regression analysis, the variable was included in the next multivariate logistic regression analysis. These statistical analyses were carried out using IBM SPSS Statistics version 22 software (IBM Japan, Tokyo, Japan). A *P*-value less than 0.05 is considered statistically significant.

Results

The mean postoperative follow-up period was 1131 days (79–2880). Vesico-urethral anastomosis leakage was observed in 16 cases (8%) and catheter removal was delayed in these patients. Thereafter, repeat cystography was performed every week until the leakage resolved. The mean catheter replacement period was 19.7 days (11–36) in the patients with anastomosis leakage. A

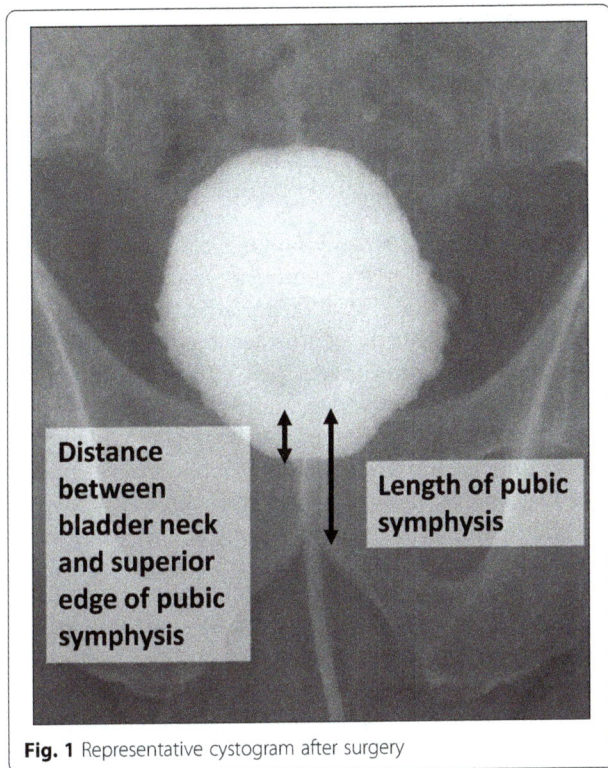

Fig. 1 Representative cystogram after surgery

Distance between bladder neck and superior edge of pubic symphysis

Length of pubic symphysis

cumulative continence recovery curve of all patients is presented in Fig. 2. The continence status at 1, 3, 6 and 12 months after surgery was evaluated in an interview by the physician during regular follow-up visits and the numbers of evaluable patients were 203 (100%), 202 (99%), 190 (93%) and 171 (84%), respectively. Continence recovery rates at 1, 3, 6 and 12 months were 25, 53, 68 and 81%, respectively. At each evaluation point, several clinical parameters, including the patient's age, surgical procedure, BMI, initial PSA value, D'Amico risk

criteria, nerve-sparing procedure, operative time, estimated blood loss, prostate volume, positive surgical margin, anastomosis leakage and BNPS ratio were compared between continent and incontinent patients (Table 2 and Additional file 1: Tables S1-S4). At 1 month after surgery, the patient's age, operation procedure and BNPS ratio differed significantly between the continent and incontinent groups. At 3 and 6 months, the patient's age and BNPS ratio were significantly different. However, at 12 months, only the BNPS ratio was differed significantly between the groups. The difference of mean BNPS ratio between the continent and incontinent groups was significant at all evaluation points (Fig. 3).

Next, in order to elucidate the risk factors for delayed recovery of continence, we evaluated our patients' data by logistic regression analysis. According to the risk factors reported previously in the literature, we chose several variables for analysis, including the patient's age, BMI, nerve-sparing technique, prostate volume, vesico-urethral anastomosis leakage and BNPS ratio. In addition, we included the surgical procedure, because this showed a significant difference at one month in our cohort. Continuous variables, including age, BMI, prostate volume and BNPS ratio, were divided into two categories according to the median values. The median values of age, BMI, prostate volume and BNPS ratio were 68y, 23.4 kg/m^2, 38 mL and 0.59, respectively. In order to determine whether other clinical factors were confounding the BNPS ratio, we compared these factors between the high (> 0.59) and low (≤ 0.59) BNPS ratio

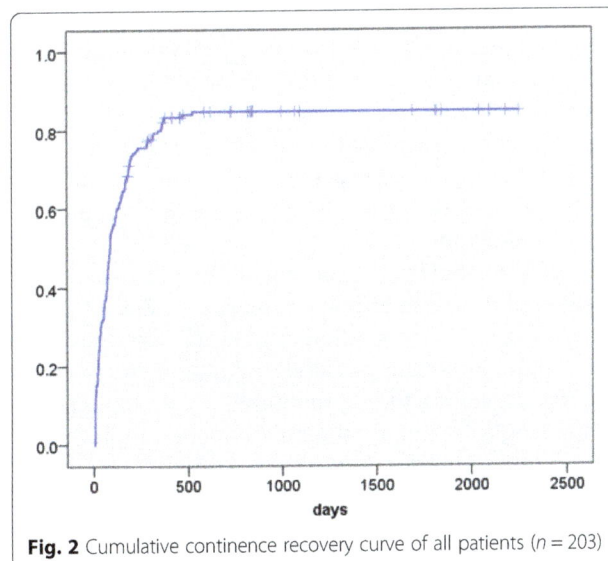

Fig. 2 Cumulative continence recovery curve of all patients ($n = 203$)

Table 2 Results of statistical analysis of perioperative characteristics between continent and incontinent patients at 1, 3, 6 and 12 months

Follow-up	1 m	3 m	6 m	12 m
Continent (n)	51	107	130	139
Incontinent (n)	152	95	60	32
	P-Value			
Age	0.0020	0.0056	0.0031	0.0512
Procedure	0.0010	0.6601	0.9215	0.3073
BMI	0.5920	0.7470	0.6147	0.8844
PSA	0.3154	0.8596	0.2856	0.7107
D'Amico risk criteria	0.1437	0.4865	0.2614	0.0919
Nerve-sparing	0.2318	0.4737	0.4744	0.3259
Operative time	0.8303	0.7510	0.4918	0.5753
Estimated Blood loss	0.3971	0.2866	0.2039	0.4344
Prostate volume	0.4027	0.5929	0.3245	0.3158
Positive resection margin	0.9801	0.8345	0.3967	0.8450
Anastomosis leakage	0.9906	0.4413	0.1902	0.1285
BNPS ratio	< 0.0001	0.0006	< 0.0001	0.0003

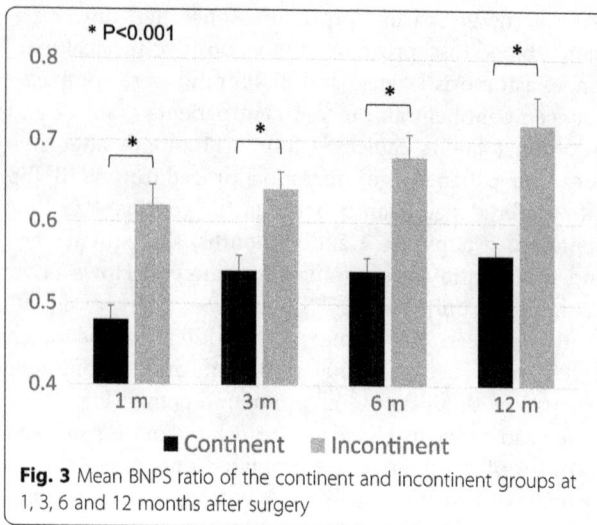

Fig. 3 Mean BNPS ratio of the continent and incontinent groups at 1, 3, 6 and 12 months after surgery

groups (Additional file 1: Table S5). The BNPS ratio did not correlate with any other factors.

At one month, the univariate logistic regression analysis showed that the older age, RARP and higher BNPS ratio correlated with persistent incontinence (Table 3). Similarly, a multivariate logistic regression analysis showed that older age (OR 2.171, 95% CI 1.011–4.663), RARP (OR 3.131, 95% CI 1.528–6.417) and higher BNPS ratio (OR 2.867, 95% CI 1.49–5.831) were significant risk factors. At three months, the univariate logistic regression analysis showed that the older age and higher BNPS ratio correlated significantly with prolonged recovery of continence. Multivariate logistic regression analysis showed that older age (OR 2.009, 95% CI 1.127–3.581) and higher BNPS ratio (OR 2.245, 95% CI 1.265–3.983) were significant independent variables. However, at 6 and 12 months, only the BNPS ratio was a significant predictor in uni- and multivariate logistic regression analyses. Therefore, the BNPS ratio was the only constant predictor, not only in short-term but also long-term continence recovery within a year of prostatectomy.

Discussion

Urinary incontinence is a frequent negative outcome of radical prostatectomy and postoperative incontinence rates of 8~20% have been reported in large series [13, 14]. For patients, recovery of urinary continence is one of the most important concerns with respect to quality of life [15]. Several predictive preoperative characteristics have been reported to correlate with recovery of continence [1, 2, 7]. In particular, older age, obesity and large prostate volume have been reported as the worst predictors of continence convalescence. The preoperative urethral length, measured by magnetic resonance imaging, was suggested to be a prognostic factor [16, 17]. Intra-

or postoperative factors were also analyzed as predictors of post-prostatectomy incontinence and were as follows: nerve-sparing techniques, posterior/anterior reconstruction, bladder neck preservation, periurethral suspension, pelvic floor muscle exercise, incontinence volume at a very early phase after catheter withdrawal, and so on [7].

Postoperative cystography findings also were reported as a predictive factor for continence recovery by a few groups [9–12]. Jeong et al. reported a correlation between VUAL and early continence recovery in a large cohort [9]. They categorized their 678 cases into three groups, based on the vesico-urethral anastomosis location (VUAL), as determined by postoperative routine cystography: group I - above the upper margin of the symphysis pubis, group II – between the upper margin and the middle of the symphysis pubis, and group III – below the middle of the symphysis pubis. Group I showed the best recovery rate, while group III had the worst continence convalescence. They concluded that a higher VUAL leads to a higher rate of early continence recovery. In their study, they mentioned that the critical point of VUAL was the middle of the symphysis pubis. Olgin and colleagues also reported that the higher bladder neck position correlated with good continence recovery after RARP [10]. They devised a new quantitation parameter, the BNPS ratio, which was calculated on the basis of a postoperative cystogram. The BNPS ratios derived from the postoperative cystograms of 215 patients who underwent RARP were evaluated and compared with their continence status. At three months after surgery, continent patients had a mean BNPS ratio of 0.39, while incontinent patients had a mean BNPS ratio of 0.49 ($p = 0.01$). At 12 months, the mean BNPS ratio was 0.40 for continent patients, whereas incontinent patients had a mean BNPS ratio of 0.60 ($p = 0.001$). The authors concluded that the BNPS ratio on cystogram correlates with continence rates and the lower position of the bladder neck may predict a risk for prolonged incontinence. These two studies and the data presented here confirm that the correct suspension of the bladder neck predicts good recovery of continence and the critical position is around the middle of the symphysis pubis on a postoperative cystogram.

What contributes to achieving a higher bladder neck position after prostatectomy? Extensive studies of pelvic anatomy have been carried out and much effort has been devoted to improving surgical techniques. A common concept pervading these procedures is the conservation of the original anatomical structure. The restoration of the posterior rhabdosphincter, reported by Rocco et al., was a landmark in the progress of surgical technique [18, 19]. The authors emphasized that reconstruction of the posterior musclofascial plate and suspension of the

Table 3 Uni- and multivariate logistic regression analysis of the parameters for incontinence status at 1, 3, 6 and 12 months

Follow-up	1 m	3 m	6 m	12 m	1 m	3 m	6 m	12 m
	Univariate logistic regression				Multivariate logistic regression			
Parameters	OR (95% CI) P-value				OR (95% CI) P-value			
Age (< 68 vs. > 68)	2.442 (1.222–4.881) P = 0.011	2.102 (1.193–3.704) P = 0.010	1.826 (0.983–3.392) P = 0.057	1.527 (0.706–3.305) P = 0.282	2.171 (1.011–4.663) P = 0.047	2.009 (1.127–3.581) P = 0.018	1.690 (0.898–3.180) P = 0.104	–
Procedure (LRP vs. RARP)	3.008 (1.534–5.898) P = 0.001	1.132 (0.651–1.968) P = 0.660	1.031 (0.559–1.901) P = 0.921	1.492 (0.690–3.227) P = 0.309	3.131 (1.528–6.417) P = 0.002	–	–	–
BMI (< 23.4 vs. > 23.4 kg/m2)	0.843 (0.447–1.592) P = 0.599	1.041 (0.599–1.808) P = 0.888	0.798 (0.432–1.473) P = 0.470	0.483 (0.219–1.064) P = 0.071	–	–	–	0.449 (0.198–1.017) P = 0.055
Nerve-sparing (Yes vs. No)	1.474 (0.779–2.791) P = 0.233	1.228 (0.700–2.154) P = 0.474	1.256 (0.672–2.347) P = 0.475	1.493 (0.669–3.332) P = 0.328	1.323 (0.634–2.763) P = 0.456	–	–	–
Prostate volume (< 38 vs. > 38 mL)	1.040 (0.551–1.961) P = 0.904	0.921 (0.530–1.601) P = 0.772	1.143 (0.619–2.109) P = 0.669	0.895 (0.415–1.933) P = 0.778	–	–	–	–
Anastomosis leakage (No vs. Yes)	1.007 (0.310–3.274) P = 0.991	1.495 (0.534–4.183) P = 0.444	2.014 (0.695–5.839) P = 0.197	2.389 (0.756–7.551) P = 0.138	–	–	1.817(0.609–5.426) P = 0.285	2.747(0.820–9.198) P = 0.101
BNPS ratio (< 0.59 vs. > 0.59)	3.127 (1.581–6.188) P = 0.001	2.333 (1.326–4.106) P = 0.003	2.060 (1.103–3.850) P = 0.023	2.371 (1.063–5.290) P = 0.035	2.867 (1.409–5.831) P = 0.004	2.245 (1.265–3.983) P = 0.006	1.989 (1.056–3.745) P = 0.033	2.338 (1.034–5.288) P = 0.041

urethral sphincteric complex is the key to the early recovery of continence. They reported that their procedure with posterior reconstruction dramatically shortened recovery periods (72, 79 and 86% at 3, 30 and 90 days compared with 14, 30 and 46%, respectively, without posterior reconstruction) [18]. Another pivotal modification is the anterior reconstruction. Various procedures were reported by a number of surgeons, including periurethral suspension stitch [20], preservation of puboprostatic collar [21] and puboprostatic ligament preservation [22]. Later, some authors reported on the importance of the total reconstruction procedure, which includes both anterior and posterior reconstructions. Tewari et al. presented the results of a prospective study to compare continence recovery rates of no reconstruction, anterior reconstruction only and total reconstruction [8]. They reported that total reconstruction enabled a statistically significant early return to continence (38, 83, 91, and 97% at 1, 6, 12, and 24 weeks, respectively) compared with no reconstructive procedure (13, 35, 50, and 62%) or with only anterior reconstruction (27, 59, 77, and 86%). They also presented typical cystograms of these three groups and the bladders of the total reconstruction group showed the highest vesico-urethral junctions [8]. Therefore, the suspension and stabilization of the bladder neck by anatomical reconstruction was believed to contribute to an early return of continence. All of our cases were performed with both posterior and anterior reconstructions. Consequently, it was not possible to differentiate these cases from patients without the use of these techniques. A lower bladder neck position after surgery might reflect unsuccessful anatomical preservation.

After prostatectomy, most patients achieve final continence status within 1 year; therefore, we choose the postoperative observation points of 1, 3, 6 and 12 months for our cases. Interestingly, the mean BNPS ratios of both the continent and incontinent groups increased gradually over the postoperative period (Fig. 3). Olgin et al. evaluated their patients at 3 and 12 months and reported that the mean BNPS ratios of the incontinence group were 0.49 and 0.60, respectively. Similar to our result, the BNPS ratio at 12 months was higher than at 3 months. Taking their and our findings into account, patients with a BNPS ratio of 0.6 or more might constitute the poorest group in terms of postoperative incontinence. Naturally, the postoperative bladder neck position cannot constitute a predictive factor before prostatectomy, therefore, the BNPS ratio is not valuable as a preoperative predictor of incontinence. However, the BNPS ratio can be useful as a prognostic factor which may be obtained easily by a routine postoperative cystogram and may be useful, for example, to identify patients who require strict instructions for postoperative recovery of continence, such as pelvic floor muscle exercise. For surgeons, the BNPS ratio might be used as a surrogate predictor for the degree of achievement of preservation of anatomical support of the bladder neck/sphincter complex. Further research on this point is needed.

Our study has some limitations. First, our data were obtained from the experience at a single institution and the number of patient is relatively small. Second, we evaluated the position of the bladder neck in a restricted condition, in that cystography was performed in the supine position without straining or standing. With increased abdominal pressure, the bladder neck presumably will present in a lower position. Third, we did not evaluate various other parameters which may correlate with incontinence. Pre- and/or post-operative membranous urethral length, preoperative LUTS, preoperative incontinence, and the surgeon's extent of experience were not evaluated in our series, because of a lack of adequate data. However, regardless of these limitations, the location of the bladder neck visualized by a cystogram may become a helpful predictor of post-prostatectomy incontinence.

Conclusion

A lower location of the bladder neck in postoperative routine cystography predicts incontinence, not only in the short term but also in the long term. According to previous reports of reconstruction techniques, it is assumed that stabilization and suspension of the urethral sphincteric complex by total reconstruction is an important procedure to achieve a higher bladder neck position.

Abbreviations

LRP: Laparoscopic radical nephrectomy; PSA: Prostate specific antigen; RARP: Robot assisted radical prostatectomy

Acknowledgements

No financial support was received for this study.

Authors' contributions

SKa has made substantial contributions to the conception and design, acquisition of data and data analysis. He has drafted the manuscript and approved the submitted version. TY, NM, SKu, KT, TT, EH, KJ and NM have made contribution to the acquisition of data. AK has made substantial contributions to study design and revision of the manuscrip. All authors have read and approved the final manuscript.

Competing interests

The authors declare that they have no competing interests.

References

1.   Novara G, Ficarra V, D'elia C, Secco S, Cioffi A, Cavalleri S, et al. Evaluating urinary continence and preoperative predictors of urinary continence after robot assisted laparoscopic radical prostatectomy. J Urol. 2010;184:1028–33.
2.   Kim JJ, Ha YS, Kim JH, Jeon SS, Lee DH, Kim WJ, et al. Independent predictors of recovery of continence 3 months after robot-assisted laparoscopic radical prostatectomy. J Endourol. 2012;26:1290–5.
3.   Greco KA, Meeks JJ, Wu S, Nadler RB. Robot-assisted radical prostatectomy in men aged ≥70 years. BJU Int. 2009;104:1492–5.
4.   Ahlering TE, Eichel L, Edwards R, Skarecky DW. Impact of obesity on clinical outcomes in robotic prostatectomy. Urology. 2005;65:740–4.
5.   Takenaka A, Soga H, Kurahashi T, Miyake H, Tanaka K, Fujisawa M. Early recovery of urinary continence after laparoscopic versus retropubic radical prostatectomy: evaluation of preoperative erectile function and nerve-sparing procedure as predictors. Int Urol Nephrol. 2009;41:587–93.
6.   Patil N, Krane L, Javed K, Williams T, Bhandari M, Menon M. Evaluating and grading cystographic leakage: correlation with clinical outcomes in patients undergoing robotic prostatectomy. BJU Int. 2009;103:1108–10.
7.   Kojima Y, Takahashi N, Haga N, Nomiya M, Yanagida T, Ishibashi K, et al. Urinary incontinence after robot-assisted radical prostatectomy: pathophysiology and intraoperative techniques to improve surgical outcome. Int J Urol. 2013;20:1052–63.
8.   Tewari A, Jhaveri J, Rao S, Yadav R, Bartsch G, Te A, et al. Total reconstruction of the vesico-urethral junction. BJU Int. 2008;101:871–7.
9.   Jeong SJ, Yi J, Chung MS, Kim DS, Lee WK, Park H, et al. Early recovery of urinary continence after radical prostatectomy: correlation with vesico-urethral anastomosis location in the pelvic cavity measured by postoperative cystography. Int J Urol. 2011;18:444–51.
10. Olgin G, Alsyouf M, Han D, Li R, Lightfoot M, Smith D, et al. Postoperative cystogram findings predict incontinence following robot-assisted radical prostatectomy. J Endourol. 2014;28:1460–3.
11. Ha YS, Bak DJ, Chung JW, Lee JN, Kwon SY, Choi SH, et al. Postoperative cystographic findings as an independent predictor of urinary incontinence three months after radical prostatectomy. Minerva Urol Nefrol. 2017;69:278–84.
12. Chang LW, Hung SC, Hu JC, Chiu KY. Retzius-sparing robotic-assisted radical prostatectomy associated with less bladder neck descent and better early continence outcome. Anticancer Res. 2018;38:345–51.
13. Catalona WJ, Carvalhal GF, Mager DE, Smith DS. Potency, continence and complication rates in 1,870 consecutive radical retropubic prostatectomies. J Urol. 1999;162:433–8.
14. Begg CB, Riedel ER, Bach PB, Kattan MW, Schrag D, Warren JL, et al. Variations in morbidity after radical prostatectomy. N Engl J Med. 2002;346:1138–44.
15. Hara I, Kawabata G, Miyake H, Nakamura I, Hara S, Okada H, et al. Comparison of quality of life following laparoscopic and open prostatectomy for prostate cancer. J Urol. 2003;169:2045–8.
16. Mendoza PJ, Stern JM, Li AY, Jaffe W, Kovell R, Nguyen M, et al. Pelvic anatomy on preoperative magnetic resonance imaging can predict early continence after robot-assisted radical prostatectomy. J Endourol. 2011;25:51–5.

The location of the bladder neck in postoperative cystography predicts continence convalescence...

233

17. Paparel P, Akin O, Sandhu JS, Otero JR, Serio AM, Scardino PT, et al. Recovery of urinary continence after radical prostatectomy: association with urethral length and urethral fibrosis measured by preoperative and postoperative endorectal magnetic resonance imaging. Eur Urol. 2009;55: 629–37.

18. Rocco F, Carmignani L, Acquati P, Gadda F, Dell'Orto P, Rocco B, et al. Restoration of posterior aspect of rhabdosphincter shortens continence time after radical retropubic prostatectomy. J Urol. 2006;175:2201–6.

19. Rocco B, Cozzi G, Spinelli MG, Coelho RF, Patel VR, Tewari A, et al. Posterior musculofascial reconstruction after radical prostatectomy: a systematic review of the literature. Eur Urol. 2012;62:779–90.

20. Patel VR, Coelho RF, Palmer KJ, Rocco B. Periurethral suspension stitch during robot-assisted laparoscopic radical prostatectomy: description of the technique and continence outcomes. Eur Urol. 2009;56:472–8.

21. Tewari AK, Bigelow K, Rao S, Takenaka A, El-Tabi N, Te A, et al. Anatomic restoration technique of continence mechanism and preservation of puboprostatic collar: a novel modification to achieve early urinary continence in men undergoing robotic prostatectomy. Urology. 2007;69: 726–31.

22. Stolzenburg JU, Liatsikos EN, Rabenalt R, Do M, Sakelaropoulos G, Horn LC, et al. Nerve sparing endoscopic extraperitoneal radical prostatectomy–effect of puboprostatic ligament preservation on early continence and positive margins. Eur Urol. 2006;49:103–11.

32

Ki-67 expression predicts biochemical recurrence after radical prostatectomy in the setting of positive surgical margins

Mohammed Shahait[1†], Samer Nassif[2†], Hani Tamim[3], Deborah Mukherji[3], Maya Hijazi[2], Marwan El Sabban[4], Raja Khauli[1], Muhammad Bulbul[1], Wassim Abou Kheir[4] and Albert El Hajj[1*]

Abstract

Background: Positive surgical margin (PSM) is a predictor of biochemical recurrence (BCR) following radical prostatectomy (RP). Attempts to stratify PSM based on linear length, Gleason score, location and number have failed to add to predictive models using margin status alone. We evaluated the prognostic significance of Ki-67 expression in this setting.

Methods: Immunohistochemical staining for Ki-67 was done on prostatectomy specimens from 117 patients who had a PSM. Ki67 expression was measured at the margin and in the index lesion. Patients were dichotomized based on Ki-67 expression into three groups. Group 1 with no Ki-67 expression, Group 2 with Ki-67 ≤ 2%, and Group 3 with Ki-67 ≥ 3%. To eliminate the impact of the adjuvant treatment (AT) on the outcome, data were analyzed by the Cox proportional hazards in which AT was Considered as a time-dependent covariate.

Results: The discordance rate of Ki-67 expression between matched index lesion and margin specimens was 44/117 (37.6%). There was a trend for higher risk of BCR (HR:2.06, (0.97–4.43), $P = 0.06$) in patients expressing high Ki67 at the surgical margin although this was not statistically significant. However High Ki-67 expression in the index lesion was an independent predictive factor for BCR in this subset of patients. (HR:4, (1.64–9.80), $P = 0.002$).

Conclusion: High Ki67 expression in the index prostate cancer lesion is an independent predictor of BCR in patients with positive surgical margin following radical prostatectomy. Our findings need to be validated in a larger cohort.

Keywords: Ki-67, Positive surgical margin, Radical prostatectomy, Biochemical recurrence, Prostate cancer

Background

Prostate cancer is the second most common cancer to affect men worldwide, with an estimate 1.1 million new cases and 307,000 deaths in 2012 [1]. Radical prostatectomy (RP) is still the most common treatment for localized prostate cancer and has benefited from several refinements in surgical technique and technological advancements. A true measure of the oncological quality of RP remains the positive surgical margin which is considered an adverse prognostic feature that can predict biochemical recurrence (BCR). Many attempts at risk stratification of the positive margins have failed. Neither the number nor the sites of positive margins were found to have a significant impact on PSA recurrence [2]. More recently, Udo et al. showed that the linear length of positive surgical margins (PSM) in millimeters (LLOM) and highest Gleason grade or score at PSM are associated with progression. However, subcategorization of surgical margins based on these parameters failed to add to predictive models using margin status alone [3].

Ki67-LI is a proliferation marker that is determined via a rapid, cheap and simple immunohistochemical method. The Ki67-LI, measured using MIB-1 antibody provides an estimate of the growth fraction of the tumor. Although not strongly expressed in prostate cancer cells,

---
* Correspondence: Ae67@aub.edu.lb
†Equal contributors
[1]Division of Urology, Faculty of Medicine, American University of Beirut Medical Center, P.O. Box 11-0236, Riad El-Solh, Beirut 1107 2020, Lebanon
Full list of author information is available at the end of the article

several studies have shown its potential role in predicting BCR and even prostate cancer-specific mortality. High Ki67-LI was an independent predictor of increased disease specific mortality and biochemical recurrence in primarily intermediate-risk prostate cancer patients treated with RT or Radical prostatectomy [4, 5]. More recently, Tollefson et al. found that each 1% increase in Ki-67 expression was associated with a 12% increased risk of prostate cancer-specific death [6].

The aim of our study was to measure the Ki67 at the surgical margin and index lesion in a radical prostatectomy series and correlate Ki-67 expression with BCR.

Methods

Patient population:

All studies were undertaken with the approval and oversight of the Institutional Review Board for the Protection of Human Subjects at the American University of Beirut. The consent for tissue processing was waived by the IRB. The study comprised of 117 patients who underwent open radical prostatectomy between 1998 and 2012 and had a positive surgical margin at the final pathology.

No patient had clinical lymph node involvement or distant metastatic disease at the time of prostatectomy. Exclusion criteria were patients with pathologic lymph node involvement, patients treated with neoadjuvant therapy, patients with persistent PSA level, and those for whom original pathology slides were unavailable.

Tissue processing

For every patient, all slides from the prostatectomy specimen were reviewed separately by two pathologists to identify the sections/block showing a positive surgical margin, and to re-assess the Gleason score based on the most up-to-date Gleason scoring method. In cases where margins were positive multifocally, sections harboring the largest focus of tumor were selected. The lengths of the positive margin, as well as the Ki-67 proliferation index, were noted for all cases. The Ki-67 index was also assessed independently by the same two pathologists using the following method: 1-the tumor area was screened to identify the foci with the highest nuclear staining; 2-these foci were divided into quadrants and examined at high power magnification (400×); 3- tumor nuclei were counted in each quadrant, and the percentage of positive tumor nuclei was determined. For each case with a positive margin, the Ki-67 index was assessed at the margin and in the index tumor.

Immunohistochemistry

Immunostaining for Ki-67 was performed using the DAKO MIB-1 antibody. Staining was performed on the Ventana immunostainer using protocols established by the manufacturer and approved for clinical practice. With each staining run, positive control tissues were used to ensure adequate staining performance.

Follow-up

The 117 patients were followed from 10 to 106 months with a median of 48 months (mean 58.2 months). Biochemical recurrence was defined as a PSA greater than 0.2 ng/ml confirmed on two consecutive PSA examinations. A total of 62 patients received adjuvant radiotherapy (AT) with concomitant hormonal therapy (6–18 months) before evidence of biochemical or clinical recurrence.

Statistical analysis

Categorical variables were compared by the chi-square test. Cox proportional hazards regression analysis was used to test the association of various pathological and clinical features with recurrence. To eliminate the impact of the adjuvant treatment (AT) on the outcome, data were analyzed by the Cox proportional hazards in which AT was considered as a time-dependent covariate as described previously by Swindle et al. [7].

Patients were stratified based on Ki-67 expression into three groups based on the distribution of the original variables. Group 1 with no Ki-67 expression, Group 2 with Ki-67 expression less than or equal to 2%, and Group 3 with Ki-67 expression $\geq$3% (Fig. 1).

Univariable and multivariable Cox regression models were carried out to determine independent predictors of PSA failure in patients with positive surgical margin. The variable that was significant at $p < 0.2$ at the univariable level was entered into the multivariable model. Age of patients, PSA, Gleason score, SVI, and EPE, were forced into the multivariable model. Hazard ratios (HR) and their 95% confidence intervals (CI) were reported.

Results

Clinicopathological parameters

Mean age at radical prostatectomy was 62.01 years ($\pm$ 6.06). Sixteen patients (13.68%) had a Gleason score < =6, 79 (67.52%) had a Gleason score equal to 7 and 22 patients (18.8%) had a Gleason score > =8. Fifty-two patients (44.4%) had an extraprostatic extension, 23 patients (19.6%) had a seminal vesicle involvement. Adjuvant treatment was administered in 62 (52.99%) of the cases. Fifty-seven patients of the 117 (48.7%) developed biochemical recurrence during the follow-up period (Table 1).

Margin status

Of the patients 62 (52.99%) had multiple margins and the linear length of the margin (LLOM) was greater than

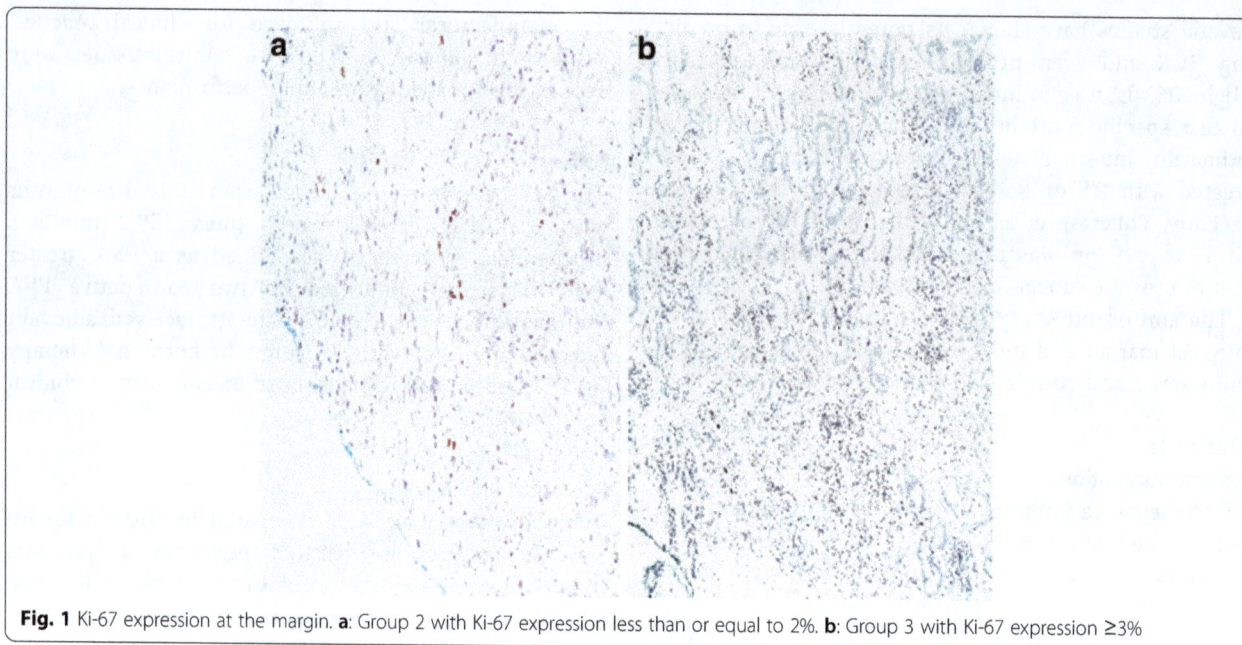

Fig. 1 Ki-67 expression at the margin. **a**: Group 2 with Ki-67 expression less than or equal to 2%. **b**: Group 3 with Ki-67 expression ≥3%

3 mm in 68 (58.62%). Ki-67 was expressed in 53 of 117 (45.3%) of the surgical margin.

Immunohistochemistry

Ki-67 was expressed in 25 of 117 (21%) of the index lesion and 53 of 117 (45%) of the matched margins. The discordance rate of Ki-67 expression between matched index lesion and margin specimens was 44/117 (37.6%) with a trend of higher Ki-67 expression at the margin compared to the index lesion (Fig. 2). The mean Ki-67 expression at the margin was 1.32% (±2.16).

Cox proportional hazards regression analysis

Higher Ki-67 expression at the margin showed a trend toward significant association with higher risk of BCR (HR:2.06, (0.97–4.43), $P = 0.06$). On the other hand, LLOM and number of the margin were not correlated with biochemical recurrence (Table 2).

High Ki-67 expression in the deep tumor was an independent predictor of biochemical recurrence (HR:4, (1.64–9.80), $P = 0.002$).

Discussion

In this cohort of patients with positive surgical margin after radical prostatectomy, our results show that high Ki-67 expression in the deep tumor was a significant predictor of BCR and high Ki-67 expression at the margin showed a trend toward significant association with BCR. We also found that there is no correlation between LLOM and extent of margin on the biochemical recurrence.

PSM is an established adverse pathological feature correlated with biochemical progression [7]. Indeed, this correlation has impacted urologist practice by utilizing adjuvant treatment in patients with PSM; Grossfeld et al. using the CaPSURE database found that patients with a positive margin were much more likely to receive adjuvant treatment (p 0.0011) [2].BCR rate in our cohort is in line with previously observed rate in PSM patients (32%–74%) [8, 9]. In the observation arm of the European Organisation for Research and Treatment of Cancer 22,911, which compared the administration of AT versus patient observation, 41% of the patients were disease-free at five years. Therefore, it is evident that there is overtreatment of patients with positive surgical margin, which might have an adverse impact on patient care, given that the use of AT is not without acute and late gastrointestinal and genitourinary toxicities [10].

Several studies attempted to classify surgical margins based on different features, such as length of the margin, the extent of the margin, and Gleason score at the margin. Sofer et al. found that there is no correlation between surgical margin site and biochemical progression. Moreover, he demonstrated that there was no statistically significant difference in time to progression between patients with single margin and patients with multiple margins [11]. Additionally, Epstein et al. failed to demonstrate any difference in the progression between patients with single margin and those with multiple margins [12]. In the current study, there was no statistically significant difference in prognosis between men with a single site of a positive margin or

Table 1 Summary of the clinical and pathological data

		Total N = 117	PSA failure Negative N = 60	Positive N = 57	p-value
Age	Mean (±SD)	62.01 ± 6.06	62.35 ± 5.98	61.65 ± 5.21	0.53
PSA-PRE surgery	0–10	69 (61.1)	42 (72.4)	27 (49.1)	0.04
	10–20	31 (27.4)	11 (19.0)	20 (36.4)	
	> 20	13 (11.5)	5 (8.6)	8 (14.6)	
GS	6	16 (13.68)	9 (15.00)	7 (12.28)	0.39
	7	79 (67.52)	43 (71.67)	36 (63.16)	
	8	17 (14.53)	7 (11.67)	10 (17.54)	
	9	5 (4.27)	1 (1.67)	4 (7.02)	
Tumor volume	Mean (±SD)	26.52 ± 20.80	26.29 ± 19.30	26.78 ± 22.62	0.90
EPE	No	65 (55.56)	37 (61.67)	28 (49.12)	0.17
	Yes	52 (44.44)	23 (38.33)	29 (50.88)	
SVI	No	94 (80.34)	49 (81.67)	45 (78.95)	0.71
	Yes	23 (19.66)	11 (18.33)	12 (21.05)	
Linear Length of the Margin	< 3 mm	48 (41.38)	28 (46.67)	20 (35.71)	0.23
	> = 3 mm	68 (58.62)	32 (53.33)	36 (64.29)	
KI67 at the Margin	1 (no expression)	64 (54.70)	31 (51.67)	33 (57.89)	0.42
	2 (weak expression)	31 (26.50)	19 (31.67)	12 (21.05)	
	3 (strong expression)	22 (18.80)	10 (16.67)	12 (21.05)	
Number of Margin	Single	55 (47.01)	30 (50.00)	25 (43.86)	0.51
	Multiple	62 (52.99)	30 (50.00)	32 (56.14)	
KI67-deep tumor	1 (no expression)	92 (78.63)	49 (81.67)	43 (75.44)	0.71
	2 (weak expression)	11 (9.40)	5 (8.33)	6 (10.53)	
	3 (strong expression)	14 (11.97)	6 (10.00)	8 (14.04)	
Adjuvant treatment	No	55 (47.01)	31 (51.67)	24 (42.11)	0.30
	Yes	62 (52.99)	29 (48.33)	33 (57.89)	

multiple sites, supporting results from previous studies. However, while LLOM more than 3 mm have been shown to confer a worse prognosis compared to margins < 3 mm, we were unable to validate this finding in our cohort [13, 14].

Ki-67 is an established marker of cell proliferation, which has been previously studied in prostate cancer and was correlated with biochemical progression, prostate cancer-specific survival and overall survival [4, 15, 16]. No study to our knowledge has examined the importance of Ki-67 expression in the setting of positive surgical margins.

Mesko et al. demonstrated a significant heterogeneity in intraprostatic and intralesional expression of Ki-67 [17]. We found that there is high heterogeneity of Ki-67 expression between the index lesion and the margin, with a discordance rate of 37.6%. This has stirred us to measure ki-67 expression at the margin and the index lesion.

Intriguingly, the mean Ki-67 expression in our cohort was 0.5% (±1.32) which is lower than the levels reported in the literature [17, 18]. There was no significant difference in overall Ki-67 proliferation values when comparing stains performed on old tissue blocks (more than five years old) to stains carried out on more recent blocks. The difference between our results and previously published results is unclear at this point, but could be attributed to the racial differences in the prostate cancer biology [19–22].

In the current study we assessed the significance of Ki-67 at margin accounting for the patients who received AT. Our study has shown that there was a trend towards biochemical recurrence in PSM patients with higher Ki-67 expression at the margin however statistical significance was not attained (HR 2.06, CI 0.97–4.43 $P = 0.06$). On the other hand, Ki67 expression in the index tumor was an independent predictor of BCR ($p = 0.002$). This finding may help in the

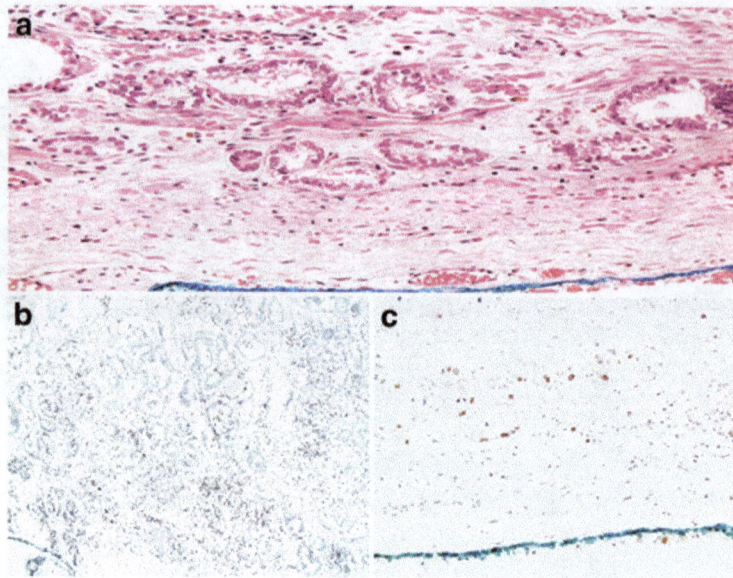

Fig. 2 Ki-67 expression at the margin and at the index lesion. **a**: Prostate Adenocarcinoma at the inked margin. **b**: High Ki-67 expression at the margin. **c**: Low Ki-67 expression at the index lesion

discussion of post-prostatectomy treatment for patients with PSM.

We acknowledge that the present study has some limitations that warrant discussion. First, the data analyzed are retrospective and included patients operated on before the 2005 International Society of Urological Pathology modified Gleason score system. For this reason all pathology slides were reviewed by two expert pathologists and the Gleason score was revised according to the new classification. Second, there are inherent limitations

to the reliability and reproducibility of the immunohistochemical techniques.

Conclusion

Ki67 expression at the margin is a potential tool to predict biochemical recurrence in patients with positive surgical margins following radical prostatectomy. There is a need to validate this finding in a larger prospective trial and determine reference Ki-67 values. In the era of genetic testing, this cost effective and simple marker can be an additional tool to determine the optimal care in this subset of patients.

Table 2 Predictors of biochemical recurrence on multivariable cox regression analysis

	HR	95% CI	P value
Ki 67 in deep tumor			
Group 1	Reference		
Group 2	1.41	(0.57–3.52)	0.46
Group 3	4	(1.64–9.80)	0.002
Ki 67 at margin			
Group 1	Reference		
Group 2	1.12	(0.55–2.31)	0.75
Group 3	2.08	(0.97–4.43)	0.06
Length of the margin			
< 3 mm	Reference		
> =3 mm	1.28	(0.70–2.37)	0.42
Number of margin			
Single margin	Reference		
Multiple margins	0.83	(0.45–1.51)	0.54

Abbreviations

AT: Adjuvant Therapy; BCR: Biochemical recurrence; CI: Confidence intervals; EPE: Extra-prostatic extension; GS: Gleason score; HR: Hazard ratios; LLOM: Linear length of the margin; PSA: Prostate specific antigen; PSM: Positive surgical margin; RP: Radical prostatectomy; SVI: Seminal Vesicle Invasion

Acknowledgments

We would like to thank Ms. Aurelie Mailhac for her assistance in the statistical analysis.

Funding

Funded by MPP fund in the American University of Beirut, Faculty of Medicine, Beirut, Lebanon.

The American University of Beirut MPP Funding program played no part in the design or conduct of the study; collection, management, analysis, or interpretation of the data; preparation, review, or approval of the manuscript; or decision to submit the manuscript for publication.

Authors' contributions

The First Authors MS and SN contributed equally to the study. MS Protocol/project development, Data collection or management, Data analysis, Manuscript writing/editing. SN Protocol/project development, Data collection or management, Manuscript writing/editing, Pathology reading. DM Protocol/project development, Data analysis, Manuscript writing/editing. HT Protocol/project development, Data collection or management, Data analysis, Manuscript writing/editing. MH Data collection or management, Manuscript writing/editing, Pathology reading. ME Protocol/project development, Data collection or management, Manuscript writing/editing, Pathology reading.
RK Protocol/project development, Manuscript writing/editing. MBI Protocol/project development, Manuscript writing/editing. WAK Protocol/project development, Manuscript writing/editing, Pathology reading. AEH Protocol/project development, Data collection or management, Data analysis, Manuscript writing/editing. All authors read and approved the final manuscript.

Competing interests

Albert El-Hajj is a member of the editorial board (Associate Editor) of BMC Urology. All other authors declare that they have no conflict of interest.

Author details

[1]Division of Urology, Faculty of Medicine, American University of Beirut Medical Center, P.O. Box 11-0236, Riad El-Solh, Beirut 1107 2020, Lebanon. [2]Department of Pathology, Faculty of Medicine, American University of Beirut Medical Center, P.O. Box 11-0236, Riad El-Solh, Beirut 1107 2020, Lebanon. [3]Department of Internal Medicine, Faculty of Medicine, American University of Beirut Medical Center, P.O. Box 11-0236, Riad El-Solh, Beirut 1107 2020, Lebanon. [4]Department of Physiology, Faculty of Medicine, American University of Beirut Medical Center, P.O. Box 11-0236, Riad El-Solh, Beirut 1107 2020, Lebanon.

References

1. Ferlay J, Soerjomataram I, Dikshit R, Eser S, Mathers C, Rebelo M, et al. Cancer incidence and mortality worldwide: sources, methods and major patterns in GLOBOCAN 2012. Int J Cancer. 2015;136(5):E359–86.
2. Grossfeld GD, Chang JJ, Broering JM, Miller DP, Yu J, Flanders SC, et al. Impact of positive surgical margins on prostate cancer recurrence and the use of secondary cancer treatment: data from the CaPSURE database. J Urol. 2000;163(4):1171–7. quiz 1295
3. Udo K, Cronin AM, Carlino LJ, Savage CJ, Maschino AC, Al-Ahmadie HA, et al. Prognostic impact of subclassification of radical prostatectomy positive margins by linear extent and Gleason grade. J Urol. 2013;189(4):1302–7.
4. Verhoven B, Yan Y, Ritter M, Khor LY, Hammond E, Jones C, et al. Ki-67 is an independent predictor of metastasis and cause-specific mortality for prostate cancer patients treated on radiation therapy oncology group (RTOG) 94-08. Int J Radiat Oncol Biol Phys. 2013;86(2):317–23.
5. Bubendorf L, Sauter G, Moch H, Schmid HP, Gasser TC, Jordan P, et al. Ki67 labelling index: an independent predictor of progression in prostate cancer treated by radical prostatectomy. J Pathol. 1996;178(4):437–41.
6. Tollefson MK, Karnes RJ, Kwon ED, Lohse CM, Rangel LJ, Mynderse LA, et al. Prostate cancer Ki-67 (MIB-1) expression, perineural invasion, and Gleason score as biopsy-based predictors of prostate cancer mortality: the Mayo model. Mayo Clin Proc. 2014;89(3):308–18.
7. Swindle P, Eastham JA, Ohori M, Kattan MW, Wheeler T, Maru N, et al. Do margins matter? The prognostic significance of positive surgical margins in radical prostatectomy specimens. J Urol. 2005;174(3):903–7.
8. Mithal P, Howard LE, Aronson WJ, Terris MK, Cooperberg MR, Kane CJ, Amling C, Freedland SJ. Positive surgical margins in radical prostatectomy patients do not predict long-term oncological outcomes: results from the shared equal access regional cancer hospital (SEARCH) cohort. BJU Int. 2016;117(2):244–8.
9. Seo WI, Kang PM, Yoon JH, Kim W, Chung JI. Correlation between postoperative prostate-specific antigen and biochemical recurrence in positive surgical margin patients: single surgeon series. Prostate Int. 2017;5(2):53–8.
10. Daly T, Hickey BE, Lehman M, Francis DP, See AM. Adjuvant radiotherapy following radical prostatectomy for prostate cancer. Cochrane Database Syst Rev. 2011;12:CD007234.
11. Sofer M, Hamilton-Nelson KL, Civantos F, Soloway MS. Positive surgical margins after radical retropubic prostatectomy: the influence of site and number on progression. J Urol. 2002;167(6):2453–6.
12. Epstein JI, Pizov G, Walsh PC. Correlation of pathologic findings with progression after radical retropubic prostatectomy. Cancer. 1993;71(11):3582–93.
13. Shikanov S, Song J, Royce C, Al-Ahmadie H, Zorn K, Steinberg G, et al. Length of positive surgical margin after radical prostatectomy as a predictor of biochemical recurrence. J Urol. 2009;182(1):139–44.
14. Ochiai A, Sotelo T, Troncoso P, Bhadkamkar V, Babaian RJ. Natural history of biochemical progression after radical prostatectomy based on length of a positive margin. Urology. 2008;71(2):308–12.
15. Cattoretti G, Becker MH, Key G, Duchrow M, Schlüter C, Galle J, et al. Monoclonal antibodies against recombinant parts of the Ki-67 antigen (MIB 1 and MIB 3) detect proliferating cells in microwave-processed formalin-fixed paraffin sections. J Pathol. 1992;168(4):357–63.
16. Kim SH, Park WS, Park BR, Joo J, Joung JY, Seo HK, et al. PSCA, Cox-2, and Ki-67 are independent, predictive markers of biochemical recurrence in clinically localized prostate cancer: a retrospective study. Asian J Androl. 2016;19(4):458–62.
17. Mesko S, Kupelian P, Demanes DJ, Huang J, Wang PC, Kamrava M. Quantifying the ki-67 heterogeneity profile in prostate cancer. Prostate Cancer. 2013;2013:717080.
18. Li R, Heydon K, Hammond ME, Grignon DJ, Roach M 3rd, Wolkov HB, et al. Ki-67 staining index predicts distant metastasis andsurvival in locally advanced prostate cancer treated with radiotherapy: an analysis of patients in radiation therapy oncology group protocol 86-10. Clin Cancer Res. 2004;10(12 Pt 1):4118–24.
19. Pollack A, DeSilvio M, Khor LY, Li R, Al-Saleem TI, Hammond ME, et al. Ki-67 staining is a strong predictor of distant metastasis and mortality for men with prostate cancer treated with radiotherapy plus androgen deprivation: radiation therapy oncology group trial 92-02. J Clin Oncol. 2004;22(11):2133–40.
20. Guo Y, Sigman DB, Borkowski A, Kyprianou N. Racial differences in prostate cancer growth: apoptosis and cell proliferation in Caucasian and African-American patients. Prostate. 2000;42(2):130–6.
21. Kinseth MA, Jia Z, Rahmatpanah F, Sawyers A, Sutton M, Wang-Rodriguez J, et al. Expression differences between African American and Caucasian prostate cancer tissue reveals that stroma is the site of aggressive changes. Int J Cancer. 2014;134(1):81–91.
22. Wallace TA, Martin DN, Ambs S. Interactions among genes, tumor biology and the environment in cancer health disparities: examining the evidence on a national and global scale. Carcinogenesis. 2011;32(8):1107–21.

33

Seminal vesicle abnormalities following prostatic artery embolization for the treatment of benign prostatic hyperplasia

Jin Long Zhang[1,2], Kai Yuan[2], Mao Qiang Wang[1,2*], Jie Yu Yan[2], Yan Wang[2] and Guo Dong Zhang[2]

Abstract

Background: Prostatic artery embolization (PAE) has been proved effective in the treatment of lower urinary tracts (LUTS) secondary to benign prostatic hyperplasia (BPH) with low complications, and most of the them are due to non-target embolization of adjacent organs, such as bladder, rectum, seminal vesicles and penis. Aim of this study was to present seminal vesicle (SV) abnormalities following prostatic artery embolization (PAE) for the treatment of symptomatic benign prostatic hyperplasia.

Methods: We reviewed 139 BPH patients who received PAE during the period of February 2009 and January 2015 at a single institution, highlighting seminal vesicle abnormalities and their clinical relevance after PAE. PAE was performed using 90~ 180-μm (mean 100-μm) polyvinyl alcohol foam particles.

Results: Nine of 139 patients with SV abnormalities (6.5%) were identified by magnetic resonance imaging (MRI), including subacute haemorrhage in 3 patients and ischaemia in 6 patients. Using cone-beam computed tomography (CB-CT), the seminal vesicle arteries were identified 8 of the 9 patients. All 9 patients complained of a few episodes of mild haematospermia during the 1–4 weeks after PAE; the haematospermia disappeared spontaneously without any treatment.

Conclusion: SV haemorrhage and ischaemia may occur after PAE, and these patients may present with transient and self-limited haematospermia.

Keywords: Angiography, Benign prostatic hyperplasia, Prostate artery embolization, Seminal vesicle haemorrhage, Seminal vesicle ischaemia

Background

Prostatic artery embolization (PAE) has been adopted as a minimally invasive therapeutic modality for the treatment of lower urinary tract symptoms (LUTS) following benign prostatic hyperplasia (BPH) [1–10]. However, a recent systematic review suggest that PAE is inferior to standard treatment methods, such as open prostatectomy (OP) or transurethral resection of the prostate (TURP), and PAE is still considered an experimental treatment modality [11]. Complications of PAE are low and are primarily related to non-target embolization of other arteries, such as the vesical, rectal, and dorsal arteries of the penis. Major complications have been rare, with only two cases of bladder focal necrosis [1, 7]. Minor adverse events after PAE have occurred in, cumulatively, 11% of patients [1, 2, 7–10] and have included urinary tract infections, transient haematuria, transient haematospermia, a small amount of rectal bleeding, ischaemic rectitis, and balanitis.

Haematospermia, an uncommon clinical event, has occurred in 5.9–16% of cases after PAE [1, 3, 5, 10]. We hypothesize that haematospermia secondary to PAE may be associated with seminal vesicle (SV) ischaemia and haemorrhage, resulting from non-target embolization. Herein, we report nine cases of SV abnormalities after PAE, including SV ischaemia in 6 patients and SV haemorrhage in 3 patients, identified by magnetic resonance imaging (MRI) follow-up.

* Correspondence: wangmq@vip.sina.com
[1]School of Medicine, Nan Kai University, 94 Wei-jin Rd, Tianjin 300071, People's Republic of China
[2]Department of Interventional Radiology, Chinese PLA General Hospital, 28 Fu-xing Rd, Beijing 100853, People's Republic of China

Methods

Patients

Between February 2009 and January 2015 in our institution, a total of 139 patients (mean age, 72.0 years±10.5 [standard deviation]) diagnosed with moderate or severe LUTS (International Prostate Symptoms Score [IPSS] > 18 points, quality of life [QoL] score > 3, and/or urinary retention with urinary catheter removal failure) due to BPH who were refractory to medical treatment for at least 6 months underwent PAE.

PAE protocols

The selection criteria included patients with a diagnosis of severe LUTS, negative screening for prostate cancer, prostate volume (PV) > 40 mL measured by MRI, and bladder outlet obstruction (BOO) confirmed by urodynamic examination, peak urinary flow rate (Qmax) < 12 mL/sec, and PVR post-void residual urine (PVR) > 150 mL evaluated by ultrasound, biopsy was performed to rule out prostate malignant if PSA level > 4.0 ng/mL. The patient selection was evaluated by a multidisciplinary team that included urologists, anaesthesiologists, and interventional radiologists. Exclusion criteria included pelvic malignancy, chronic renal failure, large bladder diverticula (> 5 cm), active urinary tract infection, large bladder stones (> 2 cm), unregulated coagulation parameters, neurogenic bladder, allergy to intravenous contrast media, detrusor failure and urethral stricture diagnosed through pressure flow studies or urethrography [1, 9].

The preparative clinical observation included IPSS, QoL, peak urinary flow rate (Qmax), post-void residual volume (PVR), international index of erectile function short form (IIEF-5) score, and PV before PAE and at 1, 3, 6 and every 6 months after the procedure. All patients underwent 1.5-T multiparametric enhanced MRI (GE Healthcare, Milwaukee, Wisconsin, USA) of the prostate to measure PV and to rule out cancer before PAE using a phased-array 12-channel body coil. For each patient, the MRI protocol was the same, including axial, coronal, and sagittal T2-weighted imaging (T2WI) and contrast- and non-contrast enhanced T1-weighted imaging (T1WI).

Embolization technique

The details of the procedure of PAE have been described previously [10]. The PAEs were performed by two senior interventional radiologists (M.Q.W. and K. Y., with 26 and 12 years of vascular and interventional radiology experience, respectively), using a therapeutic angiography unit equipped with a digital flat-panel detector system (INNOVA 4100 IQ; GE Healthcare, Milwaukee, Wisconsin, USA). PAE was performed under local anaesthesia through a single right femoral approach using a 4-Fr vascular sheath (Radifocus, Terumo, Japan). Digital subtraction angiography (DSA) and cone-beam computed tomography (CB-CT) were performed to identify prostatic arteries (PAs). Embolization was performed with 100-μm non-spherical PVA particles (90~ 180-μm, PVA, Cook Incorporated, Bloomington, IN, USA). The endpoint of embolization was occlusion of the identifiable vessels supplying the prostate.

Follow-up

Follow-up was performed at 1, 3, 6, and every 6 months after PAE by the interventionalists and the urologists. IPSS, QoL, IIEF-5, PSA, Qmax, PVR, and PV on MRI were evaluated at those dates to measure clinical and radiological changes after PAE.

Imaging evaluation

All MR images were assessed independently by two radiologists (reader 1 and reader 2, with 11 years and 15 years of experience in interpreting body MR images, respectively) without knowing the outcomes of the PAE. If there was disagreement, the relevant MR images were reassessed by a third independent reader (reader 3, with 20 years of experience in interpreting body MR) to reach a consensus.

The procedural angiographic images, including DSA, rotational angiography, and CB-CT, were reviewed retrospectively by two interventional radiologists (G. D. Z. and M.Q.W., with 16 and 25 years of vascular and interventional radiology experience, respectively), highlighting the possibility of the blood supplying the SV ("vesiculo-deferential artery"). After independent interpretations were achieved, the differences in evaluations between the two radiologists were resolved by consensus.

Results

Peri-procedural outcomes

Nine cases of SV abnormalities (6.5%) after PAE, including SV ischaemia in 6 patients and SV haemorrhage in 3 patients, were identified by MRI follow-up. The baseline characteristics of the nine patients are provided in Table 1. PAE was performed bilaterally in the 9 patients, identifying a total of 13 prostatic arteries. Of these prostatic arteries, six were originated from the internal pudendal artery, and seven were originated from the gluteal-pudendal trunk. No immediately procedural complications occurred.

Imaging findings

Subacute SV haemorrhage was presented in 3 patients (Patient No. 1, 2, and 3). MRI at 1 month following PAE showed high-intensity signals on T1WI with low-intensity signals on T2WI in the SVs, suggesting typical subacute haemorrhage (Fig. 1a-b). These findings were not presented on the pre-procedural MRI. During the 3- to 12-month follow-up, these high-intensity signals on T1WI within the SVs became iso-intensity signals, with a reduction in the

Table 1 Clinical Data Obtained before and at 12 Months after PAE (N = 9)

Patient	IPSS		QoL		PV(ml)		PSA(ng/ml)		Q_{max}(ml/s)		PVR(ml)		IIEF-5	
	Pre	Post	Pre	Post	Pre	Post	Pre	Post	Pre	Post	Pre	Post	Pre	Post
1	28	6	6	1	79	39	4.6	3.4	7.0	15.0	70	0	16	18
2	26	5	5	0	72	44	3.9	3.0	8.5	16.0	50	0	19	19
3[a]	32	5	6	1	127	58	8.0	3.9	–	14.0	–	10	9	10
4	30	7	6	2	90	47	3.0	3.4	6.0	14.0	80	10	17	15
5	27	5	5	0	67	37	2.0	1.5	8.0	16.0	60	0	16	18
6	29	8	6	2	116	64	7.1	5.7	5.0	13.0	100	10	7	7
7	28	6	6	1	87	46	4.5	3.0	7.0	15.0	90	0	11	12
8	27	4	6	1	84	52	7.0	2.0	10.0	19.0	70	0	18	19
9	30	6	6	2	122	66	2.9	1.5	8.5	17.0	110	0	15	16
mean	28.6	6	5.8	1	93.8	50.3	4.8	3.1	7.5	15.4	74.3	3.8	14	15

[a]Patient with urinary retention before PA

size of the SV, suggestive of SV atrophy (Fig. 1c). With retrospective analysis of the intra-procedural angiographic images, the CB-CT images showed that the small arteries branched proximally from the prostate arteries supplied to the SV (i.e., the seminal vesicle arteries) in 3 patients; however, these small arterial branches could not be identified on DSA (Fig. 1d-f).

SV ischaemia was presented in 6 patients (Patient Nos. 4–9). Contrast-enhanced T1WI images at 1 month following PAE showed obvious hypoperfusion in the seminal vesicles, suggestive of ischaemia (Figs. 2, 3 and 4). SV atrophy was also noted in those patients during the follow-up. The SV arteries could be identified in 5 of the 6 patients on the CB-CT but were difficult to identify on DSA.

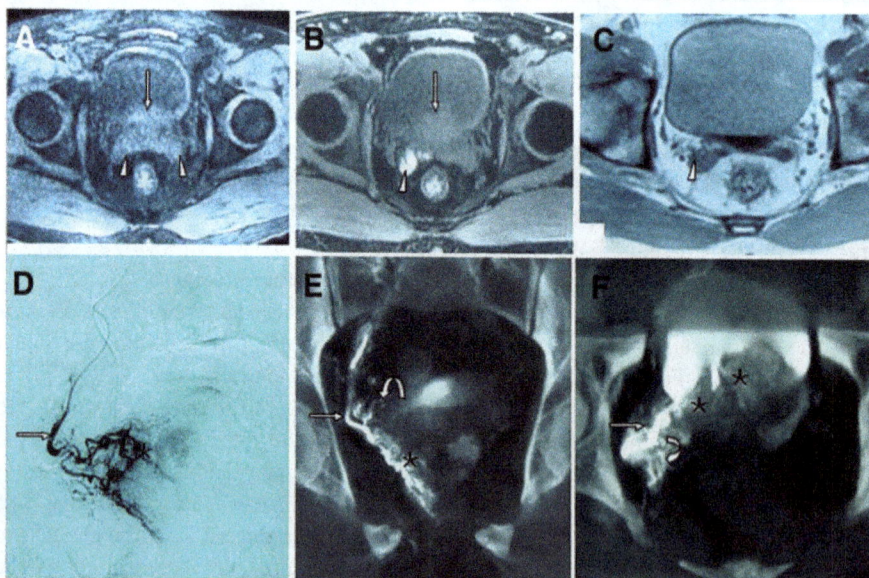

Fig. 1 Seminal vesicle haemorrhage. Image from a 65-year-old man with lower urinary tract symptoms due to benign prostatic hyperplasia (BPH). He presented with mild haematospermia at 1 week after PAE that disappeared 4 weeks later without specific treatment. **a** Axial T1-weighted MR image obtained before PAE shows the normal appearance of the seminal vesicles (arrowheads) and BPH (straight arrow). **b** Axial T1-weighted MR image obtained 1 month after PAE shows high-intensity signals on the right side of the seminal vesicles (arrowhead), suggestive of haemorrhage, and BPH (straight arrows). **c** Axial T1-weighted MR image (without fat suppression) obtained 12 months after PAE shows iso-intensity signals on the right side of the seminal vesicles (arrowhead) and reduction in the size of the SVs. **d** Digital subtraction angiography (DSA) of the right prostatic artery (straight arrow) with same-side anterior oblique projection (35°) demonstrates contrast medium staining in the right prostate lobe (asterisk). **e** Cone-beam CT (CB-CT) with coronal view after catheterization of the right prostatic artery (straight arrow) demonstrates the small branches (curved arrow) supplying the seminal vesicles and contrast medium staining in the right prostate lobe (asterisk). **f** CB-CT with axial view after catheterization of the right prostatic artery (straight arrow) demonstrates the small branches (curved arrow) supplying the seminal vesicles (the seminal vesicle artery) and contrast medium staining in the right prostate lobe (asterisks)

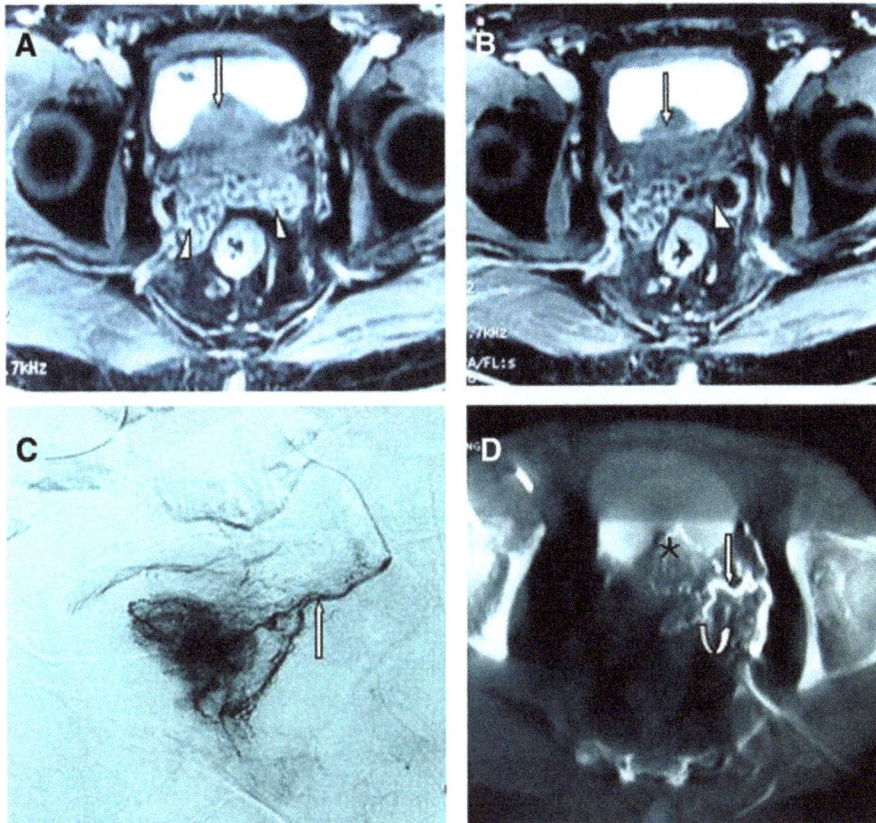

Fig. 2 Seminal vesicle ischaemia. Image from a 72-year-old patient with lower urinary tract symptoms due to a large BPH (120 mL). **a** Axial contrast-enhanced T1-weighted MR image obtained before PAE shows a large benign prostatic hyperplasia (straight arrow) and normal seminal vesicles (arrowheads). **b** Axial contrast-enhanced T1-weighted MR image obtained 1 month after PAE shows reduction of the prostate (straight arrows) and hypoperfusion in the seminal vesicles (arrowhead), suggestive of ischaemia. **c** DSA of the left prostatic artery (straight arrow) with same-side anterior oblique projection (35°) demonstrates contrast-medium staining in the left prostate lobe (asterisk). **d** CB-CT with axial view after catheterization of the left prostatic artery (straight arrow) demonstrates the small branches (curved arrow) supplying the seminal vesicles (the seminal vesicle artery) and contrast medium staining in the left prostate lobe (asterisk)

The relevant clinical findings

At the 1-month follow-up visit, all 9 patients complained a few episodes of mild haematospermia during 1–4 weeks after PAE; the haematospermia disappeared spontaneously without any treatment. Four of them had co-occurring mild macroscopic haematuria, but without evidence of bladder ischaemia on the MRI follow-up. Three cases had temporary anxiety due to the haematospermia. The remaining 130 patients had no complaints of haematospermia or haematuria; no abnormalities of the SVs were presented on the follow-up MRI.

The mean follow-up time of the 9 patients was 22 months (range, 14–36 months). The mean IPSS (pre-PAE vs post-PAE 28.6 vs 6.0; $P < 0.01$), QoL (5.8 vs 1.0; $P < 0.05$), Qmax (7.5 vs 15.4; $P < 0.01$), PVR (74 mL vs 4 mL; $P < 0.01$), PV (94 mL vs 40 mL; $P < 0.05$), and PSA (4.8 ng/mL vs 3.1 ng/mL; $P < 0.05$) had significant differences compared with baseline, as shown in Table 1. The mean IIEF-5 had no significant difference from baseline ($P = 0.8$).

Discussion

PAE is a safe and effective procedure with low morbidity in most cases [1, 7–13]. Although various complications of PAE, such as bladder ischaemia, urinary tract infections, balanitis, and ischaemic rectitis, have been reported, seminal vesicle abnormality after PAE is rare [1, 7, 14, 15]. In the present study, the incidence of SV abnormalities (haemorrhage and ischaemia) after PAE, identified by MRI follow-up, was 6.5%. Clinically, patients with SV haemorrhage or ischaemia usually present with haematospermia [16]. Pisco JM et al. [1] reported that transient haematospermia occurred in 7% of cases after PAE. De Assis AM et al. [5] reported that transient and self-limited haematospermia occurred in 5.9% of cases after PAE. Recently, Amouyal G et al. [12] evaluated 32 patients treated with PAE and reported that 3 patients (9%) experienced haematospermia during 3 days to 1 month after PAE. Bagla et al. [3] reported an incidence of 16% (3 of the 19 patients) self-limited haematospermia even using CB-CT.

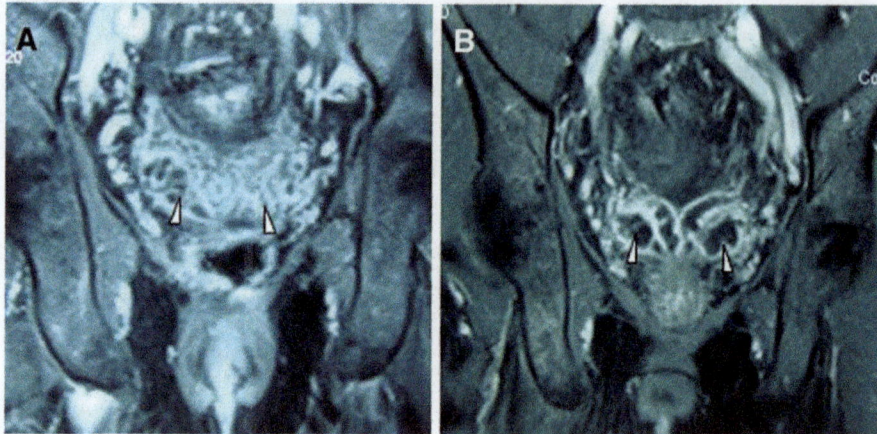

Fig. 3 Seminal vesicle ischaemia. Image from a 69-year-old patient with lower urinary tract symptoms due to a large BPH (132 mL). **a** Coronal contrast-enhanced T1-weighted MR image obtained before PAE shows normal seminal vesicles (arrowheads). **b** Coronal contrast-enhanced T1-weighted MR image obtained at 1 month after PAE shows significant hypoperfusion in the seminal vesicles (arrowheads), suggestive of ischaemia

Haematospermia secondary to PAE may be related to seminal vesicle ischaemia and haemorrhage resulting from non-target embolization. In the present cases, the SV abnormalities could be explained by embolic particle reflux, existence of a common trunk between the prostate capsule branch and the seminal vesicle artery, misidentification of the seminal vesicle artery as a capsular artery, or a prostato- seminal vesicle arterial anastomosis not detected angiographically at the time of embolization.

There is no specific therapeutic option in the treatment of seminal vesicle haemorrhage or ischaemia after PAE. However, bacterial inflammation may occur after bleeding in the seminal vesicles [16]. Therefore, antibiotic treatment is recommended once seminal vesicle haemorrhage or ischaemia has been confirmed by MRI. In addition, haematospermia after PAE may cause the psychological

anxiety for the patient; therefore, it is necessary to explain the complication to patients before the procedure.

Knowledge of the detailed anatomy of the pelvic arteries is crucial for a safe and effective PAE and to avoid complications from non-targeted embolization of surrounding organs to yield better outcomes [1, 2, 17]. The blood supplies to the prostate, bladder, rectum, and penis have been reported previously in the literature [18–22]. However, little work appears to have been performed on the anatomy of the arterial circulation in the seminal vesicles; most of the standard textbooks even ignore the existence of a blood supply to this organ. In early studies in cadaveric specimens by Clegg EJ [23], he described that the seminal vesicle arteries were supplied by the "vesiculo-deferential artery"; the origin of this vessel is highly variable and includes the umbilical artery, internal pudendal artery, superior vesical

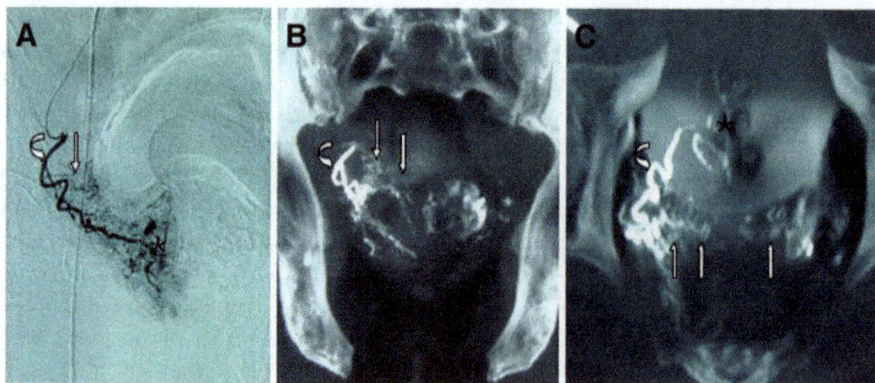

Fig. 4 Images from the same patient as Fig. 3. **a** DSA of the right prostatic artery (curved arrow) with same-side anterior oblique projection (35°) demonstrates contrast-medium staining in the right prostate lobe (asterisk) and the small branches (straight arrow), which were suspected to be the seminal vesicle arteries. **b** CB-CT with coronal view after catheterization of the right prostatic artery (curved arrow) demonstrates the small branches (straight arrows) supplying the seminal vesicles. **c** CB-CT with axial view after catheterization of the right prostatic artery (curved arrow) demonstrates the small branches (straight arrows) supplying the seminal vesicles (the seminal vesicle arteries) and contrast medium staining in the prostate (asterisks)

artery, and prostato-vesical artery. Currently, there are no in vivo studies published in the literature documenting the imaging findings of SV artery anatomy.

In the present study, with retrospective reviews using DSA and CB-CT, we could identify the SV arteries, which presented with very small branches on the CB-CT images in 8 of the nine patients, which originated proximally from the prostatic artery. To prevent PAE-related SV complications, more studies are needed to understand the detailed anatomy of the SV arteries. From our experience, CB-CT performed intraoperatively using a three-dimensional arteriography with maximum-intensity projection is a useful tool for PAE procedures. Although the result is a low-quality image compared with that of conventional computed tomography, it provides good vessel identification when vessels cannot be visualized on arteriography [24].

Conclusions

Although the SV abnormalities after PAE were not significant consequences, interventionalists should be aware of that non-targeted embolization of the seminal vesicles may be the cause of haematospermia. Long-term follow-up is needed to understand the long-term effects of seminal vesicle haemorrhage or ischaemia.

Abbreviations
BPH: Benign prostatic hyperplasia; CB-CT: Cone-beam computed tomography; DSA: Digital subtraction angiography; IIEF-5: International Index of Erectile Function; IPSS: International Prostate Symptom Score; LUTS: Lower urinary tract symptoms; MRI: Magnetic resonance imaging; PAE: Prostatic artery embolization; PSA: Prostate-specific antigen; PV: Prostate volume; PVA: Polyvinyl alcohol particles; PVR: Post-void residual volume; Q_{max}: Peak urinary flow rate; QoL: Quality of life

Acknowledgements
The authors thank all of our participants for their gracious participation in this study.

Funding
This study was supported by grants from the National Scientific Foundation Committee of China (No. 81471769), the Central Health Research Project (2013BJ09) and the Chinese PLA Scientific Foundation of the Twelve-Five Programme (BWS11J028).

Authors' contributions
JLZ and KY: Contributed equally to this work and are joint first authors on this article. JLZ and MQW: Study concept and design and interpretation of the imaging data. KY: Acquisition of data. GDZ: Interpretation of clinical and angiographic data. JYY and YW: Analysis and interpretation of clinical data. All authors read and approved the final manuscript.

Competing interests
The authors declare that they have no competing interests.

References
1. Pisco J, Campos Pinheiro L, Bilhim T, Duarte M, Rio Tinto H, Fernandes L, Vaz Santos V, Oliveira AG. Prostatic arterial embolization for benign prostatic hyperplasia: short- and intermediate-term results. Radiology. 2013;266(2):668–77.
2. Carnevale FC, da Motta-Leal-Filho JM, Antunes AA, Baroni RH, Marcelino AS, Cerri LM, Yoshinaga EM, Cerri GG, Srougi M. Quality of life and clinical symptom improvement support prostatic artery embolization for patients with acute urinary retention caused by benign prostatic hyperplasia. J Vasc Interv Radiol. 2013;24(4):535–42.
3. Bagla S, Martin CP, van Breda A, Sheridan MJ, Sterling KM, Papadouris D, Rholl KS, Smirniotopoulos JB, van Breda A. Early results from a United States trial of prostatic artery embolization in the treatment of benign prostatic hyperplasia. J Vasc Interv Radiol. 2014;25(1):47–52.
4. Russo GI, Kurbatov D, Sansalone S, Lepetukhin A, Dubsky S, Sitkin I, Salamone C, Fiorino L, Rozhivanov R, Cimino S, Morgia G. Prostatic arterial embolization vs open prostatectomy: a 1-year matched-pair analysis of functional outcomes and morbidities. Urology. 2015;86(2):343–8.
5. de Assis AM, Moreira AM, de Paula Rodrigues VC, Yoshinaga EM, Antunes AA, Harward SH, Srougi M, Carnevale FC. Prostatic artery embolization for treatment of benign prostatic hyperplasia in patients with prostates > 90 g: a prospective single-center study. J Vasc Interv Radiol. 2015;26(1):87–93.
6. Sun F, Crisóstomo V, Báez-Díaz C, Sánchez FM. Prostatic artery embolization (PAE) for symptomatic benign prostatic hyperplasia (BPH): part 1, pathological background and clinical implications. Cardiovasc Intervent Radiol. 2016;39(1):1–7.
7. Lebdai S, Delongchamps NB, Sapoval M, Robert G, Amouyal G, Thiounn N, Karsenty G, Ruffion A, de La Taille A, Descazeaud A, Mathieu R. Early results and complications of prostatic arterial embolization for benign prostatic hyperplasia. World J Urol. 2016;34(5):625–32.
8. Carnevale FC, Iscaife A, Yoshinaga EM, Moreira AM, Antunes AA, Srougi M. Transurethral resection of the prostate (TURP) versus original and PErFecTED prostate artery embolization (PAE) due to benign prostatic hyperplasia (BPH): preliminary results of a single center, prospective, urodynamic-controlled analysis. Cardiovasc Intervent Radiol. 2016;39(1):44–52.
9. Wang MQ, Wang Y, Yan JY, Yuan K, Zhang GD, Duan F, Li K. Prostatic artery embolization for the treatment of symptomatic benign prostatic hyperplasia in men ≥75 years: a prospective single-center study. World J Urol. 2016;34(9):1275–83.
10. Wang MQ, Guo LP, Duan F, Yuan K, Zhang GD, Li K, Yan JY, Wang Y, Kang HY. Prostatic arterial embolization for the treatment of lower urinary tract symptoms caused by benign prostatic hyperplasia: a comparative study of medium- and large-volume prostates. BJU Int. 2016;117(1):155–64.
11. Shim SR, Kanhai KJ, Ko YM, Kim JH. Efficacy and safety of prostatic arterial embolization: systematic review with meta-analysis and meta-regression. J Urol. 2017;197(2):465–79.
12. Amouyal G, Thiounn N, Pellerin O, Yen-Ting L, Del Giudice C, Dean C, Pereira H, Chatellier G, Sapoval M. Clinical results after prostatic artery embolization using the PErFecTED technique: a single-center study. Cardiovasc Intervent Radiol. 2016;39(3):367–75.
13. McWilliams JP, Kuo MD, Rose SC, Bagla S, Caplin DM, Cohen EI, Faintuch S, Spies JB, Saad WE, Nikolic B. Society of InterventionalRadiology. Society of interventional radiology position statement: prostate artery embolization for treatment of benign disease of the prostate. J Vasc Interv Radiol. 2014;25(9):1349–51.
14. Moreira AM, Marques CF, Antunes AA, Nahas CS, Nahas SC, de Gregorio Ariza MA, Carnevale FC. Transient ischemic rectitis as a potential complication after prostatic artery embolization: case report and review of the literature. Cardiovasc Intervent Radiol. 2013;36(6):1690–4.
15. Pisco JM, Rio Tinto H, Campos Pinheiro L, Bilhim T, Duarte M, Fernandes L, Pereira J, Oliveira AG. Embolisation of prostatic arteries as treatment of moderate to severe lower urinary symptoms (LUTS) secondary to benign hyperplasia: results of short- and mid-term follow-up. Eur Radiol. 2013;23(9):2561–72.
16. Furuya S, Furuya R, Masumori N, Tsukamoto T, Nagaoka M. Magnetic resonance imaging is accurate to detect bleeding in the seminal vesicles in patients with hemospermia. Urology. 2008;72(4):838–42.
17. Carnevale FC, Antunes AA. Prostatic artery embolization for enlarged prostates due to benign prostatic hyperplasia. How I do it. Cardiovasc Intervent Radiol. 2013;36(6):1452–63.

18. Garcia-Monaco R, Garategui L, Kizilevsky N, Peralta O, Rodriguez P, Palacios-Jaraquemada J. Human cadaveric specimen study of the prostatic arterial anatomy: implications for arterial embolization. J Vasc Interv Radiol. 2014; 25(2):315–22.

19. Bilhim T, Pisco JM, Rio Tinto H, Fernandes L, Pinheiro LC, Furtado A, Casal D, Duarte M, Pereira J, Oliveira AG, O'Neill JE. Prostatic arterial supply: anatomic and imaging findings relevant for selective arterial embolization. J Vasc Interv Radiol. 2012;23(11):1403–15.

20. de Assis AM, Moreira AM, de Paula Rodrigues VC, Harward SH, Antunes AA, Srougi M, Carnevale FC. Pelvic arterial anatomy relevant to prostatic artery embolisation and proposal for angiographic classification. Cardiovasc Intervent Radiol. 2015;38(4):855–61.

21. Bilhim T, Tinto HR, Fernandes L, Martins Pisco J. Radiological anatomy of prostatic arteries. Tech Vasc Interv Radiol. 2012;15(4):276–85.

22. Carnevale FC, Soares GR, de Assis AM, Moreira AM, Harward SH, Cerri GG. Anatomical variants in prostate artery embolization: a pictorial essay. Cardiovasc Intervent Radiol. 2017;40(9):1321–37.

23. CLEGG EJ. The arterial supply of the human prostate and seminal vesicles. J Anat. 1955;89(2):209–16.

24. Bagla S, Rholl KS, Sterling KM, van Breda A, Papadouris D, Cooper JM, van Breda A. Utility of cone-beam CT imaging in prostatic artery embolization. J Vasc Interv Radiol. 2013;24(11):1603–7.

The application rate for urology specialty compared with other specialties from 2007 to 2014 in Korea: is it influenced by social interest manifested by internet trends?

Hwa Yeon Sun[1], Young Myoung Ko[2], Seung Wook Lee[3], Bora Lee[4*] and Jae Heon Kim[1*] (iD)

Abstract

Background: Reduced clinical exposure to urology at the undergraduate or internship level is the main explanation for the marked decrease in applicants to urology residencies. This manuscript was to access the application rate for urology specialty compared with that of other specialties and to investigate the relationship between the decreasing trend in urology applications and social interest using internet trend tests.

Methods: We reviewed data collected by the Korean Hospital Association from 2007 to 2014. We assessed internet trends using Naver Trend for domestic social interest and Google Trends for international social interest (2007 to 2014). Trend tests and Spearman correlations were used for statistical analyses.

Results: Among the all specialties, the application rates to obstetrics and gynecology, emergency medicine, and occupational medicine are significantly increasing ($p = 0.015$, 0.012, and 0.048, respectively). Application to other specialties is mostly decreasing. The decreasing trend is highest for urology (beta $= -12.21$ and $p < 0.001$). The application rate and domestic social interest revealed by Naver trends were significantly correlated ($r = 0.786$ and $p = 0.021$). No correlation was found between Naver trends and Google trends ($r = -0.19$ and $p = 0.651$).

Conclusions: The rate of application to urology specialty is decreasing the fastest, and this trend is related to domestic social interest. An attempt should be made to increase the number of urologic applicants.

Keywords: Clinical clerkship, Trends, Employment, Supported, Urology, Education

Background

Urology has been perceived as a competitive specialty for the last decade, but its popularity is decreasing worldwide. A recent report from Canada demonstrated the current status of the reduced popularity of urology using data from the Canadian Residency Matching Service from 2002 to 2011 [1]. Although the number of urology positions has increased, the number of applicants to medical residency specialty who make urology their first choice is decreasing [1, 2].

Considering that the popularity of surgery is also decreasing worldwide, it is not surprising that the popularity of urology is decreasing. However, amongst all surgical specialties, the pattern is most critical in Urology [1, 2].

There is growing concern about this issue because the prevalence of urological diseases, including prostate hyperplasia, overactive bladder, and urological cancers, is increasing [3] and more urologists are necessary from the perspective of public health and the health of individual communities. Reduced clinical exposure to urology at the undergraduate or internship level is the main explanation for the marked decrease in applicants to urology residencies [4].

Although several factors to explain this phenomenon have been noted, including lower early exposure to urology, demand for less difficult specialties associated

---

* Correspondence: mintbora0125@gmail.com; piacekjh@hanmail.net
[4]Department of Statistics, Graduate School of Chung-Ang University, 84, Heuksukro, Seoul 156-756, South Korea
[1]Department of Urology, Soonchunhyang University Hospital, Soonchunhyang University College of Medicine, 59, Daesagwan-ro, Yongsan-gu, Seoul 140-743, South Korea
Full list of author information is available at the end of the article

with greater work-life balance, and a gender shift to female predominance among medical students [1, 2], more explanations are needed to fully account for this sharp decrease, especially in Korea.

The aim of our study is to assess the decrease in the application rate to urology specialty compared with that to other specialties and to investigate the relationship between the decreasing trend in urology applicants and social interest using internet trend testing, which is a validated tool that has been used to explore social interest.

Methods

Application rates for medical specialties

We reviewed data collected by the Korean Hospital Association from 2007 to 2014. The application rates to medical specialties, including total applications, internal medicine, pediatrics, neurology, psychiatry, dermatology, rehabilitation, and family medicine were reviewed. The application rates to surgical specialties including overall surgical specialties, general surgery, thoracic surgery, orthopedic surgery, neurosurgery, plastic surgery, obstetrics and gynecology, ophthalmology, otorhinolaryngology, and urology were reviewed. The application rates to other specialties, including the overall rate, anesthesiology, radiology, radiation oncology, laboratory medicine, pathology, emergency medicine, nuclear medicine, occupational medicine, and preventive medicine were reviewed.

Social interest

Social interest was identified by researching internet trends using Naver Trend and Google Trends. After accessing Naver Trend (http://trend.naver.com/), we searched for each specialty in Korean. The classification was 'PC version'. The period analyzed was from 2007 to 2014. The trends for the search words were calculated from January to December of each year.

The trend scores were defined as relative indexes. The highest trend score in each year was 100, representing peak search interest and the lowest score was 0, indicating no search entries. The medical specialties investigated were family medicine, neurology, digestive medicine, nephrology, pulmonology, hemato-oncology, rheumatology, endocrinology, infectious disease, cardiology, neurosurgery, orthopedic surgery, thoracic surgery, vascular surgery, plastic surgery, pediatrics I (terminology in Korean before 2007), pediatrics II (terminology in Korean after 2007), obstetrics and gynecology, psychiatry I (terminology in Korean before 2011), psychiatry II (terminology in Korean after 2011), anesthesia, pain medicine, emergency medicine, dermatology, ophthalmology, otorhinolaryngology I (real terminology in Korean), otorhinolaryngology II (similar terminology in Korean), urology, radiology I, radiology II, occupational medicine, preventive medicine, laboratory medicine, and pathology.

These were identical as searching terminologies used during trend test.

After accessing Google Trends (http://www.google.com/trends/), we searched for each specialty using the English language and did not limit the geographical region other than to exclude Korea. The category was chosen the 'All category', the classification was selected as 'web search' among 'web search', 'Image search', 'News search', 'Google shopping, and 'YouTube search'. The method for calculating trend scores was conducted as for Naver trends.

Statistical analysis

To investigate whether Google and Naver Trend data were related to the application rates in the period from 2007 to 2014, we used a linear regression model; we also used Pearson correlation analysis to analyze the association between Naver trends and the rate of application to urology departments. The trend score is not an absolute value from searched amounts, but rather relative value depending on the flows. Hence, newly calculated calibrated index was adopted using percentage scales: the highest trend score of each period (year) as 100 for retaining objectivity. R (ver3.1.2) was used to analyze and plot data using linear regression and Pearson correlation test. During linear regression test, beta was defined as regression coefficient which represents the estimates of impact. During Pearson correlation analysis, r was defined as correlation coefficient. All tests were two-tailed and statistical significance was set at $p < 0.05$.

Results

Application rates to medical residency specialty in Korea from 2007 to 2014

The application rates to obstetrics and gynecology, emergency medicine, and occupational medicine programs significantly increased over the study period ($p = 0.015$, 0.012, and 0.048, respectively) (Fig. 1). The application rates to other specialties mostly decreased (Fig. 1). The extent of the decrease is greatest for urology (beta = − 12.21 and $p < 0.001$) (Additional file 1: Table S1).

Trend for each specialty as assessed using Naver trend

Naver Trend was used to investigate the domestic social interest for each specialty within Korea (Fig. 2). Among the medical specialties, significantly increasing social interest was noted in hemato-oncology, rheumatology, endocrinology, cardiology, and psychiatry, whereas only dermatology showed significantly decreasing social interest (Additional file 2: Table S2). Among the surgical specialties, ophthalmology and urology showed significantly decreasing social interest. For urology, the beta value was highest, − 7.10 ($p = 0.01$) (Additional file 2: Table S2). For other specialties, significant increasing

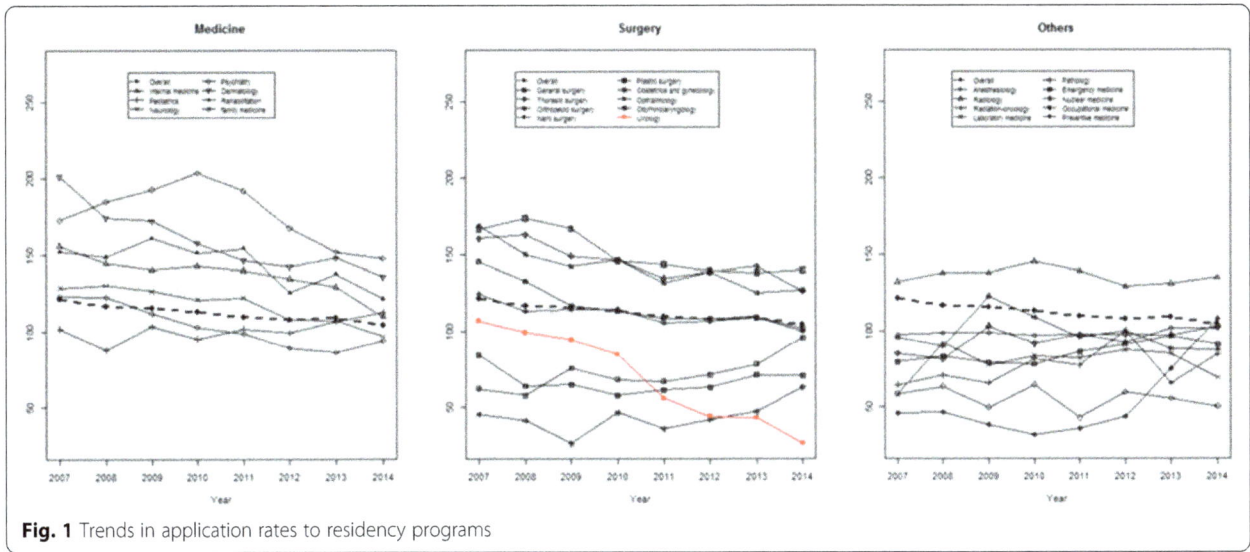

Fig. 1 Trends in application rates to residency programs

trends were noted in radiology, occupational medicine, and preventive medicine (Additional file 2: Table S2).

Trend for each specialty as assessed using Google trends

Google Trend was used to investigate the international social interest for each specialty (Fig. 3). For medical specialties, a significant increasing trend was noted in family medicine, infectious diseases, and dermatology (Additional file 3: Table S3). A significant decreasing trend was noted in neurology, nephrology, rheumatology, endocrinology, cardiology, and pediatrics (Additional file 3: Table S3). Among the surgical specialties, a significant decreasing trend was noted in neurosurgery, orthopedic surgery, thoracic surgery, and vascular surgery (Additional file 3: Table S3). Only chest

surgery showed a significant increasing trend. For other specialties, a significant increasing trend was noted in pain medicine and dermatology, whereas a significant decreasing trend was noted in anesthesia, radiology, preventive medicine, occupational medicine, laboratory medicine, and pathology (Additional file 3: Table S3). For urology, no significant trend was noted.

Correlation between application rate and social interest

For urology, the application rate and domestic social interest as revealed by Naver Trend were significantly correlated ($r = 0.786$ and $p = 0.021$) (Fig. 4). Out of all specialties, only pain medicine was similar in Naver and Google trends, revealing a significant increase in domestic and worldwide social interest.

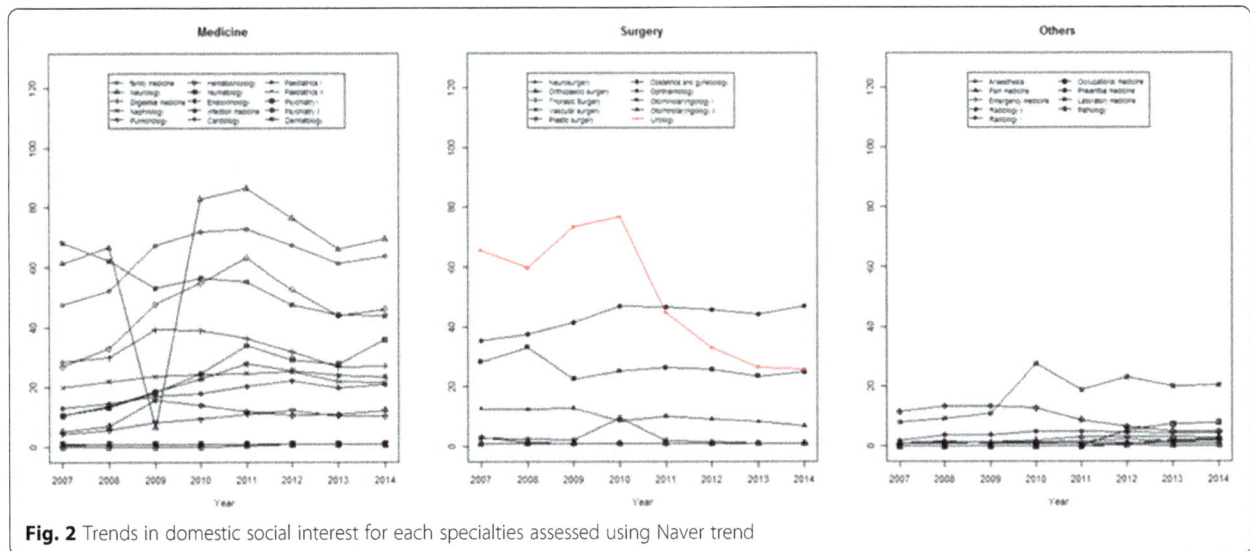

Fig. 2 Trends in domestic social interest for each specialties assessed using Naver trend

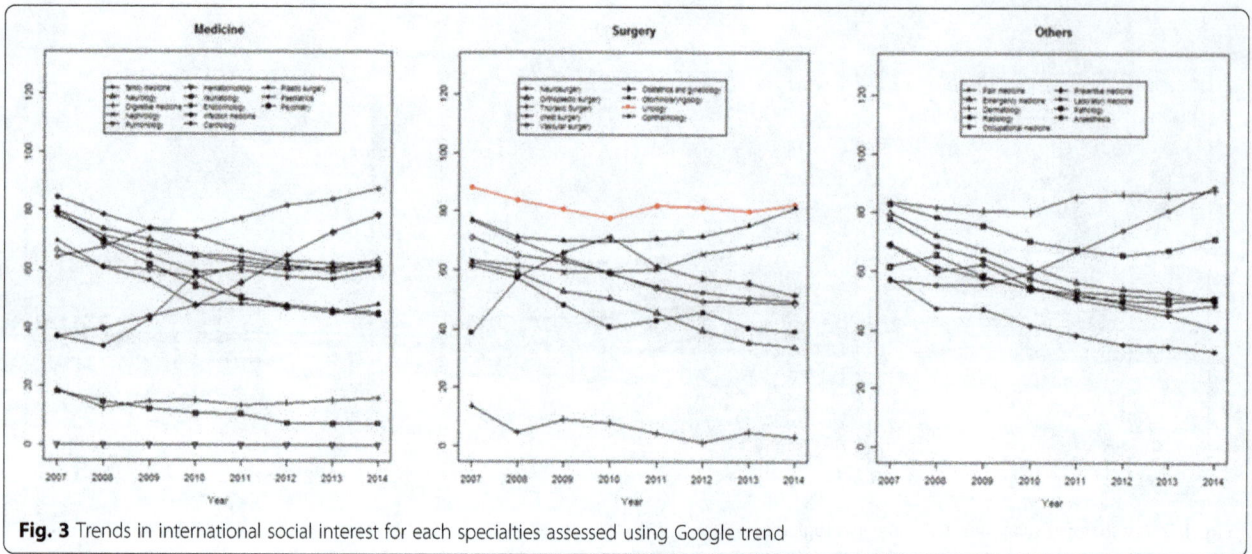

Fig. 3 Trends in international social interest for each specialties assessed using Google trend

Discussion

The hypothesis of this study was that application rate could be associated with social interest, which was confirmed by our analysis. Basic assumption of this hypothesis was that general interest regarding urologic specific disease is decreasing. To prove this basic assumption, we also investigated the social trend using Naver and Google trend about urologic cancers, which showed the decreasing trend as basic assumption (Additional file 4: Figure S1).

Traditionally, urology has been perceived as a competitive and popular surgical specialty. The main attraction of urology for prospective trainees was that urology consists of a mixture of medical and surgical specialties and those trainees can begin working in a clinical setting earlier than they would in other disciplines [5]. However,

today, there is a decrease in the number of applicants to surgical specialty specialty in general [6–8], and the competitiveness and popularity of urology are decreasing [1]; this phenomenon is happening extremely quickly in Korea.

In recent years, surgical specialties have become less competitive and less popular among medical students [6–8]. Lind et al. reported that the number of medical students that chose to enter surgical fields decreased from 22% in 1982 to 15% in 2002 [9]. This large shift is attributable to the increasing interest in lifestyle factors [10]. More and more students are concentrating on their lives outside of work [11], so they enter fields that provide more flexible work hours and allow them to enjoy their private lives [10].

Before the 2000s, although there was a decreasing trend in surgery as a career choice, surgical specialties were still competitive and popular because they were associated with good career opportunities and prestige [12]. However, in the early 2000s, lifestyle factors became more important and negatively affected the number of individuals choosing surgery as their careers [10, 12]; other factors that influence this decreasing trend include long work hours during residency and the quality of the patient/physician relationship [12].

Nowadays, because of the effect of the negative factors mentioned above, the rate of applications to surgical fields is decreasing. Applications to urology specialty are decreasing at the fastest rate. Like in other countries, the application rate to urology specialty in Korea is decreasing with the highest slope (Fig. 1). The application rate to urology specialty in Korea is the lowest out of surgical specialties and all specialties.

One important factor in this change is the increasing percentage of female medical students. In Canada,

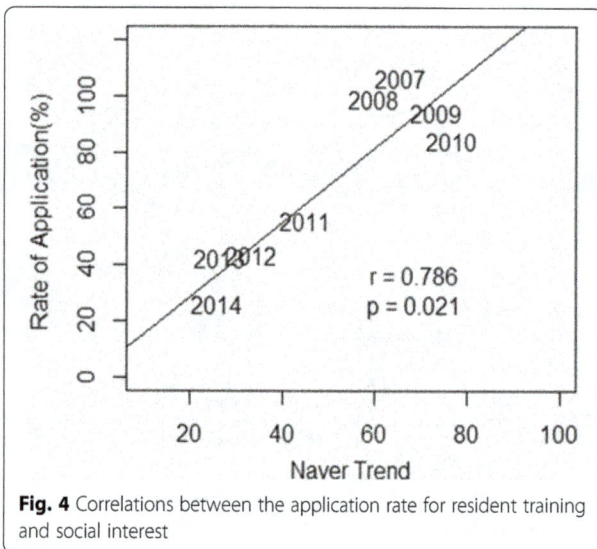

Fig. 4 Correlations between the application rate for resident training and social interest

among all medical students enrolled in 2010, more than half were female [1]. The percentage of female students is increasing; it went from 50.1% in 2002 to 57.1% in 2011 [1]. A review of application data from 2002 to 2011 revealed that, although female applicants to surgical specialties almost doubled (21 to 41%), there was no change in the percentage of medical students going into urology [1].

Besides the gender shift, there are several other factors that help to explain the rapid decrease in urology applicants. First, although there are benefits of urology, including earlier experience in the clinical field and a diversity of procedures, Kerfoot et al. found that the pathology of disease aspect of the specialty could be perceived as having a repetitive nature and that urology residencies are demanding of students' time [5, 13]. Second, during medical school, there is too little exposure to urology. Malde et al. reported that 26.6% of medical students in the UK had no urology experience throughout their clinical clerkship period. Only 30.5% of medical students were exposed to urology during their clerkships; also, the clerkship period for urology was limited to 1 week [14]. The same phenomenon was noted in the US: medical students in the US can complete their clinical clerkships without being exposed to urology. Kutikov et al. reported that length of clinical experience in urology strongly correlated with the number of students choosing urology for their careers [15].

However, even the reasons mentioned above, including gender shift, repetitive nature of some of the work, and scanty exposure to urology during the medical clerkship period, do not fully explain the extraordinary rate at which the number of urology applicants is decreasing. To identify reasons having to do with social interest, we investigated domestic and international internet trends. Korea has a high population density, and social interest may be more uniform than it is in other countries [16]. Internet trend testing is a validated method used to investigate social interest. For example, it has been used to assess the interest in bariatric surgery [17]. Internet search volume is based on social interest and several analyses have revealed that search volume trends reflect real-world events. Therefore, Google Trend is a useful tool to investigate the social interest in various clinical fields [18–21]. Moreover, Naver is more popular searching engine in Korea and Naver trend is a good tool to reflect the general social interest in Korea [22]. One more factor that may impact the near future is the system of limitation of resident working time. Limitation of resident working hours is still and will continue to be a hotly controversial topic. One hopeful study showed that increasing the time medical students are exposed to urology and decreasing the size of academic units, which makes the units more comfortable for the students, can increase students' interest level and, therefore, the number of applicants [23].

Limitations

Although our study represents a novel pilot research, it has several limitations. First, the medical education system is not uniform and each country has its own medical curriculum. However, even though the time at which students must choose their medical specialty differs between countries (in some countries it is during medical school, whereas in others it is during the internship period), students everywhere still must make that decision by themselves. Second, competition rate and application rate are different concepts. Some specialties have become more competitive because they reduced the quota for the number of applicants. However, the absolute application rate is far more important than the competition rate. Third, those data used in this study is not an individual unit data, rather a panel data based by year, which yield limitation during expansion of analysis. Lastly, this study did not consider specific social factors including the state of the job market or financial compensation. However, several studies have already documented such factors, including lifestyle factors, career ambitions, family status, finances, travel conditions, and research [2, 10, 12, 24]. Personal factors including life style or working hours are becoming an important deterrent factor to choose surgery including urology as a career choice [11, 12, 25].

Conclusions

In summary, the application rate for urology is decreasing at the fastest rate, and this trend is related to a decrease in domestic social interest. Various attempts must be made to determine the total number of urologic specialties using scientific method are needed.

Funding
This research was supported by Soonchunhyang University Research Fund.

Authors' contributions
JHK conceptualize and design the study. HYS, YMK, SWL and BL involved in data collection, analyses. All authors read and approved the final manuscript and agreed to be accountable for all aspects of the work in ensuring that questions related to the accuracy or integrity of any part of the work are appropriately investigated and resolved.

Competing interests
The authors declare that they have no competing interests.

Author details
[1]Department of Urology, Soonchunhyang University Hospital,
Soonchunhyang University College of Medicine, 59, Daesagwan-ro,
Yongsan-gu, Seoul 140-743, South Korea. [2]Department of Industrial and
Management Engineering, Pohang University of Science and Technology,
Pohang, South Korea. [3]Department of Urology, Hanyang University Guri
Hospital, Hanyang University College of Medicine, Seoul, South Korea.
[4]Department of Statistics, Graduate School of Chung-Ang University, 84,
Heuksukro, Seoul 156-756, South Korea.

References
1. Melnyk M, Nelson H, Mickelson J, Macneily AE. Trends in matching to
    urology residency in Canada: are we becoming noncompetitive? J Surg
    Educ. 2013;70(4):537-43.
2. Jones P, Rai BP, Qazi HA, Somani BK, Nabi G. Perception, career choice and
    self-efficacy of UK medical students and junior doctors in urology. Can Urol
    Assoc J. 2015;9(9-10):E573-8.
3. Song W, Jeon HG. Incidence of kidney, bladder, and prostate cancers in
    Korea: an update. Korean J Urol. 2015;56(6):422-8.
4. Slaughenhoupt B, Ogunyemi O, Giannopoulos M, Sauder C, Leverson G.
    An update on the current status of medical student urology education in
    the United States. Urology. 2014;84(4):743-7.
5. Kerfoot BP, Nabha KS, Masser BA, McCullough DL. What makes a medical
    student avoid or enter a career in urology? Results of an international
    survey. J Urol. 2005;174(5):1953-7.
6. Deedar-Ali-Khawaja R, Khan SM. Trends of surgical career selection among
    medical students and graduates: a global perspective. J Surg Educ.
    2010;67(4):237-48.
7. Ek EW, Ek ET, Mackay SD. Undergraduate experience of surgical teaching
    and its influence and its influence on career choice. ANZ J Surg.
    2005;75(8):713-8.
8. Minor S, Poenaru D, Park J. A study of career choice patterns among
    Canadian medical students. Am J Surg. 2003;186(2):182-8.
9. Lind DS, Cendan JC. Two decades of student career choice at the University
    of Florida: increasingly a lifestyle decision. Am Surg. 2003;69(1):53-5.
10. Grigg M, Arora M, Diwan AD. Australian medical students and their choice
    of surgery as a career: a review. ANZ J Surg. 2014;84(9):653-5.
11. Creed PA, Searle J, Rogers ME. Medical specialty prestige and lifestyle
    preferences for medical students. Soc Sci Med. 2010;71(6):1084-8.
12. Azizzadeh A, McCollum CH, Miller CC 3rd, Holliday KM, Shilstone HC,
    Lucci A Jr. Factors influencing career choice among medical students
    interested in surgery. Curr Surg. 2003;60(2):210-3.
13. Kerfoot BP, Masser BA, Dewolf WC. The continued decline of formal
    urological education of medical students in the United States: does it
    matter? J Urol. 2006;175(6):2243-7. discussion 2247-2248.
14. Malde SSN. Undergraduate urology in the UK: does it prepare doctors
    adequately? Br J Med Surg Urol. 2012;5:20-7.
15. Kutikov A, Bonslaver J, Casey JT, et al. The gatekeeper disparity--why do
    some medical schools send more medical students into urology? J Urol.
    2011;185(2):647-52.
16. Mok JY, Choi SW, Kim DJ, et al. Latent class analysis on internet and
    smartphone addiction in college students. Neuropsychiatr Dis Treat.
    2014;10:817-28.
17. Linkov F, Bovbjerg DH, Freese KE, Ramanathan R, Eid GM, Gourash W.
    Bariatric surgery interest around the world: what Google trends can teach
    us. Surg Obes Relat Dis. 2014;10(3):533-8.
18. Johnson AK, Mehta SD. A comparison of internet search trends and
    sexually transmitted infection rates using Google trends. Sex Transm Dis.
    2014;41(1):61-3.
19. Davis NF, Breslin N, Creagh T. Using Google trends to assess global interest
    in 'Dysport(R)' for the treatment of overactive bladder. Urology.
    2013;82(5):1189.
20. Rossignol L, Pelat C, Lambert B, Flahault A, Chartier-Kastler E, Hanslik T.
    A method to assess seasonality of urinary tract infections based on
    medication sales and google trends. PLoS One. 2013;8(10):e76020.
21. Linkov F, Ardalan A, Hennon M, Shubnikov E, Serageldin I, Laporte R. Using
    Google trends to assess interest in disasters. Prehosp Disaster Med.
    2010;25(5):482-4.
22. Kang DH, Cho KS, Ham WS, Choi YD, Lee JY. The possibilities as a prediction
    tool for cancer research of big data. Korean J Urol Oncol. 2015;13(1):35-42.
23. Hoag NAHR, Macneily AE. Undergraduate exposure to urology : impact of
    the distributed model of medical education in British Columbia. Can Urol
    Assoc. 2011;7(1-2):20-5.
24. Brundage SI, Lucci A, Miller CC, Azizzadeh A, Spain DA, Kozar RA. Potential
    targets to encourage a surgical career. J Am Coll Surg. 2005;200(6):946-53.
25. Schmidt LE, Cooper CA, Guo WA. Factors influencing US medical students'
    decision to pursue surgery. J Surg Res. 2016;203(1):64-74.

Permissions

All chapters in this book were first published in UROLOGY, by BioMed Central; hereby published with permission under the Creative Commons Attribution License or equivalent. Every chapter published in this book has been scrutinized by our experts. Their significance has been extensively debated. The topics covered herein carry significant findings which will fuel the growth of the discipline. They may even be implemented as practical applications or may be referred to as a beginning point for another development.

The contributors of this book come from diverse backgrounds, making this book a truly international effort. This book will bring forth new frontiers with its revolutionizing research information and detailed analysis of the nascent developments around the world.

We would like to thank all the contributing authors for lending their expertise to make the book truly unique. They have played a crucial role in the development of this book. Without their invaluable contributions this book wouldn't have been possible. They have made vital efforts to compile up to date information on the varied aspects of this subject to make this book a valuable addition to the collection of many professionals and students.

This book was conceptualized with the vision of imparting up-to-date information and advanced data in this field. To ensure the same, a matchless editorial board was set up. Every individual on the board went through rigorous rounds of assessment to prove their worth. After which they invested a large part of their time researching and compiling the most relevant data for our readers.

The editorial board has been involved in producing this book since its inception. They have spent rigorous hours researching and exploring the diverse topics which have resulted in the successful publishing of this book. They have passed on their knowledge of decades through this book. To expedite this challenging task, the publisher supported the team at every step. A small team of assistant editors was also appointed to further simplify the editing procedure and attain best results for the readers.

Apart from the editorial board, the designing team has also invested a significant amount of their time in understanding the subject and creating the most relevant covers. They scrutinized every image to scout for the most suitable representation of the subject and create an appropriate cover for the book.

The publishing team has been an ardent support to the editorial, designing and production team. Their endless efforts to recruit the best for this project, has resulted in the accomplishment of this book. They are a veteran in the field of academics and their pool of knowledge is as vast as their experience in printing. Their expertise and guidance has proved useful at every step. Their uncompromising quality standards have made this book an exceptional effort. Their encouragement from time to time has been an inspiration for everyone.

The publisher and the editorial board hope that this book will prove to be a valuable piece of knowledge for researchers, students, practitioners and scholars across the globe.

Contributors

Dehui Lai and Meiling Chen
Urology Department, Fifth Affiliated Hospital, Guangzhou Medical University, 621 Gangwan Road, Huangpu District, Guangzhou 510700, China

Shifang Zha
2Urology, Citic Huizhou Hospital, Huizhou, Guangdong, China
Shawpong Wan
3Urology, First People's Hospital of Xiaoshan, Hangzhou, Zhejiang, China

Margaret Fitch, Kittie Pang
Sunnybrook Health Sciences Centre, 2075 Bayview Ave, Toronto, ON, Canada

Veronique Ouellet
Institut du cancer de Montréal and Centre de recherche du Centre hospitalier de l'Université de Montréal, 900 St Denis St, Montreal, QC, Canada

Jean-Baptiste Lattouf and Fred Saad
Institut du cancer de Montréal and Centre de recherche du Centre hospitalier de l'Université de Montréal, 900 St Denis St, Montreal, QC, Canada
Department of Surgery Université de Montréal, 2900 Edouard Montpetit Blvd, Montreal, QC, Canada

Anne-Marie Mes-Masson
Institut du cancer de Montréal and Centre de recherche du Centre hospitalier de l'Université de Montréal, 900 St Denis St, Montreal, QC, Canada
Department of Medicine, Université de Montréal, 2900 Edouard Montpetit Blvd, Montreal, QC, Canada

Simon Tanguay, Carmen Loiselle and Simone Chevalier
McGill University and McGill University Health Centre, 1001 Decarie Blvd, Montreal, QC, Canada

Shabbir Alibhai and Antonio Finelli
University Health Network, 610 University Ave, Toronto, ON, Canada

Darrel E. Drachenberg
Manitoba Prostate Centre, 675 McDermot Ave, Winnipeg, MB, Canada

Simon Sutcliffe
Terrry Fox Research Institute, 675 West 10th Avenue, Vancouver, BC, Canada

Alan So
Vancouver Prostate Centre, 2660 Oak St, Vancouver, BC, Canada

Wu Xiaobing, Gong Wentao, Liu Guangxiang, Zhang Fan, Gan Weidong, Guo Hongqian and Zhang Gutian
Nanjing University Medical School Affiliated Nanjing Drum Tower Hospital, Nanjing 210008, China

Sarah H. M. Reuvers, Jeroen R. Scheepe, Lisette A. 't Hoen and Bertil F. M. Blok
Department of Urology, Erasmus MC, Wijtemaweg 80, Room Na 1724, 3015, CN, Rotterdam, The Netherlands

Ida J. Korfage
Department of Public Health, Erasmus MC, Rotterdam, The Netherlands

Tebbe A. R. Sluis
Department of Rehabilitation, Rijndam Rehabilitation, Rotterdam, The Netherlands

Yichun Wang, Chen Chen and Chuanjie Zhang
The First Clinical Medical College, Nanjing Medical University, Nanjing, China

Chao Qin and Ninghong Song
Department of Urology, The First Affiliated Hospital of Nanjing Medical University, 300 Guangzhou Road, Nanjing 210029, China

Yunyan Wang, Bing Zhong, Xiaosong Yang, Gongcheng Wang, Peijin Hou and Junsong Meng
Department of Urology, Huai'an First People's Hospital, Nanjing Medical University, No. 6 West Beijing Road, Huai'an, Jiangsu 223300, China

Yang Xun, Qing Wang, Henglong Hu, Yuchao Lu, Jiaqiao Zhang, Baolong Qin and Shaogang Wang
Department of Urology, Tongji Hospital, Tongji Medical College, Huazhong University of Science and Technology, No.1095 Jiefang Avenue, Wuhan, China

Yudi Geng
Reproductive medicine center, Tongji Hospital, Tongji Medical College, Huazhong University of Science and Technology, Wuhan, China

Henrik Grönberg and Martin Eklund
Department of Medical Epidemiology and Biostatistics, Karolinska Institutet, S-171 77 Stockholm, Sweden

Tobias Nordström
Department of Medical Epidemiology and Biostatistics, Karolinska Institutet, S-171 77 Stockholm, Sweden
Department of Clinical Sciences at Danderyd Hospital, Karolinska Institutet, S-182 88 Stockholm, Sweden

Jan Adolfsson
Department of Clinical Science, Intervention and Technology, Karolinska Institutet, Stockholm, Sweden
Swedish Agency for Health Technology Assessment and Assessment of Social Services, Stockholm, Sweden

Yinglong Xiao and Jun Lu
Department of Urology, Shanghai General Hospital of Nanjing Medical University, No.100, Haining Road, Hongkou District, Shanghai 200080, China

Yi Shao
Department of Urology, Shanghai General Hospital of Nanjing Medical University, No.100, Haining Road, Hongkou District, Shanghai 200080, China
Department of Urology, Shanghai Jiao Tong University School of Medicine, Shanghai General Hospital, No.100, Haining Road, Hongkou District, Shanghai 200080, China

Deng Li and Lei Chen
Department of Urology, Shanghai Jiao Tong University School of Medicine, Shanghai General Hospital, No.100, Haining Road, Hongkou District, Shanghai 200080, China

Yaoting Xu
Department of Urology, Branch of Shanghai General Hospital, No. 1878, Middle Sichuan Road, Hongkou District, Shanghai 200081, China

Dingguo Zhang
Department of Urology, Shanghai Pudong New Area People's Hospital, No. 490, South Chuanhuan road, Shanghai Pudong New Area, Shanghai 201200, China

Arif Demirbas, Demirhan Orsan Demir, Erim Ersoy, Mucahit Kabar, Serkan Ozcan, Mehmet Ali Karagoz and Omer Gokhan Doluoglu
Department of Urology, Ankara Training and Research Hospital, 06340, Sukriye, Altındağ Ankara, Turkey

Ozgecan Demirbas
Department of Pediatrics, Ankara Dr. Sami Ulus Women Health, Children's Training and Research Hospital, 06340 Ankara, Turkey

Emily M. Mader
Department of Family Medicine, SUNY Upstate Medical University, 475 Irving Ave., Suite 200, Syracuse, NY 13210, USA

Hsin H. Li
Department of Family Medicine, SUNY Upstate Medical University, 475 Irving Ave., Suite 200, Syracuse, NY 13210, USA
Department of Public Health and Preventive Medicine, SUNY Upstate Medical University, 766 Irving Ave., Rm. 2262, Syracuse, NY 13210, USA

Christopher P. Morley
Department of Family Medicine, SUNY Upstate Medical University, 475 Irving Ave., Suite 200, Syracuse, NY 13210, USA
Department of Public Health and Preventive Medicine, SUNY Upstate Medical University, 766 Irving Ave., Rm. 2262, Syracuse, NY 13210, USA

Department of Psychiatry and Behavioral Sciences, SUNY Upstate Medical University, 750 E Adams St., Syracuse, NY 13210, USA

Margaret K. Formica and Telisa M. Stewart
Department of Public Health and Preventive Medicine, SUNY Upstate Medical University, 766 Irving Ave., Rm. 2262, Syracuse, NY 13210, USA

Kathleen D. Lyons and Terry Mosher
Department of Psychiatry, Geisel School of Medicine at Dartmouth, Dartmouth-Hitchcock Medical Center, 1 Medical Center Dr., Lebanon, NH 03756, USA

Mark T. Hegel
Department of Psychiatry, Geisel School of Medicine at Dartmouth, Dartmouth-Hitchcock Medical Center, 1 Medical Center Dr., Lebanon, NH 03756, USA
Cancer Control Program, Norris Cotton Cancer Center, Dartmouth-Hitchcock Medical Center, 1 Medical Center Dr., Lebanon, NH 03756, USA

Scott D. Perrapato and Brian H. Irwin
Division of Urology, Department of Surgery, University of Vermont College of Medicine, Fletcher House 301, 111 Colchester Ave., Burlington, VT 05401, USA

John D. Seigne and Elias S. Hyams
Urology Section, Geisel School of Medicine at Dartmouth College, Dartmouth-Hitchcock Medical Center, 1 Medical Center Dr., Lebanon, NH 03756, USA

Fan Zhang and Limin Liao
Department of Urology, China Rehabilitation Research Center, Beijing 100068, China

Department of Urology, Capital Medical University, Beijing, China

Frank Waldbillig, Abdallah Abdelhadi, Annette Steidler, Jost von Hardenberg, Maurice Stephan Michel and Philipp Erben
Department of Urology, University Medical Centre Mannheim, University of Heidelberg, Theodor-Kutzer-Ufer 1-3, 68167 Mannheim, Germany

Thomas Stefan Worst
Department of Urology, University Medical Centre Mannheim, University of Heidelberg, Theodor-Kutzer-Ufer 1-3, 68167 Mannheim, Germany
Institute of Pathology, University Medical Centre Mannheim, University of Heidelberg, Theodor-Kutzer-Ufer 1-3, 68167 Mannheim, Germany

Cleo-Aron Weis and Maria Gottschalt
Institute of Pathology, University Medical Centre Mannheim, University of Heidelberg, Theodor-Kutzer-Ufer 1-3, 68167 Mannheim, Germany

Tommy Kjærgaard Nielsen and Jørgen Bjerggaard Jensen
Department of Urology, Hospitalsenheden Vest, Holstebro, Denmark

Xia-cong Lin
Department of Urology, the 175th Hospital of PLA (Dongnan Affiliated Hospital of Xiamen University), Zhangzhou, Fujian 363000, People's Republic of China

Xiang Gao and Qing-hua Zhang
Department of Obstetrics and Gynecology, Daping Hospital, Third Military Medical University, Chongqing 400038, People's Republic of China

Gen-sheng Lu and Bo Song
Urological Research Institute of PLA, Southwest hospital, Third Military Medical University, Chongqing 400038, People's Republic of China

Alexander P. Glaser, Ilina Rosoklija, Emilie K. Johnson and Elizabeth B. Yerkes
Department of Surgery, Division of Urology, Ann and Robert H. Lurie Children's Hospital of Chicago, 225 E. Chicago Ave, Chicago, IL 60611, USA

L. Topazio, C. Perugia, G. Gaziev, V. Iacovelli and D. Bianchi
School of Specialization in Urology, University "Tor Vergata", Rome, Italy

C. De Nunzio
Department of Urology, Sant'Andrea Hospital, University "La Sapienza", Rome, Italy

G. Vespasiani and E. Finazzi Agrò
Department of Experimental Medicine and Surgery, University "Tor Vergata", Rome, Italy

Martin L. Brady and Raghu Raghavan
Therataxis, LLC, Baltimore, MD, USA

King Scott Coffield and Belur Patel
Department of Surgery, Division of Urology, Scott and White Medical Center, Temple, TX, USA
Texas A&M Health Science Center College of Medicine, Temple, TX, USA

Thomas J. Kuehl
Department of Obstetrics and Gynecology, Scott and White Medical Center, Temple, TX, USA

Departments of Obstetrics and Gynecology, Pediatrics, and Molecular and Cellular Medicine, Texas A&M Health Science Center College of Medicine, Temple, TX, USA

V. O. Speights Jr
Department of Pathology, Scott and White Medical Center, Temple, TX, USA
Texas A&M Health Science Center College of Medicine, Temple, TX, USA

Scott Wilson and Mike Wilson
Twin Star TDS, LLC, Lexington, KY, USA

Rick M. Odland
Twin Star TDS, LLC, Lexington, KY, USA
Department of Otolaryngology, Hennepin County Medical Center, University of Minnesota, Minneapolis, MN, USA

Atsushi Okada, Shuzo Hamamoto, Kazumi Taguchi, Rei Unno, Teruaki Sugino, Ryosuke Ando, Kentaro Mizuno, Keiichi Tozawa, Kenjiro Kohri and Takahiro Yasui
Department of Nephro-urology, Nagoya City University Graduate School of Medical Sciences, 1 Kawasumi, Mizuho-cho, Mizuho-ku, Nagoya, Aichi 467-8601, Japan

Andrea Schlegel and Philipp Kron
Division of Visceral and Transplantation Surgery, University Hospital, Zurich, Switzerland

Markus K. Muller
Division of Visceral and Transplantation Surgery, University Hospital, Zurich, Switzerland
Department of Surgery, Kantonsspital Frauenfeld, 8500 Frauenfeld, Switzerland

Jeannette D. Widmer
Department of Surgery, Kantonsspital Frauenfeld, 8500 Frauenfeld, Switzerland

Marc Schiesser
Department of Surgery, Kantonsspital St. Gallen, St. Gallen, Switzerland

Jens G. Brockmann
Department of Surgery, Kidney and Pancreas Transplantation, King Faisal Specialist Hospital, Riyadh, Kingdom of Saudi Arabia

Xujun Sheng, Ding Xu, Yu Wu, Yongjiang Yu, Jianhua Chen and Jun Qi
Department of Urology, School of Medicine, Xinhua Hospital, Shanghai Jiao Tong University, 1665 Kongjiang Rd, XinHua Hospital, Shanghai 200092, China

Ning Shao
Department of Urology, Fudan University Shanghai Cancer Center, Shanghai, China

Gui Ma
Department of Urology, Second People's Hospital of Wuxi, Nanjing Medical University, Wuxi, China

Jinying Zhang and Wei Zhu
Department of Oncology, First Affiliated Hospital of Nanjing Medical University, Nanjing 210023, China

Helen Quirk
Centre for Sport and Exercise Science, Sheffield Hallam University, S10 2BP, Sheffield, UK

Derek J. Rosario
Department of Oncology, University of Sheffield, Sheffield, UK

Liam Bourke
Faculty of Health and Wellbeing, Sheffield Hallam University, Sheffield, UK

Chengwei Zhang, Xiaozhi Zhao, Changwei Ji, Wei Wang and Hongqian Guo
Department of Urology, Nanjing Drum Tower Hospital, Medical School of Nanjing University, 321 Zhongshan Rd., Nanjing 210008, People's Republic of China

Suhan Guo
School of Public Health, Nanjing Medical University, Nanijng 210029, People's Republic of China

Yin-Chien Ou, Che-Yuan Hu, Hong-Lin Cheng and Wen-Horng Yang
Department of Urology, National Cheng Kung University Hospital, No.138, Sheng Li Road, Tainan 704, Taiwan, Republic of China

Le-Ye He
Department of Urology, Third Xiangya Hospital, Central South University, Changsha, Hunan, China

Ming Zhang
Department of Urology, the Second Hospital of Jilin University, Changchun, China

Zhi-Wen Chen
Department of Urology, Southwest Hospital, Third Military Medical University, Chongqing, China

Jian-Lin Yuan
Department of Urology, Xijing Hospital, the Fourth Military Medical University, Xi'an, China

Ding-Wei Ye
Department of Urology, Fudan University Shanghai Cancer Center, Shanghai, China

Lu-Lin Ma
Department of Urology, Peking University Third Hospital, Beijing, China

Hui Wei
Department of Urology, Shenzhen Zhongshan Urological Hospital, Shenzhen, China

Jiang-Gen Yang
Department of Urology, Shenzhen People's Hospital, The Second Clinical Medical College of Ji'nan University, Shenzhen, China

Shan Chen
Department of Urology, Beijing Tongren Hospital Capital Medical University, Beijing, China

Ben Wan
Department of Urology, Beijing Hospital of the Ministry of Health, Beijing, China

Shu-Jie Xia
Department of Urology, Shanghai First People's Hospital Affiliated to Shanghai Jiaotong University, Shanghai, China

Zhi-Liang Weng
Department of Urinary Surgery, the First Affiliated Hospital of Wenzhou Medical College, Wenzhou, China

Xiang-Bo Kong
Department of Urology, China-Japan Union Hospital, Jilin University, Changchun, China

Qiang Wei
Departmentof Urology, West China Hospital, Sichuan University, Chengdu, Sichuan, China

Feng-Shuo Jin
Department of Urinary Surgery, Institute of Surgery Research, Daping Hospital, Third Military Medical University, Chongqing, China

Xiang-Hua Zhang
Department of Urology, Shougang Hospital of Peking University, Beijing, China

Wei-Qing Qian
Department of Urology, Huadong Hospital, Fudan University, Shanghai, China

Shu-Sheng Wang
Department of Urology, Guangdong Provincial Hospital of Chinese Medicine, Guangzhou University of Chinese Medicine, Guangzhou, China

Ying-He Chen
Department of Urology, Second Affiliated Hospital of Wenzhou Medical College, Wenzhou, China

Hong-Shun Ma
Department of Urology, Tianjin First Central Hospital, Tianjin, China

Ying-Hao Sun and Xu Gao
Department of Urology, Changhai Hospital, Second Military Medical University, 168 Changhai Road, Shanghai 200433, China

Eshani Sharan and Kelly Hunter
Institute of Biomaterials and Biomedical Engineering, University of Toronto, 164 College Street, Room 407, Toronto, ON M5S 3G9, Canada

Paul B. Yoo
Institute of Biomaterials and Biomedical Engineering, University of Toronto, 164 College Street, Room 407, Toronto, ON M5S 3G9, Canada
Department of Electrical and Computer Engineering, University of Toronto, Toronto, ON, Canada

Magdy Hassouna
Division of Urology, Toronto Western Hospital, Toronto, ON, Canada

Dmitry Enikeev, Petr Glybochko, Leonid Rapoport, Natalya Potoldykova, Roman Sukhanov, Mikhail Enikeev, Ekaterina Laukhtina and Mark Taratkin
Institute for Urology and Reproductive Health, Sechenov University, Moscow, Russia

Zhamshid Okhunov and Mitchel O'Leary
Department of Urology, University of California, Irvine; Orange, CA, USA

Qingmei Huang, Ping Jiang, Lina Feng, Liping Xie, Shuo Wang, Dan Xia, Baihua Shen, Baiye Jin, Li Zheng and Wei Wang
Department of Urology, The First Affiliated Hospital, College of Medicine, Zhejiang University, 79 Qingchun Road, Hangzhou 310003, Zhejiang, China

Gustavo R. Bechara, Waldemar S. Costa, Francisco J. B. Sampaio and Diogo B. De Souza
Urogenital Research Unit, Rio de Janeiro State University, Rio de Janeiro, RJ, Brazil

José A. Damasceno-Ferreira
Urogenital Research Unit, Rio de Janeiro State University, Rio de Janeiro, RJ, Brazil
Department of Veterinary Clinical Pathology, Fluminense Federal University, Niterói, RJ, Brazil

Leonardo A. S. Abreu
Urogenital Research Unit, Rio de Janeiro State University, Rio de Janeiro, RJ, Brazil
Faculty of Medicine, Estacio de Sá University, Rio de Janeiro, RJ, Brazil

Marco A. Pereira-Sampaio
Urogenital Research Unit, Rio de Janeiro State University, Rio de Janeiro, RJ, Brazil
Department of Morphology, Fluminense Federal University, Niteroi, RJ, Brazil

Susumu Kageyama, Tetsuya Yoshida, Masayuki Nagasawa, Shigehisa Kubota, Keiji Tomita, Kenichi Kobayashi, Ryosuke Murai, Teruhiko Tsuru, Eiki Hanada, Kazuyoshi Johnin, Mitsuhiro Narita and Akihiro Kawauchi
Department of Urology, Shiga University of Medical Science, Seta Tsukinowa-cho, Otsu, Shiga 520-2192, Japan

Mohammed Shahait, Raja Khauli, Muhammad Bulbul and Albert El Hajj
Division of Urology, Faculty of Medicine, American University of Beirut Medical Center, Riad El-Solh, Beirut 1107 2020, Lebanon

Samer Nassif and Maya Hijazi
Department of Pathology, Faculty of Medicine, American University of Beirut Medical Center, Riad El-Solh, Beirut 1107 2020, Lebanon

Hani Tamim and Deborah Mukherji
Department of Internal Medicine, Faculty of Medicine, American University of Beirut Medical Center, Riad El-Solh, Beirut 1107 2020, Lebanon

Wassim Abou Kheir and Marwan El Sabban
Department of Physiology, Faculty of Medicine, American University of Beirut Medical Center, Riad El-Solh, Beirut 1107 2020, Lebanon

Jin Long Zhang and Mao Qiang Wang
School of Medicine, Nan Kai University, 94 Wei-jin Rd, Tianjin 300071, People's Republic of China
Department of Interventional Radiology, Chinese PLA General Hospital, 28 Fu-xing Rd, Beijing 100853, People's Republic of China

Jie Yu Yan, Yan Wang, Guo Dong Zhang and Kai Yuan
Department of Interventional Radiology, Chinese PLA General Hospital, 28 Fu-xing Rd, Beijing 100853, People's Republic of China

Hwa Yeon Sun and Jae Heon Kim
Department of Urology, Soonchunhyang University Hospital, Soonchunhyang University College of Medicine, 59, Daesagwan-ro, Yongsan-gu, Seoul 140-743, South Korea

Young Myoung Ko
Department of Industrial and Management Engineering, Pohang University of Science and Technology, Pohang, South Korea

Seung Wook Lee
Department of Urology, Hanyang University Guri Hospital, Hanyang University College of Medicine, Seoul, South Korea

Bora Lee
Department of Statistics, Graduate School of Chung-Ang University, 84, Heuksukro, Seoul 156-756, South Korea

Index